Global Handbook of Health Promotion Research, Vol. 1

Louise Potvin • Didier Jourdan
Editors

Global Handbook of Health Promotion Research, Vol. 1

Mapping Health Promotion Research

With Contributions by Catherine Chabot and Valérie Ivassenko

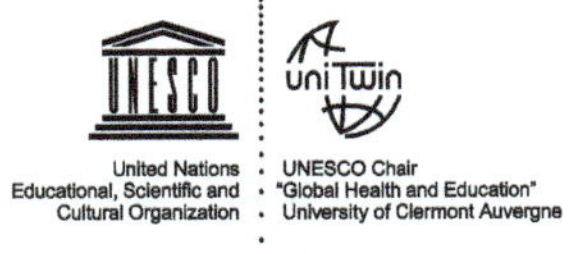

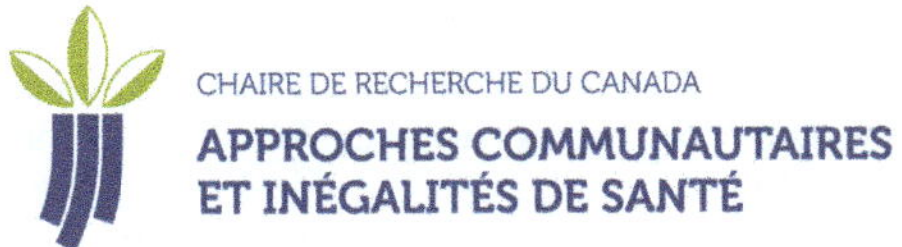

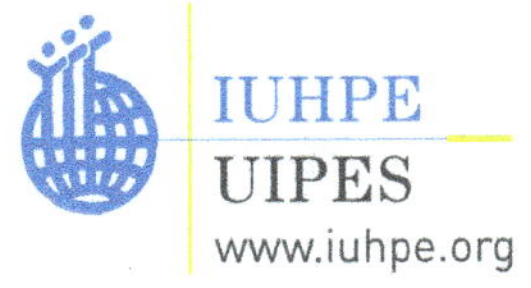

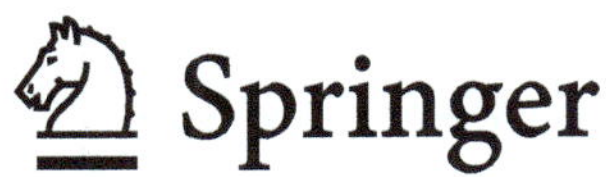

Editors
Louise Potvin
School of Public Health
University of Montreal
Montreal, QC, Canada

Centre de recherche en santé publique (CReSP)
Université of Montreal and CIUSSS du Centre-Sud-de-l'Île-de-Montréal
Montréal, QC, Canada

Didier Jourdan
UNESCO Chair and WHO Collaborating Centre in Global Health & Education
University of Clermont Auvergne
Clermont-Ferrand, France

ISBN 978-3-030-97211-0 ISBN 978-3-030-97212-7 (eBook)
https://doi.org/10.1007/978-3-030-97212-7

This Springer imprint is published by the registered company Springer Nature Switzerland AG
The registered company address is: Gewerbestrasse 11, 6330 Cham, Switzerland

Foreword

Recent history, and how it motivated the current proposal, cannot be omitted in writing this foreword. The first call to send letters of interest to participate in the current project was on April 15, 2020. Does this date have any meaning for you? On March 11, 2020, just a month before, the WHO declared a global pandemic due to COVID-19. This context encourages us to consider the global consequences of the pandemic, the importance of generating knowledge during this historical era, and the role of health promotion research in the current world.

There are no excuses for not inquiring into current realities, and how to transform them, as public health promotion has gone from being in a comfort zone to being in that most uncomfortable of places: the real world.

The field has ceased to be a catalog of descriptions of benefits, of neat, aseptic, conformist recipes for achieving the unattainable. We are learning a new way of understanding health promotion, living, and building the field in a questioning way, with sensitivity and accepting contradictions.

The science of health promotion conforms to a speleological way of investigating and confronting living spaces. We cannot understand or accept health promotion without adopting a questioning stance. Would it be possible not to be skeptical in a world that, now and in the immediate future, exposes us to a worrying panorama? Can certain forms of constructive critical skepticism flourish alongside remnants of a sense of humor, and allow us to traverse this dark, tangled jungle without falling into the temptation of declaring it an apocalypse?

Several authors question the prevailing medical-health model. For instance, Petr Skrabanek, in *Death of Humane Medicine and the Rise of Coercive Healthism*, 1994, encourages skepticism of medical dogma and critical thinking so as to protect us against errors, delusions, myths, and frauds in medicine and healing. He says that the goal is no longer to help sick individuals but to have a positive influence on the entire population. Health ceases to be something private and individual; instead, it becomes a moral duty, a new religion with priests and dogmas. He also underlines the fact that states try to interfere with ways of life, even against the wishes and interests of citizens. Part of Skrabanek's criticism addresses what he sees as the obsession with super health—maximum prolongation of life, healthism, and lifestylism—and, especially, the coercion of citizens to achieve these ideals. He disagrees with prohibitions of all kinds, and restrictions, confinements, threats to freedom, and limits to rights have become common during these turbulent times.

During the period of neoliberal techno-capitalism, there was growing criticism that health industries systematically exaggerate the benefits of health care, and of technologies for diagnosis, treatment, and disease prevention. This approach was called "persecutory health" by Luis David Castiel and Carlos Álvarez-Dardet in *La Salud Persecutoria. Los Límites de la Responsabilidad*, 2021. It leads to an enormous burden of human suffering through what Ivan Illich called social iatrogenesis; in *Medical Nemesis*, 1974, he discussed the complexities and subtleties of this approach, pointing outside effects that result from the interplay between biopolitics and necropolitics.

Faced with these realities, research into health promotion assumes the need to accelerate the processes of knowledge generation in order to stimulate responses, catalyze social mechanisms, and improve global reconstruction of population networks and social cohesion.

Although thinking about the future is not synonymous with futurology, health promotion research does add value by expanding the time horizons of prospective scenarios. The current global crisis—climate change, armed conflicts, forced migrations, the pandemic itself, growing inequities, and economic recession affecting the development of vast sectors of the planet—tends to encourage scenarios in which the possibility of thinking prospectively is truncated. This book encourages us to look beyond existing uncertainties, to build futures worth exploring and living in.

Health promotion research requires inspiration and creativity, breaking down the barriers of clichés and labels, creating new epistemic bridges. It requires sensitivity and dialectical realism. One of its characteristics is the implicit need to expand the notion of health, to think outside the box, to challenge epistemic boundaries and disciplinary limits, and to rethink old questions in transepistemic and disruptive ways. This book invites us to break down boundaries in searching to explain health complexities.

Health promotion becomes one of the few "woke" disciplines; it maintains a prudent distance from interests that go against people's rights. As described in this book, it considers a kaleidoscope of realities so as to investigate the contexts, problems, environments, methodologies, ideas, research questions, population groups, and life courses of individuals and communities.

Each of the chapters of this book serves as a brick added to a complex building. Research groups contributed information on the modes and paradigms that explain their realities. In doing so—in co-constructing knowledge, in their acts of true academic citizenship—they exemplify the best of globalization, and deserve recognition for intellectual honesty and solidarity.

One of the global dimensions of this project, and a major challenge, was organizing a collaboration between people from the global South and the global North.

Some groups find that academic global health is geared to their interests, while others find the field gives less priority to what they know, to how they see the world, and to what they consider important. Some people are recognized as credible knowers within global health, while the knowledge of others is accorded less value or recognition. This situation has led to what is called "epistemic injustice," an expression of the imbalance generated by top-down approaches to research and to the implementation of interventions.

It is known that structural and epistemic exclusion exists in academic global health, and that knowers, producers, and recipients of knowledge belonging to marginalized groups in HIC countries and LMICs suffer the consequences of these epistemic divides.

This is nothing more than a new interpretation from the field of ethics and philosophy, one which deals with colonial and postcolonial influences in the generation of knowledge (testimonial injustice) and in its reception (interpretive injustice). These credibility differentials are rooted in historical patterns of social relations (racism, sexism, colonization), in which excess epistemic credibility of dominant groups appears at the expense of the credibility of marginalized groups.

In this book, we struggle to break with these historical epistemic injustices by appealing to an emancipatory and inclusive form of knowledge generation, integrating the global South and North within a single dimension.

The pandemic has left us naked and helpless. It has led to an increase in existing structural inequalities, an increase in poverty, loss of sources of work, lack of education, and new forms of discrimination and social exclusion. It has revealed several realities, one of which is the small space that health promotion occupies as a field of research and policy formulation. The reparative-care model prevails over health constructive and salutogenic approaches. The epidemiology of this tragedy has subsumed societies and perhaps needs to be reconsidered through the "epistemology of hope."

In present times, people are subject to the so-called "algorithmic society." Algorithms have become the main mediator through which power is exercised over people. Governments are increasingly turning towards algorithms to predict criminality, deliver public services, allocate resources, and calculate recidivism rates. Health promotion is subject to the forces shaping social behavior: penetrating marketing strategies, commercial determinants of health, imposing distorted needs, and demands that disguise themselves as rights. Materialistic behaviors are shaped by powerful interests which health promotion tries to confront or balance, in certain circumstances, in idyllic, naive, and compassionate ways.

The introduction to this book says: "Researchers are social actors whose behaviors are shaped by structuring forces." One of the questions that could be asked is: "What type of forces can be generated from health promotion research so as to sensitize audiences, to translate science into decision-making, to empower knowledge so that it induces ethical behaviors in sectors of power, encouraging health to be considered in the rules of the market?" This book constitutes an excellent point of departure for formulating answers to these and other questions.

Beyond the identified practices of health promotion (Chap. 2)—the interventions of the professionals from health and other sectors aimed at improving the health of individuals or populations; the decisions taken by politicians and others to change norms; the distribution of resources in various contexts; and the work of those who study health promotion practices, share their findings, and systematically experiment with new ways of promoting health—there is a field of counterinsurgency subverting the salutogenic field so as to protect the interests of market economies, consumerism, and unhealthy models of life.

Readers may wonder what led the authors of this book to mobilize such generous intellectual effort on a planetary scale. Unlike other similar scientific literature projects, this commendable effort is imbued with ethical qualities aimed at achieving coherence between discourse and praxis and recognizing knowledge as a common good and a right.

What type of mortar would be necessary for the integration of linguistic roots (The Tower of Babel, circa 3000 BC), the growth of knowledge (Alexandria Library, 306 BC), and the ephemerality of social relations (Zygmunt Bauman and the *Liquid Modernity*[1])? Health promotion research can be considered as a science integrating externalities, identifying how each sector of society contributes to health.

Perhaps, in this book on health promotion research, we will encourage a different experience, a way of understanding science through academic generosity and cognitive altruism, and thus overcoming impositions that result from the interplay of the forces that run through our societies.

Coordinator, Program of Social Sciences and Health, Raúl Mercer
FLACSO (Latin American Faculty of Social Sciences)
Buenos Aires, Argentina

[1] Bauman, Z. (2000). *Liquid Modernity.* Polity Press.

Preface

A Need to Strengthen the Knowledge Base

Since the adoption of the Ottawa Charter in 1986, many countries have adopted and implemented a health promotion strategy understood as a set of coordinated intersectoral actions that aims to orient and support social change in order to improve health for all and reduce health inequalities. This expansion of health promotion practices and policies is linked to the evolution of our understanding of the conditions that influence the health of populations and individuals and generate, reduce or mitigate health inequalities. The knowledge base for this strategy relies on the broad determinants of health and on programmes and policies—their planning, implementation and impact—aimed at changing the distribution of these determinants. While research teams, some of them high level, are producing relevant and valid data to enhance this knowledge base, evidence production remains insufficient and scattered.

Thus, the challenge is not just whether research is carried out. It is also essential to adopt a comprehensive approach that will enable the development of a structured field of research that is likely to meet the need for scientific knowledge to inform health promotion. That's why the ambition of this handbook is not only to describe but also to contribute to organizing health promotion research as a specific and clearly identified field of research and to strengthen the global research community.

A Collective Endeavour

The project was spearheaded by the UNESCO chair and WHO Collaborating Centre "Global Health and Education" and the Canada Research Chair in Community Approaches and Health Inequalities in partnership with the International Union for Health Promotion and Education (IUHPE). The UNESCO chair and WHO Collaborating Centre "Global Health and Education" was launched in 2018. Among the objectives shared with the United Nations agencies, the contribution to the strengthening of the research community and the epistemological renewal of the field hold a central place. For 20 years, the Canada Research Chair in Community Approaches and Health Inequalities has been a driving force behind the development and recognition of health promotion and population health intervention research as key contributors to increasing population health and reducing health inequality. The International Union for Health Promotion and Education is the only global NGO with a membership composed of decision makers, practitioners and researchers in the field of health promotion.

A meeting focused on "Re-examining and deepening the epistemological foundations of health promotion research; Structuring the research field" in Montreal, in January 2019, acted as a trigger for the development of the handbook. A call for contributions was launched in April 2020. It was open to the global community of health promotion researchers, defined as individuals and groups interested in advancing health promotion research by reflecting and sharing their research practices. One hundred and sixty-five people from 26 countries from the 5 continents contributed to this collective endeavour!

An Open Project

Beyond the publication of this handbook, our ambition is to contribute to create a global and sustainable community of health promotion researchers involved in knowledge production and sharing. Recognizing that we cannot pretend to be an exhaustive coverage of all relevant approaches of health promotion research, this handbook is conceived of as an opening for the future and a steppingstone for an ongoing global initiative. As a continuation of the publication of the handbook, a section entitled "Doing health promotion" in the journal *Global Health Promotion* has been launched. This section will publish introductory-level presentations of paradigms, approaches and methods relevant for health promotion research, making the handbook you hold in your hand the cornerstone of a worldwide effort to strengthen and structure the research field.

With Catherine Chabot, Montréal, Québec, Canada, and Valérie Ivassenko, Clermont-Ferrand, France

Montréal, Québec, Canada Louise Potvin
Clermont-Ferrand, France Didier Jourdan

Contents

Part IV Researching the Practices of Researchers and Innovators

About the Editors

Louise Potvin is currently professor in the Department of Social and Preventive Medicine, School of Public Health (ESPUM), Université de Montréal, Canada. She is the scientific director of the Centre de recherche en santé publique, the largest grouping of researchers dedicated to public health in Québec, Canada. She holds the Canada Research Chair in Community Approaches and Health Inequalities. She is a founder of Population Health Intervention Research, a domain of scientific endeavour that seeks to develop a cumulative body of knowledge on public health interventions, their planning, implementation, scaling up and sustainability. She is also a leading figure in health promotion research, more specifically through her work on the role of local environments in health inequality and local intersectoral action.

Didier Jourdan is the chair holder of the UNESCO Chair "Global Health & Education" and head of the WHO Collaborating Centre for "Research in Education & Health". He is full professor, former dean of the Faculty of Education and vice president of University of Clermont Auvergne in Clermont-Ferrand, France. He used to be president of the "prevention, education and health promotion" commission of the French High Council for Public Health and director of the Health Promotion Division of the French National Public Health Agency. His research activities focus on the impact of health promotion interventions, particularly with regard to health inequalities, implementation mechanisms, professional activity and ethical issues.

About the Contributors

Jens Aagaard-Hansen has a double training background as medical doctor (specialized in general medicine) and social anthropologist. He has worked in the field of prevention and health promotion in relation to communicable as well as non-communicable diseases for the past four decades and on four different continents. His work encompasses practical public health programmes as well as research, with a track record of 100+ scientific publications. His double background has led to a special interest in cross-disciplinary research. He is working as a senior researcher at Steno Diabetes Center Copenhagen, Denmark, with special focus on health promotion in a life-course perspective.

Caroline Adam holds a doctorate in Public Health from the University of Montreal. She is teaching Social Work at the Cégep du Vieux Montreal and also performs research in a college setting. Dr Adam has extensive professional experience in social intervention. She is particularly interested in population health interventions, especially in connection with social health inequalities. Her main research interests are food insecurity, social housing, social inequalities in health and the interventions that attempt to address these issues.

Alix Adrien is a Community Medicine specialist at the Montreal Regional Public Health Department. He is also an assistant professor at McGill University's Department of Epidemiology and Biostatistics and at Université de Montréal's Département de médecine sociale et préventive. He has led the development and undertaking of HIV-related behavioural research and surveillance projects in Canada, Haiti, Morocco, India and Pakistan. He emphasizes participatory approaches for the design and implementation of these projects. Dr Adrien is a founding member of Groupe d'action pour la prévention de la transmission du VIH et l'éradication du sida (GAP-VIES), a community-based AIDS organization serving the Haitian community in Quebec.

Marco Akerman is a full professor at the School of Public Health, University of São Paulo, Brazil; Latin America Vice President of the International Union of Health Promotion and Education (2010–2016); Chair of the Working Group on

Health Promotion and Sustainable Development of the Brazilian Association of Public Health (2011–2016); and former PAHO Regional Consultant on Local Development and Health and Focal Point on Social Determinants of Health. Marco Akerman focuses his consulting activities, teaching and research in the areas of evaluation of public policies, intersectoral action for health equity and social determinants of health. In 2014, he led a review process of the National Health Promotion Policy in Brazil, activating multiple simultaneous movements with intense social participation.

Tassawar Ali is working as a country health promotion manager with MSF (Médecins sans frontières/Doctors Without Borders) in Pakistan. He is mainly responsible for formulating a health promotion strategy on malnutrition, mother and child health, and cutaneous leishmaniasis (CL) programme. He has expertise in community engagement and in designing and implementing health promotion initiatives. Previously, he worked with Rutgers International in an HIV and harm reduction project. He also worked as a mental health expert in a global vision organization. He frequently wrote field blogs on the MSF page and previously on a communication initiative network. He is also a member of the HepC movement.

François Alla is Professor of Public Health at the University of Bordeaux, France, where he leads a research team dedicated to prevention at the Inserm (Institut National de la Santé et de la Recherche Médicale) U1219 "Bordeaux Population Health" Research Centre. With an MD and a PhD, he is also Head of the Department of Prevention, University Hospital of Bordeaux. His research fields include health services research and population health intervention research. His research is informed by his field experience as a population health practitioner and expert at the local and national levels. He has authored or co-authored more than 300 articles, books, book chapters and national reports.

Joshua Amo-Adjei is presently a senior lecturer at the Department of Population and Health, University of Cape Coast, Ghana. He was a postdoctoral and associate research scientist at the African Population and Health Research Center (a recipient of the 2015 UN Population Award), Nairobi, Kenya, between 2016 and 2018. His research interests are in health systems for maternal health, abortion care, and sexual and reproductive health of young people. He leads two studies on adolescent sexual and reproductive health: an implementation research on comprehensive sexuality education for vulnerable (children living with HIV and AIDS children in detention), out-of-school young people and child sexual exploitation in mining, oil, fishing, agricultural and e-waste enclaves of Ghana.

Julia Anaf is a research fellow in Public Health at the Southgate Institute for Health, Society and Equity, Flinders University, Adelaide, South Australia. In 2012 she completed a PhD on the "implications for health and well-being arising from mass job loss at a transnational automotive corporation". Her main research interests concern the growth and power of transnational corporations and the ways in which they act as commercial determinants of health and health equity. She has undertaken research on the health impacts of fast food, extractives and alcohol corporations using a corporate health impact assessment (CHIA) framework and on civil society activism against negative health impacts arising from the products and operations of transnational corporations.

Kirsti Sarheim Anthun is an associate professor at the Department of Neuromedicine and Movement Science, Norwegian University of Science and Technology. She is also a senior researcher at the Department of Health Research at SINTEF, one of Europe's largest independent research organizations. She has a PhD in Social Anthropology and years of experience in applied public health research aiming to improve health equity for citizens. Anthun's research spans topics such as citizen involvement in public health, organization studies, governance research, implementation science and digital health research.

Ioanna Antoniadou-Koumatou has been Head of the Department of Social and Developmental Pediatrics, Institute of Child Health, Athens, Greece, since 1989. She has extensive experience in developmental paediatrics and in the administration of various developmental tests, which she has also used in research or clinical practice. Her fields of interest and expertise include: developmental and behavioural paediatrics, diagnostic and screening tests, primary health care and health promotion programmes, training of paediatricians in the field of developmental and social paediatrics. Her special areas of interest include the effects of toxins or heavy metals on pre-natal development and intra-uterus brain development. She has participated in about 40 research programmes as a main researcher and has supervised five doctoral theses. She is the president of the Medical Ethics Committee of the Institute of Child Health, a member of the scientific committees of the Ministries of Health and Education, and has also served as an expert adviser to the Minister of Education (2015–2016).

Cecilie Høj Anvik is Associate Professor of Sociology and Vice-Dean for Research & Development at the Faculty of Social Sciences, Nord University, Norway. She has a PhD in Social Anthropology. Anvik has more than 20 years of experience and expertise in qualitative research on youth in vulnerable transitions, mental health issues and school dropout processes. She has participated in comprehensive national, as well as international, collaborations within the research field of education, school absence and dropout, marginalization of youth from education and working life, as well as welfare policy, institutions and services.

Bridget Ira C. Arante is a registered nurse, who obtained her Bachelor of Science degree from the University of the Philippines, Manila. She is passionate about enhancing her skills in clinical research and aims to enhance her knowledge and participate in studies regarding patient safety and quality-of-care improvement in her future practice.

Achilleas Attilakos is Associate Professor of Paediatrics at National and Kapodistrian University of Athens, "Attikon" University Hospital, Athens, Greece. He is a general paediatrician, interested in primary paediatric care, childhood dyslipidemia and antiepileptic drug safety. He was the coordinator of and main contributor to the Institute of Child Health's (Athens, Greece) programme "Development of Guidelines for the Systematic Follow-up of Health and Development of Greek Children and Adolescents, 0–18 Years Old". Also, in 2016, he participated in reforming the Greek Child Health Booklet, a parent-held health record focusing on regular follow-up of children's health and development, health education and support of parents in raising their children. He participates in educational seminars for healthcare practitioners regarding paediatric primary care and dyslipidemia.

Ioanna Bakogianni is Project Officer, Health in Society Unit, European Commission's Joint Research Centre, Ispra, Italy. She works in the Health Promotion team. Ioanna is a nutritionist and dietitian by training and works on providing evidence and knowledge in order to inform public health policies in the areas of nutrition, non-communicable diseases, mental health and well-being.

Margaret M. Barry holds the Established Chair in Health Promotion and Public Health and is Head of the World Health Organization Collaborating Centre for Health Promotion Research, National University of Ireland Galway. Professor Barry has his research published widely in health promotion and works closely with policymakers and practitioners on the development, implementation and evaluation of mental health promotion interventions and policies at national and international levels. She has served as a project leader on WHO projects and European research initiatives and has acted as an expert adviser on mental health promotion policy and research development in a number of countries around the world. Professor Barry was elected as global president of the International Union for Health Promotion and Education in 2019.

Nina Bartelink is a postdoctoral researcher at the Department of Health Promotion, Maastricht University, the Netherlands. During her PhD she focused on the process and effect evaluation of a Dutch health-promoting school initiative, called "The Healthy Primary School of the Future". In this research study, she used a contextual action-oriented research approach to be able to deal with the complex and adaptive nature of school systems. Nina has presented her work at several (inter)national conferences and had several work visits abroad. She finished her PhD Cum Laude in 2019. As a postdoctoral researcher, she kept her focus on school health promotion. She is conducting and involved in several (inter)national research projects (e.g. in collaboration with the Schools for Health in Europe [SHE] network foundation).

Jean-Charles Basson is a political scientist. Within the University of Toulouse, France, he is Director of the Institut Fédératif d'Etudes et de Recherches Interdisciplinaires Santé Société (IFERISS, FED 4142—"Federative Institute for Interdisciplinary Studies and Research in Health and Society"), Deputy Director of the Centre de Recherches Sciences Sociales Sports et Corps (CreSco, EA 7419—"Social Science Research Centre on Sports and the Body"), a member of the Centre d'Epidémiologie et de Recherche en Santé des Populations (CERPOP, UMR Inserm [Institut National de la Santé et de la Recherche Médicale] 1295—"Centre for Epidemiology and Population Health") and a member of the Laboratoire des Sciences Sociales du Politique (LaSSP, EA 4175—"Laboratory of Political Social Sciences"). He is also a member of the Global Working Group on Health Impact Assessment at the International Union for Health Promotion and Education (IUHPE) and an expert to the Haut Conseil de la Santé Publique (HCSP—French Public Health Council). His work focuses on the ways in which populations are governed in the fields of public health, public order, public space and education.

Fran Baum, AO (Officer of the Order of Australia) is Matthew Flinders Distinguished Professor of Public Health at Flinders University, Adelaide, Australia. She is a fellow of the Academy of the Social Sciences in Australia, the Australian Academy of Health and Medical Sciences and the Australian Health Promotion Association. She is a past national president and life member of the Public Health Association of Australia. She is co-Chair of the Global Steering Council of the People's Health Movement—a global network of health activist (www. phmovement.org). She served as a Commissioner on the World Health Organization's Commission on the Social Determinants of Health. Her two books *The New Public Health* and *Governing for Health: Advancing Health and Equity Through Policy and Advocacy* are widely quoted.

Marianne Beaulieu is an associate professor at the Faculty of Nursing, Laval University, Quebec, Canada. Through the various research projects in which she has been involved, she has been and still is deeply concerned by the injustices experienced by vulnerable groups. For this reason, she has developed expertise in participatory research to work with these groups. Given the complexity of the issues she is interested in, she combines participatory approaches with advanced quantitative methods of multidimensional analysis (structural equation modelling; exploratory and confirmatory factor analysis). Adopting an atypical position of engaged researcher, she proposed a conceptualization of the emerging notion of "engaged scholarship".

Angèle Bilodeau holds a PhD in Applied Human Sciences from l'Université de Montréal, Québec, Canada, and a Master in Sociology from Université Laval, Québec. She is a full researcher/professor at the School of Public Health, l'Université de Montréal. She is also a researcher at the Canada Research Chair Community Approaches and Health Inequalities and at the Centre InterActions, CIUSSS du Nord-de-l'Île-de-Montréal. Her research contributions include intersectoral collaborations and governance, action in partnership and social innovation, and effects of intersectoral action on local neighbourhoods.

Miranda Blake is a research fellow at the Global Obesity Centre (GLOBE), Deakin University, Victoria, Australia, where she finished an Institute for Health Transformation postdoctoral fellowship to investigate business outcomes of healthy food retail initiatives (2019–2021). Her research focuses on implementation of healthy food policy and retail interventions, with an emphasis on novel and mixed-method approaches. She has led projects to enhance our knowledge of effective and feasible healthy food retail initiatives, including capacity-building interventions with council-owned sporting facilities, online food pricing and labelling experiments, and healthy vending machine and retail pricing interventions. She works closely with translational partners within local, state and national governments, NGOs and public health groups. She is a leader in producing translational outputs for engaging retailers and health promotion practitioners, and research-practice collaborations.

Laurence Boulaghaf is a philosopher. She is a member of the Institut Fédératif d'Etudes et de Recherches Interdisciplinaires Santé Société (IFERISS, FED 4142—"Federative Institute for Interdisciplinary Studies and Research in Health and Society") and a doctoral student in Sociology at the Centre de Recherches Sciences Sociales Sports et Corps (CreSco, EA 7419—"Social Science Research Centre on Sports and the Body"), University of Toulouse, France. Her thesis focuses on the biographical trajectories of patient-users at the Case de Santé in Toulouse.

Eric Breton is Assistant Professor of Health Promotion at the EHESP School of Public Health, Rennes, France, and a researcher at the Arènes research unit (UMR CNRS 6051). His main research interests focus on policy advocacy strategies in the prevention of NCDs, evaluation of complex community-based interventions and local capacity-building strategies for health and equity. An associated editor for the journal *Health Education and Behavior*, he also sits on different national and regional expert groups such as the High Council for Public Health (HCSP). In 2020, he had, with three other editors, his second edition of the first health promotion handbook in French published, a publication that has mobilized contributions from 40 authors from six countries.

Amy Brown is the Executive Officer of Healthy Greater Bendigo, a community movement for better health, working to influence systems, structures and environments to make it easier for Central Victorians to eat well and move more. She has been involved in the "Eat Well @ IGA" project and the preceding pilot project since inception, playing a brokerage and stakeholder liaison role, supporting the design, implementation and evaluation of the project, as well as ensuring the findings are communicated and translated into policy and practice. Amy leads the Australian Healthy Supermarkets Community of Practice, supporting health promotion practitioners to work in partnership with supermarket retailers to enable healthier shopping environments. With ten years in health promotion, planning and policy development, and research and evaluation in the local government sector, she works with wide-ranging partners, holding a philosophy that health is everyone's business.

Bjarne Bruun Jensen has been Professor and manager of Health Promotion Research at Steno Diabetes Center Copenhagen and at the Danish University of Education in Denmark. He has been the Regional Vice President of Europe at the International Union for Health Promotion and Education (IUHPE), where he also served on its executive board. Bjarne was the national coordinator for Health-Promoting Schools in Denmark for more than ten years and has been coordinating many European projects on school health promotion—such as the EU-funded project "Shape Up—Towards a Healthy and Balanced Growing Up". Bjarne has his research published 30 books, 110 articles in journals and 98 chapters in books. He is the editor of 33 books.

Anne Bunde-Birouste is an adjunct senior lecturer at the School of Population Health at the University of New South Wales, Professor of Leadership at the international Football Business Academy and a member of the Academic Board of the Australian College of Physical Activity. Anne is internationally recognized for her expertise in health promotion, sport for development and social change, and innovative community-based approaches for working with disadvantaged groups. Anne specializes in fostering the nexus between practice-based research, teaching, and social impact. Anne is the founding director of Football United (http://footballunited.org.au/), Director of the Creating Chances social enterprise (http://creatingchances.org.au/) and an elected member of the Streetfootballworld international football for good network, https://www.streetfootballworld.org/

Jimryan Ignatius B. Cabuslay obtained his Bachelor of Science in Nursing degree from the College of Nursing, University of the Philippines, in 2019. He graduated Cum Laude, UP College of Nursing, Class 2019, Valedictorian, and was the recipient of the Bienvenido M. Gonzales Award for Academic Excellence. Imbued with dedication to render selfless service to fellow Filipinos, he aims to contribute and work for the Philippine healthcare system, with his advocacies on maternal and child health, disease surveillance and epidemiology. He is dedicated in his career in public health, as he serves as City Epidemiology and Surveillance Unit Support Coordinator under the Department of Health Philippines—Epidemiology Bureau, providing technical assistance and epidemiology and surveillance support related to the COVID-19 response.

Sandra Caldeira is Deputy Head of the Health in Society Unit at the European Commission's Joint Research Centre (JRC). Sandra and the JRC team tease out the science in the areas of public health to inform and ensure better and healthier policies in the EU, grounded on solid evidence. The Unit works on aspects such as cancer, rare diseases and health promotion. Ever since she joined the European Commission in 2010, she has worked broadly and heartily on the prevention of non-communicable diseases, with a focus on food-related policies. Sandra holds degrees in Microbiology and Biotechnology as well as a PhD in Biomedical Sciences.

Mirela Castro Santos Camargos is an adjunct professor at the Department Health Management, School of Nursing, Federal University of Minas Gerais, Brazil. Evaluation of public health policies, demography and management are some of the objects of her study. She also works as a researcher at the Health Management Centre (NUGES, Brazil).

Adrian Cameron is an epidemiologist and Assistant Director of the Global Obesity Centre, Institute for Health Transformation at Deakin University, Victoria, Australia. His research is focused on influencing retail food environments to promote healthier eating at scale, particularly in the supermarket food environment, where most food is purchased. He led the "Eat Well @ IGA" supermarket intervention trials described in this handbook, together with the City of Greater Bendigo, and is a chief investigator of both the Australian government–funded Centre for Research Excellence in Food Retail EnvironmentS for Health ("RE-FRESH") and the annual, multi-country International Food Policy Study.

Daniela Souzalima Campos is a career servant at the State Health Department of Minas Gerais (SES-MG), Brazil, in charge of the Health Promotion Board, with experience as Municipal Health Secretary in the city of Cajuri-MG. She has a degree in Nutrition from the Federal University of Viçosa, with specialization in the area of public health and in food and nutrition policy management. She is a Master's student in Health Management and Service at the Federal University of Minas Gerais (UFMG), having the State Health Promotion Policy as the object of her study.

Viola Cassetti is a health promotion researcher and anthropologist, specialized in community health initiatives, in particular with a focus on qualitative and participatory methodologies. She has worked in community development in Latin America and in applied research in primary care and public health in the United Kingdom and Spain. She co-coordinated an interdisciplinary project to adapt the NICE guidelines for community engagement in health to the Spanish context. With a PhD in Public Health obtained from the University of Sheffield, UK, researching asset-based approaches in communities, she works in a project to evaluate the implementation of community engagement guidelines in Spain and collaborates with local authorities to promote community action in health from a participatory and interdisciplinary approach.

Catherine Chabot is a research professional and coordinator for the Canada Research Chair Community Approaches and Health Inequalities (CACIS). With a Master's degree in Urban Studies and a Bachelor's degree in Geography, her research interests include planning, nature in the city and community action. Her collaborations with the Léa-Roback Center, Montreal, Canada, as well as with CACIS have led her to explore questions of intersectoral action and social innovation.

Venkatesan Chakrapani is Chairperson of the Centre for Sexuality and Health Research and Policy (C-SHaRP), a non-profit research agency in Chennai, India, and DBT/Wellcome Trust India Alliance senior fellow hosted in the Humsafar Trust, Mumbai. He is an STI/HIV physician, a public health researcher and a health policy analyst. He has his work published in several peer-reviewed research articles and book chapters that documented and explained health inequalities among sexual and gender minorities in India. His research interests include stigma, discrimination and structural violence; barriers to HIV prevention and treatment services and gender transition; effect of intersectional stigmas on mental health and HIV risk; acceptability of new and forthcoming HIV prevention products; and designing and evaluating theory-based health promotion interventions.

Nance Cunningham is a PhD student at the University of British Columbia, Canada, and works at the British Columbia Centre for Excellence in HIV/AIDS in Vancouver, British Columbia, leading research institutions in the delivery of testing and treatment for HIV and hepatitis C. She has experience in a range of roles in humanitarian work in protection and health promotion, mainly in conflict contexts in Asia. She has particular interests in health literacy and in primary and secondary prevention in silent epidemics such as viral hepatitis, HIV and diabetes.

Obrillant Damus Born into a traditional peasant family, Obrillant Damus is a full professor at the University of Quisqueya and the State University of Haiti. He is an associate professor at the University of Sherbrooke (Centre d'études du religieux contemporain, Faculté de droit). He holds the international chair "Epistemologías del Sur: fortalecimiento de los saberes locales e indígenas" (Centro Universitario Autónomo Comunal Ndaniguia, Mexico). His research interests include disability, solidarity, human vulnerability, peace education, traditional childbirth, local and indigenous knowledge, women's rape, breastfeeding, the role of local knowledge in health promotion and so on. He is the author and co-author of numerous works. He has been an invited lecturer and professor in many countries.

Clément Dassa is a retired professor, senior statistician and psychometric specialist in the Département de médecine sociale et préventive, School of Public Health (ESPUM), Université de Montréal, Canada. He acted as a consultant to groups that require complex multidimensional statistical analysis. He had a known expertise in measurement, evaluation, statistics and psychometry in health research. His interdisciplinary approach and his work in developing innovative quantitative methodologies have led him to promote the integration of advanced statistical methods and techniques into related disciplines.

Vanessa de Almeida Guerra is an associate professor at the Department of Health Management, School of Nursing, Federal University of Minas Gerais, Brazil. She is coordinator of the Thematic Group on Health Promotion and Sustainable Development (HPSD Group) of the Brazilian Association of Collective Health (ABRASCO). Health promotion is object of her study. She is also a researcher at the Health Management Centre (NUGES).

Charlotte Decroix is a PhD Student at the Department "Methods for Population Health Intervention Research", Bordeaux Population Health Research Center (BPH), Inserm (Institut National de la Santé et de la Recherche Médicale) U1219, University of Bordeaux, France. She is conducting a thesis titled "From the Development of a Complex Public Health Intervention to Its Scaling Up: Conceptual and Methodological Aspects of Viability Studies". At the same time, her work focuses on the evaluation of complex interventions in health promotion, especially in the field of early childhood (childcare centres; maternal and child protection). She has a particular interest in qualitative methods and in taking into account social inequalities in health in population health interventions.

Evelyne de Leeuw is operating at the interface of health research, policy and practice at the University of New South Wales (UNSW), the South Western Sydney Local Health District/Population Health and the Ingham Institute, Liverpool, New South Wales, Australia. She is Director of the HUE (Healthy Urban Environments) Collaboratory, a Maridulu Budyari Gumal partnership, run by three universities (UNSW, University Technology of Sydney (UTS) and Western Sydney University (WSU)) and two large Local Health Districts. She has glocal roles in Healthy Cities development with the WHO and several NGOs. She serves on the Board of the International Union for Health Promotion and Education (IUHPE) and is active in the scientific health promotion arena, as Chair of IUHPE 2022 and Editor-in-Chief of Health Promotion International. She (co)leads initiatives to establish a health political science disciplinary effort.

Bhimsen Devkota obtained his PhD from Aberdeen University, Scotland. He is involved in various researches in Nepal, as well as in South Asia and the United Kingdom. His research interests include applied and participatory action research in education, public health, nutrition, health service, adolescent and sexual health, WASH, behaviour change communication, disaster management, peace and conflict, humanitarian assistance, child rights, social inclusion and evidence-based programming. He has worked with many different international agencies, UN agencies, and governmental and many non-governmental organizations. He has his work published in over 50 original articles in peer-reviewed journals, in addition to a dozen books.

Danilo Di Emidio is completing his PhD at the University of East London, UK. After moving to the United Kingdom as a migrant worker and English-language learner, Danilo experienced a number of life-changing experiences as a result of travelling around the world, mastering several languages and obtaining a degree in Social Anthropology and qualified teacher status in the Humanities. After 20 years in education, as a teacher and school leader, Danilo moved into research through the UCL, Bloomsbury and East London Doctoral Training Partnership, an ESRC-funded organization which brings together five leading social science institutions. Danilo's personal history matched the doctoral training partnership's strategic vision. The latter is driven by a shared emphasis on interdisciplinary research, a multiplicity of existing connections within and across the partners, a joint appetite for engagement with non-academic partners and a collective embedding in London, where Danilo has lived on and off for the past 27 years. Danilo continues to be engaged with the secondary education sector by working as a part-time supply teacher.

Dieinaba Diallo is a research assistant at the Institut National de la Santé et de la Recherche Médicale (Inserm), Paris, France. She has worked as a research engineer at the Department of Social and Human Sciences, EHESP School of Public Health, Rennes, France, on the CLoterreS project and on a case study project on local health contracts in the Bretagne and Pays de Loire regions, with a focus on health promotion and environmental health. She is working on the Long_COCO project to analyse the long-term consequences of SARS-CoV-2, particularly its impact on healthcare consumption and the associated risk factors.

Lea Dippon is working on her PhD at the Department of Sport and Sport Science, Friedrich-Alexander-University Erlangen-Nürnberg, Germany, where she previously received her MA in Physical Activity and Health. Her thesis was part of the KaziAfya project examining the effectiveness of a school-based intervention programme on the growth, physical health and mental well-being of African primary school children. She is working as a research assistant in the nationwide project KOMBINE (Community-based physical activity promotion for the implementation of the National Recommendations) aiming to implement the German physical activity recommendations in local communities, with a focus on structural change and health equity. Her research focus is on intersectoral collaboration and good practice in community-based physical activity promotion.

Katherine Dowling is a postdoctoral researcher at the National University of Ireland Galway. Her research interests are around the development, implementation and evaluation of mental health and well-being programmes for young people across educational and youth settings. Katherine played a lead role in the development of a national mental well-being programme (MindOut) for young people in Ireland for both post-primary schools and youth settings. She completed her doctoral studies at the World Health Organization Collaborating Centre for Health Promotion Research at NUI Galway. Her PhD focused on a large-scale evaluation of the effectiveness and implementation of the MindOut programme in Irish post-primary schools, and her postdoctoral research focuses on monitoring and enhancing implementation support systems for schools delivering MindOut.

Eric Dugas A university full Professor of Education Sciences and Training and charged with the "disability mission" at the University of Bordeaux, Eric Dugas is a member of the LACES EA7437 Laboratory and a co-responsible of the "Diversities, cultures and societies" axis. Withal, he is the president of the "Carry-on" association, and his applied research is part of a systemic approach through the prism of an individual and a collective well-being and empathy (professional and relational).

Dugas' applied researches are more particularly related to the fields of school/university inclusion (alterities, handicaps, serious illnesses), physical and sports activities and game theory (situation of dilemmas), and the physical environment (e.g. architecture and facilities school and care spaces) and its impact on life quality. He is Director of the scientific collection "S@nté in context" at the Bordeaux University presses.

Karyn Dugas Working in cancerology for 30 years, Karyn Dugas pursued studies in the field of health information and mediation, then, a second Master's in Health Ethnomethodology. She was, particularly, interested in informational parents' care in paediatric oncology. The Gustave Roussy Institute, Paris, France, and Dr Olivier Hartmann have entrusted her with the responsibility of a pilot meeting information space (ERI) to support parents whose children were undergoing treatment at the Department of Childhood and Adolescent Cancer. She had created in this service a system to help students with cancer return to class, a precursor to the "PAS CAP" system, and it was an answer to parents' demands. Karyn Dugas is working at the Bordeaux University Hospital at the MARADJA house and supports adolescents and young adults suffering from cancer or rare chronic disabling diseases. She is also a member of the board of directors of the association Groupe Onco-hématologie Adolescents et Jeunes Adultes (GO-AJA).

Sandro Echaquan is a nurse practitioner specializing in primary care, from the Atikamekw community of Manawan. He is practising at the Masko-Siwin Health Center, as well as at the Mihawoso Social Pediatrics Center (Manawan), where he works to continuously improve the health care and services offered in Manawan. Mr. Echaquan has contributed to advancing the field of Indigenous nursing practice and is the recipient of numerous distinctions, such as the 2019 Personality of the Year of the "Top 20 de la Diversité". His leadership has also led him to hold several management positions, including that of Director of Masko-Siwin Health Services in Manawan and of the Mihawoso Center.

Nada El Osta is a dentist, with a Master's degree in Prosthodontic Sciences and a PhD from the University of Clermont Auvergne, France. She is a lecturer/clinical professor at the Department of Removable Prosthodontics, Faculty of Dental Medicine, Saint Joseph University of Beirut, Lebanon. She is co-leader of the "Oral health" unit within the craniofacial research laboratory (LRCF) of the Saint Joseph University Dental School. Nada has conducted several epidemiological studies and questionnaire surveys evaluating oral health-related quality of life and nutritional impacts of oral diseases or anxiety, in various populations namely older individuals or patients with cancer. The majority of these studies are being conducted in connection with the CROC EA4847 research group.

Geir Arild Espnes is Mayor of the Oppdal Municipality, Norway, and Professor of Public Health Sciences at the Department of Public Health and Nursing (ISM), Norwegian University of Science and Technology (NTNU). He is founder of the

NTNU Center for Health Promotion Research, the European Forum for Health Promotion Research and the International Forum for Health Promotion Research. Espnes has been a professor at Australian National University (ANU) and holds an honorary professorship at the National University of Singapore (NUS). His main research interest concerns health promotion research as part of public health, especially with regard to community tools for health promotion and working with the young. For an update on his research and activities see: https://www.ntnu.no/ansatte/geir.arild.espnes

Shannen G. Felipe has a Bachelor of Science in Nursing from the University of the Philippines Manila. While reviewing for the upcoming Philippine Nursing Licensure Examination, she is working as a research associate for the external accreditation project of the Quality Assurance Committee at the Manila College of Nursing, University of the Philippines Manila.

Matt Fisher is a senior research fellow in Public Health at the Southgate Institute for Health, Society and Equity, Flinders University, Adelaide, Australia. His research over 12 years has focused on the intersection between public policy and social determinants of health and health equity in Australia. Since completing his PhD in 2010, Matt has had a particular interest in understanding the social factors that affect chronic stress and mental illness, and what they mean for public policy and social change to prevent mental ill-health and promote human well-being. In 2019 his work "A Theory of Public Wellbeing" was published in *BMC Public Health*, which defined seven well-being abilities and showed how these can be promoted or inhibited by social conditions.

Maria Cristina Franceschini has a BA in Anthropology from the University of Maryland, an MHS in International Health from Johns Hopkins University and a PhD in Public Health from the University of São Paulo, Brazil. She is a programme manager at the Institute for Health Policy Research (IEPS) in Sao Paulo, Brazil. Between 2015 and 2021, she was the Executive Secretary for CEPEDOC-Healthy Cities, a research centre at the University of Sao Paulo and a World Health Organization Collaborating Centre. Previously, she worked as a technical officer for the Pan American Health Organization and a consultant for the World Bank Institute. She has worked in Brazil, Cape Verde, Ecuador, Mozambique and Washington DC.

Ruth Freeman is Professor of Dental Public Health Research and an honorary consultant in Dental Public Health. She is Director of the Oral Health and Health Research Programme and co-Director of the Dental Health Services Research Unit at the University of Dundee, Scotland. Ruth completed her PhD from the Queen's University of Belfast. She also studied at the University of London, where she completed her training in Dental Public Health. She is a member of the British Psychoanalytic Council and a fellow at the Faculty of Public Health, Royal College of Physicians, UK.

Katherine L. Frohlich is a professor at the Département de médecine sociale et preventive, École de Santé Publique, l'Université de Montréal (ESPUM), Canada, as well as a research associate at the Centre de Recherche en Santé Publique (CReSP). She co-holds the Myriagone McConnell-UdM Chair on Youth Knowledge Mobilisation. Katherine has dedicated her career to researching social inequalities in youth health in urban contexts, particularly with regard to health practices such as smoking and free play. Katherine has been running the Health Promotion option of the PhD programme at the Université de Montréal for over ten years and is one of the co-editors of the fourth edition of the book *Health Promotion in Canada*.

Sabrina Galella is the Policy and Influencing Coordinator of A Way Home Scotland, a coalition of individuals, organizations and authorities dedicated to ending youth homelessness in Scotland. A Way Home focuses on prevention, partnership and innovation achieved through working together, sharing best practice, influencing decision-makers and shaping policy. Sabrina and her partners aim to inspire and facilitate change by promoting and developing preventative strategies to end youth homelessness. Previously a researcher with the Scottish Parliament, Sabrina has a BA in Politics and International Relations and an LLM in Human Rights and International Law.

Patrizia Garista holds a BA in Educational Sciences and a PhD in Health Education, and has been a researcher in General Pedagogy at the National Institute of Documentation, Innovation and Educational Research (INDIRE), Italy, since 2014. She is Adjunct Professor of Social Pedagogy and Lifelong Learning at the University of Perugia, Italy, where she has been collaborating in the health promotion publishing, research, and training activities of the Research Centre on Health Promotion and Education since 2001. She has been also collaborating with the European Training Consortium (ETC). Her research interests are focused on the connection between well-being and lifelong learning; resilience and salutogenic pedagogy; social justice, empowerment and sustainability; and narrative and art-based research methods for teaching and learning.

Kate Garvey is a leader and manager within the Tasmanian Department of Health and is responsible for the promotion of public health action across functional boundaries. She has worked in the public health sector for over 20 years in a variety of leadership and policy roles. Her responsibilities include building public health translational research capacity as well as supporting a comprehensive policy and programme response to promote community health and well-being. Kate has been involved in the design and implementation of a large number of research projects as well as in supporting researchers to communicate findings to maximize policy impact. Kate is motivated by the belief that access to conditions for health and well-being is a human right.

Peter Gelius is a research associate at the Department of Sport Science and Sport at Friedrich-Alexander University Erlangen-Nürnberg (FAU), Germany. He is also co-Director of the Department's WHO Collaborating Centre for Physical Activity and Public Health. His main research interests include physical activity policy, knowledge co-production in health promotion and health promotion theory. He has been involved in several projects related to policy monitoring and participatory physical activity promotion, including the transdisciplinary Capital4Health consortium. He regularly consults the World Health Organization on issues of physical activity policy.

Sylvie Gendron is a professor and Vice-Dean of Graduate Studies, Faculté des sciences infirmières, University of Montreal. She is also a nurse and holds a PhD in Public Health from the same university. Since the early 1990s, her research activities have evolved around health promotion practices and programmes with/for socially marginalized populations, with a view towards generating equity in health practice. She has been teaching qualitative research and collaborative methods to graduate students for more than 25 years. She enjoys exploring social theories with her graduate students as they engage in their doctoral research to advance nursing and health promotion science and practice.

Sudha Ghimire is a PhD scholar at NORHED, Rupantaran Project under the Graduate School of Education, Tribhuvan University (TU), Nepal. Her study is based on participatory action research with early adolescents in the Chitwan district of Nepal. She is an assistant professor at TU under the Faculty of Health Education. She has also done a degree in Nursing and has worked as a registered nurse (RN) for more than 17 years in different hospitals and communities of Nepal. Her research interests include participatory action research in education, public health, adolescent sexual health and gender. She has worked as a research consultant for different developmental projects and international agencies.

Lisa Gibbs is Professor of Public Health at the University of Melbourne, Australia, where she is Director of the Child and Community Wellbeing Unit in Melbourne School of Population and Global Health. Her research interests are disaster resilience and child health and well-being, with a focus on practice-informed evidence and evidence-informed practice achieved through community-based participatory research approaches. She is a consortium member (leadership team) for the International Collaboration for Participatory Health Research (ICPHR), with specific responsibility for leading initiatives relating to participatory approaches with children.

Linda Gibson is Professor of Public Health, Institute of Health & Allied Professions, Nottingham Trent University (NTU), UK. She has over 20 years of experience in health promotion and working with local communities in the United Kingdom and internationally, and her work is informed by the social model of health. She is involved in several research partnerships, networks and teaching projects in Europe, Eastern Africa (Uganda, Malawi, Ethiopia) and the United States. Linda's research focus is on health systems' strengthening in low- and middle-income countries, community health workforce in primary care in Uganda, non-communicable diseases, antimicrobial stewardship and patient safety. Linda is the UK lead of the ten-year successful partnership between NTU and Makerere University, Uganda.

Dan Grabowski is a sociologist and health promotion researcher employed as a senior researcher at Steno Diabetes Center Copenhagen, Denmark. He leads a research team that conducts health promotion research in the areas of children, young people and families living with diabetes and/or obesity. His main areas of expertise within this field include: (1) Family involvement: What constitutes genuine family involvement and how is it achieved in families confronted with chronic illness or serious health problems? How do we develop or motivate settings that allow for and encourage positive involvement, and how do we furthermore help families develop the preconditions for mutual involvement in their everyday life? (2) Health and illness identities: Why do people understand themselves in significantly different ways in relation to health and illness, and how can we develop health-promoting interventions and new ways of communicating health and illness that do not generate negative self-perceptions?

Nicola Gray is an affiliated researcher within the UNESCO Chair and WHO Collaborating Centre in "Global Health and Education" at the Université Clermont Auvergne, France. She is also Senior Lecturer in Pharmacy Practice at the University of Huddersfield, England, UK. Her research interests include how people access and use health information and services. She has specialized in young people's health, but retains a keen interest in the lives of adults as well, adopting a life-course approach to health and well-being. Her research also highlights the intersection between lay and medical representations of health and medicines, including information obtained in online environments, and the health promotion/public health roles of community pharmacists.

Cyrille Harpet is an anthropologist (University Lyon 2 and University of the Mediterranean—Marseille) with a diploma in Environmental Management (Institute for Applied Engineering—Lyon), Professor at the EHESP School of Public Health, Rennes, France, and accredited to supervise PhD Research in Space Planning and Urbanism. His main field of research concerns Public Health and Urban planning, with an integrative approach of the determinants of health (social, environmental). This research agenda brought him to look at the challenges for public health agencies to adopt a cross-sector perspective to address climate change.

Nadine Haschar-Noé is a sociologist. She is a university lecturer, member of the Institut Fédératif d'Etudes et de Recherches Interdisciplinaires Santé Société (IFERISS, FED 4142—"Federative Institute for Interdisciplinary Studies and Research in Health and Society"), member of the Centre de Recherches Sciences Sociales Sports et Corps (CreSco, EA 7419—"Social Science Research Centre on Sports and the Body") and member of the Laboratoire des Sciences Sociales du Politique (LaSSP, EA 4175—"Laboratory of Political Social Sciences") at the

University of Toulouse, France. Her work centres on the social processes and methods that govern sport, culture and health. She is more particularly interested in the construction, implementation and evaluation of public action programmes and their instrumentation.

Natalie Helsper is working on her PhD at the Department of Sport Science and Sport, Friedrich-Alexander University Erlangen-Nürnberg, Germany. She did her MA in the field of Physical Activity and Health and completed her thesis in cooperation with the Victoria University, Melbourne. In her thesis she focused on an asset-based participatory approach and evaluated a health- and physical activity–promoting integration programme among the CALD (culturally and linguistically diverse) community in West Melbourne. As research assistant, she has supported the nationwide implementation of the National Recommendations for Physical Activity and Physical Activity Promotion in local communities as part of the project KOMBINE (Community-based physical activity promotion for the implementation of the National Recommendations). Her research focuses on the assessment of urban and rural municipal structures to embed physical activity–based health promotion, improving health equity systematically and sustainably.

Alfons Hollederer is Professor of Theory and Empirics of Health at the Faculty of Human Sciences (FB 01), University of Kassel, Germany. He graduated with a degree in Public Health and a degree in Social Work. He completed his doctorate in Public Health at the University of Bielefeld and his habilitation in Public Health at the University of Bremen. The professorship focuses on analyses at the healthcare system level (macro level), of institutions and actors in the healthcare system (meso level) and of the health of affected human beings (micro level). Special research interest is directed towards questions of health promotion among unemployed people.

Ingrid Holsen is Professor of Health Promotion at the Department of Health Promotion and Development, Faculty of Psychology, University of Bergen, Norway. She is leading the Master's programme in Health Promotion and Health Psychology at the respective department. She has for many years been involved in and leading health promotion research in the educational field in close collaboration with schools, municipalities and counties, with a special focus on planning and implementation of programmes, youth participatory action research, psychosocial learning environments and youth mental health.

Hervé Hudebine is Senior Lecturer in Sociology (Social Policy) at the Department of Sociology and the Sociology Research Centre (LABERS), Université de Bretagne Occidentale, Brest, France. He is researching public health and long-term care policies at the subnational level, focusing on governance issues and participatory processes. His research interests have also focused on the meaning and uses of vulnerability in old-age policy, on harm reduction policies and on social inequalities issues in health policy in the United Kingdom.

Efrelyn A. Iellamo is an assistant professor at the College of Nursing, University of the Philippines Manila. She is the Specialty Head Course Coordinator of the Maternal and Child Nursing Program. She teaches Maternal and Child Nursing courses, with specialization on Human Lactation and Breastfeeding. She is one of the national trainers of the Essential Intrapartum Newborn Care and Infant and Young Child Feeding. She is a member of the University of the Philippines Manila Chancellor's Committee on Culture and Arts. Moreover, she is the Board of Trustee and Chairperson of the Research and Scholarship Committee of the Mother and Child Nurses Association of the Philippines. She is a clinical instructor handling Obstetrics and Gynaecology wards and Intensive Maternal Unit at UP-Philippine General Hospital.

Deborah Ikhile is a research fellow at the Department of Primary Care and Public Health, Brighton and Sussex Medical School, UK. She is the postdoctoral researcher for the National Institute for Health Research Applied Research Collaboration (NIHR ARC) for Kent, Surrey and Sussex, one of the 15 NIHR ARCs in England. Prior to this, she worked as a research assistant at Nottingham Trent University (NTU), where she supported the international health partnership between NTU and Makerere University (Uganda), focusing on capacity building of community health workers, antimicrobial resistance and stewardship, and non-communicable diseases. Deborah coordinates, with NTU, a newly established Pan-African Network for Mental Health and Society Research comprising seven countries: Burkina Faso, Ghana, England, Uganda, Zimbabwe, Nigeria and South Africa.

Siw Tone Innstrand is Professor of Occupational Health Psychology at the Department of Psychology and Director of the Center for Health Promotion Research, Norwegian University of Science and Technology. The Center takes part in the scientific exploration of what promotes, maintains and restores good health—in healthy, vulnerable and diseased populations. Innstrand has a PhD from NTNU on the "interaction between work and family". Her research interests include, among others, occupational health, health promotion, healthy universities, work-family balance, work engagement and burnout, interventions and implementation research. Innstrand has initiated and developed ARK, which is a comprehensive implementation programme to promote a psychosocial work environment in academia. Over 19 universities and university colleges in Norway N>30.000, and two in Sweden, are using ARK regularly in their systematic health, work and safety efforts.

Valérie Ivassenko is Project Officer at the UNESCO Chair Global Health and Education and coordinates the development and monitoring of the Chair's various activities. A nurse for 15 years, with a Master's in Practical Philosophy and a degree in Ethnology, she is particularly interested in the ethical and anthropological issues of health and care, and especially in vulnerabilities related to old age. She is involved in the implementation of several international capacity-building and knowledge-sharing projects in health promotion.

Maria Jansen is Professor of Population Health at the Department of Health Services Research, Maastricht University, the Netherlands, and programme leader of Academic Collaborative Centre for Public Health, a network organization of science, policy and practice. Her expertise is population health by means of intersectoral implementation of public health (policy) interventions to prevent avoidable chronic diseases and socio-economic health inequalities. School health promotion research has been one of its focus areas for many years. She leads a consortium of researchers that study the effectiveness of school-based health interventions in the Netherlands. She has supervised more than 20 PhD students, (co-) authored more than 200 books, reports and articles in national and international journals (including *Health Promotion International* and the *European Journal of Public Health*), and has been awarded many grants.

Kim Jose is a senior research fellow at the Menzies Institute for Medical Research, University of Tasmania, Australia. She is the president of the Tasmanian branch of the Public Health Association of Australia. Her primary research interest is in promoting health and well-being and the prevention and management of chronic disease across the life course. She has extensive experience in conducting evaluations of programmes (school breakfast programmes), services (Child and Family Centres) and systems (Tasmanian Child Safety System), knowledge translation and implementation. Her research includes participatory research methods and has focused on working with children, young people and vulnerable families. Kim is recognized for conducting high-quality collaborative research in partnership with the government, service providers, health service consumers and the community.

Manmeet Kaur is Professor of Health Promotion at the Department of Community Medicine and School of Public Health, Post Graduate Institute of Medical Education and Research (PGIMER), Chandigarh, India, and an honorary professorial fellow at the George Institute for Global Health, Sydney, Australia. She is a council member of the Global White Ribbon Alliance and a regional coordinator of the White Ribbon Alliance, India. She is a member of the Board of Studies, Central University of Himachal Pradesh, Dharamshala, and Technical Advisory Group on Respectful Maternity Care, Indian Council of Medical Research, New Delhi. She is a member of the State Appropriate Authority and Advisory Committee of Prenatal Diagnostic Techniques Act of two states and the Gender-Based Violence, State Health System Resource Center, Haryana, India.

Jasvir Kaur is a senior nursing officer at the Post Graduate Institute of Medical Education and Research (PGIMER), Chandigarh, India. She holds a postgraduate degree in Psychology and completed her PhD (Health Promotion) in 2019. Her doctoral work presents a theory-guided novel nutrition intervention in community settings implemented using information technology. She has her work published in several peer-reviewed articles in international journals and chapters in books. She specializes in mediational analyses of longitudinal and observational data. She is in charge of the vaccination centre at PGIMER and actively involved in preventive and health-promoting services and related research. Health promotion for all, including HIV prevention among sexual gender minorities, in clinical as well as community settings, constitutes her research interest.

Peter Kelly is Professor of Education and the Head of the UNESCO's UNEVOC Centre, School of Education, RMIT University. UNEVOC is UNESCO's global network for promoting learning for the world of work. Peter's research interests include a critical engagement with young people, their well-being, resilience and enterprise, and the challenges associated with the emergence of the Anthropocene. In the context of the COVID-19 pandemic, these interests are framing the development of a research agenda titled "COVID-19 and Young People's Well-being, Education, Training and Employment Pathways: Scenarios for Young People's Sustainable Futures". Peter has a significant international publishing and research profile. He has his research published in 13 books and more than 75 book chapters and journal articles on young people, marginalization, education, training and work pathways, and well-being.

Charlotte Kervran is a postdoctoral researcher at the Bordeaux Population Health (BPH) Center of the University of Bordeaux, France. Her research focuses on the evaluation of the effectiveness, conditions of effectiveness and viability of complex prevention and health promotion interventions in the fields of early childhood and tobacco use during pregnancy. Over the past seven years, his research has focused on the study of sleep, addiction, craving and harm reduction interventions. Charlotte Kervran's doctoral research has explored the stability of craving as an etiologic (predictive) marker of substance use using EMA and its psychometric stability as a diagnostic criterion within the DSM-5 Substance Use Disorder using the Item Response Theory (IRT).

Edith Kieffer is an emeritus professor at the School of Social Work, University of Michigan, and conducts qualitative formative and intervention research addressing health inequities using community-based participatory research approaches. She holds an MPH (Master's in Public Health) and a doctoral degree. She and collaborators have evaluated the effectiveness of Detroit community health worker (CHW) programmes addressing type 2 diabetes prevention and management, including among pregnant and postpartum women. Kieffer is a founder of the CHW Common Indicators Project, which seeks to identify and put into practice a multi-level set of common CHW evaluation indicators and measures. She helped found the Michigan Community Health Worker Alliance, which promotes sustainability of CHW programmes and careers through policy change and workforce development. Kieffer leads the qualitative component of Michigan's Medicaid expansion evaluation.

Simone Kohler is a nutritionist with an MSc in Public Health. She completed her respective theses at the German Cancer Research Center and the World Health Organization. Through her work at the Robert Koch Institute as part of the KiGGS study (German Health Interview and Examination Survey for Children and

Adolescents) and later at the University Hospital Regensburg in the context of the German National Cohort, she has six years of work experience in surveillance and monitoring of health across Germany. She is working on her PhD at the Department of Sport and Sport Science, Friedrich-Alexander-University Erlangen-Nürnberg, Germany. Since 2018 she has supported the nationwide implementation of the National Recommendations for Physical Activity and Physical Activity Promotion through the project KOMBINE (Community-based physical activity promotion for the implementation of the National Recommendations) in local communities. Her work aims to provide evidence regarding effective interventions for physical activity promotion in metropolises.

S. Kremers is Professor of Health Promotion at Maastricht University, the Netherlands. His research focus is on the study of determinants of dietary behaviour and physical activity and on the evaluation of comprehensive interventions regarding these behaviours for different target groups (e.g. children, adolescents, young adults, (pre-)diabetics). Research lines have additionally focused on methodological and theoretical approaches to the study of determinants of energy balance–related behaviours as well as to the evaluation of preventive interventions.

Maja Kuchler works as a research assistant at the Department of Applied Health Sciences, University of Applied Sciences (HS Gesundheit), Bochum, Germany. Originally an occupational therapist, she has been involved in various research projects on participation and participatory methods in health promotion since her Master's degree and is planning a dissertation in this field. For this purpose, she is an active member of PartGroup, a German working group of young scientists who deal with participatory research in the health sector.

Rajesh Kumar is Executive Director, State Health Systems Resource Center, Department of Health & Family Welfare, Govt. of Punjab, India; honorary professor, London School of Hygiene & Tropical Medicine, UK; visiting professorial fellow, School of Public Health & Community Medicine, University of New South Wales, Sydney, Australia; associate editor, *Journal of Epidemiology & Community Health*; and member of the WHO Technical Advisory Group on Mother and Newborn Information Tracking of Outcomes and Results. He has worked as an emeritus scientist in the Indian Council of Medical Research and as Dean (Academic) & Head of the Department of Community Medicine and School of Public Health, Post Graduate Institute of Medical Education and Research, Chandigarh. He is a fellow of the National Academy of Medical Sciences, New Delhi, India.

Tuuli Kuosmanen works as a postdoctoral researcher at the WHO Collaborating Centre for Health Promotion Research (HPRC) at the National University of Ireland Galway. She has a particular interest in promoting the mental health and well-being of more vulnerable groups of young people. Her PhD examined the effectiveness and implementation of the SPARX-R computerized cognitive behavioural therapy intervention with young people attending alternative education centres across

Ireland. She has been the lead researcher on several international research projects aiming to enhance the translation of research into practice, including developing an evidence-based framework for promoting mental health in the European youth sector and a review commissioned by the WHO European Regional Office on the implementation of effective interventions for promoting adolescents' mental health and well-being and for preventing mental health and behavioural problems in the WHO European region.

Thierry Lang specializes in Social Epidemiology. He is Professor of Public Health, the founding director of the Institut Fédératif d'Etudes et de Recherches Interdisciplinaires Santé Société (IFERISS, FED 4142—"Federative Institute for Interdisciplinary Studies and Research in Health and Society") from 2009 to 2019, and a member of the Centre d'Epidémiologie et de Recherche en Santé des Populations (CERPOP, UMR Inserm [Institut National de la Santé et de la Recherche Médicale] 1295—"Centre for Epidemiology and Population Health") at the University of Toulouse, France. He is also a member of the Haut Conseil de la Santé Publique (HCSP—French Public Health Council); he serves on the council's board and is the president of the task force on social inequities in health and on children.

Torill Larsen has a PhD in Health Promotion and is a professor at the Department for Health Promotion and Development, University of Bergen, Norway. She has more than ten years' experience in teaching Health Promotion at Bachelor's and Master's levels. She has been the Vice Dean for Research at the Faculty of Teacher Education, Arts and Sport, Western Norway University of Applied Science, and was the project leader for the Complete project on behalf of the Ministry of Education. She has extensive experience in leading health promotion research in the educational field in close collaboration with schools, NGOs and counties, with a special focus on planning and implementation of programmes, school leadership, psychosocial learning environments and positive youth development.

Deana Leahy is Associate Professor of Health Education, School of Education, Culture and Society, Faculty of Education, Monash University, Victoria, Australia. Deana's research draws on interdisciplinary perspectives to critically study health education—from policy formations to their translations into everyday pedagogies. Whilst her work has a strong school focus, she has recently begun to explore the possibilities of other pedagogical spaces and approaches that seek to teach us something about health, including museums/exhibits, festivals and various digital technology platforms and gamification. Deana is known for her innovative use of social theory and creative methodologies to forge new directions in both research and teaching.

Yann Le Bodo is a research fellow at the Department of Social and Human Sciences, EHESP School of Public Health, Rennes, France. Recently, he coordinated the CLoterreS study aimed to analyse the disease prevention and health promotion action plans of the "local health contacts" in France (2018–2020) and now coordinates the Soda-Tax interdisciplinary research project on the development, implementation and effects of the soda tax applied in France since July 2018 (2019–2023). Over the last years, his research interests have focused on healthy eating and physical activity policies as well as health promotion at the community level in France and in the Canadian province of Québec.

Janna Leimann studied Physiotherapy in Utrecht, the Netherlands, and Evidence-Based Health Care in Bochum, Germany. She worked as a physiotherapist for many years. Since 2017 she works as a research assistant at the Department of Applied Health Sciences, University of Applied Sciences (HS Gesundheit), Bochum, Germany, in various national and international research projects. Her focus is on health promotion in the municipal setting and public health. In 2021 she started to set up a student health management programme at the HS Gesundheit, which focuses on the participatory involvement of the students.

Monica Lillefjell is a professor at the Department of Neuromedicine and Movement Science, Norwegian University of Science and Technology (NTNU). She is an Occupational Therapist (Reg. OT) and has a PhD from NTNU on "occupational rehabilitation and work participation". She is previous head of the Norwegian Network for Research and Education in Health Promotion and has extensive research leadership experience in developing knowledge on complex public health interventions and their planning, implementation and sustainability. Lillefjell's research spans topics such as health promotion research, applied public health research, salutogenesis, citizen involvement in public health, public governance research, implementation science, digital health research and occupational rehabilitation research.

Ivan Rene G. Lim (RN, SO2) is a registered nurse who obtained his Bachelor of Science degree from the College of Nursing, University of the Philippines. He strongly believes in the principles of holistic care and never fails to provide this kind of care to all of his patients. Concurrently as a certified safety officer, his aim is to ensure a safe, clean and supportive work environment for all employees in any kind of company. With a passion for teaching, he truly believes that educating the next generation on health, wellness and disease prevention is a vital step in improving the healthcare system as a whole.

Daniel López-Cevallos serves as Associate Professor of Latinx Studies, Ethnic Studies & Health Equity; Assistant Vice Provost for Undergraduate Education and affiliated faculty with the Center for Global Health, Oregon State University, with an MPH (Master's in Public Health) and a doctoral degree. For well over a decade, he has worked towards addressing health equity issues in Ecuador and the United States. His research takes a socio-ecological approach to tackle the intersections of race/ethnicity, gender, class and other socio-economic and socio-cultural factors, and their relationship to health and healthcare outcomes. Furthermore, he is involved in the development and implementation of community-, institution- and policy-level strategies to improve the health and well-being of marginalized communities.

Ruca Maass is an Associate professor at the Norwegian University for Science and Technology, Trondheim, Norway. Her professional background includes Occupational Therapy (OT reg.), a Master's degree in Community Psychology and a PhD in Public Health. Her research and teaching focus on how to create salutogenic settings that provide individuals and communities with appropriate resources and coherent experiences, and enable them to tackle life's ups and downs. She has been an appointed member of the International Union for Health Promotion and Education (IUHPE)'s working group on salutogenesis since 2018. She is also an active member of the Norwegian Network for Research and Education in Health Promotion, as well as the Nordic Health Promotion Research Network (NHPRN).

Colin Macdougall is Emeritus Professor of Public Health at Flinders University, Adelaide, Australia, with honorary appointments at the University of Melbourne and the Centre for Health Equity and at Pokhara University, Nepal. Before academic life, he was a child psychologist, founded a community health service for children and families, and was a chief planning officer in a health system. Experienced in capacity building in Australia, Nepal, South Africa and Papua New Guinea, he has strong research links in France. Colin's research contributes to social and climate justice, healthy public policy, rights approaches to childhood and linking public health, disasters and climate change. He is co-editor of the new fifth edition of *Understanding Health*.

Andrew Macnab is Professor of Paediatrics in Vancouver and a visiting fellow at the Stellenbosch Institute for Advanced Study, Stellenbosch, South Africa. Highly respected as a clinician, he is also a distinguished scholar and award-winning researcher and a global health project director with a reputation for innovation and excellence. Many of his initiatives involving novel educational approaches and application of leading-edge technology to improve healthcare delivery have been adopted nationally and internationally. He is a Grand Challenges Canada "Star in Global Health" and the founder of the school-based programme Brighter Smiles Africa (a Rose Charities Canada project), which is committed to developing initiatives that engage young people in sub-Saharan Africa effectively in health promotion and lead to a positive lifestyle choice.

Kenny Maes (he/him) is an associate professor, faculty union organizer and Director of the Applied Anthropology Graduate Program at Oregon State University. He is a member of the leadership team of the Community Health Worker (CHW) Common Indicators (CI) Project and author of *The Lives of Community Health Workers: Local Labor and Global Health in Urban Ethiopia* (2017), in addition to many research articles. As a medical anthropologist, he trains graduate students in mixed-methods research in healthcare settings, and carefully documents the process of the CI Project. His previous research focused on the work and well-being of unpaid CHWs in Ethiopia, and the development of culturally responsive measures of household food and water insecurity.

Fabien Maguin is the administrative and financial coordinator of the Case de Santé in Toulouse, France. He oversees this experimental project geared towards health autonomy.

Josephine Marshall is an associate research fellow at the Global Obesity Centre (GLOBE), a designated World Health Organization Collaborating Centre for Obesity Prevention, Institute for Health Transformation at Deakin University, Victoria, Australia. She is also a member of the Australian government–funded Centre for Research Excellence in Food Retail EnvironmentS for Health ("RE-FRESH"). Josephine is a dietitian working on research to address the impact of the food environment on population diet. Her work is focused on the policies and practices of food retailers and food manufacturers, and how these contribute to poor diets and socio-economic inequalities in obesity. In addition, she is involved in several projects highlighting opportunities for government food policy to improve the accountability and practices of the food industry to equitably support healthier diets.

Rosilda Mendes is a professor at the Federal University of São Paulo, Brazil (since 2008) of the Professional Master's Program in the Family Health Network and of the Graduate Program in Social Work and Social Policies. She is Director of the Center for Research, Studies and Documentation in Healthy Cities—CEPEDOC, Collaborating Centre of the World Health Organization (WHO), which has been dedicated to implementing professional training courses for managers and health professionals in Brazil in the areas of promotion health and Sustainable Development Goals. It has been dedicated to studies and research on the following topics: collective health; health promotion; health training and social participation; evaluation of policies, programmes and services; and social determination of the health–disease–care process.

Birgit Metzler is a health expert and coordinator of the Competence Center for Health Promotion in Hospitals and Health Care (CC-HPH), Department of Health Literacy and Health Promotion, Austrian National Public Health Institute, Wien, Austria. She is responsible for the management of projects in the field of health-promoting healthcare organizations at regional, national and international levels. She provides scientific and strategic support to the Austrian Network of Health Promoting Hospitals and Health Services and the Vienna Alliance for Health Promotion in Health Care Facilities. Furthermore, she is responsible for the scientific coordination of the International Conferences on Health Promoting Hospitals and Health Services.

Alain Meunier is a research and development adviser for the organization Communagir. He has a degree in Indigenous Studies (Community Development) from Trent University, Peterborough, Ontario, Canada, and holds a Master's in Human Systems Intervention from Concordia University, Montreal, Quebec, Canada. He is also trained in the theory and practice of open systems and is a graduate of the Gestalt Institute in Toronto. He has over 25 years of experience in community development. He is interested in community planning and the application of the principles of participatory democracy in collective development processes. Convinced that acting together is a powerful way to meet the critical challenges facing our societies, Alain is committed to practices leading to systemic change. He collaborates on various partnerships to make collective development more equitable, inclusive and sustainable.

Kerry Montero is a freelance academic with an interest in youth health, health promotion and education, and young road user safety promotion and policy. Formerly Programme Manager of the Bachelor of Social Science Youth Work programme at RMIT University, Melbourne, Australia, Kerry has an extensive background in youth work, youth work education, and adolescent health promotion, education and service delivery. A focus of Kerry's research and practice over the past 20 years has been the development of targeted road safety education programmes and initiatives for young road users, with a particular emphasis on peer education and community-based approaches. She has worked with industry partners, NGOs and business to develop and deliver successful road safety peer education programmes targeting industrial workers, community and tertiary students in Australia and international settings, most recently, Cambodia.

Shea Moran is the coordinator of Aff the Streets, the national youth steering group for the A Way Home Scotland Coalition, dedicated to ending youth homelessness in Scotland. He works to bring together young people from across Scotland to have a unified voice on homelessness issues that will inform policy and practice. Shea recently contributed to the A Way Home's Youth Homelessness Prevention Pathways, in partnership with the Scottish government: "Youth Homelessness Prevention Pathway—Improving Care Leavers Housing Pathway, 2019".

Conceição Aparecida Moreira is a career servant at the State Health Department of Minas Gerais (SES-MG), Brazil, working in the coordination of health promotion and tobacco control programmes. Throughout his career at SES, she worked with health promotion programmes. She has a degree in Physiotherapy and a Master's in Management and Health Service, and is a specialist in health promotion.

Michelle Morgan is a policy officer at the Tasmanian Department of Health and a doctoral candidate at the University of Tasmania, Australia. In these integrated roles, Michelle's research is exploring how systems thinking can support communities to improve health and well-being, which is informing state-based preventive health policy as insights are generated. Michelle has worked in a variety of health promotion and leadership roles in the Tasmanian government over the past 15 years. Recently, this work has included building systems thinking capacity in public health—both within the workforce and through the development and teaching of postgraduate curriculum. Michelle's work is motivated by trying to find ways to create positive, meaningful and lasting change to improve health and well-being for all.

Samuel Jorge Moysés holds a PhD in Epidemiology and Public Health from the University of London, England (1999). He is a full professor at the Pontifical Catholic University of Paraná, Brazil, and adjunct professor at the Federal University of Paraná. He has experience in the field of public health, with an emphasis on epidemiology, working mainly on the following themes: social determination of the health–disease–care process, social inequities in health, healthy public policies, urban health, health promotion and primary health care.

David Musoke is a lecturer at the Department of Disease Control and Environmental Health, Makerere University School of Public Health, Kampala, Uganda. He is co-Chair of the Community Health Workers Thematic Working Group of Health Systems Global. He is also a senior visiting fellow at Nottingham Trent University (NTU), UK, and Uganda lead of the ten-year partnership between NTU and Makerere University that has supported over 750 community health workers in the Wakiso district. He spearheaded the organization of the first-ever International Symposium on Community Health Workers held in Uganda in 2017. He is also an academic editor for *PLOS Global Public Health*, *BMC Public Health*, B*MC Health Services Research* and the *Journal of Environmental and Public Health*.

Júlia Aparecida Devidé Nogueira is a professor at the Physical Education School, University of Brasilia, Brazil. She coordinates the Research Group on Health Promotion and Equity, certified by the Brazilian National Council for Scientific and Technological Development, a scientific endeavour group that works with local environments' public health, by intersectoral actions, fighting health inequalities. She is also a member of the executive committee of the Working Group on Health Promotion and Sustainable Development at the Brazilian Association of Collective Health (ABRASCO), a group that supports and articulates training, teaching and research in public health. Her research projects involve mainly the role of physical education on health promotion in cities, universities and schools.

Mathew Nyashanu is a senior lecturer and admissions tutor on the MA programme in Public Health at Nottingham Trent University, UK. He teaches on the postgraduate courses, including supervising PhD students. Dr Nyashanu also collaborates with community groups working in public health development and education in the United Kingdom and is involved in international research collaboration with colleagues in South Africa, Uganda, Zambia and the United States. Dr Nyashanu has his research published widely in the area of global public health.

Lily O'Hara is Associate Professor of Public Health at Qatar University, Doha, Qatar. Lily is a public health and health promotion educator, researcher and practitioner with experience in Australia, United Arab Emirates (UAE) and Qatar. She has worked in health promotion practice roles with governmental, non-governmental and private sector organizations. Lily has worked on community-, workplace-, school- and health service–based programmes addressing a broad range of health and well-being issues. Her research focuses on analysing public health approaches to body weight and their inequitable impact on people with larger bodies. She develops and evaluates ethical, evidence-based, salutogenic health promotion initiatives for body liberation, drawing on the social justice–based Health at Every Size approach. Lily's research also focuses on developing the ethical and technical competencies of the health promotion workforce.

Ebenezer Owusu-Addo is a senior research fellow at the Bureau of Integrated Rural Development, Kwame Nkrumah University of Science and Technology, Kumasi, Ghana. He has a PhD in Health Promotion (Programme Evaluation) and over 15 years of work experience in the health and social sectors. He is a co-principal investigator for the USAID Analytical Support Services and Evaluations for Sustainable Systems (ASSESS) Project in West Africa. He is a leading figure in health promotion research and evaluation, more specifically through his work on the role of public policies and intersectoral action in addressing the social determinants of health and health inequality. His research interests are in the social determinants of health, health equity, social protection, rural health systems and the interface between public health and town planning.

Joan J. Paredes-Carbonell is a Doctor of Medicine, a Master's in Public Health and a specialist in Family and Community Medicine. He started working as a health promotion doctor in several public health centres, becoming Deputy Director General of Health Promotion of the Valencian government. He is Deputy Director of Primary Care in the Health Department of La Ribera (Alzira, Spain) and researcher in the area of health inequalities of the FISABIO Foundation, promoting various health promotion and community action projects. He coordinated an interdisciplinary project to adapt the National Institute for Clinical Excellence (NICE) guidelines for community engagement in health to the Spanish context and is the principal investigator of a project funded by the Carlos III Institute of Spain to evaluate the implementation of this guide.

Estelle Pegon-Machat is a dentist, has a PhD and a Master's degree in Health Ethics, and is full Assistant Professor of Public Health, at the Dental faculty, University of Clermont Auvergne, France. She is working within a research group (CROC EA4847), and her research interests relate to ethics and public health. She has experience in qualitative research methodologies and has particularly explored the issue of access to oral health services for deprived populations. The integration of oral health issues within general health, by the development of the common risk factor approach, is also a common trait of her research activities.

Klaus Pfeifer holds a Chair for Physical Activity and Health at Friedrich-Alexander University Erlangen-Nürnberg (FAU), Germany. He is Head of the Department of Sport Science and Sport at FAU, which is designated as a WHO Collaboration Centre for Physical Activity and Health. He is leading several transdisciplinary research projects in the field of physical activity promotion, health promotion and health care. He has co-coordinated the development of the National

Recommendations for Physical Activity and Physical Activity Promotion in Germany as well as projects for their dissemination and implementation. He serves as a scientific consultant for the German Federal Ministry of Health for physical activity promotion.

Helene Pichot is a dentist, and has a Master's degree in Nutrition and a PhD from the University of Clermont Auvergne in France. She is Deputy Director of the New Caledonian Health and Social Agency. She has developed, set up and still manages the oral health promotion programme and works with the CROC EA4847 research team on the evaluation of the programme under a partnership agreement.

Christina Plantz completed her diploma studies in Health Promotion at the University of Applied Sciences Magdeburg, Germany, and then her Master's degree in Public Health at the University of Düsseldorf, Germany. She has 15 years of professional experience as a technical officer in the field of prevention and health promotion in different settings and at different political levels (local, federal, European), with a focus on community-centred approaches and health equity. Since 2016, she works at the Federal Centre for Health Education (BZgA) in Germany. Since 2018, she has been leading the "Healthy Living Environments" work package in the EU Joint Action Health Equity Europe (JAHEE) and coordinating its implementation in Germany.

Giancarlo Pocetta holds an MD, an MA and a PhD in Health Education; and is a leading researcher in health promotion and Aggregate Professor of Hygiene and Public Health, University of Perugia, Italy, where he is teaching Health Promotion, Hygiene and Epidemiology. He is a board member of the University's Research Centre for Health Promotion and Education. Dr Pocetta is Scientific Director of the Master's degree "Planning Management and Evaluation of Health Promotion in the Community", and represents the University of Perugia in the European Training Consortium (ETC) PHHP Consortium, where he regularly carries out lecturing and tutoring activities. His research is oriented towards the application of quantitative and qualitative methods to organizational development and capacity-building of health promotion services and professionals.

Alexia Prasouli is a developmental paediatrician. She has been working at the Department of Developmental and Social Pediatrics, Institute of Child Health (ICH), Athens, Greece, since September 2006. She is strongly interested in the early recognition of developmental disorders and in early intervention. She has worked on this topic in several scientific projects. She has an extensive experience in the clinical evaluation of children with developmental difficulties as well as in the administration of various developmental tests, applying the relevant knowledge in a Child Health Center founded by the ICH (1992). Recently, she has participated in the scientific team that has issued the guidelines for developmental surveillance in the context of primary paediatric care in Greece and in reformation of the *Greek Child Health Booklet*. She participates in educational seminars for primary healthcare practitioners regarding developmental surveillance and assessment.

Eike Quilling is Professor of Health Education and Communication at the Department of Applied Health Sciences and is Vice President for Research and Transfer at the University of Applied Sciences (HS Gesundheit), Bochum, Germany. Her research focuses on community- and setting-oriented health promotion and prevention. In addition, she leads the research group on setting-based health promotion and prevention and creating healthy living environments.

Alex Richmond is a doctoral candidate at the School of Population Health, University of New South Wales, Sydney, Australia. She has a background in non-profit programme development and sustainability, with particular focus to build capacity in the field of sport for development and social change (S4SC). She is increasingly experienced in fourth-generation evaluation, an evaluation protocol designed to put the voice of the stakeholders at the centre of research and development challenges. She holds dual BA/BS degrees from the University of Georgia, Athens, Georgia, and an MSc in Sport Management, Policy, and International Development from the University of Edinburgh, UK.

Therese Riley is Associate Professor of Complex Community Interventions at the Mitchell Institute, Victoria University, Australia. Therese has held appointments in universities in Australia and Canada, along with the not-for-profit sector. Therese has been an active member of collaborations that have led the field in the application of complexity theory and systems science in public health and health promotion research and evaluation. Her interests lie in understanding the social processes that enable or constrain our capacity to act systemically at the community level.

Dais Gonçalves Rocha is Professor of Health Promotion and Health Equity; Human Rights, Culture and Society at the Department of Public Health, Faculty of Health Science, University of Brasília, Brazil. She coordinates the Research Group on Health Promotion and Equity, certified by the Brazilian National Council for Scientific and Technological Development. Her research projects involve intersectoral cooperation and health promotion as a strategy for local sustainable development and promotion of equity on health. She is also a member of the Working Group on Health Promotion and Sustainable Development at the Brazilian Association of Collective Health (ABRASCO), a group that supports and advocates democracy and social political approach of health promotion at municipal, state and federal levels.

Keara Rodela (she/they) is a community health worker (CHW) and CHW supervisor. She obtained her Master of Public Health in Global Maternal Child Health from the School of Public Health and Tropical Medicine, Tulane University, New Orleans, Louisiana, and holds a Bachelor of Science in Community Health Education from Portland State University, Oregon. Keara is a Black, queer woman who is committed to redressing the social determinants of health affecting her communities, utilizing the CHW model, popular education philosophy and a racial equity lens. She has held various roles in her 19 years in the health field and is a strong advocate for the CHW profession. Keara is a member of the CHW Common Indicators Project's leadership team.

Andrea Rodriguez is Lecturer in Dental Public at University of Dundee, Scotland. She leads the Scottish Oral Health Improvement Research Programme, Smile4life, to promote oral health and psycho-social well-being for people experiencing homelessness. She is an invited member of Scottish government commissions to reduce homelessness at local (Dundee City Council) and national (Health and Homelessness steering group) levels. Andrea is an associated researcher at the Observatory of Favelas, Brazil. She has over 20 years of experience working in favelas in Rio de Janeiro and doing community-based participatory research. She has a Master's in Psycho-sociology of Communities and a PhD in Social Psychology from Federal University of Rio de Janeiro, Brazil. Her academic and professional experience has a strong connection with third-sector organizations working with popular education, health promotion and community development.

Leticia Rodriguez Avila (she/her) is a community health worker (CHW) and leads a CHW Capacity-Building Program in Los Angeles County. She obtained her Master of Public Health from Portland State University, Oregon. Leticia's experiences as an immigrant from Michoacán, Mexico, and from a farmworker family inform her work in addressing the social determinants of health in her communities. She has held various roles in the public health field and is honoured that most of those have been in working alongside other CHWs. Leticia's roles include CHW, evaluation and capacitation assistant, capacity-building facilitator and capacity-building director. Leticia is a member of the CHW Common Indicators Project and a stakeholder in the Community Health Workers & *Promotores* in the Future of Medi-Cal Project.

Daniela Rojatz holds a PhD in Sociology from the University of Vienna, Austria. She is a health expert at the Department of Health Literacy and Health Promotion, Austrian National Public Health Institute, Vienna. Her work focuses on the implementation of health promotion, prevention and health literacy in primary care units and patient participation. Within the Austrian National Public Health Institute, she is co-coordinator of the internal Task Force on Primary Care and the Community of Practice Participation. In addition, she is a lecturer at the Institute of Sociology at the University of Vienna in the field of health and organizational sociology. She is voluntarily involved in the board of the Austrian Society for Public Health and as one of the spokespersons of the competence group Participation of the organization.

Zoé Rollin is a lecturer at the Department of Educational Sciences, University of Paris, France. She is a researcher at Centre de recherche sur les liens sociaux (CERLIS, Paris), Paris, and associated with Laboratoire interdisciplinaire d'évaluation des politiques publiques (LIEPP, Paris). She is Scientific Director of the "Carry-on association" and co-Director of Giscop 93. After her doctoral thesis, she has focused most of her work onto intervention research with adolescents and young adults followed up for cancer or exposed to carcinogenic risks.

Alfred Rütten is a senior fellow at Friedrich-Alexander University (FAU) Erlangen-Nürnberg, Germany. He served as Head of the FAU Division of Public Health and Physical Activity and has been Director of the first WHO Collaborating Centre on Physical Activity and Public Health in Europe. He has led several cross-national research and development projects on behalf of the European Commission and served as a temporary adviser of the WHO in various contexts (e.g. policy development, health inequality). He has been a leading scientific consultant for the development and implementation of the WHO European Physical Activity Strategy. He has also coordinated the development of National Recommendations for Physical Activity and its promotion in Germany and is leading several demonstration projects and a scaling-up approach on the implementation of the German physical activity recommendations.

Gary Sacks is an associate professor and Heart Foundation's Future Leader fellow, Global Obesity Centre, Deakin University, Victoria, Australia. Gary's research focuses on policies for improving population diets and preventing obesity. Gary has co-authored several international reports on obesity prevention, including the Lancet Commission on Obesity, and several reports for the World Health Organization. Gary led the first-ever studies to benchmark progress on obesity prevention by Australian governments and food companies, for which he was awarded a prestigious VicHealth Award for research translation. Gary co-founded INFORMAS (International Network for Food and Obesity/non-communicable diseases Research, Monitoring and Action Support)—a global network for monitoring food environments. Gary leads the component of INFORMAS dedicated to monitoring the actions of food companies in relation to obesity prevention and population nutrition.

Fernando Sacoto is Director of the Master's degree in Public Health at the International University of Ecuador and President of Ecuadorian Society of Public Health. He is a health policy, systems and services consultant, and is managing a community COVID-19 surveillance programme and monitoring essential maternal and child services with support from UNICEF. He has experience in the management of health promotion programmes and prevention of non-communicable diseases, as part of international networks of healthy cities.

Hans Savelberg is Professor of Evolving Academic Education at the Department of Nutrition and Movement Sciences, Maastricht University, the Netherlands. One of his areas of interest is assessing daily physical activity and understanding the impact of physical activity on health and cognitive performance. He performs studies in varying populations, from primary school children to elderly and people with diabetes. Study designs comprise both large cohort field studies and smaller controlled trials and everything in between. In this way he tries to link the understanding of underlying biological mechanisms to real-life implementations of physical activity interventions.

Jana Semrau is a postdoctoral researcher and the coordinator of the project KOMBINE (Community-based physical activity promotion for the implementation of the National Recommendations) at the Department of Sport and Sport Science, Friedrich-Alexander-University Erlangen-Nürnberg, Germany. She holds the position of Vice President at the Bavarian Association for Health Promotion and Disease Prevention. She is also engaged Lecturer in Health Promotion at the FOM University of Applied Sciences, Essen, Germany. Her work is located at the intersection of health promotion science and practice related to the nationwide implementation of the German Prevention Act in local communities. Her transdisciplinary research focuses on the sustainable implementation and scaling-up of population-based health promotion interventions in local communities, with a specific focus on health equity.

Andy Sharma is a faculty member in Public Policy Studies and Global Health at Northwestern University. His research interests are in aging, older adult health disparities and minority health, and older adult disability. His overall research theme is in the areas of applied demography and population health. Andy's research can be read in *Applied Geography, Ageing and Society, Health Promotion International*, the *Journal of Aging and Health*, the *Journal of Applied Gerontology*, *The Journals of Gerontology: Series B*, *Obesity Research and Clinical Practice,* and *Women's Health Issues.* His most recent work examines mortality risk from COVID and this research was featured both in *The Journals of Gerontology* and the Gerontological Society of America (GSA) special webinar on COVID conversations. Andy was granted a PhD in Public Policy, with a minor in Sociology, from the University of North Carolina at Chapel Hill and was a pre-doctoral trainee with the Carolina Population Center.

William Sherlaw is an honorary professor at the EHESP School of Public Health, Rennes, France. Prior to retirement in June 2019, he worked both at the Department for International Relations and at the Department of Social Sciences, specializing in the fields of health promotion, health anthropology, health inequities, disability studies and migrant health. After retirement he continues to write and teach, contributing to research projects, publications and initiatives founded on participatory research methods highlighting inclusive practice and policy. He is an active member of the French-speaking network of disability specialists, the GIFFOCH (https://giffoch.org/), involved in training on participation for professionals and people with disabilities.

Charlyn Khrysse I. Sia is a registered nurse, who obtained her Bachelor of Science degree from the College of Nursing, University of the Philippines in 2019. For more than a year, she spent her career dedicated to the COVID-19 response of the Philippines. Ms. Charlyn previously served as City Epidemiology and Surveillance Unit Support Coordinator for the COVID-19 response of the Philippines at the World Health Organization—Philippines. She works as a Regional Epidemiology and Surveillance Unit Support Coordinator for the COVID-19 response at the Department of Health, Philippines Epidemiology Bureau. Moreover, she is an upcoming medical student at the College of Medicine, University of the Philippines.

Lucas Sivilotti After an initial nursing training, a Master's degree in Health Education and a doctorate degree in Education Sciences and Training defended in December 2019, Lucas Sivilotti is a postdoctoral researcher on the research project affiliated with "Carry on". He prepared a thesis on mediation with students suffering from cancer or rare diseases. It is through surveys by questionnaires, interviews and ethnographic follow-ups that he had studied the concepts of disability and inclusion through the prism of professional support co-constructed via a systemic approach. At the same time, he teaches particularly at the INSPé of the Académie de Bordeaux and the University of Paris, France, about inclusion thematic, health education, school climate, family education and intervention analysis.

Amal Skandrani is a dentist, has a Master's degree in Public Health and is a PhD student at the Dental faculty of University of Clermont Auvergne, France, within the research group (CROC EA4847) and under the supervision of Stephanie Tubert-Jeannin. Her PhD will participate in evaluating the impact on children's health of the oral health promotion programme conducted in New Caledonia. She will use mixed methods to identify changes that need to be made to improve the programme within an overall health equity approach.

Marjorita Sormunen is Adjunct Professor of Health Promotion and works as a senior lecturer at the Institute of Public Health and Clinical Nutrition, Faculty of Health Sciences, University of Eastern Finland. Her research focuses largely on the area of school health promotion, particularly related to health partnership development between home and school, and children's health learning. She is a qualified educator of health education and a teacher trainer. She serves as the Chair of the Schools for Health in Europe (SHE) research group, is a co-convenor of the Health Education network of the European Educational Research Association and is a Fulbright alumna of the Department of Health Education and Behavior, University of Florida.

Kate St-Arneault is a PhD candidate in the School of Public Health, University of Montreal (ESPUM), Canada. She also has a Master's in Nursing and is a lecturer at the Nursing Department of the Université du Québec en Outaouais. Her PhD focuses on how parents' health, well-being and practices are affected by health promotion interventions that target children. Specifically, she is interested in better understanding how outdoor free-play promotion strategies can also promote or hinder parents' mental health and quality of life in the current context of the rise of intensive parenting practices.

Marie-Pier St-Louis holds a Master's in Sociology from the Université du Québec à Montréal, Canada. She works as a professional researcher at the Canada Research Chair in Community Approaches and Health Inequalities (CACIS) and the Centre of Applied Social Research. She has extensive experience supporting concerted action processes in social development and fight against poverty. Working for several years with Angèle Bilodeau, Marie-Pier participated in the development of the "Tool for Assessing the Effects of Local Intersectoral Action", a knowledge transfer tool developed in partnership with local actors.

Mikael St-Pierre is an urban planner and designer at the Montréal Urban Ecology Centre, Canada. His practice is centred on community town planning and social innovation. Mikael is National Coordinator for the Active Neighbourhoods Canada network, an initiative that aims for equitable access to healthy built environments for all Canadian communities. In 2016, Mikael was identified as one of Canada's 20 Emerging Innovators by the American Express Leadership Institute and Ashoka. He is also a lecturer at the Department of Urban Studies, Université du Québec à Montréal.

Jane Taylor is Associate Professor of Public Health at the University of the Sunshine Coast (USC), Australia, where she is the Discipline Leader for Public Health. Jane has worked as a health promotion practitioner in community and government sectors on a range of community-based health promotion programmes, including women's health, Aboriginal and Torres Strait Islander health, school health promotion and public health service delivery in rural and remote Queensland. Jane teaches philosophical and technical health promotion courses at undergraduate and postgraduate levels. Jane's health promotion research focuses on strengthening the theoretical foundations of health promotion to support a critical practice approach using values and principles to design, implement, evaluate and critique health promotion policies and programmes, and undertake research.

Eric Y. Tenkorang is Associate Professor of Sociology, cross-appointed to the Division of Community Health and Humanities at Memorial University, Newfoundland, Canada. He is a member of the Royal Society of Canada (the College of New Scholars, Artists and Scientists) and a fellow of the Carnegie African Diaspora Programme. Dr Tenkorang served as a member of the Institute Advisory Board for Gender and Health of the Canadian Institutes of Health Research (CIHR), Ottawa. He has broad research interests in population health, especially in limited-resource settings. This includes an investigation of the sexual and reproductive health of vulnerable and marginalized populations in HIV-endemic parts of the world, mostly sub-Saharan Africa. His most recent research has explored links between gender-based violence and health outcomes.

Irene Torres is a researcher specialized in health promotion, working from Fundación Octaedro in Quito, Ecuador. Her studies focus on the social determinants of health, school food, nutrition education and health education, children's well-being, health policy, migration and health, and, more recently, the impact of COVID-19 and related government responses in Latin America. She is a board member of the Ecuadorian Society of Public Health and is an active advocate against inequity.

Marie-Claude Tremblay is Associate Professor at the Department of Family Medicine and Emergency Medicine, Université Laval, Québec, Canada. She is also a co-responsible of the expertise in Indigenous health of the Quebec Strategy for Patient-Oriented Research Support Unit and an associate editor of the academic journal *Health Promotion International*. Tremblay's research expertise includes qualitative methods, cultural safety, patient engagement and participatory research approaches. Her research programme includes various projects realized in partnership with patients and communities that address cultural safety of health care, racism issues in the health system, patient participation in research and health education, as well as reflexivity as a mode of transformation of healthcare practices.

Stéphanie Tubert-Jeannin is a dentist, full Professor of Public Health and former Dean of the Dental faculty, University of Clermont Auvergne, France. She is a past president of the Association for Dental education (ADEE) in Europe. She is a member of the "Platform for Better Oral Health in Europe" and coordinator of the European Erasmus ¬+ "O-Health-Edu" project. She is part of the steering comity of the UNESCO Chair "Global Health and Education". Her research interests within the CROC EA4847 team include various aspects of public health interventions, such as the evaluation of health needs, the development and validation of health indicators, and the implementation and evaluation of (oral) health promotion programmes. The integration of oral health issues within general health, by the development of the common risk factor approach, is a common trait of those research activities.

Helga Bjørnøy Urke has a PhD in Health Promotion from the University of Bergen, Norway. She is an associate professor at the Department of Health Promotion and Development, University of Bergen, and has several years of experience in teaching health promotion. She is leading a large research project on mental health inequalities among the youth in Norway. She also held the position of project coordinator in Complete for two years. Her main area of research is related to social aspects of child and adolescent health and well-being.

Patricia van Assema is an associate professor at the Department of Health Promotion, Maastricht University, the Netherlands. She has ample experience as a research project leader, has supervised more than ten PhD students and co-authored more than 125 articles in international peer-reviewed journals and articles/chapters in Dutch scientific journals, professional journals and books. She has been a project leader of research projects regarding determinants of nutrition behaviours, and the development, evaluation and dissemination of health-promoting programmes in schools and the wider community, especially targeting people with a low social-economic status. Her work includes implementation studies in schools and municipalities.

Helen Vaneyk is a senior research fellow at Flinders University, Adelaide, Australia. Her research focuses on effective healthy public policy and addresses the social determinants of health and health equity. She was a project manager during the five-year Australian National Health and Medical Research Council–funded evaluation of South Australia's Health in All Policies approach and has had key papers from that research published. She is also interested in research translation into policy and has supported this within her research activities. Prior to her research role, she spent 28 years working on health policy development and analysis, including in senior executive positions in population and social health policy in an Australian state public service.

Maude Vézina is a PhD candidate in Population Health at the University of Ottawa, Canada. Her research focuses primarily on maternal health and mental health, with an emphasis on the complementarity between biomedical and traditional approaches to health care. In 2017, she stayed in Laos as part of her Master's project, to conduct research exploring the association between a traditional postnatal practice (called the *hot bed*) and the occurrence of postpartum depression symptoms. She works as a research evaluation coordinator for a community health clinic and is collecting data for her thesis project, around the theme "Factors influencing the use of midwifery services among parents in Quebec".

Ragnhild Holmen Waldahl is a senior researcher at Nordland Research Institute, Bodo, Norway. Her research includes welfare innovation and the organization and cooperation between different welfare services. Empirically, her projects range from youth, dropout and exclusion to welfare technology and health and care services for the elderly. She has extensive experience in developing and implementing innovation and research projects in close collaboration with public actors.

Marcia Faria Westphal graduated in Political and Social Sciences from Catholic University in São Paulo (1965), Brazil, and has a Master's in Public Health (1974) and a PhD in Public Health (1982) from the University of São Paulo. She is a full senior professor at the University of São Paulo, with special training in public health/health promotion. In her long experience of over 50 years working in the field of public health, she has acted on the following subjects: health promotion, health education, social participation, Healthy Cities and public health in general. She was Vice-president for the Latin American Chapter of the International Union for Health Promotion and Education between 1998 and 2007. She is also a researcher at the Center for Studies, Research and Documentation on Health Cities, a

Collaborating Centre of the World Health Organization (WHO) and of the National Health Department of Brazil.

Noelle Wiggins (she/her) is Principal at Wiggins Health Consulting LLC and co-principal investigator for the Community Health Worker (CHW) Common Indicators Project. She served as Associate Director of the landmark National Community Health Advisor Study and lead author on the chapter on Core Roles and Competencies of CHWs. Noelle founded and directed the Community Capacitation Center in Portland, Oregon, and was taught community organizing and research paradigms and methods at Portland State University. She has her research published in numerous peer-reviewed journals and presented at over 60 state and national conferences on topics including CHWs, popular (people's) education and community-based participatory research and evaluation. Noelle holds a BA from Yale University, a Master of Science from the Harvard School of Public Health and an EdD from Portland State University.

Carmel Williams is Director of the Centre for HiAP Research Translation, South Australian Health and Medical Research Institute, and co-Director of the WHO Collaborating Centre for Advancing Health in All Policies. Carmel has overseen the establishment and sustainability of South Australia's Health in All Policies approach, which works across the government to influence public policy decisions to improve health and well-being. She led numerous collaborative projects on the social and environmental determinants of health, drawing research, policy and practice together to deliver evidence informed public policy outcomes. Carmel has significant experience in health promotion and public health. She works extensively with the WHO and other international organizations, undertaking knowledge translation and capacity-building programmes with researchers, policymakers and practitioners.

Jan Wollgast is Scientific Officer, Health in Society Unit, European Commission's Joint Research Centre, Ispra, Italy. He leads a team on health promotion and, with his colleagues, provides knowledge, assessments and tools towards developing and implementing effective policies to promote physical and mental health and well-being. Jan's scientific work has focused on how to promote healthy, and more recently sustainable, diets, thereby increasing the evidence base for European food and public health nutrition policies and helping to reduce preventable burden of diseases, such as cancer, heart disease, obesity and diabetes. His interest is in scientific approaches to complex and systemic societal challenges such as public health as well as the food system. Jan is a nutritionist by training and holds a PhD in Nutritional Sciences from the Justus-Liebig University in Giessen, Germany.

Adamandia Xekalaki is a paediatrician at the Department of Social and Developmental Pediatrics, Institute of Child Health (ICH), in Athens, Greece, for the last 25 years. The main fields of her scientific interest are primary paediatric health care and health education and health promotion programmes. The main focus of interest is holistic care of children and support of their families, by the healthcare system and health professionals, and effective work of the healthcare team in primary healthcare settings. She has participated in many health education programmes in the community, through work in a Child Health Center, founded by the ICH. She was a member of the scientific team that has issued national guidelines for the follow-up of children and adolescents in the context of primary care (2015) and a member of the team that has reconstructed the *Greek Child Health Booklet* (2017). She has participated in several training seminars and postgraduate lectures for paediatricians and other health professionals.

Keli Bahia Felicíssimo Zocrato is an adjunct professor at the Department Health Management, School of Nursing, Federal University of Minas Gerais, Brazil. Law and health is the object of her study. She is also a researcher at the Health Management Centre (NUGES, Brazil).

Chapter 1
A Global Participatory Process for Structuring the Field of Health Promotion Research: An Introduction

Louise Potvin and Didier Jourdan

With the exception of the Bangkok Charter, which calls to anchor health promotion practices on the best available evidence (WHO, 2005), there is no mention of research and of relevant scientific knowledge in health promotion founding documents. In these documents, health promotion is mostly framed as a discourse and as a professional practice based on a set of values and principles that promotes changes at the individual, community and global levels (Potvin & Jones, 2011). There is no well-defined knowledge base and no distinctive, widely agreed knowledge production approach for health promotion research. Nevertheless, during the past decades, health promotion research has developed and gained recognition as witnessed through various signs of scientific institutionalization (scientific journals, graduate research-oriented programmes, departments in higher education institutions and research units in universities). In many knowledge institutions, health promotion research has gained the status of "a name on the door" (Potvin & McQueen, 2007).

Like all other research domains related to professional practice, health promotion research started its development following what we would call a potluck model. Researchers from various disciplinary backgrounds, attracted to the values and transformative vision underpinning the health promotion discourse, have used their disciplinary-based theories and methods to conduct studies on the various practices associated with health promotion (Jourdan, 2013; MacDonald & Bunton,

L. Potvin (✉)
School of Public Health, University of Montreal, Montreal, QC, Canada

Centre de recherche en santé publique (CReSP), Université of Montreal and CIUSSS du Centre-Sud-de-l'Île-de-Montréal, Montréal, QC, Canada
e-mail: louise.potvin@umontreal.ca

D. Jourdan
UNESCO Chair and WHO Collaborating Centre in Global Health & Education, University of Clermont Auvergne, Clermont-Ferrand, France

L. Potvin, D. Jourdan (eds.), *Global Handbook of Health Promotion Research, Vol. 1*,
https://doi.org/10.1007/978-3-030-97212-7_1

2002). A question arises as to whether health promotion research is still at its potluck stage or is it now a constituted, distinctive field of scientific enquiry. In other words, is health promotion research simply a crossroads where researchers from different disciplines temporarily meet, or is it a constituted field of research on its own with its specific objects, epistemological frameworks, methods and specialists? This question has been raised in all research fields founded on social practices (see, for example, Fischer & Miller, 2007, on political science or Wyse, 2016, on education science) and not on a specific approach to reality (physics, sociology and so on). We created this *Global Handbook of Health Promotion Research* project to make visible that health promotion research has come of age and has become a distinct field of scientific enquiry. It can be distinguished from other fields through its distinctive objects and a unique configuration of ethical and epistemological perspectives that shape the research practices of those who identify as health promotion researchers.

However, as of yet, these ethical and epistemological foundations have not been explicitly formulated and articulated into a coherent structuring framework for health promotion research. This is the project of this global handbook, for which the process of achieving the framework itself was a stepping stone for structuring the field, mobilizing a community of health promotion researchers and contributing to the capacity building of the newly minted researchers.

To our knowledge, there exist only a couple of books entirely dedicated to presenting health promotion research (Goodson, 2009; Salazar et al., 2015). Both these references discuss health promotion research from the perspective of researching health behaviour changes and are blind to researching health-promoting systems and policies. Neither makes extensive references to the broader perspective on health promotion as a practice aimed at influencing the social, political, environmental and economic determinants of health. Although there is room in health promotion research for researching individual practices and heath behaviours, we conceive of health promotion research as a much broader field of enquiry. To contribute to the sustainability of health promotion, health promotion research needs to encompass the entire transformative agenda proposed in the Ottawa Charter (WHO, 1986).

Developing knowledge on such a broad range of practices involving a diversity of social actors requires a pluralist view of science that makes room for and integrates diverse relevant paradigms. With this handbook, our ambition is threefold.

(1) To map the various health promotion research practices, to make visible their diversity and distinctive characteristics
(2) To provide a reference tool and a usable resource for researchers, practitioners and students to navigate and conduct health promotion research
(3) To contribute to the creation of a shared and recognized identity for health promotion researchers

1.1 The Need for a Solid and Relevant Knowledge Base

Health promotion was institutionalized in the mid-1980s through a WHO-EURO effort to operationalize the goal of "achieving health for all in 2000" (Kickbusch, 2003). With the recognition towards the end of the twentieth century that non-communicable diseases and modifiable lifestyle risk factors were major causes of disease and mortality in not only high- but also low- and middle-income countries (Murray & Lopez, 1994), health promotion has become global. The Bangkok Charter for Health Promotion in a Globalized World (WHO, 2005) made this explicit. However, to survive and thrive as a global professional activity, health promotion must develop a solid and relevant knowledge base to buttress other elements of professional sustainability such as training programmes, accreditation processes and competency frameworks.

Parallel to this geographical expansion, health promotion has also penetrated the academic domain. The fact that a growing number of scientific journals, research infrastructure and specialized academic degrees include health promotion in their titles is a sure sign of a thriving scientific enterprise. While research teams are capable of producing scientific knowledge, the field of health promotion research is yet to be recognized as distinct and associated with a coherent body of knowledge anchored in shared paradigms, approaches and methods (Jourdan, 2019). In comparison to well-established, theory-based fields of research such as psychology, sociology or epidemiology, for example, health promotion research could appear to be weak from an epistemological point of view: its objects are somewhat ill-defined and the epistemic boundaries with established fields of research are blurred (Jourdan et al., 2012). The field is still in search of a proper niche as witnessed by the fact that the health promotion research infrastructure and degrees are associated with various scientific disciplines that range from psychology, education, social work and various allied health sciences, such as public health, nutrition and others, depending on university traditions (Van den Broucke, 2017).

The key question is then: What are the criteria to define a research field, and does health promotion research meet these criteria? In reference to Bourdieu's notion of a social field (Bourdieu, 1980), a field of research is a structured space of relationships for social actors, both individual and institutional (in our case, people and organizations involved in health promotion research). It is defined by its boundaries with other related fields (such as public health research, political science or health psychology), and it defines an identity for those within. Actors in the field struggle to obtain significant shares of various types of capital from which they can position themselves favourably within this space. In the case of a scientific field, these are mainly peer recognition, role in scientific journals or funding organizations or other authoritative instances for knowledge production and dissemination (Jourdan et al., 2012). Given the volume of scientific publications, journals, research teams, graduate degrees and other metrics of scientific activity, we consider that health promotion research has many of the attributes of a distinct research field. What is missing is an explicit and shared structuring framework that will facilitate the development of other attributes such as a clear identity of health promotion researchers, recognition of the value of their work in their academic careers, funding processes and scholarly associations. Developing such a framework for health promotion research is the next step in the development of a mature field of the health promotion process that will support the maturing of health promotion research and the sustainability of health promotion. This work could only be accomplished by mobilizing the forces of health promotion research at a global level. This is why we launched the initiative to create a global handbook.

1.2 A Collaborative Process for Structuring Health Promotion Research

The overarching ambition of this global handbook is to contribute to structuring the field of health promotion research based on the actual research practices. From the work of Ludwig Fleck (2005) in the early twentieth century to that of Thomas Kuhn (1962) and Bruno Latour (1989), empirical investigations of the activity of scientists have demonstrated that science is a sociological enterprise. Over and above the philosophical considerations about the thinking process foundational to all knowledge, scientific knowledge is the product of the social practices of researchers whose work cannot be reduced to applying methods. Science is a social activity. Researchers are social actors whose behaviours are shaped by structuring forces related to the community of researchers to which they belong. Scientific activity is rooted in the worldviews, paradigms, methods and tools elaborated by those recognized as contributing to the discipline in which the activity is embedded and that, conversely, shapes the discipline. Although every research project is a singular original activity, it is related to an identifiable scientific field through a configuration of characteristics that are shared by the community of researchers in the discipline.

To structure the field of health promotion research, we opted to work from the bottom up, i.e. to start by taking stock of the research practices of those who compose the field and who identify as health promotion researchers. After having carefully mapped these practices, their analysis should allow the identification of underlying principles and their organization into a coherent framework.

The second objective of this handbook is to help structure a distinctive community of health promotion researchers and to support its expansion by providing the next generation of researchers with a tool to situate their own contributions to the field. We also want to expose these future researchers to a coherent framework to organize the breadth and depth of valid health promotion research practices. Coming from a variety of disciplinary perspectives, those involved in health promotion research often operate at the margin of their own discipline. Providing a structured and recognized space in the form of a scientific field will strengthen and legitimate the label of "health promotion researcher" and will provide criteria and directions to further develop tools (journals, graduate programmes, funding mechanisms) adapted to the specificities of the practices of health promotion researchers. In order to ensure the relevance of the proposed structuring framework to the global community of health promotion researchers, we framed the project as a participatory enterprise in which those who identify as health promotion researchers contribute to creating the framework through sharing and discussing their own research practices. The intent is to base this handbook on the collective experiences of health promotion researchers globally about how they create and share health promotion knowledge.

This is why a call for contributions was launched in 2020. It was open to the global community of health promotion researchers, defined as individuals and groups interested in advancing health promotion research by reflecting on and sharing their practices. To reach these researchers, we associated with the International Union of Health Promotion and Education (IUHPE), the only NGO with a global membership composed of decision-makers, practitioners and researchers in the field of health promotion, and posted our call on their website and in their journal *Global Health Promotion*. The call was also disseminated through the community of the UNESCO Chair Global Health and Education. We also sent invitations to authors who had published research articles between January 2017 and February 2020 in two flagship journals: *Global Health Promotion* and *Health Promotion International*. Finally, we issued personalized invitations to a number of prominent colleagues and researchers in health promotion. The call asked for outlines of potential chapters detailing research practices as implemented in specific research projects or more comprehensive research programmes. We provided the following headings for guidance.

1: *The specific health promotion practices investigated*: Who were the actors? What were they doing? For what purposes?
2: *The purpose of the research project or programme*: What were the objectives? In which context were they defined? Who participated in their definition? Were values other than knowledge production pursued through this research? Which ones? Who defined them?
3: *The research framework*: Which research paradigm was used to frame the research and why? Which theories were used and how?
4: *The relationship with those whose practices were investigated*: How were research participants involved in the planning and conducting of the research? Were research results shared with non-researchers? If yes, how and for what purpose?
5: *The methods used*: What kinds of data were collected? How were they collected and analyzed?
6: *Specific challenges of health promotion research enlightened by the project or programme*: How does the research contribute to advancing health promotion research?

We received more than 108 outlines from all continents encompassing a wide range of research practices and methods reporting on research that were clearly about issues related to health promotion. The authors were diverse as well, with some of them just graduating from a doctorate programme and some being seasoned researchers. We interpreted this highly positive response to our call as a real need of the field to reflect on research practices and as a genuine willingness from researchers to contribute to shaping and structuring health promotion research. We invited a total of 95 individuals or groups to contribute a full chapter, eliminating outlines that did not report on research or on the dissemination of research results. We also rejected outlines that reported research on a subject that could not be linked to the health promotion discourse and practice as delineated by the Ottawa Charter of Health Promotion (WHO, 1986) or related documents.

At this very early stage, we noted two types of outlines. The majority of outlines described a research project or programme and discussed the ways in which it contributed to addressing distinctive challenges in health promotion research. Taken together, these contributions would constitute the first volume of this handbook aiming to answer the question: how is health promotion research conducted globally? To further guide the authors in their reflexive task, we asked them to organize their chapters in a way that would provide evidence to answer the following four questions.

1: What makes the research objects distinctive of health promotion?
2: What kind of knowledge does the research generate?
3: What makes this research approach distinctive of health promotion research?
4: How does this research contribute to advancing and structuring the field of health promotion research?

There was a second type of outline. Mostly written by more seasoned researchers, these contributions presented a high-level reflection on how a specific research approach or method, which the authors had championed as either a developer or main adapter from another field, was contributing to shaping health promotion research because it addresses the fundamental challenges inherent to studying health promotion. We asked these authors to write a chapter for didactic purposes. These chapters would provide an overview of the approaches, strategies of inquiry and methods for generating knowledge about health promotion practices. To complement these chapters, we also issued more personalized invitations to colleagues known for their work in a specific area. All these contributions would constitute the third volume of this handbook aiming to guide researchers on conducting health promotion research. This volume would be more akin to a textbook in which more junior researchers and graduate students could find accurate introductions to approaches and innovative practices in health promotion research. We asked the authors to structure these contributions around the following questions:

1: Which general health promotion research issues does this approach address?
2: How does this approach solve that issue?
3: What are the approach's fundamentals and key references?
4: How does this approach structure the field of health promotion research?

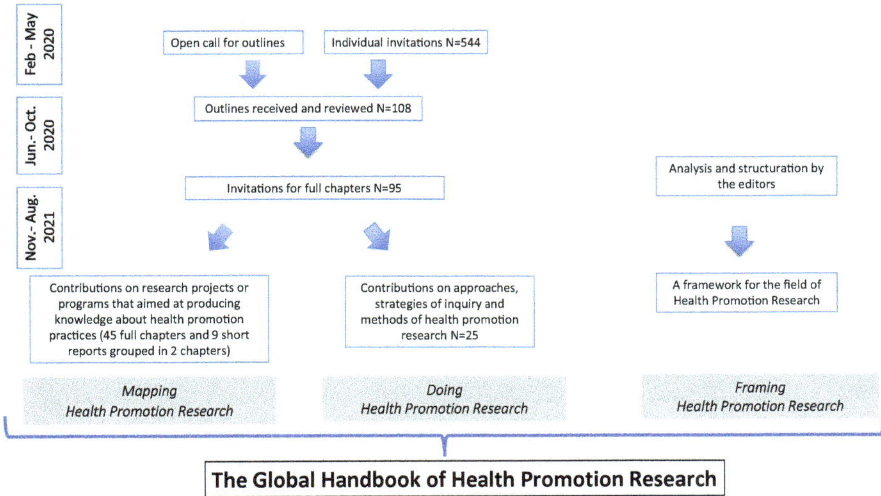

Fig. 1.1 Collaborative process of creating *Global Handbook of Health Promotion Research*

Based on our experience with similar projects, we expected that about half the number of invitations we issued would lead to full chapters. To our amazement, almost all the authors and groups of authors invited produced a full-fledged chapter. We received, reviewed and commented on 85 full chapters! The chapters have gone through several rounds of exchanges between the authors and the editors. In addition to describing research practices, all of them include an epistemological and ethical analysis that contributes to the construction of the field of health promotion research. A genuine process of maturation occurred, which enabled the authors to make the foundations of their work more explicit and the editors to acquire a global vision of health promotion research practices in all their diversity. Finally, although this is not a systematic collection, the topics, approaches, strategies of inquiry and practices, disciplines and research settings presented and discussed in this wide selection of chapters offer a valid and realist perspective on the breadth and variety of health promotion research globally. Figure 1.1 provides a schematic representation of the process.

1.3 Content of This Global Handbook: An Open Project

Given the amount of contributions received, this handbook comprises three distinct volumes. Each volume has a unique scope and format, providing a unique perspective for structuring the field of health promotion research. The mapping of practices is the first phase of our work. It has led to the publication of the present book, the first volume of this handbook. Based on this material, the second part of the work consists of a systematic description of the epistemological and ethical frameworks

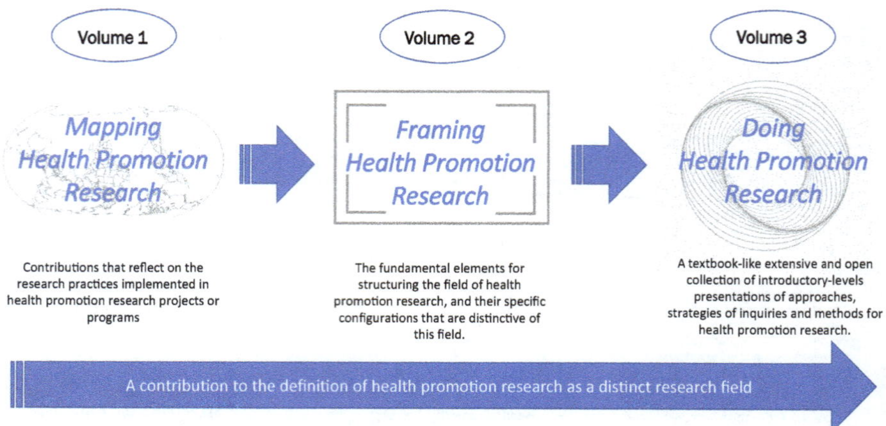

Fig. 1.2 Structure of the *Global Handbook of Health Promotion Research*

of health promotion research. It constitutes the second volume of this handbook. Finally, the third part, corresponding to the third volume, proposes a systematic collection of approaches, strategies of inquiry and methods (see Figure 1.2).

Volume 1 (this volume) is subtitled *Mapping Health Promotion Research.* The main body of the book is composed of 47 original chapters that reflect on research projects or programmes that are aimed at producing knowledge about health promotion practices. These chapters offer an overview of the range of health promotion practices studied by health promotion researchers, on the one hand, and of the research practices carried out to do so, on the other hand. Following this introduction, those chapters are organized into four parts according to the health promotion practices studied, as we consider that, due to the nature of health promotion, this is a fundamental dimension for structuring the research field. The fifth part is composed of our analysis of this material to derive some shared elements from the actual practices in health promotion research that will inform our effort to structure the field.

Volume 2 is subtitled *Framing Health Promotion Research.* It is entirely written by Jourdan and Potvin and proposes our view of what makes health promotion research a distinct field. It is composed of short chapters with a didactic aim that describe and discuss what we consider as the fundamental elements for structuring the field and their specific configurations that make this field of research distinct. The argument is organized into four parts. The first part defines what constitutes a research field and why it is relevant and useful to distinguish health promotion research from other related research fields. The second part discusses the objects and questions that delineate the range of health promotion practices studied by health promotion research. Part III discusses the values and the ethical framework that we consider is the main characteristic of health promotion research. Part IV proposes a comprehensive epistemological framework for health promotion research.

Volume 3 is subtitled *Doing Health Promotion Research.* It is composed of short chapters written by authors who have developed a recognized expertise with regard to either a paradigm, a strategy of inquiry or a method associated with health promotion research. These chapters are written as introductions to these paradigms, approaches or methods in relation to the specific health promotion research challenge each addresses. The volume is structured in three parts. Part I addresses the various paradigms as sets of beliefs, worldviews or epistemologies that guide health promotion research practices. Part II presents strategies of inquiry implemented in health promotion research and that provide specific directions for designing studies. Part III discusses the various methods that are used in or adapted to the conduct of health promotion research. These are related to the collection, analysis and interpretation of the empirical material used in a study.

Recognizing that: (1) we cannot pretend to have an exhaustive coverage of all the relevant paradigms, strategies of inquiry and methods for health promotion research and (2) the field is evolving rapidly, this handbook, especially the third volume, is conceived of as an opening for the future and as a stepping stone to an ongoing global initiative. In collaboration with the editorial board of *Global Health Promotion,* the official journal of the International Union for Health Promotion and Education, we will create a section in the journal entitled "Doing health promotion research". This section will publish introductory-level presentations of paradigms, approaches and methods relevant to health promotion research and will be written by health promotion researchers.

References

Bourdieu, P. (1980). Quelques propriétés des champs. In P. Bourdieu (Ed.), *Questions de sociologie* (pp. 113–120). Éditions de Minuit.

Fischer, F., Miller, G., & H. (2007). *Handbook of public policy analysis. Theory, politics, and methods*. Routledge.

Fleck, L. (2005). *Genèse et développement d'un fait scientifique*. Les belles lettres.

Goodson, P. (2009). *Theory in Health Promotion Research and Practice*. Jones & Bartlett.

Jourdan, D. (2013). Evaluating effects of HP programs in complex systems. Keynote lecture in the satellite event Strengthening health promotion research, 21st IUHPE World Conference on Health Promotion. Pattaya (Thailand), 25–29 August 2013.

Jourdan, D. (2019). Réinterroger et approfondir les fondements épistémologiques de la recherche en promotion de la santé: un enjeu de structuration du champ. Retrived on March 1st 2022 from: https://www.facebook.com/espumudem/videosconf%C3%A9rence-magistrale-de-didierjourdan/358804024712326/

Jourdan, D., O'Neill, M., Dupéré, S., Stirling, J. (2012). Quarante ans après, où en est la santé communautaire? *Santé Publique, 24*, 165–178.

Kickbusch, I. (2003). The contribution of the World Health Organisation to a new public health and health promotion. *American Journal of Public Health, 93*, 383–388.

Kuhn, T. (1962). *The structure of scientific revolution*. University of Chicago Press.

Latour, B. (1989). *La science en action. Introduction à la sociologie des sciences*. La Découverte.

MacDonald, G., & Bunton, R. (2002). Health promotion: Disciplinary developments. In R. Bunton & G. MacDonald (Eds.), *Health promotion. Disciplines, diversity and development* (pp. 9–27). Routledge.

Murray, C. J. L., & Lopez, A. D. (1994). Global and regional cause-of-death patterns in the 1990. *Bulletin of the World Health Organization, 72*, 447–480.

Potvin, L., & Jones, C. M. (2011). Twenty-five years after the Ottawa Charter: The critical role of health promotion for public health. *Canadian Journal of Public Health, 102*(4), 244–248.

Potvin, L., & McQueen, D. M. (2007). Modernity, public health and health promotion: A reflexive discourse. In D. M. McQueen, I. Kickbusch, L. Potvin, J. M. Pelikan, L. Balbo, & T. Abel (Eds.), *Health & modernity. The role of theory in health promotion* (pp. 12–20). Springer.

Salazar, L. F., Crosby, R. A., & DiClemente, R. J. (2015). *Research methods in health promotion* (2nd ed.). Jossey-Bass.

Van den Broucke, S. (2017). Strengthening public health capacity through a health promotion lens. *Health Promotion International, 32*(5), 763–767. https://doi.org/10.1093/heapro/dax064

WHO. (1986). *Ottawa Charter for health promotion*. World Health Organization. Retrieved in December 2020 from: https://www.euro.who.int/__data/assets/pdf_file/0004/129532/Ottawa_Charter.pdf

WHO. (2005). *Bangkok Charter for health promotion in a globalized world*. World Health Organization. Retrieved in December 2020 from: https://www.who.int/healthpromotion/conferences/6gchp/hpr_050829_%20BCHP.pdf?ua=1

Wyse, D., Selwyn, N., Smith, E., & Suter, L. E. (Eds.). (2016). *The BERA/SAGE Handbook of educational research*. Sage.

Chapter 2
Mapping Health Promotion Research: Organizing the Diversity of Research Practices

Louise Potvin and Didier Jourdan

As evidenced by the amount of scientific activity, and by the strong response to our call for contributions, there is a significant number of researchers who identify as health promotion researchers. The venues in which they publish and those from which they nurture their own research are diverse and cover a wide range of disciplinary perspectives (Gagné et al., 2018). The overarching goal of this handbook is to propose a framework to structure the field based on researchers' practices. The objective of this first volume is to map the field, while ensuring that we would capture the broadest possible range of research practices. To organize this diversity, we took the object of the research, i.e. what exactly is the research producing knowledge about, as the entry point.

2.1 Health Promotion as a Social Practice

The knowledge produced by health promotion research is about ordinary activities of individuals and populations, policies and interventions implemented with the aim to promote health. In an effort to determine a set of core concepts to define health promotion 20 years ago, Rootman and collaborators (2001) identified up to 11 different definitions that roughly cover 2 decades around the time the Ottawa Charter

L. Potvin (✉)
School of Public Health, University of Montreal, Montreal, QC, Canada

Centre de recherche en santé publique (CReSP), Université of Montreal and CIUSSS du Centre-Sud-de-l'Île-de-Montréal, Montréal, QC, Canada
e-mail: louise.potvin@umontreal.ca

D. Jourdan
UNESCO Chair and WHO Collaborating Centre in Global Health & Education, University of Clermont Auvergne, Clermont-Ferrand, France

L. Potvin, D. Jourdan (eds.), *Global Handbook of Health Promotion Research, Vol. 1*,
https://doi.org/10.1007/978-3-030-97212-7_2

was elaborated (from 1974 to 1992). The number of definitions is still growing (Rootman & O'Neill, 2017). They found some commonalities in all these definitions. They all propose a positive orientation for health and are all action-oriented, involving a large spectrum of primary actors, from individuals to organizations, to the community up to the state and global actors. These actions address a broad range of determinants of health rooted in everyday life going well beyond individual risk factors (Breslow, 1999). So, health promotion is about the practices (what people do in context) of individuals and of various social actors that contribute to promoting health. Doing health promotion research is thus producing knowledge about the practices of a variety of social actors that have the potential to improve the health of individuals and groups.

Putting the social practices of health promotion actors at the core of health promotion research requires defining what is meant by practice. In general, practices, as blocks of activities, meanings, competences and things, are a heuristic entry point to understand the social world (Latour, 2006). In the context of evaluation research, which he argues is concerned with practice, Schwandt (2005) defines social practice "not as an object or thing-like entity or system but as an event (or a series of events) that is always developing, unfolding and being accomplished. Hence, practice is concerned primarily with activities and relationships, with the manners in which people change and develop, and the ways they continually interact with others" (Schwandt, 2005, p. 100). Practice is a way to conceive of the recursive relationships between human action and its context. While practice is both enabled and constrained by contextual conditions, it also produces and reproduces context (Frohlich et al., 2001; Poland et al., 2008).

An example of this context–practice recursive relationship can be found in tobacco-control efforts. In most Western countries, legislators were able to roll out a series of increasingly severe tobacco restrictions to the extent that a growing number of citizens were stopping smoking and the norm for a smoke-free environment was strengthening. Conversely, it has been shown that stopping smoking (or not taking up the habit) is facilitated by tobacco-control legislations, albeit not for all citizens (Cummings, 2002). There are contexts and conditions (e.g. low-paying jobs, low education) that enable and support smoking habits and make it more difficult for people to stay away from tobacco (Marmot, 2015).

Health promotion as a social practice involves focusing on what actors do in context to affect their own health in the case of individuals' practices or that of groups or entire populations in the cases of actors whose role is to intervene to change the conditions that affect health. Thus, researching health promotion is to create knowledge about social practices, understood as what people do in relation to others and to structural constraints to achieve health goals for themselves or for groups of people.

2.2 Four Practices of Health Promotion

We identify four types of practices (what people actually do) as fundamental to, and distinctive of, health promotion (Charlot, 2008; Jourdan, 2019). They are defined as a function of the categories of actors they relate to and the type of goals pursued.

- *The practices of individuals and populations to promote their own health.* It encompasses what people do as individuals and groups in relation to their health. Health promotion proposes that these practices, like all practices, are shaped by the conditions in which people and groups live, the so-called determinants of health. These practices are anchored in different cultures, knowledge and social contexts.
- *The practices of the professionals from the health and other sectors* who intervene in health promotion/health education/prevention to improve the health of individuals or that of populations. This group also includes activists, associations, forums and communities engaged in social change. These practices are most often in the form of programmes or interventions targeting health determinants.
- *The practices of politicians and institutions' decision-makers* to change norms and the distribution of resources in various contexts. These practices often take the form of the implementation and advocacy of policies at the national, regional and local levels, not only in the health sector but also in all sectors that influence the determinants of health.
- *The practices of researchers and innovators* who study health promotion practices and share research findings or systematically experiment new ways of doing health promotion. These actors comprise a network of scholars and international agencies through which a continued investment in research and the production of evidence-based guidelines are made.

We make a distinction between ordinary practices and programmes or policies. The former refers to what people and communities do in their everyday life to influence the determinants of their health. The latter are deliberate, planned actions operated by people holding a legitimate mandate to change social and/or material conditions for other peoples' lives. This also includes the practice of professionals in relation to their clients.

2.3 Describing Research Practices as Configurations

Research is an intellectual activity aimed at producing new and cumulative knowledge using scientifically recognized methods within a social and political context. It introduces intelligibility and rationality into complex practical–ethical discussions

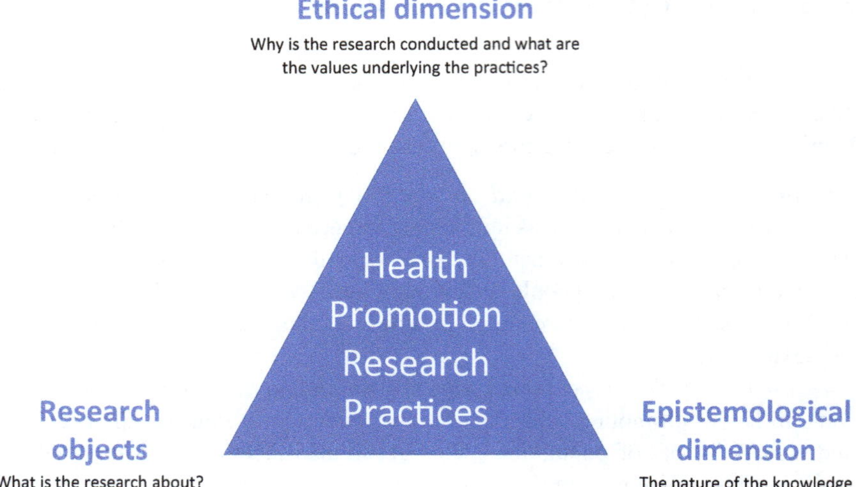

Fig. 2.1 Three structuring dimensions for the field of health promotion research

such as those that characterize the field of health promotion (Tannahill, 2008). We also conceive of research as a social practice. It is the "doing" of researchers as social actors, operating through a series of constraints and enablers in the pursuit of a knowledge creation-related goal.

As a social practice, research takes different forms to compose unique research fields. These fields are associated with distinct bodies of knowledge, paradigms and rules of methods. Valid knowledge in sociology, for example, is not about the same phenomenon as valid knowledge in physics. It is not produced with the same tools nor does it serve the same purposes. To define a research field, three structuring dimensions must be considered (see Fig. 2.1).

- The objects of research. It relates to the question: What is the research about?
- The epistemological dimension is about the nature of knowledge and the ways in which it is generated. It relates to the question: What is knowledge and how is it acquired?
- The ethical dimension is about the values, aims and purpose of the research. It relates to the question: Why is the research conducted and what are the values involved?

Although often important to the identity of a research field, we do not include strategies of inquiry and methods as a structuring dimension. Valid methodological research options are largely derived from these three structuring dimensions.

Because health promotion research practices are linked to a wide range of objects and rooted in different disciplinary backgrounds, it is not appropriate to rest the structuration of the field on a single theory. Instead, our approach is to look for markers to characterize the field. In fact, it is like placing a few fixed buoys on the sea while being aware that these buoys' positions will not tell all there is to say about the oceanic immensity. It simply enables navigators to know their own position. It marks safe channels and other important reference points and isolated dangers and other areas of special significance. Therefore, within these three dimensions, we will look for markers to characterize research practices that are described in the chapters composing this volume.

Since every research is a singular, original activity, identifiable by a set of characteristics within multiple dimensions, the definition of research configurations is more relevant than typological thinking for our purpose of structuring the field. By configuration, we mean the way in which markers for the problematization of the research objects, the purpose of the research and the modalities of knowledge production are articulated. These configurations of research objects, purpose and knowledge base/production specific to health promotion research constitute the pillars on which to anchor the field.

2.4 The Organization of This Volume

As mentioned earlier, we have organized the chapters in this volume about mapping of health promotion research based on the health promotion practices that form the object of the research described in each chapter. In addition to the introduction and this description of the approach we have used, this volume consists of five parts.

Part I has six chapters, among which the first five (Chaps. 3, 4, 5, 6 and 7) present research to study a broad range of *individuals' and populations' health practices* in a variety of contexts. They were selected either because the individuals or groups of individuals whose practices are studied present challenges that researchers deliberately address through the research they describe or because there is little research about the individuals and practices studied. As examples of the former, Adam and colleagues (Chap. 6) describe a research that addresses the issue of structure and agency for people in vulnerable situations, whereas MacDougall et al. (Chap. 7) present ways for research to listen to the children's voice, which is usually discarded in the adult-oriented world of health. Studying families living with type 2 diabetes, young adults treated for rare diseases and young people experiencing homelessness are all examples of the latter. The last chapter (Chap. 8) is a composite of five capsules presenting research projects that describe how researchers adapt research methods to respond to the needs and specific characteristics of the context in which research was implemented.

Part II comprises 12 chapters that present research on the *practices of professionals*. They all propose an innovative perspective for studying professional practices. For example, the first four chapters (Chaps. 9, 10, 11 and 12) are about researching or adapting caring practices with non-Western populations for which medical care practices and research are usually designed. The next five chapters (Chaps. 13, 14, 15, 16 and 17) present studies on the practices of lay people (community health workers) or professionals deliberately engaged in health promotion in the community setting. Altogether, these chapters make a strong case that the necessary interactions between researchers and practitioners in conducting research can be harnessed and taken advantage of to improve professional practices and ultimately population health. The final group of three chapters (Chaps. 18, 19 and 20) is about conducting research to study health promotion programmes in schools.

Part III includes 14 chapters, 13 of which reflect on research studying how social changes occur through the planned actions of various *politicians and institutions' decision-makers* within or outside of the health sector. Here, the focus is not on the practices of professionals or individuals in their health-promoting professional activity. Instead, the objects of these studies are complex systems and their transformation to improve health or health equity. The first two chapters (Chaps. 21 and 22) propose approaches to research interventions that aim at schools as whole systems, embedded in their communities. The following two chapters (Chaps. 23 and 24) propose reflections on conducting research with non-institutional organizations such as NGOs and supermarkets, whose missions, contrary to that of institutions, are not primarily concerned with the public good (Moore, 2000). The challenges of these partnerships are unique and require a different kind of work from the researchers in order to align the research objectives with those of the host organizations. The following three chapters (Chaps. 25, 26 and 27) take local communities as settings for changes through intersectoral action or local policy. The following four chapters (Chaps. 28, 29, 30 and 31) are about researching state-wide changes through scaling up of programmes. Finally, the chapter from Frohlich et al. (Chap. 32) and that from Anaf and her colleagues (Chap. 33) propose a critical reflection on context as a key issue in evaluating complex systems interventions. The last chapter (Chap. 34) comprises short descriptions of initiatives to support the use of evidence for policy changes.

Part IV has 15 chapters that propose reflections and approaches to improve various aspects in conducting *health promotion research*. Our conceptualization of the practices of health promotion researchers as contributing to the field of health promotion makes it clear that research and the knowledge it produces play a critical reflexive role in health promotion practices. It situates the research activity within the field of health promotion, in interaction with those engaged in health promotion. The chapters composing Part IV offer in-depth discussions on how the practices of researchers contribute to shaping and strengthening the field of health promotion.

Finally, in the conclusion in Part V, we propose our analysis of this material in terms of the objects of health promotion research and the epistemological and ethical dimensions of researching health promotion. Every research is a singular, original activity, identifiable by a set of characteristics within multiple dimensions. As previously stated, the definition of research configurations is more relevant than typological thinking. Although this collection is not exhaustive or even representative of all the research practices, its very diversity allows to identify potential markers (related to the objects studied, the epistemological and ethical frameworks) that characterize the specific configurations of health promotion research.

References

Breslow, L. (1999). From disease prevention to health promotion. *JAMA, 281*, 1030–1033.

Charlot, B. (2008). La recherche en éducation entre savoirs, politiques et pratiques: spécificités et défis d'un champ de savoir. *Recherches et Éducations* (online), 1 retrieved on October 11, 2021. https://doi.org/10.4000/rechercheseducations.455

Cummings, K. M. (2002). Programs and policies to discourage the use of tobacco products. *Oncogene, 21*, 7349–7364.

Frohlich, K. L., Corin, E., & Potvin, L. (2001). A theoretical proposal for the relationship between context and disease. *Sociology of Health & Illness, 23*(6), 776–797.

Gagné, T., Lapalme, T., & McQueen, D. V. (2018). Multidisciplinarity in health promotion: A bibliometric analysis of current research. *Health Promotion International, 33*, 610–621. https://doi.org/10.1093/heapro/dax002

Jourdan, D. (2019). *Réinterroger et approfondir les fondements épistémologiques de la recherche en promotion de la santé: un enjeu de structuration du champ de recherche.* Conférence magistrale organisée par l'École de santé publique de l'Université de Montréal. Retrieved on October 11, 2021 from: https://it-it.facebook.com/espumudem/videos/conf%C3%A9rence-magistrale-de-didier-jourdan/358804024712326/

Latour, B. (2006). *Changer de société, refaire de la sociologie.* La Découverte.

Marmot, M. (2015). *The health gap. The challenges of an unequal world.* Bloomsbury.

Moore, M. (2000). Managing for value: Organizational strategy in for-profit, non-profit, and governmental organizations. *Nonprofit and Voluntary Sector Quarterly, 29*, 183–204.

Poland, B., Frohlich, K., & Cargo, M. (2008). Context as a fundamental dimension of health promotion program evaluation. In L. Potvin & D. McQueen (Eds.), *Health promotion evaluation practices in the Americas* (pp. 299–317). Springer.

Rootman, I., & O'Neill, M. (2017). Key concepts in health promotion. In I. Rootman, A. Pederson, K. L. Frohlich, & S. Dupéré (Eds.), *Health promotion in Canada. New perspectives on theory, practice, policy and research* (pp. 20–43). Canadian Scholars.

Rootman, I., Goodstadt, M., Potvin, L., & Springett, J. (2001). A framework for health promotion evaluation. In I. Rootman, M. Goodstadt, B. Hyndman, D. V. McQueen, L. Potvin, J. Springett, & E. Ziglio (Eds.), *Evaluation in health promotion. Principles and perspectives* (pp. 7–38). WHO regional publications. European series; No 92.

Schwandt, T. A. (2005). The centrality of practice to evaluation. *American Journal of Evaluation, 26*, 95–105. https://doi.org/10.1177/1098214004273184

Tannahill, A. (2008). Beyond evidence-to ethics: A decision-making framework for health promotion, public health and health improvement. *Health Promotion International, 22*, 380–390.

Part I
Researching the Practices of Individuals and Populations

Chapter 3
Design-Based Research on Active Family Involvement: Developing a Family Toolbox to Support Health Care Professionals Working with Diabetes Management

Dan Grabowski, Jens Aagaard-Hansen, and Bjarne Bruun Jensen

3.1 Introduction

In both research and practice, there is a general need to investigate how we can make use of a family-focused health promotion approach to motivate and co-create a heightened level of positive involvement and support – while simultaneously acknowledging that this involvement must be sensitive to a myriad of potential family characteristics. In this chapter, we will describe and elaborate on a comprehensive family health promotion design-based research project and use it as an exemplary case to illustrate why the family is an important setting for health promotion. The project serves as a prime example of how focusing on the different ways of involving complex target groups in the various phases of the research process should be a central concern when planning, executing and implementing health promotion research initiatives.

The project was based on a comprehensive and integrated health promotion approach, including a set of five evidence-based principles: (1) a broad and positive health concept; (2) participation and involvement; (3) action and action competence; (4) a settings perspective and (5) equity in health (Grabowski et al., 2017a). The five principles derive from widespread critique of the so-called moralizing paradigm that has long characterized much of the work conducted within the field of health promotion, prevention and treatment. This paradigm is characterized by

D. Grabowski (✉) · B. B. Jensen
Health Promotion, Steno Diabetes Center Copenhagen, Herlev, Danmark
e-mail: dan.grabowski@regionh.dk

J. Aagaard-Hansen
Health Promotion, Steno Diabetes Center Copenhagen, Herlev, Danmark

SA MRC Developmental Pathways for Health Research Unit, Department of Paediatrics, School of Clinical Medicine, Faculty of Health Sciences, University of the Witwatersrand, Johannesburg, South Africa

L. Potvin, D. Jourdan (eds.), *Global Handbook of Health Promotion Research, Vol. 1*,
https://doi.org/10.1007/978-3-030-97212-7_3

being expert-driven as opposed to user-driven, given its narrow focus on creating predefined behavioural changes and exclusive focus on avoiding or reducing the risk of disease and death (Jensen, 1997).

The study was guided by a design-based research (DBR) process (Brown & Wyatt, 2010). The DBR approach aims at understanding the complex world of everyday settings and healthcare practices and is characterized by involving all target groups in participatory processes using dialogue and involvement (Dolmans & Tigelaar, 2012). Being situated in the context of actual target groups ensures the validity of the development and research and makes it more likely that the results can be effectively used to inform and strengthen health promotion in "real-life" healthcare practices (Anderson & Shattuck, 2012).

The DBR process is a system of overlapping spheres that recur in continuous cycles of design, research and redesign, including three overall spheres: inspiration, ideation and implementation (Brown & Wyatt, 2010; Dolmans & Tigelaar, 2012). Inspiration arises from a problem or an opportunity that motivates the search for solutions. Ideation is the process of generating, developing and testing ideas, and implementation is the path that leads from the development stage to practice (Brown & Wyatt, 2010). In the present project, the research-based creation and development of the intervention was carried out in a close collaborative arrangement that included researchers, healthcare professionals (HCPs) and families living with type 2 diabetes (T2D).

We present the background, objectives and overall purpose of the project before outlining the research design. The different forms of and methods for involving the target groups are both at the very core of this chapter and arguably the main reasons for the project's overall success, and the chapter is primarily devoted to describing in detail how this involvement played out in each phase of the development process. Finally, we present the different categories of knowledge the project produced and spend some time specifically discussing how this relates and adds to the field of health promotion.

3.2 Background

3.2.1 The Family as a Key Player in Health Promotion

Although families are receiving increased attention within health promotion research, family health systems are still generally underutilized in health promotion practices (Barnes et al., 2020; Crandall et al., 2019). Communities and populations comprise individuals and families who collectively affect the health of the community and vice versa. Because members may support and nurture one another across various life stages, the family unit is potentially a key player in maintaining health and in preventing disease. In this way, the family has the potential to work as a mediator – or a buffer – between unhealthy influences arising from the structural context (such as the local neighbourhood) and the individual. Preliminary research confirms that family-oriented health is a promising strategy because the family unit is both a resource and a priority group in need of professional supportive services throughout the life course (Barnes et al., 2020).

In most cases, the family is the place where health behaviours are developed, maintained and changed. Incorporating a genuinely participatory health promotion approach into chronic disease prevention and care has the potential to improve health outcomes (Garcia-Huidobro & Mendenhall, 2015). A review of studies on the benefits of a family-oriented approach tentatively concludes that enhancing family relationships and developing family-strengthening activities are effective strategies in the areas of physical and mental health outcomes, multiple diseases and throughout the human lifespan (Barnes et al., 2020).

Limited training in family science as well as lack of instruments to help professionals "think family" often result in HCPs feeling ill-equipped to develop and carry out interventions that support, target and/or involve a diverse range of families. Tools to help public health practitioners think in terms of the family are therefore imperative if we are to improve health promotion outcomes (Crandall et al., 2019).

3.2.2 Family Involvement and Type 2 Diabetes

Family involvement plays a key role in diabetes management, and the importance of family approaches has received increasing recognition (Kovacs Burns et al., 2013; Torenholt et al., 2014). However, family involvement is a complex matter, often characterized by unclear structural relations and contrasting needs and expectations among family members. Supportive and obstructive behaviours frequently co-occur (Khan et al., 2013; Mayberry & Osborn, 2014). For this reason, more family involvement is not always beneficial (Mayberry & Osborn, 2014; Stephens et al., 2013). People with limited resources are especially vulnerable to the harmful aspects of family involvement (Mayberry & Osborn, 2012). Close relatives often describe discomfort with the perceived need to monitor a person with diabetes as well as confusion about their role in diabetes care. These feelings may lead to family conflicts (Samuel-Hodge et al., 2013). Studies have also shown that relatives tend to have concerns about diabetes that are often not voiced (White et al., 2007). When one family member has T2D, relatives have a significantly higher risk of also developing it (Weijnen et al., 2002; Khan et al., 2013).

One major obstacle to constructive intra-familial communication about prevention, familial risk and risk reduction behaviours is a lack of perceived disease relevance (Heideman et al., 2015; Myers et al., 2015;). Godino et al. (2014) reported that people's motivation to engage in risk-reducing health behaviours or to undergo screening depends on whether they are aware of their susceptibility to a given disease. Therefore, family health promotion is a challenging task.

One way of approaching the challenges of intra-familial communication is to look at the contextual conditions for developing a shared family identity. When family members experience considerable stress associated with their caregiver roles, their mutual understanding of the roles and interconnected relationships affects how they interpret and respond to the roles (Badr et al., 2007). Viewing family identity as the feature that both differentiates the family from other important entities and constitutes a unique set of potentials and limitations enables us to focus on how identities are constructed within the family through a mutual differentiation process (Scabini & Manzi, 2011). Studies on identity have shown that familial relationships play a major role in how health is perceived and integrated into everyday life and self-perception (Grabowski, 2015).

Although it is widely recognized that family involvement is important in diabetes management (Torenholt et al., 2014) and can increase the action competence of families and individuals, few interventions, tools and approaches meant to generate family involvement exist. Consequently, both HCPs and relatives in families living with T2D have been unsupported and are unsure about how to provide support.

In Denmark, many people diagnosed with T2D are offered patient education courses. These courses are typically constructed as a series of weekly meetings with nurses, dieticians and/or physical therapists who instruct groups of patients on topics such as exercise, diet and general self-management of T2D. These courses rarely include familial involvement, although some may invite spouses to join the part of the course about healthy cooking.

3.2.3 The Case Under Study

The health promotion design-based research project under study was conducted by the Steno Diabetes Center Copenhagen, The Danish Diabetes Association, The Region of Southern Denmark and the Capital Region of Denmark. The entire project encompassing all the phases described below lasted for 3 years and included participants from two distinctly different regions of Denmark, ensuring both geographical and socio-economic diversity. The objectives of the study were:

- To generate knowledge about the value of user involvement across all phases of design-based development and research, to constantly evaluate and refine these involvement processes and to produce methodological knowledge about family involvement;
- To investigate the facilitators of and the barriers to working with health promotion in families living with T2D and to specifically gain knowledge about how to prevent the intra-familial spread of T2D;
- To develop a hands-on approach supporting HCPs in creating family involvement – and to implement and evaluate this health promotion approach.

During the various phases of the research process, workshops with families living with T2D were organized as a series of dialogue fora, during which participants were split into groups – sometimes with their own families and sometimes with other relatives/people with diabetes. In addition to people with T2D, participants were primarily their spouses and adult children. The workshops were semi-structured in the sense that the research team facilitated each group session, maintaining a focus on topics related to family issues and everyday life with T2D. The workshops with HCPs focused on participants' experiences with family involvement and used similar dialogue tools.

Data for the implementation-phase effect study were generated through semi-structured group interviews. We conducted family interviews, the most suitable method for gaining access to families' private everyday lives, while still taking ethical considerations into account (Daly, 1992; Åstedt-Kurki et al., 2001). A very loose semi-structured interview guide with questions related to families' concrete work with the tools and family-related health topics was used to explore how families experienced and managed toolbox sessions (Daly, 1992; Reczek, 2014; Åstedt-Kurki & Hopia, 1996).

In a complex project with multiple sets of data from different target groups, it is important that the analytical approach addresses this complexity by being sensitive to constantly evolving empirical, methodological and theoretical approaches. Data from all phases were iteratively analyzed and categorized using radical hermeneutics, which are guidelines for content analysis that combine hermeneutics and constructivism to ensure both empirical accuracy and theoretical complexity (Rasmussen, 2004).

Radical hermeneutics is a method for maintaining a balance between theory, method and data in an interconnected process; a constant focus on how all elements influence each other is required. The methodology entails three analytical steps. In the first step, data are read with a view to exploring how specifically selected guiding differences are observed. This observation constitutes an interpretation rather than a description, and its purpose is to reduce complexity by extracting elements from the data. In the second step, these elements are the subject of a theory-based observation of the differences used in step one. Finally, all extracted differences are interpreted individually.

Conducting the analysis with a theoretically sensitive approach ensures that the results automatically include elements that are directly relevant to: (1) practice-related barriers and facilitators when working with family involvement, (2) further development of the health promotion principles and (3) conceptual framing and reframing of the theoretical elements.

3.3 Involvement of Target Groups

Participation and involvement constitute the most essential principle of the health promotion approach discussed here. Sustainable health promotion change can only take place if the target group has the opportunity to develop ownership, which is more likely to be achieved when the target group is actively involved in the processes from the outset. The principle of participation and involvement can imply many different things among different groups of HCPs. This principle highlights the fact that development of ownership is not necessarily determined by those who take the initiative. It may begin in a subsequent process, leading to the point of decision-making. A situation in which the HCP initiates the process by proposing a range of options, which the target group (e.g. patients) then develops and modifies, allows for greater involvement and strengthened ownership and empowerment. The focus of developing ownership thus shifts from the initiative itself and bottom up to dialogue and co-creation.

Hart (1992) noted that participation varies with individual characteristics and context. People vary in terms of their types of motivation, capacity and potential for participation (Hart, 1992; Sinclair, 2004). It is therefore important to maximize the opportunity for everyone to choose to participate at the highest level of his/her ability.

In the project discussed here, a central concern was to achieve the highest level of involvement of families and HCPs at every stage of the DBR process. This caused significant challenges due to differences between the phases and in the motivation and goals of the two target groups. As researchers, we had to adjust continuously and rethink the way in which we involved the target groups with each other and in the separate project stages.

Consistency was vital across the various phases with shifting participants and different methods of involvement. It was ensured by establishing a steering group consisting of senior consultants representing the HCPs in the two participating regions of Denmark, which also provided constant access to the fields of practice and made the developed approach feasible and easy to implement.

Based on the DBR model, we decided to work with the following phases in the research project: needs assessment, ideation, prototyping, feasibility testing and implementation. In the following, we will describe how the concepts of participation and involvement of the target groups were operationalized in each.

3.3.1 Needs Assessment

In the first phase, to create the best conditions for positive involvement and peer-to-peer exchange of thoughts and experiences, we conducted separate needs assessments with the two groups. We separately met with several groups of families and HCPs in a workshop format, where we gathered qualitative research data. The workshop format continually evolved through continually evaluating it collaboratively with participants. The workshop key themes were fairly broad and were based on the five health promotion principles and the concepts of family health identity and healthcare authenticity. The semi-structured format helped us maintain a perpetual focus on the health communication aspects related to both the generated knowledge about family involvement and the constant refining of the workshop concept.

The process generated complex, in-depth data for the ongoing analysis as well as knowledge related to creating optimal involvement and ownership among the target groups (Grabowski et al., 2017b). The needs assessment was characterized by a high level of involvement on the part of both target groups. The peer-to-peer exchange of experiences created a highly constructive atmosphere within both target groups; during every workshop, participants insisted on moving from discussing needs, challenges and problems to generating ideas for resolving these issues. This meant that we started the ideation process without planning to do so – and that we had a much more focused entry into the next phase.

3.3.2 Ideation

After two separate rounds (one focusing on problem domains and the other on barriers to intra-familial prevention, as described below) of thorough analysis of the needs assessment data, we went back to the target groups to present and discuss our findings. We kicked off the ideation phase by facilitating a 2-day workshop, inviting a group of HCPs to stay with us in a hotel, where we analyzed and interpreted the initial findings and began generating possible ideas for addressing the identified challenges. The HCPs were split into working groups, and, several times over the course of the 2 days, we invited different families to come in and give feedback on the innovations the HCPs proposed within their groups. The HCPs then iteratively incorporated the feedback into their ideation processes. The sessions with both families and HCPs shared a clear theoretical focus on the degree to which the individual families perceived the HCPs as relevant to the family's specific health identity.

This phase generated a great deal of genuine involvement on several levels as the HCPs, families and researchers freely exchanged their thoughts and ideas during discussions. As in the previous phase, we discussed both the development of innovative approaches and how to approach involvement in the following project phases.

After the intense 2-day workshop, we took a step back to create a research-based overview of the status of the innovative ideas and make plans for determining how to move on with them. We decided to hold a series of additional workshops with HCPs and families who had not participated in the previous one to help us decide which innovations would move on to the next phase. This additional step ensured our confidence in the selected innovations.

3.3.3 Prototyping

We hired a graphic designer to help us develop the initial rough prototypes of the dialogue tools that we, in collaboration with the target groups, had decided to focus on developing further. In this phase, the research team facilitated dialogue sessions with groups of families to discover which elements worked well and which elements needed adjustment. In these workshop sessions, we began by simulating real-life family sessions, where we played the part of the HCPs facilitating a family session with several families. When the families had tried working with the tools, we changed the dynamics by doing a thorough element-by-element assessment of the tools with the same families, who then served as the experts on family life with T2D. We discussed the pros and cons of the tools with the families, who gave us valuable input regarding changes and adjustments. When consulting the families in this phase, the most important issue was to determine whether the tools captured how these families perceived themselves in relation to illness and health. This was an ongoing process that lasted for 5 months and included numerous iterations involving adjustments and additional family sessions.

3.3.4 Feasibility Testing

After a 5-month testing period, we ended up with a nearly finished set of four dialogue tools for HCPs working with families living with T2D. The final phase of the development process involved a feasibility test of the tools in actual healthcare practice. For this purpose, we arranged a seminar for 70 HCPs, presenting them with the background and findings of the project and instructing them in using the tools in their practice.

They then tested the tools with families and subsequently filled in a questionnaire on the tools' ease of use and implementation. Furthermore, we interviewed 13 of the HCPs to get a more nuanced picture of how the tools fit into their practices and to encourage them to reflect on issues that would be important to incorporate into plans for broader implementation of the tools (Andersen et al., 2020). The data from the questionnaires and interviews led to a few final adjustments to the Family Toolbox that was now ready to be implemented in the Danish healthcare practice when working with people with T2D.

3.3.5 Implementation

In this most recent phase, we studied the family effects of working with the tools. We contacted all HCPs who had attended the training seminar and asked them whether they had used or were planning to use the toolbox with patients' families. All families with whom the tools had been used were contacted and asked whether we could interview them, preferably in their own homes. This interview process was less involving than the other phases, but we did strive to base the interviews on what each family specifically felt was important to talk about, and we used the findings from this effect study (Grabowski et al., 2019) to make several small changes in the tools, especially in how the tools are presented to the HCPs. The implementation phase also included a process in which the HCPs and their organizations were given control over how they implemented the toolbox in their fields of practice. The research team served as consultants in this process.

Table 3.1 Categories of involvement among HCPs and families, inspired by the categories suggested by Hughes and Duffy (2018): targeted consultation (users are consulted on specific aspects), embedded consultation (users are contacted regularly during the research process), co-creation (users are involved in decisions regarding the research process) and user-led (users lead the research and invite researchers as consultants or co-creators)

	Needs assessment	Ideation	Prototyping	Feasibility	Implementation
Families	Embedded consultation Targeted consultation Project planning	Co-creation Embedded consultation Targeted consultation Project planning	Co-creation Embedded consultation Targeted consultation Project planning	Targeted consultation	Targeted consultation Embedded consultation
HCPs	Embedded consultation Targeted consultation Project planning	Co-drivers Embedded consultation Targeted consultation Co-creation Project planning	Embedded consultation Targeted consultation Project planning	Co-creation Embedded consultation Targeted consultation Project planning	Drivers Project planning

3.3.6 *Overarching Considerations*

Table 3.1 summarizes the involvement process of each target group using, and is inspired by, the categories of involvement described by Hughes and Duffy (2018).

Although the project was neither user-initiated nor user-driven, the constant high level of positive involvement ensured the development of a health promotion tool that was very sensitive to the real-life needs, barriers and potentials of both families and HCPs.

In many phases, we used different representatives from each of the target groups. Some of them were entirely embedded in the overall project and some were only consulted briefly. This further underscores the complexity of involvement across the project phases.

3.4 Knowledge and Perspectives for Health Promotion Research and Practice

The project and the developed Family Toolbox intervention have been instrumental in the ongoing further development of the principled health promotion approach. Based on this project and on other recent health promotion projects, we propose an approach to health promotion we call Version 2.0. As one of the key features, Health Promotion Version 2.0 combines bottom-up and top-down developments in a dialogue-oriented approach. Using this approach, HCPs have a crucial role to play in facilitating, stimulating and challenging the target group to develop their own health promotion strategy.

The primary outcome of the project is a set of four practical and tangible tools that are designed to promote the health of families living with T2D. The Family Mirror invites participants to construct an image of themselves and a family member using cards with pictures and quotes related to support, everyday life, worries, roles, communication and knowledge about life with T2D. It is intended to help participants reflect on and discuss the challenges and opportunities within the family. The Family Book prepares participants for interactive reflection on various aspects of everyday family life while giving them practical knowledge and information about T2D. It can be read at home or used as a communication tool in patient education for families. The Family Line enables family members to show each other how large a role diabetes plays in their daily life and how great a role they believe it should play, which can initiate dialogue about T2D in daily life. The Family Plan enables the family to identify the challenges and solutions related to T2D and to establish specific objectives and plans for how they will improve or positively maintain important elements in their daily life (Grabowski et al., 2019).

It is important to stress that two different dimensions of user involvement took place in this process. One is user involvement in the different research phases, leading to the concrete intervention and its tools. Another dimension of user involvement is reflected in the next phase as the intervention is implemented in practice and leads to user involvement. However, these two dimensions of involvement are closely interrelated because user-involving research is more effective in producing user-friendly and engaging tools and interventions.

A study of the potential effects of working with the tools (Grabowski et al., 2019) yielded several key findings. First, the tools generated better and broader intra-familial involvement. Most families mentioned that the conditions for creating mutual involvement had improved after working with the Family Toolbox. However, improved involvement took many different forms and depended substantially on the family dynamics, the level of intra-familial communication and the degree of self-reference in each family. Second, it was easier for all family members to accept new roles and self-understandings after working with the tools. The processes of identifying with peers, as well as observing and reflecting on the roles of others and themselves in the context of T2D, involved coming to identify and understand new roles or making old roles fit new circumstances. The study showed that the tools can potentially play an important part in this involvement process by making the health identification easier as well as more relevant and authentic. Third, working with the tools gave family members mutual insights into their collective thoughts and worries. The ways T2D was contextualized when working with the tools turned the disease into something relevant that was integrated positively into identities and self-understandings in new ways. The perceived authenticity of this mutual contextualization generated feelings of genuine caring that, in turn, generated instant identification and mutual involvement. Fourth, the tools made it substantially easier to discover the potential challenges to and the possibilities for behaviour change. Most families had never experienced joint approaches to T2D or healthy behaviour; these had never been part of their collective practices, resulting in diabetes becoming the sole responsibility of the person with T2D. Working with the family tools was an effective way to make diabetes a manageable issue on which to base collective practices. Finally, most family members reported having acquired concrete knowledge as well as motivation to seek more knowledge. The majority of participants liked the informal way in which the tools generated a relaxed setting for sharing experiences and knowledge about daily life with diabetes. They said they felt motivated by the authentic involvement the tools generated.

3.5 Conclusions

The principle of user involvement in health promotion is widely recognized as being valuable for creating sustainable healthy changes in real-life settings. The health promotion research project described in this chapter demonstrates that the basic idea of user involvement contributes to the development of tailored and more effective approaches in health promotion. Generally, the tools developed in this project were well received by both HCPs and families.

The project also demonstrates how the principle of user involvement can be a foundational and innovative principle in all phases of a health promotion research initiative. We encourage people working with health promotion research to involve different groups of users (end users and professionals) in all research phases and to carefully consider the range of the potential types of user involvement when planning health promotion research projects.

References

Andersen, T. H., & Grabowski, D. (2020). Implementing a research-based innovation to generate intra-familial involvement in type 2 diabetes self-management for use in diverse municipal settings: A qualitative study of barriers and facilitators. *BMC Health Services Research, 20*, 198. https://doi.org/10.1186/s12913-020-5036-7

Anderson, T., & Shattuck, J. (2012). Design-based research: A decade of progress in education research? *Educational Researcher, 41*, 16–25. https://doi.org/10.3102/0013189X11428813

Astedt-Kurki, P., & Hopia, H. (1996). The family interview: Exploring experiences of family health and well-being. *Journal of Advanced Nursing, 24*, 506–511. https://doi.org/10.1046/j.1365-2648.1996.21810.x

Astedt-Kurki, P., Paavilainen, E., & Lehti, K. (2001). Methodological issues in interviewing families in family nursing research. *Journal of Advanced Nursing, 35*, 288–293. https://doi.org/10.1046/j.1365-2648.2001.01845.x

Badr, H., Acitelli, L. K., & Taylor, C. L. C. (2007). Does couple identity mediate the stress experienced by caregiving spouses? *Psychology and Health, 22*, 211–229. https://doi.org/10.1080/14768320600843077

Barnes, M. D., Hanson, C. L., Novilla, L. B., Magnusson, B. M., Crandall, A. C., & Bradford, G. (2020). Family-centered health promotion: Perspectives for engaging families and achieving better health outcomes. *Inquiry, 57*, 1–6. https://doi.org/10.1177/0046958020923537

Brown, T., & Wyatt, J. (2010). Design thinking for social innovation. *Stanford Social Innovation Review, Winter, 2010*, 31–35.

Crandall, A., Novilla, L. K. B., Hanson, C. L., Barnes, M. D., & Novilla, M. L. B. (2019). The public health family impact checklist: A tool to help practitioners think family. *Frontiers in Public Health*. https://doi.org/10.3389/FPUBH.2019.00331

Daly, K. (1992). The fit between qualitative research and characteristics of families. In J. Gilgun, K. Daly, & G. Handel (Eds.), *Qualitative methods in family research* (pp. 3–11). SAGE.

Dolmans, D. H. J. M., & Tigelaar, D. (2012). Building bridges between theory and practice in medical education using a design-based research approach: AMEE Guide No. 60. *Medical Teacher, 34*, 1–10. https://doi.org/10.3109/0142159X.2011.595437

Garcia-Huidobro, D., & Mendenhall, T. (2015). Family oriented care: Opportunities for health promotion and disease prevention. *Journal of Family Medicine and Disease Prevention*. https://clinmedjournals.org/articles/jfmdp/journal-of-family-medicine-and-disease-prevention-jfmdp-1-009.php?jid=jfmdp. Accessed 16 Aug 2021

Godino, J. G., van Sluijs, E. M., Sutton, S., & Griffin, S. J. (2014). Understanding perceived risk of type 2 diabetes in healthy middle-aged adults: a cross-sectional study of associations with modelled risk, clinical risk factors, and psychological factors. *Diabetes Research and Clinical Practice, 106*, 412–419. https://doi.org/10.1016/j.diabres.2014.10.004

Grabowski, D. (2015). Health identity: Theoretical and empirical development of a health education concept. *Journal of Sociological Research, 6*, 141–157. https://doi.org/10.5296/JSR.V6I1.7754

Grabowski, D., Aagaard-Hansen, J., Willaing, I., & Jensen, B. B. (2017a). Principled promotion of health: Implementing five guiding health promotion principles for research-based prevention and management of diabetes. *Societies*. https://doi.org/10.3390/SOC7020010

Grabowski, D., Andersen, T. H., Varming, A., Ommundsen, C., & Willaing, I. (2017b). Involvement of family members in life with type 2 diabetes: Six interconnected problem domains of significance for family health identity and healthcare authenticity. *SAGE Open Medicine*. https://doi.org/10.1177/2050312117728654

Grabowski, D., Beatriz Rodriguez Reino, M., & Andersen, T. H. (2019). Mutual involvement in families with type 2 diabetes: Using the family toolbox to address challenges related to knowledge, communication, support, role confusion, everyday practices and mutual worries. *Social Sciences*. https://doi.org/10.3390/socsci8090257

Hart, R. (1992). Children's participation: From tokenism to citizenship. *Report*. https://www.unicef-irc.org/publications/100-childrens-participation-from-tokenism-to-citizenship.html. Accessed 16 Aug 2021

Heideman, W. H., de Wit, M., Middelkoop, B. J., Nierkens, V., Stronks, K., Verhoeff, A. P., et al. (2015). Diabetes risk reduction in overweight first degree relatives of type 2 diabetes patients: Effects of a low-intensive lifestyle education program (DiAlert) A randomized controlled trial. *Patient Education and Counseling, 98*, 476–483. https://doi.org/10.1016/j.pec.2014.12.008

Hughes, M., & Duffy, C. (2018). Public involvement in health and social sciences research: A concept analysis. *Health Expectations, 21*, 1183–1190. https://doi.org/10.1111/hex.12825

Jensen, B. B. (1997). A case of two paradigms within health education. *Health Education Research, 12*, 419–428. https://doi.org/10.1093/HER/12.4.419

Khan, C. M., Stephens, M. A. P., Franks, M. M., Rook, K. S., & Salem, J. K. (2013). Influences of spousal support and control on diabetes management through physical activity. *Health Psychology, 32*, 739–747. https://doi.org/10.1037/A0028609

Kovacs Burns, K., Nicolucci, A., Holt, R. I. G., Willaing, I., Hermanns, N., Kalra, S., et al. (2013). Diabetes Attitudes, Wishes and Needs second study (DAWN2™): cross-national benchmarking indicators for family members living with people with diabetes. *Diabetic Medicine, 30*, 778–788. https://doi.org/10.1111/DME.12239

Mayberry, L. S., & Osborn, C. Y. (2012). Family support, medication adherence, and glycemic control among adults with type 2 diabetes. *Diabetes Care, 35*, 1239–1245. https://doi.org/10.2337/DC11-2103

Mayberry, L. S., & Osborn, C. Y. (2014). Family involvement is helpful and harmful to patients' self-care and glycemic control. *Patient Education and Counseling, 97*, 418–425. https://doi.org/10.1016/J.PEC.2014.09.011

Myers, M. F., Fernandes, S. L., Arduser, L., Hopper, J. L., & Koehly, L. M. (2015). Talking about type 2 diabetes: Family communication from the perspective of at-risk relatives. *Science of Diabetes Self-Management and Care, 41*, 716–728. https://doi.org/10.1177/0145721715604367

Rasmussen, J. (2004). Textual interpretation and complexity: Radical hermaneutics. *Nordisk Pedagogik, 24*, 177–194.

Reczek, C. (2014). Conducting a multifamily member interview study. *Family Process, 53*, 318–335. https://doi.org/10.1111/FAMP.12060

Samuel-Hodge, C. D., Cene, C. W., Corsino, L., Thomas, C., & Svetkey, L. P. (2013). Family diabetes matters: A view from the other side. *Journal of General Internal Medicine, 28*, 428–435. https://doi.org/10.1007/S11606-012-2230-2

Scabini, E., & Manzi, C. (2011). Family processes and identity. In S. J. Schwartz, K. Luyckx, & V. L. Vignoles (Eds.), *Handbook of Identity theory and research* (pp. 565–584). Springer.

Sinclair, R. (2004). Participation in practice: making it meaningful, effective and sustainable. *Children & Society, 18*, 106–118. https://doi.org/10.1002/CHI.817

Stephens, M. A. P., Franks, M. M., Rook, K. S., Iida, M., Hemphill, R. C., & Salem, J. K. (2013). Spouses' attempts to regulate day-to-day dietary adherence among patients with type 2 diabetes. *Health Psychology, 32*, 1029–1037. https://doi.org/10.1037/A0030018

Torenholt, R., Schwennesen, N., & Willaing, I. (2014). Lost in translation—The role of family in interventions among adults with diabetes: A systematic review. *Diabetic Medicine, 31*, 15–23. https://doi.org/10.1111/DME.12290

Weijnen, C. F., Rich, S. S., Meigs, J. B., Krolewski, A. S., & Warram, J. H. (2002). Risk of diabetes in siblings of index cases with type 2 diabetes: Implications for genetic studies. *Diabetic Medicine, 19*, 41–50. https://doi.org/10.1046/J.1464-5491.2002.00624.X

White, P., Smith, S. M., & O'Dowd, T. (2007). Living with type 2 diabetes: A family perspective. *Diabetic Medicine, 24*, 796–801. https://doi.org/10.1111/J.1464-5491.2007.02171.X

Chapter 4
Action Research with People Being Treated for Cancer or a Rare Disease: Health Mediation Central to Their Experiences and Their Inclusion

Eric Dugas, Zoé Rollin, Lucas Sivilotti, and Karyn Dugas

4.1 Introduction

While very few studies have examined the experiences, schooling, well-being and well-becoming of adolescents and young adults with serious illnesses (Rollin, 2015; Rollin et al., 2018), our French team has conducted several research projects over the past 10 years in southwestern France. The projects aimed, first, to document the situations experienced by adolescents and young people being treated for a serious disease as well as that of their families. In addition, two action research projects were set up as part of a health promotion approach, facilitating the educational and vocational inclusion of these young people. This chapter focuses on the second research component, i.e. action research.

Unlike other disciplines, social science research on health issues does not place much value on interventional approaches. They are often regarded with thinly disguised contempt and dismissed as social intervention projects that offer no added value from a research point of view. They are also often seen as responding to an institutional demand, potentially restricting researchers.

The aim of this chapter is to show how this action research project, combined with a bottom-up approach, has made it possible to promote an understanding of the issues at stake in the inclusive processes of seriously ill pupils and students. Conducting action research makes it possible to create new observation situations

E. Dugas (✉) · L. Sivilotti
LACES EA 7437 Lab., University of Bordeaux, Bordeaux, Nouvelle-Aquitaine, France
e-mail: eric.dugas@u-bordeaux.fr

Z. Rollin
CERLIS UMR 8070 Lab., Université Paris Cité, Ile de France, France

K. Dugas
University Hospital Center of Bordeaux, Maison Aquitaine Ressource pour Adolescents et Jeunes Adultes, Bordeaux, Nouvelle-Aquitaine, France

L. Potvin, D. Jourdan (eds.), *Global Handbook of Health Promotion Research, Vol. 1*,
https://doi.org/10.1007/978-3-030-97212-7_4

and, in this sense, to access the original discourses and practices. Furthermore, in situ experimentation gives rise to exciting process studies. In this sense, it also requires a cross-fertilization of views between healthcare professionals and education professionals. Such interventions are the outcome of a co-construction process, whose effects are subsequently investigated. In addition to enabling evaluation in the field, the intervention also serves as a context conducive to the creation of new research data. All these elements contribute to shaping collective interventions that are better tailored to the needs identified.

This chapter is divided into three parts. The first part presents the context in which our research was conducted and the experiences of the target individuals. The second part describes the approaches used to conduct our field studies. Data were collected in the field as part of a co-construction process with the people concerned by the issues discussed. The third part shows how the action research projects conducted help facilitate the academic inclusion of young adults with chronic illnesses.

4.2 Research Context Related to Serious Diseases: An Innovative Interventional Mechanism

Disability is, above all, a category, the result of a meeting between a self-definition and a set of institutional expectations (Bodin, 2018). As a consequence, some real needs have not been categorized as such and remain unacknowledged. This is especially true in the case of serious illnesses that become chronic (cancer or rare diseases). Yet, promoting health and/or wellness means not reducing individuals to their illness or seeing them in purely biological terms. This is particularly true for adolescents and young adults who are in the midst of building their identity. To date, around 8000 rare diseases have been identified worldwide. Five new ones are discovered every week. As far as cancers are concerned, there are 800 new cases per year in young adults (18–25 years old). Most childhood cancers are considered to be rare diseases. It is difficult for public policies to take into account the specific needs of people with disabilities associated with chronic serious illnesses. Yet, the societal stakes are high in the field of education: pupils or students returning to school or university (after hospitalization, treatment, absences) have to cope with an educational context that puts them in difficulty and creates a situation of disability. Regardless of the illness or condition, in many cases, there is an impression of isolation and powerlessness, especially during hospitalization. These illnesses and their invasive treatments have strong physical and psychological effects. The stigma of the disease accentuates the “feeling of being invaded” (nausea, increased tiredness, alopecia (temporary hair loss), etc.). Moreover, on returning to school or university, the pupil or student has to cope with an educational context that places him or her in difficulty, which in turn creates a situation of disability (Dugas & Rollin, 2014; Dugas, 2020).

For international readers, it may be useful to clarify a few points with respect to the French system. The needs for our target public come within the scope of the various laws related to the inclusion of people with disabilities. For example, (1) Pupils may benefit from adapted teaching arrangements as part of their schooling. If these special arrangements do not involve any specific costs, the support is provided by the teaching team following consultation with the school doctor. If a pupil needs human assistance or specific equipment, administrative recognition of the disability is required. (2) The French higher education system is extremely heterogeneous. Students can also study within special programmes in small classes (institutions where they train for a specific trade or prepare for entrance exams to highly selective institutions). At university, they have access to a specific service ("disability centre/service"), which, in conjunction with the university medical service, can recommend teaching adaptations. However, the institutional and educational programmes or arrangements available to them present limitations, obstacles and barriers, despite the stated inclusion intentions (Ebersold, 2017).

So, how can we address these practices at school, at university, at work or in everyday life in order to reduce exclusion? To achieve this goal, we need to introduce specific mechanisms adapted to sensitive issues and topics. Knowledge of these situations took shape through two complementary channels that were built in the course of our research work: (1) a health mediator (specializing in adolescent oncology) was able to draw on extensive experience to identify the needs of these students and their families over the years and (2) studies identified the educational trajectories of pupils and students treated for these illnesses. Thus, there appears to be a gap in the support provided during the school/university trajectory, the specific support needs and the coordination between the players and institutions.

4.3 Research Approaches Serving Adolescents and Young Adults Treated for Chronic Serious Conditions

Having established the intervention context and environment, we now take a closer look at the creation of the health innovation mechanism, associated with our field research.

4.3.1 Cross-Disciplinary and Multi-Category Research for Health Promotion

The field research carried out required a multidisciplinary perspective and a range of expertise. It mobilized and brought together multiple players, combining two categories of interacting stakeholders. This cross-fertilization and knowledge-sharing approach can help structure research in order to promote the health of these young people with chronic serious illnesses.

A multidisciplinary research team: Not simply on the periphery, but central to the mechanism, researchers in the field of human and social science and health work together to develop a cross-disciplinary research by collating their perspectives of the subject under investigation. There is no hierarchy in the discussions between the professional players and the target population. In order to foster the inclusion of the target public, the approach is bottom-up and is also intended to be horizontal, weighting the asymmetry of the interacting players.

Healthcare and paramedical professionals and education professionals are also involved, along with association sector players in the field, and, above all, young people suffering from a chronic serious illness and their families.

The aforementioned multidisciplinary nature is a strength, while also remaining a complex challenge. On the one hand, comparing perspectives is a genuine priority, since the subject of the research and action is best approached from a variety of angles. On the other hand, examining one's own challenges remains highly complex. Implementing projects with such content, therefore, requires a great deal of time for discussions and needs to be regularly formulated and reformulated in order to maintain the intelligibility and effectiveness of the exchanges.

According to the terms of the Ottawa Charter (1986), health promotion assumes introducing a dynamic that enables individuals to better control and act on the various determinants of health. By definition, these are identified on a collective basis and are associated with social inequalities, particularly in the area of health. In line with the work of WHO (1998), health promotion is considered here as a "comprehensive social and political process, it not only embraces actions directed at strengthening the skills and capabilities of individuals, but also action directed towards changing social, environmental and economic conditions so as to alleviate their impact on public and individual health". Hence the support and mediation mechanism contribute to the reduction of social inequalities in the field of health (discrimination, institutional abuse, invisibility, socio-spatial issues) that tend to affect this group of people suffering from serious illnesses in particular. To counter such inequalities, "relationships" and "emotions" help develop the target public's capabilities (Sen, 1985) and improve their health by changing their "social and environmental situation". This approach supports full participation in social life via collective action through such health promotion actions and by creating spaces favourable to individual and collective fulfilment.

4.3.2 *Working on the Overall Health of a Vulnerable Population Implies Acting Both as a Community and for the Community*

The political and societal stakes of the education research mechanism are high: on returning to school or university (after hospitalization or treatment leading to absence), pupils or students treated for serious illnesses have to deal with an educational context that places them in difficulty and crystallizes the disability situation. The awareness raising required is global since it concerns all the players (professional and non-professional) that interact with the pupil/student patient. From hospital to school, followed by university, and even in the world of work, all are contexts that involve multiple players. Our research consequently adopts a resolutely systemic approach. The aim is to co-construct a more comfortable life trajectory, working not "on" but "with" the target population.

This approach justifies intervening in the field, where the many players, structures and services are often compartmentalized, with heterogeneous discourses and actions, despite their desire to compensate for inequalities and to improve health. The innovations introduced seek to combat isolation, dropping out and the impression of powerlessness.

In order to remain true to the co-construction approach that we are seeking to implement, it was important to build the research mechanism on the basis of what young people and their families had to say, gathered from interventions in the field of secondary and higher education as well as from exploratory interviews with the professionals concerned. Consequently, it was important that all the players were not only actively involved in the research process but also in evaluating the results and the way in which the information gathered was conveyed. During the action research project, the vulnerable target populations, researchers, professionals and players from the association sector were drawn together during two study days and an international symposium in order to compare the perspectives of all the results and to determine how to take ownership of them and exploit them together. The neutral location, mentioned earlier, used to mediate interventions, organized – and still organizes today – focus groups on specific themes (especially on school and university trajectories). It welcomes and supports young patients and their families, promoting health by providing education to vulnerable populations, delivered by healthcare and non-caregiver professionals present in the structure while at the same time creating a favourable environment for the patients' psychological and social health. This is in addition to the physical care they receive in the nearby hospital. It is also a space occupied by researchers, which gives the latter privileged access to the populations under study, wherein lies the scientific value of the action research carried out.

4.3.3 Generating Knowledge and Research Findings by Understanding the Processes Involved

The researcher's position is intrinsically modified by the research topic. Instead of adopting a position overlooking or detached from the field and stakeholders to analyze the challenges, needs and expectations, the research draws its strength from the reciprocal links forged with players in the field to understand and act on the various health determinants.

Below, we describe the action research carried out in secondary schools and universities.

Questions relating to the schooling of secondary school pupils being treated for cancer have long posed a dual challenge. First, researchers knew little about the situations experienced by these young people (Marchand & Rollin, 2015). There was a serious lack of data on back-to-school situations, with the scarce information that was available relating to only very short periods of time.

Second, in response to the challenges associated with returning to school reported by young people in hospital departments, practical experiments were set up but without the possibility of analyzing their impact at the same time.

Implementing action research, therefore, offered the dual advantage of trialling a back-to-school support system for these young people while at the same time creating situations for observing the processes at work. The experimental project was conducted between 2013 and 2015.

In concrete terms, it consisted of several key steps, with an interventional component and a research component (Fig. 4.1). After carrying out a diagnostic interview with pupils and their families, the researchers visited the patients' school. There, two types of interventions were carried out: (1) participation in educational teams with the aim of raising awareness of the specific needs of young people and (2) a 2-hour awareness-raising presentation in front of the class of the young person concerned. Each intervention was accompanied by ethnographic observations to document the situations.

Following these interventions, the young people concerned and their families were offered a debriefing session, and questionnaires were handed out and then analyzed to assess the approach undertaken. All the support measures were the subject of carefully collected ethnographic observations.

At the end of an academic year of classroom-based interventions, a "family focus group" was organized in order to offer the target families an interim analysis of the situations observed. This interactive context made it possible to discuss the initial avenues for analysis.

The different action research phases appear to make the intervention a genuine basis for the production of scientific knowledge. There are several reasons for this:

1. Action research creates observation situations that would be impossible in another context. This is particularly true with regard to going back to school. Indeed, after acute treatment for cancer, pupils tend to return to the classroom discreetly, in an often precarious and uncertain overall context of remission. It is difficult to imagine accompanying such pupils or students returning to class in the framework of a conventional ethnographic observation. Indeed, it could cause additional unease at an already difficult time. Visiting schools in the context of the intervention thus meets the conditions for ad hoc observation.
2. It allows us to observe the evolution of a pupil's attitude and that of the entire educational community over a long period of time. The various data collection cut-off points make a longitudinal observation possible.

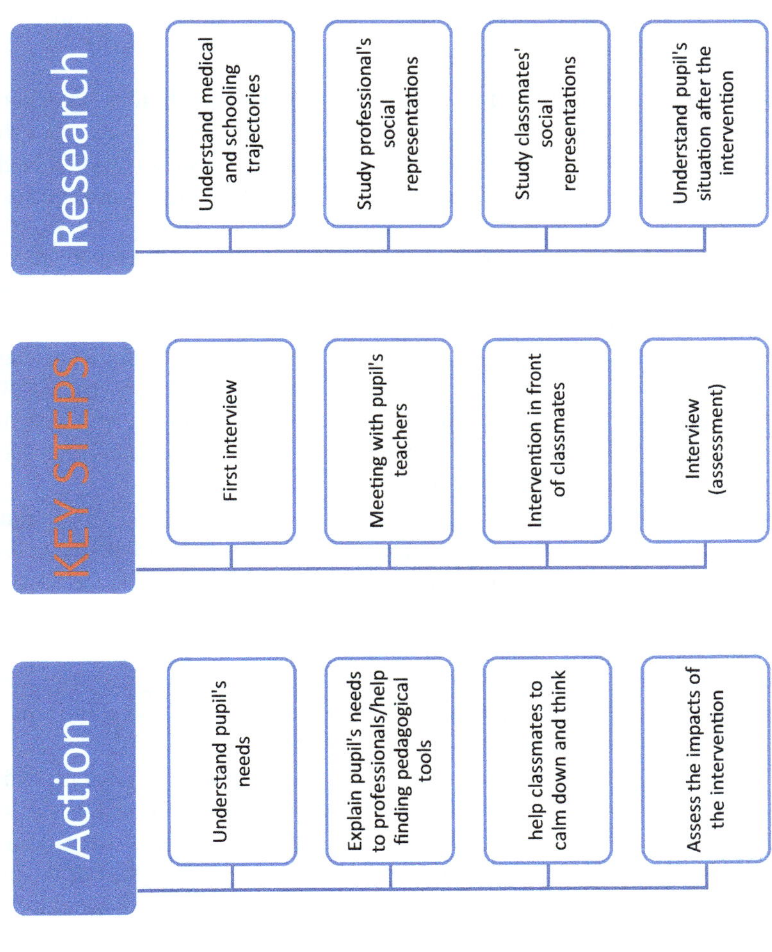

Fig. 4.1 Action research process (designed by Z. Rollin)

3. These observations are all the richer since they are produced by researchers who themselves adopt a reflexive participatory observation approach. Joining an education team with the intention of taking part in negotiating teaching adaptations is not at all the same as going there as a simple observer. Participatory observation, particularly with this dual approach, helps create a new form of empathy. Indeed, in order to report on the experiences of young people and their families, researchers need to be immersed in their outlook. For part of the research team, especially the former teachers, the evolution is heuristic since it involves shifting from a group focus to an individual focus, particularly as they are aware of the difficulties specific to everyday teaching.

The project, which was continued following the action research, aims to procure individual benefits for young people coming out of acute cancer treatments as well as more global social benefits. In addition to disseminating valuable public health information, it also helps raise awareness of disability and serious illness and seeks to combat stigmatizing attitudes.

In 2016, after observing similarities in the situations experienced by people being treated for rare diseases and cancer, it was decided to turn the first project into a tailored support and mediation system, designed to encourage continuity in school, university and medical care for adolescents and young adults affected by such health events (Courty et al., 2019). The study, called EMELCARA ("Experience of a mediation scheme for students and high school pupils with cancer or a rare disease"), was later extended and expanded due to the fact that access to higher education is more restricted for people with disabilities.

Inspired by the "PAS-CAP!" action research project, EMELCARA continues along the same lines but retains an innovative dynamic. It would not be feasible to present the specificities of a given student in lectures or tutorials, since such an approach would be completely out of sync with everyday university life. Moreover, students who find themselves in a situation of disability following a health event are eligible for specific support mechanisms (see earlier). However, they are not always aware of these mechanisms, and the teaching and research staff sometimes find it difficult to refer them to the right place.

Hence, a specific trial was set up in the context of the MARADJA centre, which is affiliated to the University Hospital in Bordeaux. It involves working with the students concerned to provide help with university administrative procedures, career guidance and help with socio-professional integration processes, all the while offering support to the family, as well as explaining the tailored support offered by the "disability" service during the student's university programme (extra time for exams, staggered study programmes, human, technological and material assistance, etc.).

All these endeavours involve frequent, almost daily, virtually invisible actions that combine to produce educational and professional continuity and, more generally, the well-being of the person concerned. To document the study carried out and its effects, we could have simply interviewed the young people in question, but this would have given just one version of the support situation, and the data might have been distorted by selective memory. To avoid this pitfall, the team opted to conduct an ethnographic follow-up with the support staff through an observation based on the dual perspectives of a MARADJA health mediator, Karyn Dugas, who carries out the actions, and a researcher in education science, Lucas Sivilotti, who faithfully monitors them.

Here again, experimentation provides us with a perfect setting for the production of data that would not exist otherwise. Beyond traditional health determinants, this "embedded" perspective also gives us a detailed analysis of the many institutional, economic, financial and social barriers that impede educational continuity and the socio-professional integration of students undergoing treatment for chronic illnesses. On the other hand, this perspective requires considerable reflexivity, an indispensable condition if the data collected and their analysis are to be relevant.

4.4 Action Research that Helps Improve the Inclusion of Young People Being Treated for Cancer or a Rare Disease

4.4.1 Facilitating the Educational Continuity of Adolescents in Secondary Education

Between 2012 and 2015, an initial survey was carried out in the context of a PhD thesis (Rollin, 2015; Rollin, 2021) in which around 60 case studies combining observations and interviews with young people and their parents were explored. In parallel, action research was conducted to trial back-to-school support for adolescents treated for cancer (see earlier). This work gave us a better understanding of the adolescents'experiences. While the school experience is different for every young cancer patient, in the short term, most of the adolescents we met had experienced a period in which schooling was put on hold to some extent during their intensive medical treatment. Even if learning continues in the hospital, it is far removed from the usual school day and reinforces the sense of overall strangeness experienced by the young people during this period of their life. For these youngsters, the return to school generally coincides with remission, i.e. the moment when the symptoms disappear. This period is particularly difficult to manage. For young people, the end of acute treatment is often synonymous with considerable fatigue, a fear of relapse and a sense of disruption. For education professionals, remission is often perceived as a "return to normal" and a resumption of ordinary school expectations. Thus, specific mediation is very useful in such situations. It gives education professionals useful insights into the young person's situation, which are essential when working on educational adaptation. A few young people continue to attend school more or less as usual during acute treatment, without waiting for remission, and their difficulties are often poorly understood by education professionals. Mediation is also extremely useful in such situations in order to shed light on the hidden difficulties and to enable the adjustments to be made.

Both during and after treatment, these adolescents often fear inappropriate questions or unpleasant comments from their peers. Classroom interventions can partially defuse this type of problem. Such interventions are generally positively received by education professionals, who are often reluctant and uncomfortable when it comes to discussing these topics with their pupils.

In addition, during the classroom interventions, other specific objectives are pursued in terms of health promotion. Classroom presentations can offer overall information about cancer risk factors to deliver public health information that is useful to everyone. Information can be given about both individual risk factors (alcohol, smoking, diet, etc.) and collective factors, such as the role of the work environment. Thus, by tackling the risk factors external to the disease, two major public health issues are addressed: prevention (the main tool in the fight against the disease) and routine screening (a tool promoting the early treatment of potential cancers, thereby ensuring more people are cured).

The classroom interventions therefore help the young people to return to school after they finish their acute treatment and raise awareness of their difficulties among the educational community as a whole.

4.4.2 Health Mediation Trials Among Sick Students

In 2016, a second investigation using a combined methodology was launched, which included:

- A survey among students (n = 8155) and higher education professionals (teaching and research staff and administrative staff) (n = 2769) by self-administered questionnaires.
- A survey by semi-directive interviews with professionals (n = 14), high school pupils and students with a rare disease (n = 32) and their parents (n = 5).
- An ethnographic follow-up carried out during the health mediation trial with four students presenting a rare disease.

The main finding from the student survey was that 65% of those with a health problem (and 73.6% of those with a rare disease) felt that the challenge to manage the time devoted to their studies was amplified by their health concerns. Lack of time forced them to prioritize their physical needs over their psychological needs. Hence, students followed up for health events tend to experience more complex study situations than the other students, something that is exacerbated in cases of cancer or rare diseases. Students being treated for a rare illness or chronic condition are among those declaring a health problem: (1) the most concerned in having to constantly repeat their problem to different parties, especially teachers and (2) the most likely to say they would like to have an intermediary to explain their needs, in other words, support in terms of student empowerment, the need to co-construct with all the stakeholders and the creation of a bond of trust in informal spaces.

As for the professionals questioned, the main challenges appear to relate to a lack of cooperation between the professionals and a lack of knowledge of the disability, requiring specific training (Sivilotti, 2020). This lack of information and training is particularly evident when it comes to rare diseases, where only 19.6% of higher education professionals consider themselves sufficiently trained and informed (Sivilotti, 2019).

The results of the ethnographic follow-up showed how health mediation can contribute to the successful inclusion of adolescents and young adults with cancer or a rare disease.

First, this professional practice helps promote health among the various players, fostering a holistic approach in order to co-construct a life course that is closer to the expectations of the people concerned.

Second, it contributes to their autonomy by relaying the message and helps the young people by doing things with them rather than for them. It gives them the keys to assimilate, understand, choose and decide. The mediator's status and the professional environment in which he or she works are "influencing factors" that help foster the inclusion of young people with serious illnesses.

4.4.3 Mediation and Avenues for Further Exploration Regarding Inclusion of These Young People

The interviews and follow-up of mediation on the ground also revealed the full value of non-caregiver support: exchanges are not constrained in terms of time (no compulsory appointment) in contrast to other health professionals in particular, and if there is an appointment, it is not time-limited. The mediator remains an available option, a recourse, a support, linked to an informal reciprocal commitment. At school, in front of the youngster's classmates, the presence of a mediator means that it is not the teacher who announces the illness or relays information on an issue that is as complex as it is delicate.

Supported by other studies (Marioni, 2014; Leprince et al., 2016; Guirimand et al., 2018), the mediator also takes the time to work on the "unexpressed needs" of these young people. In a face-to-face situation with a healthcare facility and/or a school worker, issues of dependence and autonomy come into play. The position of dominance and power embodied by the white coats, psychologists or teachers, makes the young people more aware of their challenges, shortcomings and problems. They are the mirror that reflects a situation of increased vulnerability. With a non-caregiver mediator, the caregiver/patient or teacher/learner relationship is diluted, something that is greatly appreciated by these young people. They feel legitimized and are able to discuss their needs more easily. Moreover, once the need has been expressed, it becomes plural. It may concern family, school and healthcare issues as well as access to leisure, culture and sport. If each player has a well-targeted and well-defined status, function and role, the non-caregiver mediator can intervene in all aspects of life of a developing adolescent or young adult: a role "specialized in diversity", at the crossroads between internal and external resources related to serious illness.

However, our systemic approach invites us to investigate other research avenues and other hypotheses in favour of mediation as a factor for health promotion and inclusion. This is the case with the issue of "transitions" between healthcare services (paediatric and adult) and between schools and universities. Indeed, we can easily observe that health and education professionals or teachers (whether specialized or not) change over time, depending on the establishment, structure and services attended (primary school, middle school, high school and university, integration into the workplace). This makes transitional periods difficult to cope with, potentially generating stress and problems in terms of adaptation and accessibility. However, if necessary, the non-caregiver mediator can be present in all these different scenarios and over a longer timeline (15–25 years). As the first mirror is other people, you have to trust this mirror – something that takes time when accompanying a journey marked by numerous transitions.

Another difficulty reported is that of access to services. If it is ill-adapted, the space dedicated to professionals can have a strong and negative impact on the asymmetrical relationship between young people and professionals. Indeed, the places where we live, learn and work are not simply backdrops (Moser, 2009) but affect the ways we live and behave (Fischer, 2011). They play a non-negligible role in the climate of trust, exchange of knowledge and relations with others. However, as already mentioned, the first contacts with our mediator take place in a "place of transition", carefully chosen in advance and close to the hospital. This space appears to be conducive to encounters, to free speech and to "doing things together", which are all research hypotheses and avenues currently being explored by the research team. In this respect, the lighting, colours and amenities in the spaces of the said location are also being studied (individual or collective spaces, face-to-face, kitchen, sports room, multimedia, relaxation area, etc.).

4.5 Conclusions

Nine years of action research involving two research programmes have been developed and analyzed in order to better understand and facilitate the educational, university and socio-professional continuity of adolescents and young adults treated for serious and chronic illnesses. This applied research demonstrates the value of out-of-the-box thinking for experiments with methodologies rooted in the field and the realities of the users being supported. Moreover, the approaches adopted are also marked by the desire to practise an engaged, grassroots-based science in a bid to help combat social inequality in the field of health and, more generally, to contribute to social change. This action research thus aims to create an original socio-educational support mechanism, from school to employability, supported by a web platform linked to the existing internal and external resources. This tried and tested mechanism may be partially transferable by adapting it to the target public, local policies and the wider educational, social, economic and cultural contexts of the intervention. Improving physical, mental and social health is closely linked to the ecosystem in which overall health and wellness is promoted. At the heart of the system is a place where the mediator and the mobile multi-skilled team operate alongside the researchers. It is a place of transition between school, family and healthcare institutions that facilitates access to structures and services as well as interaction with dedicated users.

Our research and associated methodologies, founded on health mediation within an ethical context, contribute to the promotion of health, offering adolescents and young people the tools to express themselves and to acquire knowledge. This makes it possible to build solutions together, with them instead of for them, rather than adopting a vertical, top-down and compartmentalized approach, as is too often the case. This innovative way of working, creating coordinated and intersectoral actions, helps structure the field of health promotion research by contributing to the development of this population's capacities. In other words, mediation and synergy between players are the factors that foster inclusion and help boost health by empowering these young people coping with serious illnesses.

In short, action research combined with an intervention mechanism can bring together researchers, professionals, young patients and their families and friends on a common, shared and non-compartmentalized ground. In these circular interactions, the parents – and, above all, the young patients – are legitimized and given responsibilities. This type of research fosters their empowerment, a genuine lever to help them improve their health and, ultimately, live fuller lives in society.

References

Bodin, R. (2018). *L'institution du handicap. Esquisse pour une théorie sociologique du handicap*. La Dispute.

Courty, B., Sivilotti, L., Rollin, Z., & Dugas, É. (2019). L'apport des éthiques du care et des théories de la médiation pour penser l'inclusion scolaire des jeunes suivis pour des maladies graves chronicisées. In É. Dugas (Ed.), *Handicap et recherches regards pluridis-ciplinaires* (pp. 91–106). CNRS Editions.

Dugas, É. (2020). Former les enseignants à l'empathie pour favoriser l'inclusion des élèves en situation de handicap? *Éducation permanente, 224*, 131–138.

Dugas, É., & Rollin, Z. (2014). Handicap et école: la formation des enseignants en question. *La revue de santé scolaire et universitaire, 29*(5), 29–32. https://doi.org/10.1016/j.revssu.2014.08.009

Ebersold, S. (2017). *L'éducation inclusive: Privilège ou droit ?* Presses Universitaires de Grenoble.

Fischer, G.-N. (2011). *Psychologie sociale de l'environnement*. Dunod.

Guirimand, N., Thouroude, L., & Leplège, A. (2018). La posture de l'entre-deux des professionnels des secteurs médico-social et sanitaire et la coordination des parcours des jeunes en situation de handicap. *Alter, 12*(1), 13–25. https://doi.org/10.1016/j.alter.2017.07.003

Leprince, T., Sauveplane, D., Ricadat, E., Seigneur, É., & Marioni, G. (2016). Aspects psychosociaux et développementaux des AJA atteints de cancer: Existe-t-il des spécificités propres aux jeunes adultes ? *Bulletin du Cancer, 103*(12), 990–998. https://doi.org/10.1016/j.bulcan.2016.10.013

Marchand, A., & Rollin, Z. (2015). Ce que l'intervention fait à la recherche dans un contexte de maladie grave. *Santé Publique, 27*(3), 331–338.

Marioni, G. (2014). Travailler avec la non-demande des adolescents atteints de cancer. In S. Pucheu et al. (Eds.), *Psychothérapies analytiques en oncologie* (pp. 117–129). Lavoisier.

Moser, G. (2009). *Psychologie environnementale. Les relations homme environnement*. De Boeck.

Rollin, Z. (2015). Comment comprendre et faciliter le retour en classe des lycéens traités pour un cancer? Retour sur une recherche-action sociologique. *Santé Publique, 27*(3), 309–320. https://doi.org/10.3917/spub.153.0309

Rollin, Z. (2021). *Le lycée à l'épreuve du cancer. Une sociologie de l'école, de ses actrices et acteurs dans le contexte de la maladie grave*. Editions INSHEA.

Rollin, Z., Courty, B., & Dugas, K. (2018). Comprendre et répondre aux besoins spécifiques des étudiants suivis pour une maladie grave: Quatre ans de recherche-action en Aqui-taine et Île-de-France. In É. Dugas (Ed.), *Les violences scolaires d'aujourd'hui en ques-tion. Regards croisés et altérités* (pp. 27–40). L'Harmattan.

Sen, A. (1985). *Commodities and capabilities*. Elsevier.

Sivilotti, L. (2019). La Médiation auprès des étudiants atteints de cancer ou de maladies rares: analyse et compréhension des enjeux. Étude en Nouvelle-Aquitaine autour de la trajectoire estudiantine et des interactions plurielles [Thesis, Université de Bordeaux]. http://www.theses.fr/2019BORD0330.

Sivilotti, L. (2020). L'accompagnement des étudiants en situation de handicap dans l'enseignement supérieur. Une recherche exploratoire auprès des professionnels de l'enseignement supérieur. *Revue Éducation, Santé, Société, 6*(1), 103–116. https://doi.org/10.17184/eac.9782813003485

World Health Organization. (1998). *Health promotion glossary*. World Health Organization.

Chapter 5
Critical Health Promotion and Participatory Research: Knowledge Production for and with Young People Experiencing Homelessness in Scotland

Andrea Rodriguez, Sabrina Galella, Shea Moran, and Ruth Freeman

5.1 Introduction

The experience of homelessness brings many challenges and has a strong impact on the overall health and well-being of a young person (Schwan, 2018). Despite people affected by homelessness being just over four times more likely to die prematurely than the general population due to health problems (Morrison, 2009), there are still many barriers to accessing and sustaining engagement with services and practitioners (Rodriguez et al., 2020a, b). Support services in general tend to see people experiencing homelessness as "difficult" to engage with. On the other side, those affected by homelessness do not feel welcomed when accessing services. Another shared perception is that services have not been designed for them and therefore are failing to provide the most adequate support at the right time of their journeys. Thus, the involvement of those with lived experience in policy design and implementation of services to prevent and to tackle homelessness is currently necessary and required by policymakers.

In this chapter, we will present a Freireian participatory research approach underpinned by the principles of critical pedagogy to increase young people's participation in the design of health promotion interventions and social participation in society.

A. Rodriguez (✉) · R. Freeman (Deceased)
School of Dentistry, University of Dundee, Dundee, Scotland, UK
e-mail: a.rodriguez@dundee.ac.uk

S. Galella
A Way Home Scotland/Rock Trust, Edinburgh, Scotland, UK

S. Moran
Aff the Streets/Rock Trust, Edinburgh, Scotland, UK

L. Potvin, D. Jourdan (eds.), *Global Handbook of Health Promotion Research, Vol. 1*,
https://doi.org/10.1007/978-3-030-97212-7_5

5.2 Youth Homelessness in Scotland

In 2018–2019, the Scottish Government released statistics on youth homelessness, which showed that 6,996 people aged between 16 and 25 years presented as homeless (Scottish Government, 2019). This represents almost 25% of all applications. Youth homelessness refers to "the situation and experience of young people between the ages of 16 and 25 who are living independently of parents and/or caregivers, but do not have the means or ability to acquire a stable, safe, or consistent residence" (Gaetz et al., 2018, p11).

However, the information gathered by the government is based on self-reporting; due to fear of discrimination or lack of incentive in disclosing the real causes of their homelessness, the official numbers do not present a true picture of the problem. The data collected do not include young people "sofa-surfing" around friends' or families' houses, for instance, or those living in overcrowded, unsafe housing conditions. Thus, young people are more likely to be part of the "hidden homeless" population (Homeless link, 2013) with limited chances of government support.

The main cause of youth homelessness remains relationship breakdown or conflict at home (Scottish Government, 2019). However, young people's journey into homelessness is rarely linear and is often the result of structural factors, system failures and individual circumstances.

Poverty is a central structural factor leading to homelessness, along with lack of accessible housing, lack of education and unemployment. Worryingly, youth unemployment rates are on the rise in the UK, and, with the impact of the COVID-19 pandemic on the economy, there are serious concerns about further deterioration of this situation.

Reducing and eradicating youth homelessness is essential to guarantee their access to and engagement with diverse services and specialized types of support according to the different stages of homelessness. These services must be designed in ways that include young people's views, needs and aspirations.

5.3 Government Responses to End Youth Homelessness: Involvement of People with Lived Experience

Scotland has highly progressive homelessness legislation, including the Housing Options approach, to prevent homelessness.

In 2018, the Ending Homelessness Together High-Level Action Plan was launched, and it emphasized that, in addition to homelessness and housing services, partners across health, education, social work, community support, justice and the third sector were necessary to ensure that homelessness would be only rare, brief and non-recurrent (Scottish Government, 2018).

New changes in homelessness policies reduced the use of unsuitable accommodation for more than 7 days for all homeless households from 2021 (Scottish

Government, 2020), which, in the past, was only reserved to pregnant women and households with children (Scottish Government, 2017). This certainly will improve the quality of life of those young people requiring an accommodation.

In these processes of designing new policies and legislation, the Scottish Government is aware of the importance of consulting people with lived experience. In 2018, the views of 425 individuals with experience of homelessness were gathered to help identify the best solutions to end homelessness (Glasgow Homelessness Network, 2018).

One of the most influential platforms seeking service user involvement to make co-production a building block in the design of policies in Scotland is "All in for Change" (Scottish Community Development Centre, 2019). This platform is making a collaborative effort in supporting the Scottish Government to tackle rough sleeping, stigma and discrimination faced by homeless people (Homelessness Network Scotland, 2020).

Another example of joint work to develop youth homelessness prevention pathways comes from *A Way Home Scotland*, a coalition of individuals, organizations and authorities dedicated to ending youth homelessness in Scotland (Way Home Scotland, 2019). Whilst the preventative approaches brought forward by these pathways and endorsed by the Scottish Government are pivotal to end homelessness, the equal, fair and meaningful involvement of people with lived experience must continue to be the voice that shapes and informs policy and legislation.

The leadership shown by the Scottish Government and the unparalleled commitment and expertise brought forward by universities and many third sector organizations are proof that positive changes can be collectively designed and implemented.

5.4 Health Promotion for Young People Experiencing Homelessness: The Use of Critical Pedagogy

Critical pedagogy is an educational approach that was developed by Paulo Freire (1972). This approach has been extensively used by education and social work disciplines, with a fruitful field still to be explored more within health promotion studies. Critical pedagogy endorses marginalized groups' ability to critically think about their life situation and to question the structures of power in society. It highlights the principles of popular education, community development (Ledwith, 2016) and emancipatory research action for health promotion (Wallerstein et al., 2018).

Participatory research processes that seek social transformation following Freire's approach start from the assumption that if we want to be more effective as agents of social change, we must be able to understand the context in which we live and the impact of the actions we take. Health promotion interventions that create good opportunities for people to critically reflect on their experiences of health care are essential. In doing this, participants are encouraged to raise their voices on issues that affect their lives and to recognize connections between their individual problems and the social contexts of inequalities in which they are embedded.

Co-designed health promotion interventions tailored for and with people and communities with lived experience are of central importance to this study, as the knowledge production "with" young people's input can contribute to reducing the health and social inequalities of those who are socially excluded.

Phelan and colleagues (2010), writing on the theory of the fundamental causes of inequality, pointed to the importance of developing health knowledge together with significant factors in health and social inequities. This study adopted Freire's approach to health promotion intervention development in which young people experiencing homelessness were invited to co-produce knowledge on eight health promotion and social participation topics.

A typical feature of the Freireian-type education used in this epistemological and ethical framework understands people as social agents of change, and, for that reason, more opportunities need to be created in community settings for them to bring their own views and experiences to the table to produce knowledge and change in issues that affect their lives. The concept of knowledge production not just "at" but "with" young people adopted in this chapter reflects our belief in health promotion interventions that must work under the principle of "no hierarchization" of knowledge. In this case, there is no space for processes that use a top-down approach. Individuals, when experiencing freedom to express themselves and receiving appropriate encouragement to develop a critical dialogue and reflection with peers and practitioners tend to make an effort to bring about change in their lives. On the other hand, when they are perceived as just recipients of policies, services and formal bodies of knowledge, their process of taking ownership of their lives and choices can be suppressed.

Knowledge production together "with" people recognizes them as the experts of their lives, and their expert knowledge and life experiences combined with other types of knowledge and information obtained from dialogues with different actors such as practitioners, policymakers, health bodies and/or formal higher educational institutions form a vital and integral part of this intervention development. The dialogue in Freire's perspective (Freire, 1996) is an act of existential creation.

The work presented in this chapter is underpinned by the principles of critical pedagogy (Freire, 1996), co-production (Walker, 2019) and community development. A joint agenda to promote the right to health of marginalized groups addressed the need to place the young person at the centre of a health promotion intervention that is inclusive, emphatic, collective and comes from their life experiences/contexts.

5.5 The Research Process: Aims and Partner Engagement

The Scottish Government's broad goal to reduce health inequalities and poverty through the health and social care integration strategy (Scottish Government, 2014) inspired this project with young people and a wider range of partners.

The main purpose of this research was to co-produce a youth-led workshop programme committed to provoke critical consciousness and collective action towards a fairer, healthier and more equal society. The workshop programme aimed to: (1) expand young people's knowledge of wider health-related homelessness topics to orient social change and to improve health; (2) collect their experiences with services from different areas of care; and (3) use critical dialogue and thinking to increase the participants' awareness on health promotion linked to socio-political engagement.

The partners involved in this research process comprised four groups from the health and social care sectors and included:

1. National Health System (NHS) Health Boards: health practitioners that provide oral health, health promotion and health education sessions for people experiencing homelessness.
2. Public health researchers working in the Smile4Life programme (the Scottish oral health and psycho-social well-being improvement programme for people experiencing homelessness, funded by the Scottish Government and located at The University of Dundee).
3. Young people aged 16–25 years, experiencing homelessness and living in temporary and supportive accommodations provided by a third sector organization in Edinburgh.
4. Front-line staff and managers from third sector organizations working in the following fields: youth housing support, professional training on substance misuse and professional training on conflict mediation for families and young people either at risk of or experiencing homelessness.

The research participants were selected and engaged by following elements of a reflexive mapping approach developed by Rodriguez, Arora, et al. (2020a). This involved a series of steps such as online searches to identify key youth organizations, followed by several informal phone calls, face-to-face meetings and visits where the principal researcher shadowed youth workers and practitioners and discussed service provision challenges and limitations in an informal and friendly way. This path of networking was a rich experience for all involved as it created a good professional and conceptual bond towards the cause of homelessness and social transformation.

The shared commitment and work to end youth homelessness helped researchers, policymakers, young people and practitioners from health and third sectors connect in varied ways during the research process. A common research agenda was agreed upon, with shared principles of empathy and collaborative work creating the perfect environment for a community-based participatory research to be developed. This work addressed the need for academics to go to communities, to interact with people with lived experience and to listen and learn from them to improve the social participation of the voiceless groups in society.

To guarantee the genuine participation of young people and other partners, a series of meetings occurred through different phases of engagement, as previously described by Rodriguez et al. (2019). A summary of these phases is presented in Table 5.1.

This research process strengthened the idea of academic environments being open to build more connection with grassroots communities and health promotion

Table 5.1 Phases of the participants' engagement

	Stage 1	Stage 2	Stage 3
Participants and partners	Researchers, managers and front-line staff from a youth housing service, NHS Boards, third sector organizations and young people living in temporary accommodation	The same as stage 1	Front-line staff and young people
Method	A series of meetings occurred to set up a common agenda of research activities, available infrastructure and co-delivery process. The key topics and the main content of four workshops on health promotion, along with ways to co-deliver it, were defined. Then, specific meetings were arranged with the NHS Boards and third sector organizations involved in delivery, to discuss the roles in delivery, appropriate resources and additional and particular information to be included in the workshops	A series of meetings occurred to define the key topics and main content of the second package of four workshops on health promotion along with ways to deliver it	Semi-structured interviews to explore the issues raised during the workshops and to evaluate the programme
Outcomes	Four workshops were delivered to young people in partnership with the NHS boards and third sector organizations with a long track record of experience in related workshop topics	The same as phase 1	Collection of data regarding the workshop programme's approach and structure, homelessness trajectories and personal experiences in accessing services to support young people
Evaluation	This first package of workshops was evaluated through post-questionnaires distributed after each workshop. Due to a highly positive evaluation, the NGOs and young participants requested one more package of four workshops	The same as phase 1, and, at this time, even with a new requirement for more workshops, the researchers had to finalize this phase	Semi-structured interviews to evaluate the workshop programme's impact on the participants, approach and structure. The highly positive feedback and acceptance of the workshop programme led to a follow-up project: a knowledge exchange programme on youth homelessness Rodriguez, Biazus, et al. (2020b)

Source: adapted from Rodriguez, A., Beaton, L., & Freeman, R. (2019). Strengthening Social Interactions and Constructing New Oral Health and Health Knowledge: The Co-design, Implementation and Evaluation of A Pedagogical Workshop Program with and for Homeless Young People. *Dentistry Journal*, 7(1), 11, Table 1. Doi:10.3390/dj7010011, licensed under the terms of the Creative Commons Attribution License (https://creativecommons.org/licenses/by/4.0/)

services that address complex social problems in society. Non-academic partners must be involved as much as possible in participatory research processes as well as in joint publications and other ways of research dissemination.

5.6 The Research Framework

Based on the principles of critical pedagogy (Freire, 1996) and using a participatory art-based approach, this research framework involved the co-production of eight workshops on the following themes: oral health, mental health, substance misuse, healthy diet, resilience, stigma, education for the future and youth homelessness trajectory. These topics were selected by the young people and their youth workers. Details of each workshop session and participant's evaluation were described in a previous publication (Rodriguez et al., 2019).

As critical pedagogy according to Freire (1974) means empowering people to question their realities and the structures of power in society that discriminate against certain groups, young participants were invited during the workshop to identify relationships between their conceptions of health promotion, their experiences with health services and their contexts of inequalities. In Freire's social theory, the practice of dialogue helps form a critical consciousness that is integrated with people's reality. Within this critical consciousness, individuals or groups begin to see themselves and their society from their own perspective and they become aware of their own potentialities. Thus, a critical attitude for change can be developed to overcome passivity related to various aspects of young people's lives, including health care and social exclusion: "Society now reveals itself as something unfinished, not as something inexorably given; it has become a challenge rather than a hopeless limitation" (Freire, 1974, p.10).

To assure equal participation in the research process, a substantial amount of time was allocated to the research timeline. This was essential to allow the participants and research partners time to get to know each other, to align their interests and to build trust. A continuous process of evaluation was put in place during and after the workshop programme delivery, with young people being consulted about each individual workshop session as well as the full programme. This allowed the researchers and workshop facilitators to make positive changes regarding the content, resources and facilitation of the workshop sessions based on the constant feedback from the participants.

The art approach used during the sessions was also used in follow-up projects (Rodriguez, 2020b, c) and was proved to achieve a positive response from the young people and helped them raise and discuss sensitive issues through drama activities, collage making, educational games, video debate, photovoice, graffiti, capoeira and cultural exchange.

The research data collection was based on participant observation during the eight workshop sessions (3 hours each), delivered at a non-governmental organization (NGO) base in Edinburgh city. Recordings of the group discussions during the sessions were also made. The evaluation of the programme included participant observation, post-workshop questionnaires (of each session and after the programme ended) and in-depth semi-structured interviews with the young participants and staff members about the key issues on homelessness trajectories, health needs and service provision. Content analysis was used to explore qualitative data.

5.7 Results

This theoretical framework, inspired by Paulo Freire (1974), created a safe and encouraging environment to form critical consciousness and critical attitude related to the participants' health choices as well as critical thinking for action and participation in society. The workshop programme increased the participants' confidence about their rights to health, expanded knowledge on health promotion issues related to homelessness and encouraged critical discussions on accessibility of youth services with staff members and their peers.

Each workshop session captured the young people's definitions, conceptions and experiences regarding the eight topics developed during the programme. Their previous knowledge on health concepts and experiences with healthcare and health practitioners were heard, legitimated and valued in each workshop, without any other health promotion-related information being transmitted. Thus, the group had enough time to think about the topic and to express themselves using their own references and ways of communication. Feeling genuinely recognized in their knowledge, they could exchange ideas and experiences inside the group with freedom and no judgement.

After this first phase, the researcher added new information related to each topic that came from formal bodies and organizations such as the WHO and scientific studies. This subsequent addition of knowledge was made in a respectful and empathic way so as to not minimize or diminish the young people's previous knowledge and experiences but to expand their horizons, opinions and health information.

In the third phase, the young people reflected together on this additional knowledge, meanings and perceptions and a new critical dialogue was generated with these two fields of knowledge, namely, a "formal" knowledge and a knowledge derived "from experience", without making any kind of hierarchical differentiation. When young people were invited to combine/merge these two types of knowledge using different methods of art, a co-produced new knowledge was then observed through their art production and collective commitment. More clarity about the structures of power in society and how contexts of poverty may prevent certain groups from achieving better health and quality of life was perceived. The participants' strategies to overcome these challenges and to combat stigma from health services were critically discussed as well. Explanations of which aspects the group had changed or increased knowledge via the workshop sessions and group interaction were shared. The most important experience for the participants seemed to be having the chance to see that similar understandings, feelings and experiences were common to other members of the group, including staff members. This generated a sense of belonging and a group identity for hope and change. At the end of each workshop, the participants made a collective and individual commitment to change certain aspects of their lives. The verbalization of these commitments for their peers and support workers produced a powerful atmosphere.

The discussions during the workshops enabled the young people to critically reflect on their views, health needs and experiences in accessing services while being affected by homelessness. There was a construction of a new knowledge of wider health promotion issues and social participation for the young people. The process of critical thinking and dialogue formulated by Freire led to the creation of a "new knowledge", which formed a strong base for their social behaviour change. Further contact with staff members after conclusion of the research confirmed adoption of new choices and attitudes related to health care. Trust building and collective engagement with the service providers were highlighted, and improvements were noted in the young people's relationships with their peers attending the NGO as well as their wider social interactions.

This research co-created knowledge that came from the common concerns and experiences of young people. It was based on the diverse experiences and knowledge of the participants rather than on the top-down dynamics of health education that make people feel like passive consumers of information. This new knowledge emerged from listening to the young people and the front-line staff working in youth services, from letting them lead the process and being comfortable to explore their own beliefs and values regarding their trajectories through services. This work shows that universities are not unique places to produce knowledge. There are infinite types of knowledge that must be acknowledged and integrated in policies and services protocols. To address this, more inclusive and safe spaces of critical dialogue should be created.

5.8 Limitations

The substantial amount of time required to fit in this type of research can be challenging for research participants and institutions. Within the homelessness context of service provision, there are complex and frequent demands that necessitate staff responses. Research timelines should respect that and be flexible, being prepared for inevitable delays. A culture of collaboration among the health and social care sectors should be strengthened as well to permit more staff involvement in interdisciplinary research.

A relatively small number of young people (13 participants distributed across 8 workshop sessions) took part, and this project does not allow wider generalization of the findings. However, while acknowledging the small sample size, this responded to the principles embedded in the theoretical and methodological approaches as the nature of these activities requires a reduced number of participants. In addition, we were not able to examine longer-term behaviour change and actions towards social transformation. This should be done in future studies.

5.9 Final Reflections

In this chapter, a methodological and theoretical framework – inspired by Freire's formulation (1974) – that fostered a common agenda for the right to health of marginalized groups was suggested and discussed.

This experience placed the young person at the centre and enabled researchers to understand health promotion linked to social justice from the perspective of young people experiencing homelessness.

The production of knowledge "with" and not just "at" young people was another key element of this research. A co-created knowledge came from the common concerns and experiences of these young people regarding health promotion and homelessness. This work highlighted the value of this knowledge in co-designed and implemented health promotion and health education programmes that used multi-agency collaboration.

The principles of critical pedagogy applied to health promotion research were perceived as essential to create good opportunities for young people to develop critical consciousness of societal inequalities, critical dialogue and change towards better engagement with health services.

In the authors' experience, one of the current challenges of health promotion research is associated with a lack of service users' involvement. Disconnections between research production and the expectations of individuals who face health and social problems in their communities without being deeply consulted regarding their priorities and what is needed from their perspective have led to disappointing results. This type of research challenges the idea that traditionalist paradigms of positivist research are capable of appropriately representing the nature and complexity of health promotion issues linked to contexts of poverty and inequities in society.

The process of conducting research that was inclusive, multidisciplinary and diverse was reflected in the writing process of this chapter. The authors came together from different sectors (two researchers from university, a young person from the third sector and a policy officer), with different professional paths, life experiences and areas of knowledge/practice, to share their views and learnings on the topic.

The culture of critical health promotion inside third sector organizations and health services should be strengthened on a daily basis.

This work permitted young people to play the role of active participants, becoming agents of social change with increased health learning capacity and critical consciousness. Future follow-up projects with young people to implement progressive change in health policies and practice can make a substantial difference to their lives.

References

A Way Home Scotland. (2019). Youth Homelessness Prevention Pathway: Improving Care Leavers Housing Pathways. https://www.awayhomescotland.org/wp-content/uploads/sites/13/2020/04/YHPP-Final-7.11.2019-digital-version.pdf

Freire, P. (1974). *Education for critical consciousness*. Bloomsbury Revelation Series.

Freire, P. (1996). *Pedagogy of the oppressed*. Penguin Books.

Gaetz, S., Schwan, K., Redman, M., French, D., & Dej, E. (2018). In A. Buchnea (Ed.), *The roadmap for the prevention of youth homelessness*. Canadian Observatory on Homelessness Press.

Glasgow Homelessness Network (2018). Can we fix homelessness in Scotland: Aye we can. https://homelessnetwork.scot/wp-content/uploads/2019/12/Aye-Report-August-2018.pdf

Homeless Link. (2013). Hidden Homelessness. Accessed 22 Sep 2020. https://www.homeless.org.uk/facts/homelessness-in-numbers/hidden-homelessness#:~:text=Many%20people%20who%20become%20homeless,squats%20or%20other%20insecure%20accommodation

Homelessness Network Scotland. (2020). Are you all in for change? A new change team for ending homelessness together. https://homelessnetwork.scot/wp-content/uploads/2019/11/eht-all-in-for-change-2.pdf

Ledwith, M. (2016). *Community development in action. Putting freire into practice*. Police Press.

Morrison, D. S. (2009). Homelessness as an independent risk factor for mortality: Results from a retrospective cohort study. *International Journal of Epidemiology, 38*, 877–883.

Rodriguez, A., Beaton, L., Fernandes, F., & Freeman, R. (2019). Strengthening social interactions and constructing new oral health and health knowledge: The co-design, implementation and evaluation of a pedagogical workshop program with and for homeless young people. Special Issue: Promoting Inclusion Oral-Health. Social Interventions to Reduce Oral health Inequities. *Dentistry Journal, 7*, 11. https://doi.org/10.3390/dj7010011

Rodriguez, A., Arora, G., Beaton, L., Fernandes, F., & Freeman, R. (2020a). Reflexive mapping exercise of services to support people experiencing or at risk of homelessness: a framework to promote health and social care integration. *Journal of Social Distress and the Homeless, Taylor and Francis Online*. https://www.tandfonline.com/doi/full/10.1080/10530789.2020.1808344

Rodriguez, A., Biazus, C., Fernandes, F., Freeman, R., & Humphries, G. (2020b). *Helping young people feel at home in Scotland. Building collaborative and integrated services for youth homeless through a reflexive mapping approach for health and social care integration*. Knowledge Exchange Programme final report. SUII, Universities of Dundee and St Andrews. https://www.scottishinsight.ac.uk/Portals/80/ReportsandEvaluation/Programme%20reports/Young%20People%20at%20Home%20Final%20Report_updated.pdf

Rodriguez, A., Fernandes, F., Swinney, A., Freeman, R., & Humphries, G. (2020c). *Helping young people feel at home: Building Collaborative and Integrated Services for Young People Affected by Homelessness. Knowledge Exchange Practitioner Training Video documentary*. University of Dundee, SUII. https://vimeo.com/447767619

Schwan, K., French, D., Gaetz, S., Ward, A., Akerman, J., & Redman, M. (2018). *Preventing youth homelessness: An international review of evidence*. Wales Centre for Public Policy.

Scottish Community Development Centre. (2019). 'All in for change' launches in Scotland – A new approach to tackling homelessness. Accessed 14 Sept 2020. https://www.scdc.org.uk/news/article/2019/12/10/all-in-for-change-launch

Scottish Government. (2017). The homeless persons (unsuitable accommodation) (Scotland) amendment order 2017. https://www.legislation.gov.uk/ssi/2017/273/made

Scottish Government. (2018). Ending homelessness together: high level action plan (2018). https://www.gov.scot/binaries/content/documents/govscot/publications/strategy-plan/2018/11/ending-homelessness-together-high-level-action-plan/documents/00543359-pdf/00543359-pdf/govscot%3Adocument/00543359.pdf

Scottish Government. (2019). Youth homelessness 2018–2019: Statistics. Accessed 4 Sept 2020. https://www.gov.scot/publications/youth-homelessness-2018-19-statistics/

Scottish Government. (2020). Homeless persons (unsuitable accommodation) (Scotland) order 2020 amendment: CRWIA. https://www.gov.scot/publications/amendment-homeless-persons-unsuitable-accommodation-scotland-order-2020-crwia/

Walker, E. (2019). What should co-production in health look like? UCL Partners. Accessed 5 Oct 2020. https://uclpartners.com/blog-post/co-production-health-look-like/

Wallerstein, N., Duran, B., Oetzel, J., & Minkler, M. (2018). *Community-based participatory research for health* (3rd ed.). Jossey-Bass.

Chapter 6
Acting-in-Context: A Methodological and Theoretical Approach to Understanding the Actions of People Living in Poverty

Caroline Adam, Sylvie Gendron, and Louise Potvin

6.1 Introduction

Despite health promotion efforts to put forward a wide range of strategies ranging from individual skills training to public policy development, health promotion programmes are still largely focused on lifestyle and behavioural modifications related to health risk factors (e.g. smoking, physical inactivity, diet) (O'Neill et al., 2006; Potvin et al., 2005, Popay et al., 2010, Schrecker, 2013, Powell et al., 2017, Carrey et al., 2017).

However, in the mid-1980s, the Ottawa Charter offered a promising avenue by laying the groundwork for health promotion as a process that gives populations greater control over their health (Nutbeam, 1998) while also establishing social

C. Adam (✉)
Département de techniques de travail social, Cégep du Vieux-Montréal, Montréal, Québec, Canada

Canada Research Chair in Community Approaches and Health Inequalities (CACIS), Montréal, Québec, Canada
e-mail: cadam@cvm.qc.ca

S. Gendron
Canada Research Chair in Community Approaches and Health Inequalities (CACIS), Montréal, Québec, Canada

Faculté des sciences infirmières, University of Montreal, Montréal, Québec, Canada

School of Public Health, University of Montreal, Montréal, Québec, Canada

L. Potvin
School of Public Health, University of Montreal, Montréal, Québec, Canada

Centre de recherche en santé publique (CReSP), Université of Montreal and CIUSSS du Centre-Sud-de-l'Île-de-Montréal, Montréal, Québec, Canada

L. Potvin, D. Jourdan (eds.), *Global Handbook of Health Promotion Research, Vol. 1*,
https://doi.org/10.1007/978-3-030-97212-7_6

inequalities in health as a priority for intervention (Breslow, 1999; Kickbusch, 2003; WHO, 1986). Much emphasis has been placed on the structural causes that create contexts unfavourable to health, particularly contexts of poverty. On the one hand, it is known that individuals are not passive: they carry out their actions in contexts in which quality is influenced by a number of factors. On the other hand, it is recognized that much of the quality of the circumstances through which people act is beyond the direct control of individuals (CSDH, 2008; Raphael, 2002). The perspective of social determinants of health leads us to acknowledge that individuals are not completely determined by factors outside themselves, but neither are they entirely in control of the circumstances in which they live. Therefore, health promotion needs theoretical and methodological tools to understand the interactions between individuals and their contexts, especially those unfavourable to health.

For this purpose, there are few theoretical tools for understanding contexts and ways in which people's actions unfold, beyond health-related behaviours. Potvin et al. (2005) state that if we support the idea that health is a resource and is constructed in daily life, it is necessary to develop theoretical and methodological tools that enable a detailed understanding of this resource. Thus, there is a need for research that looks at the interactions between individuals and their contexts outside the framework of life habits but close to everyday life. Furthermore, the sociologist Anthony Giddens (1987) points out that to adequately study these interactions, it is necessary to "destroy" the empire of interpretive sociology, which is based on imperialism of the study of the individual subject, and the empire of functionalism and structuralism, which is based on imperialism of the study of the societal object. If we want to look at individuals' ability to act while also taking into account the contexts and interactions between these two elements, we need a method capable of capturing this. How can we consider individuals' actions in unfavourable contexts?

This chapter will present the key elements of a study that allowed us to answer this question by focusing on the steps involved in using an ethical posture in empirical data collection and analysis strategies, ultimately within a process of theoretical development from the data. This chapter highlights an often-invisible process of analytical writing that has the potential to lead to theorization.

6.2 Ethical Reflection Prior to Empirical Research

This study was part of a theoretical inquiry that was also intended to be an ethical reflection with a view to developing analytical tools that avoid labelling individuals according to attributes such as smoker, obese, drug user and diabetic. Even with the best intentions, when a research project or programme is designed to target "smokers" or "obese people", labels are applied to individuals that reduce them to an individual behaviour or characteristic while failing to consider the contexts in which the attributes have emerged (Madison, 2000). The act of labelling is not without consequence: stigmatization has a negative impact on people who have been labelled (Earnshaw & Quinn, 2012; Link & Phelan, 2006).

Indeed, Mair (2011) points out that the focus on the risk factors involved in a disease rather than on the root causes of health problems is partly because it is easier to study and devise interventions from risk factors. Risk factors can be observed at the individual level, while the root causes of illness involve individuals' surroundings and contexts. Context is a source of disorder and complexity, whereas behaviours are tangible, circumscribed and more obvious aspects to target (Mair, 2011). Nonetheless, with decades of evidence consistently demonstrating the association between low socio-economic status and poor health, ignoring poverty is no longer an option if we are serious about improving the health of these populations.

6.3 Background, Paradigm and Method Used in This Study

Background The design of this study was based on the aforementioned principle to develop a method that would provide access to individuals' actions without dissociating them from their contexts. Thus, the intention was to interview individuals in a context of poverty and vulnerability. We wanted to avoid approaching people's lives through illnesses or behaviours that were considered problematic. Thus, we chose food insecurity as a theoretically and empirically relevant pretext for exploring the subject of our study. The decision to focus on individuals who attend a community food aid organization allowed us access to people who may have been experiencing food insecurity. Food insecurity manifests in situations of vulnerability in which individuals have limited access to multiple resources and demonstrate financial insecurity (Lechaume & Savard, 2015).

Paradigm This study has emphasized the active roles of individuals without denying the constraining aspect of social contexts. This choice reflects an ontological position that acknowledges a recursive relationship between the actions of individuals and the society in which they live (Giddens, 1987): individuals reproduce and transform social systems through their actions, which are both constrained and enabled by the resources and rules that constitute these systems. Social systems are reproduced and transformed through human practices, which, in turn, become embedded in structures regarded as sets of rules and resources (Giddens, 1987). This study is part of an explicit attempt to account for both the constraining and enabling forces of structures, while recognizing that, even in conditions of severe constraint, individuals continue to "choose," think about and orchestrate their actions according to the outcomes they wish to bring about (Giddens, 1987). Therefore, it was relevant to interview people who voluntarily used the services of a community food aid organization. Going to such an organization demonstrates individuals' ability to respond to adversities they encounter. This manner of conceptualizing our research field provided potential access to contexts of poverty while also having access to people who were taking action in response to challenging situations.

Method The data collection method was chosen to highlight the interactions between the individuals' actions and their contexts. We opted for a qualitative study based on undirected individual interviews based on an ethnosociological perspective. By an ethnosociological approach, we mean a type of study that follows ethnographic traditions in terms of data collection techniques used but which constructs its objects in reference to sociological problems (Bertaux, 2016). In this study, life stories were chosen as a method of investigation to study fragments of social reality situated in time and to understand individuals' actions through their experiences.

A life story interview is an interview with varying degrees of direction in which a researcher invites an individual to tell them about their life in whole or in part (Bertaux, 2016). Like Bertaux (2016), we believe that life stories offer access to perspectives that go beyond mere subjectivity or representation of a phenomenon specific to a single individual. Stories offer access to actions over time, that is, actions embodied in social contexts that can reveal the structures and dynamics at play (Bellot, 2000; Bertaux, 2016). For this study, the starting point for the collected narratives was the circumstances that led each interviewee to use the services of a community food aid organization. Twelve people who use those services were interviewed.

Thus, the choice of life stories became a way to address some challenges of studying the interactions between individuals and their contexts. First, to study this type of interaction, it is important to overcome the pitfalls of quantitative method approaches used in structuralist sociology through which one tries to determine the way in which social structures constrain and determine individuals' behaviours (Giddens, 1987). It is equally important to avoid the limitations of interpretive sociological approaches, based mainly on qualitative methods, which focus on the subjectivity and meaning making of individuals to understand their conduct with little attention to structural constraints (Giddens, 1987). Because of the ethnosociological orientation inherent in life stories, our interviews and the analysis made of them gave us access to the uniqueness of individuals and their ability to act, while at the same time allowed us to consider the contextual elements that constrain individuals' actions without totally determining them.

6.4 Qualitative Data Analysis: A Method to Focus on the Interaction Between Action and Context

The challenge of data analysis was to focus on the interaction between action and context. Thus, an original analysis method was developed. Life stories generate a considerable amount of information, not all of which is relevant to studying the interaction between action and context. Therefore, a series of analytical steps was developed to reduce the content of the interviews and to isolate elements related to the purpose of the study. Six analytical operations were used, following an iterative process (Fig. 6.1):

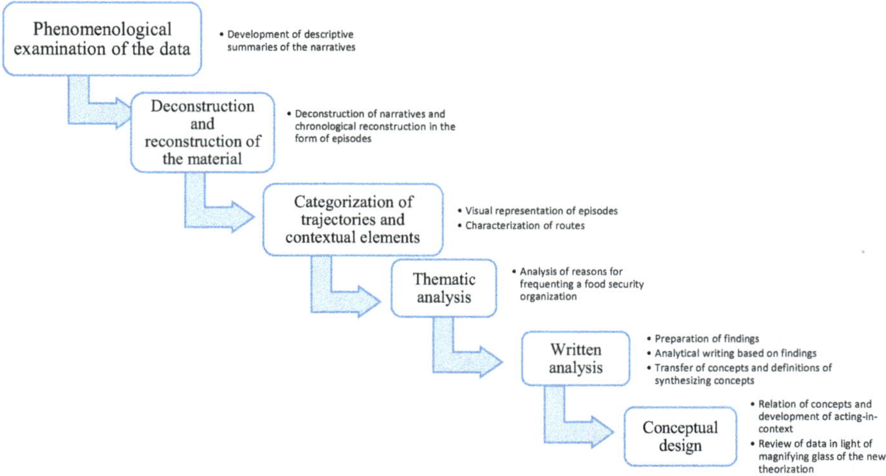

Fig. 6.1 Analytical operations used in data analysis (Adam, 2019)

6.4.1 Phenomenological Examination of the Data

The first step in the phenomenological examination of interviews (Paillé & Mucchielli, 2012) is an initial reading, where the reading exercise is oriented towards what the narratives have "to teach us before we are tempted to make them speak" (Paillé & Mucchielli, 2012, p. 141, author translation) rather than in relation to the research question. After each interview reading, a summary of each participant's situation was written. The summaries were descriptive and free of analytical objectives related to the research question. The aim was to answer the general question, "who are the participants in this study?", and to gain insight into the materials for analysis.

6.4.2 Deconstruction and Reconstruction of Episodic Narratives

After reviewing the data and organizing the material so that the narrative content could be appropriated, a "deconstruction" and "reconstruction" of the narratives was carried out to "isolate" the interaction between action and context. Deconstruction consists of undoing the initial structure of the narratives as they were delivered. Obviously, a life story from an interview does not produce a linear and chronological story (Bertaux, 2016). To capture the sequence of the course of action and its context in a participant's narrative, it was necessary to extract the relevant segments (Bertaux, 2016) and reconstruct them subsequently. This involved putting the narrative segments in a chronological order to create new summarized material that assembled meaningful data for the study.

The selected relevant segments were actions performed by individuals and the contexts in which those actions were performed. These segments were referred to as "episodes." An episode is a period of time when the participant performed actions in a given context, specifically to deal with an event or make decisions. The episodes in each story were coded alphanumerically. Each episode was identified by a brief description and a number (e.g. "Episode 6: Carl looks for work"). A descriptive memo was then written to summarize the episode according to the contextual elements involved (e.g. financial resources running out quickly); the people involved (e.g. Carl's family, who can help him in the event of financial difficulty) and their actions (e.g. sending out resumes for jobs in a desired field) and the consequences/results of the actions, if relevant (e.g. no calls for a job interview and change in job search strategy). The descriptive memos of the episodes were developed as they occurred, with an attempt to situate them chronologically in relation to each other as they were coded.

After the episodes were coded, a table representing the reconstruction of the narrative was developed for each participant. For each episode, the table displayed the following elements in a chronological order: number, assigned title, descriptive memo and associated verbatim.

The number of episodes varied among the participants: some had more episodes than others, and this in itself was information for analysis. It was then relevant to ask: Are there similarities among the participants who have many episodes? Is the nature of the episodes the same among those who have few episodes and those who have many?

6.4.3 Categorization of Trajectories and Contextual Elements

A further qualitative analysis exercise was carried out to develop a conceptual interpretation of the constituent contexts of the selected episodes and their temporal sequencing. The contextual elements of each trajectory were thus illustrated on a timeline for each participant, and each episode was situated on it to better understand the chronology of the episodes and their contexts. The resulting visual illustration provided the "background" to the events that were narrated, including, for example, the country in which the participants were living when they performed certain actions ("when this happened, I was living in [name of country]"), their occupation ("it was when I was working at [name of place]") or their marital status ("at that time, I was still with my husband"). The research questions were as follows: In which contextual elements did individuals perform actions? Are there any intersecting contextual elements that appeared in all the narratives?

Characterization of the contexts resulting from the analysis described above made it possible to identify the differences between trajectories and further consider the episodes illustrated chronologically and visually. The following questions prompted further analysis: Are there similar trajectories? Are some trajectories particularly different from others? What actions characterize these similarities and differences? Still referring to the data, a first grouping of trajectories that appeared similar was made: certain trajectories seemed much more difficult than others. Extreme cases were then compared (Miles & Huberman, 2003): the trajectory was identified that appeared to be the most difficult, in that the participant recounted episodes of constant struggle to meet basic needs. Then, it was compared to the least difficult one, where no reference to a struggle to meet the person's needs was mentioned. Our aim was to explore these questions: What is fundamentally different about the type of actions performed? What is fundamentally different about the contexts? Based on the hypotheses developed in response to these questions, the 12 trajectories were classified from the most to least difficult.

6.4.4 *Thematic Analysis*

Since the starting point for the interviews was to learn the reasons for using the services of a community food aid organization, a thematic analysis was carried out on this specific aspect (Paillé & Mucchielli, 2012). Episodes concerning the reasons for using a community food aid organization were extracted from each of the narratives while taking the previous and subsequent episodes into account. The analysis question at this stage was: what are the reasons why participants went to a community food aid organization? The analysis conducted was aimed at finding patterns (Miles & Huberman, 2003). This consisted of a careful reading of the material to identify recurrences that allowed episodes to be grouped together or otherwise distinguished. Following this identification, three reasons for using community food aid organizations were identified.

6.4.5 *Written Analysis: Development of Findings*

Through the analyses that were conducted, continuing comparisons among the narratives, episodes and trajectories led to formulating questions and then interpretations presented here under the term "Findings." A finding is expressed as "a sentence or a series of sentences that take the place of a descriptive or analytical report in relation to the understanding reached by the analyst at a given moment in their work" (Paillé & Mucchielli, 2012, p. 192, author translation). Based on these observations, written analysis took a central role in the analytical process. A written analysis represents a moment when the researcher engages in "deliberate writing and rewriting, without any other technical means, which will serve as a reformulation, explicitation, interpretation, or theorization of the material being studied" (Paillé & Mucchielli, 2012, p. 184, author translation).

Table 6.1 Summary of the findings and concepts used (Adam, 2019)

Findings	Concepts used
Finding 1: The individuals perform similar actions, but the way in which they express their agency differs.	Agency
Finding 2: Resources and capacities are used in the ways people carry out their actions, and access to these resources and capacities varies between individuals.	Resources/ capacities
Finding 3: Certain participants seem to be dealing with more threatening contexts than others.	Threats
Finding 4: The possibilities of improving one's situation or experiencing Well-being vary among individuals.	Opportunities
Finding 5: The notion of opportunity must be taken into account to understand situations of vulnerability.	Vulnerability

The first finding was concerned with reasons for using the services of a community food aid organization, which led to the second finding, which in turn led to the third finding and so on. Each finding included the previous one. Thus, the last finding contained references to the previous ones, whereas the first finding contained no reference to the others. Therefore, the findings were developed in a logical order, and that order was used to present the study results. To facilitate a summarized reading, concepts (agency, resources, capacities, threats, vulnerability and opportunities) were associated with each finding. For each concept, an initial definition was developed. Each definition was then tested against the richest and most exemplary episodes for refinement (Miles & Huberman, 2003). Next, these definitions were contrasted with the episodes with counterexamples (or negative cases) (Miles & Huberman, 2003). At the end of this phase, five stabilized findings were produced and recorded in the form of long analytical memos (Table 6.1).

6.4.6 Conceptual Design

The last phase involved connecting the findings and summarized concepts developed in the previous phases, which then led to the development of a theory (Paillé & Mucchielli, 2012) we called "acting-in-context". This stage began with the production of a visual aid to diagram the concepts developed and the action dynamics identified. Based on the findings, the diagram combined the five concepts: agency, resources, capacities, threats and opportunities (Fig. 6.2). It was validated by reviewing the stories to ensure that the diagram accounted for all the interactions, variations, similarities and differences contained in the episodes.

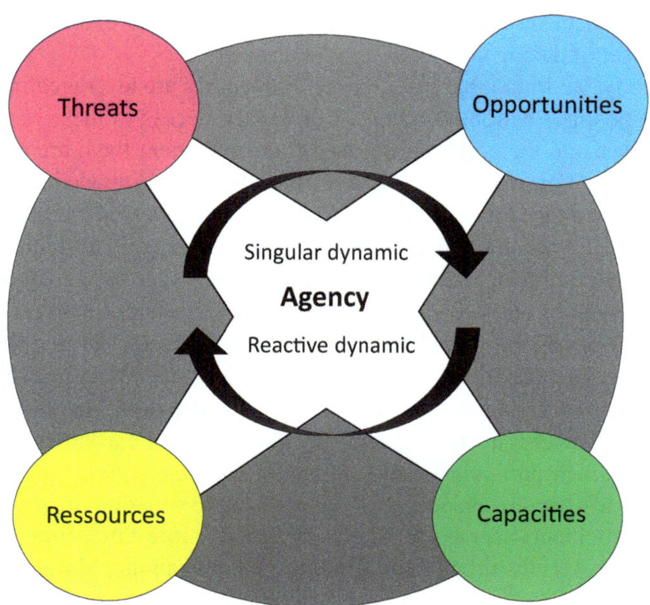

Fig. 6.2 Concept of acting-in-context (Adam, 2019)

6.5 Development of the Theoretical Model of Acting-in-Context

The iterative process of analyzing the narratives of those who took part in the study, which were reconstructed in episodes and studied in the form of trajectories, made it possible to draw up findings through which concepts were developed (see Table 6.1). This allowed us to develop an explanation for the interaction between the individuals' actions and their contexts, then add elements of understanding to the concept of vulnerability.

First, by analyzing the motives for using the services of a community food aid organization, we observed that the individuals performed similar actions but that the ways in which they expressed their agency differed (finding 1). The fact that individuals went to a community food aid organization is evidence of their agency, which is the object of interest in this study. However, not all participants had the same motivations. For some participants, going to a food cooperative is a way of demonstrating their sense of solidarity and their commitment to responsible consumption. For others, using the services of a community food aid organization was necessary to avoid going hungry. To elucidate this difference, we have proposed two dynamics of the implementation of agency: singular and reactive. The singular dynamic refers to individuals' predisposition to perform actions according to their desires, wishes, aspirations, values and principles. The reactive dynamic refers to individuals' predisposition to perform actions according to external elements to which they react or decide not to act.

Subsequently, we found that resources and capacities are leveraged in the implementation of people's actions (finding 2). However, access to these resources and capacities varies, and the opportunities to use or implement them are not the same for all individuals. For example, Madeleine[1] has resources (knowledge and skills in accounting and sewing) that enabled her to hold down a productive job in the past. However, her life was marked by a number of challenges (difficult childhood, divorce, single parenthood, financial problems). These issues seem to have seriously affected her resources and capacities, as she now experiences recurrent depressive episodes. She still has the knowledge and skills (resources), but her physical and mental issues prevent her from meeting the demands of the labour market, which in turn deprives her of financial resources. Thus, to understand how people express their agency, it is necessary to consider the resources and capacities they have at their disposal in their particular context of action implementation.

An analysis of specific episodes that occurred in the situation of poverty showed that certain participants seemed to have experienced more threatening contexts in which multiple events disturbed them (finding 3). For example, Marius, who was in a situation of homelessness for 25 years, recounts many events he has faced: the death of his friends, conflicts, physical violence, serious accidents, etc. To cope with these events, individuals attempt to use their resources and capacities. The notion of threat is therefore introduced. A threat is the potential for a disruptive event for which individuals will need to use their resources and capacities, either to avoid it or to deal with the consequences when the threat becomes a reality. For instance, for some participants, the threat of being hungry, even if it does not come to pass, leads them to take many actions: borrowing money, seeking food aid, moving, etc. The notion of threat allowed us to better identify the use of resources and capacities and to characterize precarious trajectories. However, an element was missing to properly qualify the contrast between episodes in the precarious trajectories and the more stable situations.

We then introduced the notion of opportunity. Data indicated that the possibilities of improving one's situation or quality of life also varied among the participants (finding 4). This finding led us to the notion of opportunity. An opportunity is a chance to improve one's condition or to experience well-being; when they are realized, opportunities are transformed into resources or capacities. For example, the opportunity to have a well-paid job or a decent home. Or the opportunity to travel, have fun or do a pleasant activity. Although an opportunity may exist, it does not mean that it is accessible; certain resources or capacities are necessary to access certain opportunities (e.g. a post-secondary diploma to get a job or money to travel). Therefore, resources and capacities need to be considered to understand how accessible an opportunity may be for an individual.

---

[1] All names and other personal identifiers in this chapter have been changed to protect privacy and confidentiality.

Table 6.2 The elements of acting-in-context (Adam, 2019)

Agency	The ability of humans to take action, to make choices based on what they value or the circumstances in which they find themselves.	
	Singular dynamics of agency	**Reactive dynamics of agency**
	The ability to have desires, wishes, aspirations, values and principles and to take action in accordance with them.	The ability to act and react to external elements, to make decisions and to take action (or decide not to take action).
Resources	Means that can be used to meet individuals' needs.	
Capacities	Personal and social characteristics of individuals that enable them to use or leverage resources that are available to them.	
Threats	The potential for an event to result in negative consequences for which individuals will need to use their resources and capacities to either prevent the event or deal with the consequences of it when it occurs.	
Opportunities	Favourable opportunities to improve one's situation or experience Well-being. When opportunities are realized, they become resources or capacities.	

This analysis of the interaction between opportunities, threats, resources, capacities and agency enabled us to draw an empirical outline of the notion of vulnerability used in this study. Vulnerability is understood as a situation characterized by a high probability that an individual will be exposed to a threat with little or no access to the necessary resources to cope with it without suffering any adverse consequences (Chambers, 1989). However, the interrelation of these elements and this definition of vulnerability did not allow us to explain all the episodes or to explain the differences observed between the different trajectories. The notion of opportunity allowed us to understand that vulnerability is not only the probability of being exposed to threats without having the resources and ability to deal with them but also with having access to few opportunities for improving one's living conditions (finding 5).

Thus, to enable us to characterize the composition of the immediate contexts in which individuals' actions unfold and to understand the active roles of individuals in interacting with their contexts, we propose the concept of acting-in-context (see Fig. 6.2 and Table 6.2).

6.5.1 An Example: Acting in a Context of Vulnerability

On the basis of all the elements identified above, we looked at the participants' trajectories to see if there were any particular configurations for individuals who found themselves in a trajectory of poverty. Drawing on the contrasts between the trajectories, a type of acting-in-context was identified to describe the action dynamics that were observed: constrained acting-in-context (Fig. 6.3).

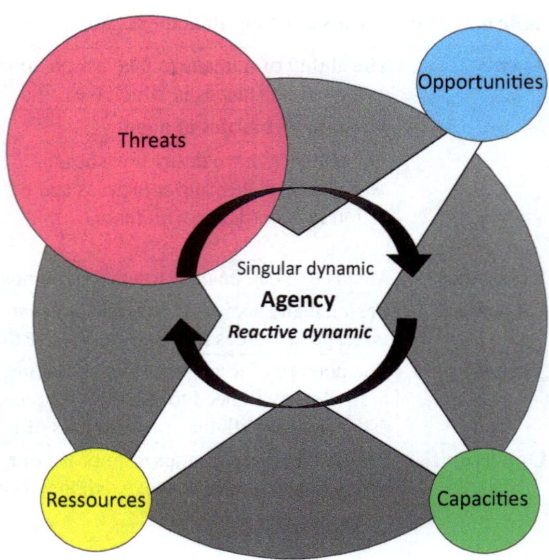

Fig. 6.3 Constrained acting-in-context (Adam, 2019)

6.5.1.1 Constrained Acting-in-Context

This type of acting-in-context is characterized by a high incidence of threats and a low incidence of opportunities, accompanied by weak resources and capacities, particularly as consequences of present and past threats. Action is mainly oriented towards threats to be managed; it is essentially reactive to the context, engaged in managing threats and their consequences. There is very little room for individuals to exercise the singular dynamics of their agency when their capacities and resources are primarily directed towards managing threats, avoiding disruptive events (i.e. the actualization of threats) or dealing with them. Desires, wishes, aspirations, values and principles have little space in the actions of individuals struggling to access opportunities. The trajectory of one study participant, Madeleine, illustrates this type of acting-in-context. Madeleine is a divorced woman in her fifties. She has three children. She had her first child at the age of 16 and experienced a separation (a disruptive event) when she had two dependent children and limited opportunities to access the labour market as she had not completed her secondary education (resources/capacities). Faced with the threat of hunger, she needed to react, take several steps to protect herself from possible financial problems and provide for her family (delaying paying her rent, seeking resources, etc.). Her capacities and resources revolved around responding to this context over a long period of time. In her trajectory, there was little room to seize opportunities to improve her living conditions or even opportunities for entertainment that could have allowed her to experience well-being. Now that her children are grown, Madeleine suffers from chronic depression, which limits her access to the labour market and keeps her in a constrained acting-in-context.

Table 6.3 Using the concept of acting-in-context

Three uses of the acting-in-context concept
At the individual level: In an individual intervention, acting-in-context can be an analytical framework for putting the actor in context (Le Bossé et al., 2009): What threats, opportunities, resources and capacities (or lack thereof) is the individual facing? What are the consequences of current or previous threats? Does the person use their agency according to the singular dynamics or is it essentially used to react to contextual aspects? What kind of intervention could reduce the threats the person is facing? These are some examples of questions that acting in context can generate to support caregivers in developing a dynamic understanding of individuals' situations and to identify the means that could be most helpful while also considering elements of acting-in-context and their interactions.
At the group or community level: Acting-in-context can be used to identify elements common to a group or community that interact with the actions of individuals within that community. An analysis of the threats common to certain so-called vulnerable populations could be a relevant avenue for developing interventions that go beyond identification of risk factors and have a dynamic understanding of the interactions between individuals and their contexts.
In research and evaluation: Acting-in-context can be used as a theoretical framework to develop research projects in terms of the context or situation rather than the behaviour or disease. Alternatively, it can support the integration of contextual elements surrounding the behaviour or disease being studied to understand the configuration and dynamics of action. Acting-in-context can also be a relevant tool to support programme development and evaluation. How do the programme's components fit into the configuration of the contextual elements of individuals participating in it? Does the programme provide access to resources? Does it reduce threats? Does it provide access to opportunities? These questions allow for broader analysis of a programme's action and enable the programme to be designed as an aspect of the individuals' contexts that has the potential to change the configuration of the contexts and the action dynamics.

This study observed that individuals in constrained acting-in-contexts spend a great deal of time and energy dealing with threats and their consequences. Time spent dealing with these threats is not spent seizing opportunities, leveraging resources and developing capacities to seize opportunities; the detrimental feedback loop continues, potentially becoming a powerful downward spiral (Table 6.3).

6.6 How This Study Contributes to Health Promotion

Several theories have provided ways to think about the mechanisms by which poverty gets under someone's skin (Link & Phelan, 2006; Marmot, 2003; Wilkinson, 2005) and influences lifestyles (Cockerham, 2005; Frolich et al., 2003). However, the ways in which poverty influences people's actions in everyday life, beyond health-related behaviours, have been underexplored. The social determinants of the health perspective lead us to acknowledge that individuals are not completely determined by factors external to themselves, but nor are they omnipotent in the face of the circumstances in which they live. Hence, there is a need for theoretical tools to understand the interactions between individuals and their contexts, particularly contexts that are unfavourable to health. To develop this type of tool, a methodological approach is central to study this type of interaction. Thus, this study's contribution is twofold: methodological and theoretical.

In terms of method, this chapter suggests that before choosing a research objective, it is important to engage in ethical reflection that goes beyond the study of health behaviour. Situations can be chosen that are manifestations of difficulties generated by contexts of poverty in which individuals take action. In this study, food insecurity was the chosen context. Situations relating to access to housing, education or certain health services could also be relevant to considering the actions of individuals in contexts of poverty. The methodological challenge was to be able to capture individual–context interactions. The choice of life stories proved to be a suitable method for this challenge. The ethnosociological approach inherent in life stories as conceived by Bertaux (2016) allowed the analysis to highlight the singularity of individuals and their ability to implement actions while considering elements of context that constrain but do not fully determine the individuals' actions.

At the theoretical level, acting-in-context offers a way of understanding how action unfolds beyond health behaviours. Our interpretations suggest that the limits of access induced by an unfavourable social position modify the configuration of contextual elements, thus creating situations of vulnerability. The latter are not only characterized by a higher possibility of exposure to threats without having the resources or capacities to cope with them but also by a limitation of the possibilities to seize opportunities for improving one's living conditions or to live according to one's desires, wishes, aspirations, values and principles. In this context, people's actions are geared towards managing threats and their consequences, allowing little space for people to act on their desires, wishes, aspirations, values and principles. The results suggest that focusing on behavioural change (capacity) without addressing the threats that drive individual action may not be effective. Thus, this study provides a theoretical tool for health promotion based on empirical research that overcomes the limitations associated with individualistic models and takes into account the constraining forces of structures while also acknowledging that individuals are not passive and take action in these contexts.

References

Adam, C. (2019). *L'agir-en-contexte: comprendre l'action des individus en situation de vulnérabilité*. Université de Montréal.

Bertaux, D. (2016). *Le Récit de vie* (3rd ed.). Colin.

Breslow, L. (1999). From disease prevention to health promotion. *Journal of American Medical Association, 281*(11), 1030–1033.

Canadian Lung Association. (2005). *Chronic obstructive pulmonary disease (COPD): A national report card*. Canadian Lung Association.

Carey, G., Malbon, E., Crammond, B., Pescud, M., & Baker, P. (2017). Can the sociology of social problems help us to understand and manage 'lifestyle drift'? *Health Promotion International, 32*(4), 755–761. https://doi.org/10.1093/heapro/dav116

Chambers, R. (1989). Vulnerability, coping and policy. *IDS Bulletin, 20*(2), 1–7.

Cockerham, W. C. (2005). Health lifestyle theory and the convergence of agency and structure. *Journal of Health and Social Behavior, 46*(1), 51–67.
CSDH. (2008). *Closing the gap in a generation: Health equity through action on the social determinant of health.* Final Report of the commission on the social determinant of health. Suisse.
Earnshaw, V. A., & Quinn, D. M. (2012). The impact of stigma in healthcare on people living with chronic illnesses. *Journal of Health Psychology., 17*(2), 157–168. https://doi.org/10.1177/1359105311414952
Frohlich, F. L., Corin, E., & Potvin, L. (2003). A theoretical proposal for the relationship between context and disease. *Sociology of Health and Illness, 23*(6), 776–797.
Giddens, A. (1987). *La constitution de la société.* Presses Universitaires de France.
Kickbusch, I. (2003). The contribution of the World Health Organization to a new public health and health promotion. *American Journal of Public Health, 93*(3), 383–388.
Laperrière, A. (2004). L'observation directe. Dans B. Gauthier (dir.), *Recherche sociale : De la problématique à la collecte de données* (p. 619). : Presse de l'Université du Québec.
Le Bossé, Y., Bilodeau, A., Chamberland, M., & Martineau, S. (2009). Développer le pouvoir d'agir des personnes et des collectivités : quelques enjeux relatifs à l'identité professionnelle et à la formation des oraticiens du social. *Nouvelles pratiques sociales, 21*(2), 175–190.
Link, B. G., & Phelan, J. C. (1995). Social conditions as fundamental causes of disease. *Journal of Health and Social Behavior*, 80–94.
Link, B. G., & Phelan, J. C. (2006). *Stigma and its public health implications* (Vol. 367). The Lancet.
Madison, A. M. (2000). Language in defining social problems and in evaluating social programs. *New Directions for Evaluation, 2000*(86), 17–28.
Mair, M. (2011). Deconstructing behavioural classifications: Tobacco control, 'professional vision' and the tobacco user as a site of governmental intervention. *Critical Public Health, 21*(2), 129–140. https://doi.org/10.1080/09581596.2010.529423
Marmot, M. G. (2003). Understanding social inequalities in health. *Perspectives in Biology and Medicine, 46*, 9–23.
Marmot, M., & Wilkinson, R. (2005). *Social determinants of health.* Oxford University Press.
Miles, M. B., & Huberman, M. A. (2003). *Analyse des données qualitatives* (2nd ed.). De Boeck.
Nutbeam, D. (1998). Health promotion glossary. *Health Promotion International, 13*(4), 349–364. https://doi.org/10.1093/heapro/13.4.349
O'Neill, M., et Stirling, A. (2006). Travailler à promouvoir la santé ou travailler en promotion de la santé? Dans M. O'Neill, A. Pederson, S. Dupéré, et I. Rootman (dir.), *Promotion de la santé au Canada et au Québec, perspectives crititques* (p. 510). : Presses de l'Université Laval.
O'Neill, M., Pederson, A., Dupéré, S., et Rootman, I. (2006). La promotion de la santé au Canada et à l'étranger: Bilan et perspectives. Dans M. O'Neill, A. Pederson, S. Dupéré, et I. Rootman (dir.), *Promotion de la santé au Canada et au Québec, perspectives crititques* (p. 510). : Presses de l'Université Laval.
OMS. (1986). *Charte d'Ottawa pour la promotion de la santé.* Genève.
OMS. (2009). *Combler le fossé en une génération : Instaurer l'équité en santé en agissant sur les déterminants sociaux de la santé.* Rapport final de la Commission des Déterminants Sociaux de la Santé. Genève, Suisse.
Paillé, P. (1996). De l'analyse qualitative en général et de l'analyse thématique en particulier. *Recherches Qualitatives, 15*, 79–194.
Paillé, P., & Mucchielli, A. (2012). *L'analyse qualitative en sciences humaines et sociales* (3rd ed.). Armand Colin.
Pederson, A. P., O'Neill, M., & Rootman, I. (1994). *Health promotion in Canada: Provincial, national and international perspectives.* W. B. Saunders Company.
Phelan, J. C., & Link, B. G. (2005). Controlling disease and creating disparities: A fundamental cause perspective. *The Journals of Gerontology, 60*(2), 27–33. https://doi.org/10.1093/geronb/60.Special_Issue_2.S27
Phelan, J. C., & Link, B. G. (2015). Is racism a fundamental cause of inequalities in health? *Annual Review of Sociology, 41*(1), 311–330. https://doi.org/10.1146/annurev-soc-073014-112305

Phelan, J. C., Link, B. G., & Tehranifar, P. (2010). Social conditions as fundamental causes of health inequalities: Theory, evidence, and policy implications. *Journal of Health and Social Behavior, 51*, S28–S40.

Popay, J., Whitehead, M., Hunter, D., & J. (2010). Injustice is killing people on a large scale – But what is to be done about it? *Journal of Public Health, 32*(2), 148–149.

Potvin, L., Gendron, S., Bilodeau, A., & Chabot, P. (2005). Integrating social theory into public health practice. *American Journal of Public Health, 95*(4), 591–595.

Powell, K., Thurston, M., & Bloyce, D. (2017). Theorising lifestyle drift in health promotion:Explaining community and voluntary sector engagement practices in disadvantaged areas. *Critical Public Health*, 1–12. ISSN 0958-1596.

Raphael, D. (2002). Adressing health inequlities in Canada. *Leadership in Health Services, 15*(3), 1–8.

Schrecker, T. (2013). Beyond 'run, knit and relax': can health promotion in Canada advance the social determinants of health agenda? *Healthc Policy, 9*(Spec Issue), 48–58. PMID: 24289939; PMCID: PMC4750152.

Watt, R. G. (2007). From victim blaming to upstream action: Tackling the social determinants of oral health inequalities. *Community Dentistry and Oral Epidemiology, 35*(1), 1–11.

Wilkinson, R. G. (2005). *The impact of inequality*. New Press.

Chapter 7
Participatory Health Promotion Research with Children

Colin MacDougall and Lisa Gibbs

7.1 Introduction to Children and Health Promotion Practices

Towards the end of the twentieth century, research emerging from developed countries showed declining children's physical activity and increasing obesity. Although it was well known that physical activity in the adult population was on a steady decline, similar trends in children were alarming – even confronting – to health authorities, education departments, governments and parents (MacDougall et al., 2004). Mainstream health promotion practitioners and researchers, often less experienced in working with children and young people, turned their attention to getting children to become more active. As public health researchers, we shared concerns about the dilemma of increasing children's activity and mobility in the face of concerns about risk and safety. Frequently, health promotion adopts adult-driven research paradigms while dealing with children, which also reflects the dominance of behavioural and lifestyle approaches in health promotion (MacDougall, 2007).

At first, in separate research programmes, we favoured the structural understandings of health promotion, informed by primary health care (MacDougall, 2009) and the 1986 Ottawa Charter for Health Promotion (World Health Organization, 1986), which agreed on the primacy of participation, empowering practice and research.

C. MacDougall (✉)
College of Medicine and Public Health, Flinders University, Adelaide, Australia

Child & Community Wellbeing Unit, Centre for Health Equity, The Melbourne School of Population and Global Health, University of Melbourne, Melbourne, Australia
e-mail: colin.macdougall@flinders.edu.au

L. Gibbs
Child & Community Wellbeing Unit, Centre for Health Equity, The Melbourne School of Population and Global Health, University of Melbourne, Melbourne, Australia

L. Potvin, D. Jourdan (eds.), *Global Handbook of Health Promotion Research, Vol. 1*,
https://doi.org/10.1007/978-3-030-97212-7_7

CM well remembers research meetings, reminiscing about "when I was a child" sprinkled with whimsical tales of a magical, free-range childhood full of adventures, high jinks and roaming the countryside and suburbia alike. The innocence of the nostalgia narrative was soon tempered by imperatives to educate parents to protect their children from the new risks of strangers, motor vehicles, television and junk food (MacDougall, 2009). After CM and LG started working on a common research programme, our reflections on the children and health promotion research led us to prepare a conference poster entitled "Six steps to ensure the failure of health promotion in the early years". Borrowing from sustainability science, we adapted an inverse approach, which "…starts by describing the ecological and health outcomes that we do not want and works backwards to identify courses of action that have the best chance of avoiding these undesirable outcomes. We can also work backwards to identify the courses of action that are more likely to result in the outcomes we don't want" (Lowe, 2011, p. 179).

The inverse logic inspired us to propose six steps to failure of health promotion with children (MacDougall et al., 2012a):

1. Focus on the responsibilities of individuals to change the powerfully and socially determined conditions of daily life.
2. Configure health promotion as adult-led short-term social marketing to parents and children, changing campaigns frequently as government departments reorganize and develop new branding.
3. Assume children are developmentally unable to participate in the research and practice about their health.
4. Justify health promotion to children in terms of their health as future adults and costs to governments if they are not active.
5. Keep the evaluation simple and tick the box.
6. Fix the gaze within the country, ignoring global perspectives.

Articulating these six steps clarified what we did not want to do and sharpened our resolve to explore alternative epistemologies referencing the United Nations Declaration on the Rights of the Child. Epistemological and methodological clarity emerged primarily from the European *sociology of childhood*, arguing that children are neither passive nor incompetent, as a result of their stage of development, rather they can and should participate productively as research participants, even to the extent of co-designing and interpreting research studies (MacDougall & Darbyshire, 2018).

In this chapter, after setting our position in health promotion research paradigms, we reflect on close to two decades of researching and theorizing about children's participation in health promotion research. We elaborate upon the underpinning values derived from critical theory, empowerment, children's rights and the primary health care participation agenda. Finally, we discuss the challenges and future prospects of health promotion with children, upending the inverse logic to increase the chances of successful participatory health promotion with children.

7.2 Research Paradigms and Theories

Modern psychology combines biological, cognitive and behavioural studies to propose developmental stages for children to navigate en route to adulthood. This developmental child theory underpins research to match policies, programmes and interventions to the most appropriate developmental stage and can be invoked to limit children's participation in research if they are seen as developmentally capable. A parallel framing, since the Industrial Revolution, identifies and reduces the risks to children, too often from adult institutions. The child at risk framing positions children as vulnerable and has made major contributions in child labour and slavery, physical abuse, sexual abuse and injury prevention. Adults fulfilling their roles as protectors can prevent children from participating in research by claiming that they are safeguarding them (MacDougall, 2009).

By contrast, a **citizen-child theory**, defined next, takes a child-centred approach and argues for the rights of children to exercise agency in their own lives (MacDougall, 2009). This theory combines a more reactive story, rejecting adultist and developmentally derived assumptions, with an aspirational story, which blends a children's rights approach with the participation and empowerment agenda (MacDougall & Darbyshire, 2018). The more reactive story rejects research and health promotion, framing children as human becomings rather than human beings, and the aspirational story builds on the new sociology of childhood and the UN Convention on the Rights of the Child (MacDougall & Darbyshire, 2018; United Nations, 1989).

The citizen-child-inspired researcher problematizes and reduces the power relationships between adults and children, understanding that there are different types of citizenships (Gibbs et al., 2013). Personally responsible citizens obey the law, pay their taxes and are kind to others. Participatory citizens join organizations, vote in elections and volunteer to help others. Socially critical citizens will investigate inequity and strive for justice. The citizen-child approach embraces discourses on rights, critiques framing children as passive and compliant citizens, encourages structures for children to become participatory citizens and – through active participation in research – invites children to consider their role in the world as advocates for social justice (MacDougall & Darbyshire, 2018; Gibbs et al., 2013; Westheimer & Kahne, 2004).

7.3 Informing Health Promotion Through Participatory Research with Children

In this section, we analyze four linked sets of studies involving the participation of children in research designed for health promotion policy and practice. The first two projects, involving CM, took place in metropolitan and rural South Australia and experimented with child-centred methodologies to understand children's perspectives on adult concerns about physical activity and health promotion. Broadly, we were interested in exploring children's perspectives about how the places, spaces and communities in which they live influence their experiences of, and engagement in, play and physical activity.

The third study occurred in Melbourne, the capital of the Australian state of Victoria where CM and LG sought to add to the evidence by including children's perspectives on how they actively participate in negotiating and developing their everyday mobility.

Again with CM and LG, the fourth international observational study of schools and their surroundings applied ethnographic methods to uncover the policies and practices in different countries that created built environments around schools, which in turn shaped the attitudes and behaviours of children and the fears of their parents. Then, we comment on the changes in health promotion research as a result of the 2020 COVID-19 pandemic.

7.4 Uncovering Children's Responses to Adult Concepts of Physical Activity Promotion for Children

One approach to the promotion of children's physical activity is for adults to take charge and direct the research on children using language and concepts with which they are comfortable. The title of the paper, *We have to live in the future*, brings a contrasting voice from a child in a focus group from a class of 9–10 year olds in Adelaide, the capital of South Australia, who wanted the children's voices to be heard. This study of 204 children aged 4–12 years, asked the following questions:

1. What are children's theories of physical activity, play and sport?
2. What do children want to tell adults?

The child was making a plea to the South Australian Department of Human Services to listen to the voices of the future generations in their commissioned research to inform a physical activity strategy for primary school-age children. The department bravely broke with the tradition of adapting strategies for adults to children and conducting adult-focused research. Instead, they commissioned us to undertake a qualitative study combining focus groups, drawing and mapping techniques and photographic methods with 204 children aged 4–12 years in metropolitan and rural South Australia. The methods of data collection, namely, focus group interviews, drawing/mapping and photovoice, which were used to provide a rich, multifaceted perspective of children's experiences, are described in detail elsewhere (MacDougall & Darbyshire, 2018).

Focus groups provide powerful ways to observe how children construct and reconstruct ideas. We have found that focus groups can move beyond the verbal to include children showing researchers what they mean, such as demonstrating a local variety of a popular game. With older children, gender can get in the way; so, depending on the question, single-sex groups could be considered. As power is inscribed in place and space researchers must do their homework and insist on using spaces in which children have had positive experiences, avoiding those in which children have experienced negative events or the demonstration of power over behaviour by adults is important. It is vital to set a culture of children being the experts of their lives so that children tell adults about their experiences. In turn, adult researchers demonstrate respect and deep listening.

Drawing and mapping provides valuable data about where children are located, how they move around and which people are important in their lives. It is not an art competition! We often provided a pencil, paper and an eraser to focus on the content – not on the art technique. In the days of film, we gave children disposable cameras and asked them to photograph aspects of physical activity that were important to them; but this is easily translated to a digital world. Crucially, for drawing, mapping and photovoice, the images are not the data. If they were, we would produce adultist interpretations of children's lives. Instead, the captions, commentaries and photographs stimulate joint discussions with children, enabling them to articulate and advocate accounts of their lives.

Children participated enthusiastically and appreciated the opportunity to communicate their views. "Physical activity" and "exercise" had little meaning for children, who described them as terms that adults use. "Play" and "sport" had powerful, contrasting meanings for children, with "play" being child-centred and "sport" being controlled by adults. Children did not respond to adult-led links between physical activity and health status.

Children's participation gives rise to critical distinctions between sport and play. Our results show that play is much more child-focused than sport, involving spontaneous decisions and rules made for and by children. Moreover, results suggest that mixing images of play and sport could be counterproductive.

Health promotion strategies will benefit from understanding how children ascribe meanings to words that adult professionals commonly use in physical activity promotion. These words matter. It is counterproductive to plan a health promotion campaign revolving around concepts and words that do not engage children. It is also fraught with danger to mix concepts such as play and sport. For example,

- Children immediately engaged with the word sport, meaning purpose, competition, organisation, and often (but not always) fun. They told us about the crucial role of adults to organise, fund participation, arrange travel and provide equipment. Sport was adult-led, pre-planned, rule-bound involving hierarchical decisions with power-over;
- Children said barriers to sport included cost, distance, travel, lack of facilities, and expense of clubs, injuries, bullying, put-downs, humiliation, gender issues;
- The word play also engaged children in focus groups where they frequently demonstrated types of play that involved fun, freedom, spontaneity, energy and physicality. While adults did not organise play, their encouragement was important. Children managed the rules to ensure high levels of inclusion and improvised with available equipment;
- Play was helped by adults fostering a culture of democratic decision-making;
- Barriers included time, space, lack of equipment, arguments and engagement reduced with age.

Unlike "sport" and "play" the words physical activity, exercise and fitness did not engage children who had trouble differentiating them from either sport or play. They said physical activity was an adult word; exercise suggested work, purpose, lack of fun (MacDougall et al., 2004).

Such child-centred research is relatively simple and should underpin expensive campaigns and policies.

The marketing company commissioned by the relevant government departments to develop a campaign used data from Table 7.1 to create television and cinema adverts focusing on children's accounts of the meaning of play. The overall campaign also included information about places for children to play. In these ways, health promotion was directly informed by children's theorizing. This illustrates the benefits of modifying tried-and-true qualitative methods to answer the simple question of understanding how children interpreted common adult health promotion language.

How is children's play influenced by geographical and parental boundary settings?.

In an Australian Research Council grant, CM and colleagues followed up the finding that children did all they could to ensure that play was child-centred,

Table 7.1 Distinctive research contributions to successful health promotion with children

Steps for successful health promotion with children	Example from studies in this chapter
Understand, map and act on the responsibilities of adults as duty bearers to change the powerfully and socially determined conditions of children's daily lives.	Children participate enthusiastically in research and state they want their voices heard. COVID-19 has illuminated the direct and indirect influences of inequity on children – Again highlighting the decisions by adults and their institutions.
Refine and design participatory and rights-based methods to encourage children's participation in the research and practice of their health, tailored to context and developmental stage.	Children's critical distinctions between the salient concepts of play and sport and less relevant adult words such as physical activity and exercise have powerful implications in research and policy. Play and sport change character as children develop, including interactions with gender.
Include the insights of children about health promotion, requiring long-term changes to natural and built environments and paradigms underlying health promotion research and practice.	The natural and built environments shape play, sport, mobility and daily physical activity. Children can contribute to diagnosing problems and suggesting solutions. Adults and adult institutions take the final decisions.
Recognize the simultaneous imperatives of improving the here and now of children's physical activity goals and contributing to their future participation as critical citizens.	Health problems from COVID-19-related decreases in activity highlight immediate and long-term consequences. The pre-existing rights-based paradigms reinforced by COVID-19 inspired concerns about the loss of rights and independence in their futures that could curtail development as citizens.
Become comfortable with nuanced evaluation and analytical frameworks.	Findings are strongly influenced by context and cannot be reduced to binary distinctions. For example, independent mobility frequently changes character and goes beyond the active–passive and independent–dependent travel.
Conduct cross-country research and reflections on practice to appreciate the importance of context and learnings from outsider perspectives.	Uncover hidden assumptions of insider researchers and learn from global policies. Great differences between city and country. Urban form varies within and between cities.

spontaneous and continually adjusted to avoid boredom, with increased access to give all children the chance to have fun (MacDougall et al., 2004). What are our boundaries, and where can we play? – This question sought children's perspectives about places, spaces and communities in which they live, which impact their experiences of, and engagement in, play and physical activity. In this study, we elicited children's perspectives on where they live and their boundaries and rules about moving through their communities (MacDougall et al., 2009).

We worked with children in an inner metropolitan school in Adelaide, the capital of South Australia, and in a rural school on Kangaroo Island off the South Australian coast known for farming and tourism. We spoke to 33 children, 8–10 year olds to find out:

1. What is the area like for you?
2. What are the rules and boundaries and who sets them?

In this project, we started with methods similar to the previous ones while paying more attention to tailoring them to the research questions, thus ensuring children retained formal ownership of their data and examining the benefits and risks of using multiple methods.

We also had to tailor methods to work efficiently in Australian rural locations that require extensive travel time. Time, cost and logistics required us to design two visits for data collection, each lasting a few days. Our focus group questions were more expansive than the previous study because they had to explore geographical and cultural boundaries. We included the drawing and mapping method within the focus group to both use time efficiently and combine verbal and visual data. Then we provided children with cameras to photograph where they played, who they played with and what they played. We returned within a month to hold workshops, where we returned the photos to the children and asked them to select four photographs and arrange them on an A4-sized worksheet page using the following prompts:

> This is my favourite photo because ...
> My favourite place to do activities is ... because ...
> This photo makes me feel ... because ...
> What I like doing best is ... because ...

During this visit, we brought resources so we could take copies of all the photographs and drawings that we needed, while returning the originals to the individual students, as well as making books of all the drawings and photographs for each year level to be used within the school curriculum. Our aim here was to demonstrate to the children that they effectively owned their data, which we were using respectfully as if on licence.

Use of multiple methods can be expensive and take up valuable time in a child's life. As a result, we compared our findings from each method and first concluded that they provided triangulation by confirming key themes from multiple data sources. Critically, each method yielded distinctive data, leaving us to conclude that multiple methods provided richer findings than single methods (Darbyshire et al., 2005).

Rural children negotiated freedom of movement by considering broad principles about safety. Those who lived on farms said that they could go anywhere as long as they could negotiate with their parents about safety in relation to risks and dangers, most of which were related to the natural environment. Rural children demonstrated the power of geographical and social contexts in their list of (relatively few) places they could not go. Children overwhelmingly supported and appreciated parental involvement in setting rules and boundaries.

We interpreted the findings using an ecological framework for physical activity comprising three factors that link human agency to structure and environment: locating in space, moving through space and relating to people in space (MacDougall, 2007). Findings raise questions about the way in which the environment is designed for social planning and the importance of children's engagement and interaction with the natural environment.

7.5 Independent Mobility and the Transition to High School

Stepping Out was funded by VicHealth, established through Victoria's visionary tobacco-control legislation in 1987 as the first health promotion body in the world to be funded by a tax on tobacco and with international recognition for health promotion and policy impact (Richardson, 2017). *Stepping out* involved CM and LG and was designed to contribute to a children's perspective on the problem of significant declines in children's independent mobility. Independent mobility is important for physical health by helping children incorporate active transport into their daily travel routines and from a rights-based perspective for providing children with the opportunities to access public spaces for play, recreation and citizenship (Gibbs et al., 2012; Nansen et al., 2015).

The study used child-centred methods to understand how children transitioning from primary to high school in inner city Melbourne, the capital of Victoria in Australia, negotiated and developed their everyday mobility in the contexts of parental rules, family routines, cultural influences, peer social connections, communication technologies and neighbourhood environments.

The first stage comprised site observations followed by child focus group discussions and then accompanying children on their travel journeys. We piloted the process with eight children in their final year of primary school who acted as research partners to help refine and shape the research design. The first stage is useful to include in grant applications for participatory research with children to help avoid reviewers critiquing the lack of detail about methods that – by their very nature – can only be finalized during data collection. Similarly, institutional ethics committees require details about interview questions and other data collection methods. By providing a sound rationale for a rigorous first stage, reviewers and ethics committees can be assured that the research plan is theoretically sound and can be reviewed as the details of each stage emerge (MacDougall & Darbyshire, 2018). Methods can be extended to multiple stages to enable children to give progressive consent as they get to know the researchers and the project. Multiple stages also open up the possibility for the children to choose or propose data collection methods they find suitable (Gibbs et al., 2013).

We conducted focus group discussions with 48 children in groups of 5–8 in schools with groups of mixed gender and diverse cultural backgrounds. The discussions were centred on two visual photo-ordering exercises (Willenberg et al., 2010) that used images depicting places and objects involved in their neighbourhood travel. Visual aids effectively stimulate children's responses, and we asked children to discuss and work together to order the importance of each image for their travel journeys.

We then used mobile methods that involved travelling with 10 children (6 boys and 4 girls) from the focus groups on an everyday travel journey. Children took the researchers on routine travel journeys, predominantly to and from the school but also to places such as shops and parks, to show how they normally travelled, with questions generated by the environments and interactions that were observed during the journey. Mobile methods position children as experts of their lives by asking them to take the researchers on a tour of a salient area. Researchers and children plan a route, work out how to collect data (e.g. the route itself, interviews, photographs, observations) and balance independence with safety. Theoretically, mobile methods are a form of visual sociology and draw upon the *new mobilities paradigm* stating that places are linked by networks of connections that stretch beyond a single locale, requiring travel for social life and connections.

Our findings suggested that a more critical engagement with the conceptual underpinnings of children's mobility can lead to new understandings. We found that children's everyday mobility is defined by interdependencies rather than a simple dichotomy between dependent and independent or active and passive. Child mobility compositions were assembled through changing relations of companionship – travel companions, companion devices and ambient companions. Children are not passive subjects of rules and environments rather they assembled relational compositions of mobility. They expressed some ambivalence about the benefits and pitfalls of 'independent mobility' and balanced independence with enjoyment of parental accompaniment, sometimes experiencing excitement and freedom alongside nervousness or fear (Nansen et al., 2015).

7.6 Culture and Place Matter

The findings from our first three studies showed the role of the natural and built environments in fostering children's activities. As a result, we designed a method for observing and analyzing the settings in four countries that influence the independent mobility of children to stimulate discussions about culture and context in children's health promotion. Both qualitative research and anthropology/ethnography distinguish between the embedded and contextual knowledge of the insider (emic) and the more detached perspective of the outsider (etic) – and of course – the interplay between the two. This rich interplay can provide outsiders with the opportunity to interrogate insiders and ask them to explain observations when outsiders observe something unusual or perplexing. In the process, insiders articulate assumptions that are taken for granted.

We conducted field observations in towns in Australia, France, Germany and Scotland using one researcher from the home country and one from another country. We observed the settings around schools, taking care not to observe or photograph people. Schools were judged to be in typical areas, and multiple observations were conducted at different times and days. Field notes and photographs were discussed immediately after observations, stimulating insider–outsider discussions of assumptions that were taken for granted, local knowledge and representative policies to consider. There was a meeting of all observers from Australia, France and Scotland to discuss the critical differences and policy and follow-up presentations with the German case, which was conducted by a student from Germany on placement in Adelaide, Australia (MacDougall et al., 2012a, b).

Illustrative findings include the surroundings of a South Australian outer suburban school characterized by a road architecture that enables parents to drop off and collect children from school during two short but congested times of the school day. Colloquially known as the "kiss and drop," this architecture reflects the distances students had to travel to schools, which are consolidating into larger schools, in a government school system which rarely enforces zones for local schools. The outsider in the research pair, from Germany, had no experience of the "kiss and drop" that was so familiar to the Australian insider. Policy observations include the need to retrofit car-based suburbs whose cul-de-sac-based design impedes walking safely. The "kiss and drop" also reflects the move to larger and larger schools driven by an efficiency agenda to compete with the significant numbers of prestigious independent and religious schools, often combining high parent fees with generous government funding.

The German observation revealed an architecture of a different type: a design to support a variety of school-based learning activities. Having observed the Australian school, the German outsider was at pains to point out a replacement of the "kiss and drop" by extensive bicycle parking for students and staff alike. The policies exemplified here prioritize active and ecologically sustainable transport over motor vehicle domination.

The French school was small, with neither a "kiss and drop" nor a bicycle park. Public transport and car parking were nearby. However, the French insider noted that the school was set in a park, linked to nearby private and social housing by a network of walking paths. The French insider pointed to a robust, well-funded government education system including local zones and the relative absence of private or religious schools. Her historical explanation was that, post revolution, France adopted the values of Liberty, Equality and Fraternity and Laïcité, producing a secular school system based on separation of the church and the state with a profound effect on education.

The Scottish school also had neither a "kiss and drop" nor a bicycle park. When the two Australian outsiders remarked curiously on the large bus stop inside the school, the Scottish insider replied that bus transport was dominant because the local government provided free transport to all within the school zone. If a bus was not feasible, children were transported by taxis. This contributed to reductions in car travel, traffic congestion and the use of fossil fuel and established independent mobility as the default.

The second Australian school, in inner city Melbourne, had more in common with the German and French schools than its Adelaide counterpart. Inner city Melbourne resisted the trends in other capital cities to make room for cars, producing multiple opportunities for composite journeys involving walking, trams and various combinations of parental supervision. Policy learnings included a specific primary-to-high-school transition including attention to children's independent mobility.

These examples illustrate the contribution of environmental observations of places – not people – as inexpensive and ethically defensible adjuncts to qualitative research. The dialectic between insider and outsider perspectives opens discussions about how culture and policy shape children's mobilities in relation to school (MacDougall et al., 2012a, b), which are typically not reported or discussed in the academic literature reporting on school-based studies. Clearly, there are environmental and contextual differences within, as well as between, countries.

7.7 Commentary on COVID-19

Early concerns about the novel coronavirus SARS-CoV-2 in Wuhan, China, in December 2019 (WHO, 2020) turned to alarm as, by March 2020, the virus had spread to all global regions. COVID-19 (the disease caused by SARS-CoV-2) was threatening to overwhelm the world's economies and strongest health systems (Editorial, 2020; Remuzzi & Remuzzi, 2020). Without an effective treatment or vaccine, public health measures including physical distancing measures became the cornerstones of global response. The scale and impact of lockdowns and physical distancing was not anticipated in epidemic planning, especially the effects on children of the widespread closures of schools, day-care centres and playgrounds and directives to stay at home. By late 2020, evidence was beginning to emerge about reductions in physical activity, increases in screen time and changed sleep patterns.

Much of the research was conceived and conducted by adults on children. For example, in relation to a broad range of physical activities, research showed how children suffer with limited social connections, which are crucial for identity and well-being, reduced physical activity, loneliness and boredom (Fegert et al., 2020; Jiao et al., 2020; Loades et al., 2020), and which may have long-term effects; children not in school do not have break-time activities or physical education classes, are not walking to school or to a bus stop and generally cannot participate in school sporting teams or clubs (Esmonde & Pollack Porter, 2020).

On the other hand, there were media stories about children taking some degree of control. The Dutch Prime Minister answered video questions by kids in the kids news (https://www.youtube.com/watch?v=wLRc6Otqs-E). Children in South Australia contributed to a guide for parents about home activities (https://dulwichcentre.com.au/creating-a-guide-for-parents-during-lock-down-by-children/) Young Indians created care packs during the pandemic (https://citizenmatters.in/wp-content/uploads/sites/2/2020/03/HELP-INDIA-PDF.pdf).

Some studies looked at the relationship between the design of neighbourhoods and children's behaviour. A Canadian study found that some children became more active and were walking/biking and playing more and had increased outdoor physical activity (Carroll et al., 2020). These children often lived in houses in lower-density neighbourhoods and lived further from a major road. Children in higher-density neighbourhoods with parks within 1 km were more likely to increase their outdoor activities. In Portugal, Pombo et al., found that children under 13 years of age with an outdoor space and who had other children in the household were significantly more active (Pombo et al., 2020). Children from families with all adults working from home showed lower levels of physical activity. A similar pattern of activity reduction was reported among high school students in Bosnia and Herzegovina between January 2020 (before COVID-19) and April 2020 (during the physical distancing).

We have discussed the role of independent mobility in children's physical activity. Riazi proposed that the value of children's independent mobility was crucial during the pandemic, offering children access to the outside world (Riazi, 2020). With many parents working from home, children's outdoor time depended on parents having time to join in physical activity outdoors after work or between meetings. Inequities in independent mobility were highlighted during the pandemic, exemplified by a lack of access to gardens for many families. Independently mobile children had more chances to be physically active by walking or biking to locations close to home.

Children's right to play, their need for play and independent mobility or the need for changes in urban design were highlighted mostly through opinion pieces in independent journalist platforms.

A rights perspective is evident in opinion articles in *The Conversation*, an Australian social media site reporting research to a broader audience. These emphasized the critical need and right for children to play during confinement and restrictions of the COVID-19 pandemic. McLean made a plea for a focus on play-based learning during confinement, noting the pandemic as a time in history where child rights and responsibilities as human beings come into clear focus (McLean, 2020). Alden noted the lack of acknowledgement by cities and authorities of the impacts of restrictions upon children's right to play as part of healthy development (Alden, 2020). This is of particular concern where families do not have access to high-quality play opportunities or access to public open spaces and green spaces. When playground equipment is also closed, children's play naturally increases in other community spaces, including neighbourhood streets. Reflecting on the existing research about children's need for collaborative play, Alden called for a balancing of the risks of limiting social play beyond households and the benefits of closing streets and empty parking spaces where green space is scarce.

In the reimagination of space following the pandemic, there are arguments for reallocating road space for collaborative play, walking and cycling, opening up green spaces and initiating car-free zones and redefining the usefulness of space for children's play in a post-pandemic era. Garau and Annunziata (2020) used a theory of affordances, similar to our independent mobilities study, to analyze the potential of public spaces to enable and support children's independent activities in Sardinia, Italy. Another study described the likely health inequities experienced by under-resourced communities and families and proposed supporting physical activity in unused school yards and through 'play street' initiatives (Esmonde & Pollack Porter, 2020).

The research reviewed in this section reinforces the importance of taking a children's rights and participation approach to understand how health promotion can conceptualize how physical activity, sport and play are influenced by natural and built environments. Health promotion can play an important role in reversing the rapid loss of environments and the opportunities for children to be active during the early stages of the pandemic. It can also generate debates about ways in which distancing measures reduce children's rights for activity and mobility.

7.8 Conclusions about Child Health Promotion Research

In this chapter, we have shown how qualitative and ethnographic research methods are ideally placed to guide health promotion research with children underpinned by participation and empowerment. Methodological development enabled us to work with children whose voices have until recently been silenced in health promotion research that concerns their lives. Findings from this study led directly to a South Australian health promotion campaign to increase children's participation in play and organized activities. Adding an ethnographic focus illustrates the responsibility of *adult duty bearers* who control policies to adopt a healthy settings approach linking structure and agency, particularly in relation to equity, the built and natural environments and the political and cultural practices that shape the daily conditions of living that determine children's health.

The citizen-child paradigm has the potential to link health promotion with children to a broader discourse of rights and citizenship, thereby bringing to bear broader social and political theories to advance our understandings of health promotion. We see this starkly in the ways in which the existing inequities shaped the experiences and consequences of physical distancing measures at the start of the COVID-19 pandemic.

Writing from Australia, we well know that health policies about children reflect *the individualized approaches to health promotion*, defined as privileging individualized actions about healthcare service delivery and access, with little attention to the social determinants of health (Phillips et al., 2016). The analysis of theories and methods in this chapter is designed to assist researchers to challenge the enduring power of the biomedical paradigm to crowd out rights-based and social models of health promotion.

We started this chapter by proposing six steps to ensure the failure of health promotion with children, theoretically informed by the literature critiquing biomedical and behavioural constraints on health promotion.

We close this chapter by reimagining these six steps and combining empirical data from our review of studies with theory and propose how adopting the inverse of these steps opens possibilities for a structural and participatory approach to health promotion with children.

Table 7.1 shows how research helps health promotion challenge dominant adultist and biomedical health promotion paradigms and benefits from being rights-based rather than pathogenic. Distinctively, health promotion researchers have the tools to involve children as much as possible in research, rejecting assumptions that particular developmental stages invalidate children's capacity to participate.

Acknowledgements CM acknowledges the work on the COVID-19 literature by his partners in the South Australian studies, Professors Philip Darbyshire' and Wendy Schiller and Dr. Tahna Pettman. CM and LG acknowledge the contribution of Dr. Bjorn Nansen from the University of Melbourne to the *Stepping Out* study and our international ethnographic collaborators Dr. Isabelle Danic (France), Professor John McKendrick (Scotland) and Jessica Schneider (Germany). Studies were partially funded by grants from the Australian Research Council, Flinders University, University of Melbourne, South Australian Government, VicHealth and University of Magdeburg-Stendal in Germany.

References

Alden, C. (2020). *Coronavirus spotlights equity and access issues with children's right to play*, in *The Conversation*. The Conversation.

Carroll, N., et al. (2020). The impact of COVID-19 on health behavior, stress, financial and food security among middle to high income Canadian families with young children. *Nutrients, 12*(8), 2352.

Darbyshire, P., MacDougall, C., & Schiller, W. (2005). Multiple methods in qualitative research with children: More insight or just more? *Qualitative Research, 5*(4), 417–436.

Editorial. (2020). COVID-19 in the USA: A question of time. *The Lancet, 395*(10232), 1229.

Esmonde, K., & Pollack Porter, K. (2020). *Distance learning makes it harder for kids to exercise, especially in low-income communities*, in *The Conversation*. 2020, The Conversation.

Fegert, J. M., et al. (2020). Challenges and burden of the coronavirus 2019 (COVID-19) pandemic for child and adolescent mental health: A narrative review to highlight clinical and research needs in the acute phase and the long return to normality. *Child Adolesc Psychiatry Ment Health, 14*(20) https://link.springer.com/article/10.1186/s13034-020-00329-3

Garau, C., & Annunziata, A. (2020). Supporting Children's independent activities in smart and playable public places. *Preprint, 12*(20), 8352.

Gibbs, L., et al. (2012). Stepping out: Children negotiating independent travel. In *Final report to VicHealth, Jack Brockhoff child health and wellbeing program, McCaughey VicHealth Centre for community wellbeing*. University of Melbourne. https://www.vichealth.vic.gov.au/media-and-resources/publications/stepping-out

Gibbs, L., et al. (2013). Research with, by, for, and about children: Lessons from disaster contexts. *Global Studies of Childhood, 3*(2), 129–141.

Jiao, W. Y., et al. (2020). Behavioral and emotional disorders in children during the COVID-19 Epidemic. *Pediatr, 221*, 264–266.

Loades, M. E., et al. (2020). Rapid systematic review: The impact of social isolation and loneliness on the mental health of children and adolescents in the context of COVID-19. *Journal of the American Academy of Child and Adolescent Psychiatry, 59*(11), 1218–1239.

Lowe, I. (2011). Environment, sustainability and health. In H. Keleher & C. MacDougall (Eds.), *Understanding health* (3rd ed., pp. 171–182). Melbourne.

MacDougall, C. (2007). Reframing physical activity. In H. Keleher, C. MacDougall, & B. Murphy (Eds.), *Understanding health promotion* (pp. 326–342). Melbourne.

MacDougall, C. (2009). Understanding twenty-first century childhood. In H. Keleher & C. MacDougall (Eds.), *Understanding health: A determinants approach* (pp. 287–307). Oxford University Press.

MacDougall, C., & Darbyshire, P. (2018). Collecting qualitative data with children. In U. Flick (Ed.), *The SAGE handbook of qualitative data collection* (pp. 617–631). California.

MacDougall, C., Schiller, W., & Darbyshire, P. (2004). We have to live in the future. *Early Child Development and Care, 174*(4), 369–388.

MacDougall, C., Schiller, W., & Darbyshire, P. (2009). What are our boundaries and where can we play? Perspectives from eight to ten year old Australian metropolitan and rural children. *Early Child Development and Care, 179*(2), 189–204.

MacDougall, C., Gibbs, L. and Phillips, C. (2012a). *Six steps to ensure the failure of health promotion in the early years*, in *Poster Presentation.* 1st Biennial Australian implementation conference, ARACY and Parenting Resource Centre: Melbourne.

MacDougall, C., et al., (2012b). *Stepping out: Comparing Children's mobility settings in Australia, France, Germany and Scotland to see how culture matters*, in *conference presentation: Population health congress*: Adelaide.

McLean, C. (2020). *Let the children play: 4 reasons why play is vital during the coronavirus*, in *The Conversation*. The Conversation.

Nansen, B., et al. (2015). Children's interdependent mobility: Compositions, collaborations and compromises. *Children's Geographies, 13*(4), 467–481.

Phillips, C., et al. (2016). To what extent do Australian child and youth health policies address the social determinants of health and health equity?: A document analysis study. *Public Health, 16*(512).

Pombo, A., et al. (2020). Correlates of Children's physical activity during the Covid-19 confinement in Portugal. *Public Health, 189*, 14–19.

Remuzzi, A., & Remuzzi, G. (2020). COVID-19 and Italy: What next? *The Lancet, 395*(10231), 1225–1228.

Riazi, N. (2020). *Free-range kids: Why a child's freedom to travel and play without adult supervision matters*, in *The Conversation*. The Conversation.

Richardson, N. (2017). *30 years of VicHealth 1987–2017*. Melbourne, Victoria. https://www.vichealth.vic.gov.au/media-and-resources/publications/30-years-of-vichealth

United Nations. (1989). *United Nations Convention on the Rights of the Child*. G.A. res. 44/25, annex, 44 U.N. GAOR Supp. (No. 49) at 167, U.N. Doc. A/44/49 (1989), entered into force September 2 1990. /C/93/Add.5 of 16 July 2003.

Westheimer, J., & Kahne, J. (2004). What kind of citizen? The politics of educating for democracy. *American Educational Research Journal, 41*(2), 237–269.

Willenberg, L., et al. (2010). Exploring the relationship between playground environmental characteristics, children's perceptions and playground activity levels. *Journal of Science and Medicine in Sport, 13*, 210–216.

World Health Organization. (1986). *Ottawa charter for health promotion*. Department of Health and Welfare, World Health Organization.

Chapter 8
Engaging with People and Populations in Health Promotion Research: A Snapshot on Participatory Processes

Valérie Ivassenko, Andrew J. Macnab, Danilo Di Emidio, Alfons Hollederer, Efrelyn A. Iellamo, Jimryan Ignatius B. Cabuslay, Ivan Rene G. Lim, Shannen G. Felipe, Bridget Ira C. Arante, and Andy Sharma

8.1 Introduction

Valérie Ivassenko

Research on the practices of individuals and populations implies specific methods, approaches and aims. As it seeks to understand the different determinants of these practices and focuses on individuals (or groups of individuals) not taken isolated,

---

Authorship is ordered by appearance of the section in this chapter.

V. Ivassenko (✉)
UNESCO Chair and WHO Collaborating Center in Global Health & Education, Clermont-Auvergne University, Clermont-Ferrand, France
e-mail: valerie.ivassenko@uca.fr

A. J. Macnab (✉)
Stellenbosch Institute for Advanced Study, Wallenberg Research Centre at Stellenbosch University, Stellenbosch, South Africa
e-mail: andrew.macnab@ubc.ca

D. Di Emidio (✉)
University of East London, London, UK
e-mail: d.diemidio@uel.ac.uk

A. Hollederer (✉)
Faculty of Human Sciences, University of Kassel, Kassel, Germany
e-mail: alfons.hollederer@uni-kassel.de

E. A. Iellamo (✉) · J. I. B. Cabuslay · I. R. G. Lim · S. G. Felipe · B. I. C. Arante
College of Nursing, University of the Philippines Manila, Manila, Philippines
e-mail: eaiellamo@up.edu.ph

A. Sharma (✉)
Northwestern University, Chicago, IL, USA
e-mail: Andy.Sharma@Northwestern.edu

L. Potvin, D. Jourdan (eds.), *Global Handbook of Health Promotion Research, Vol. 1*,
https://doi.org/10.1007/978-3-030-97212-7_8

but inserted into their spatial, social, economic and cultural environments, its tools and approaches must be constantly re-questioned and adapted according to the context. Based on various themes, the five snapshots that follow show the dynamics of the research in action in an extremely concrete way. The importance of the involvement of the different actors in the development of the research project, including those not initially anticipated by the research team, is the main thread.

The participatory dynamic is at the heart of the school-based malaria and oral health programmes developed in South Africa and presented by A.J. Macnab. Community engagement is both an ethical and a scientific priority, and it is a prerequisite for the effectiveness, relevance and sustainability of the programmes. It implies placing the community at the very heart of programme development, based on the priorities identified by the actors themselves. Ultimately, it allows for the most fruitful dialogue between scientific knowledge, professional or experiential knowledge and community knowledge, generating an innovative and promising transfer of knowledge.

Stakeholder participation in research has multiple implications in the development of research programmes. It leads to a reformulation of the research questions (i.e. the objectives and purposes that the programme aims to address): describing a participatory research programme in a primary school, the second snapshot shows very well how crucial it is to reformulate the research questions so that they respond to the needs felt and expressed by the actors. The very purpose of research is highlighted here: beyond the production of knowledge as such, the researcher's methods and knowledge must also serve the concrete needs of the actors.

It is therefore not a question of a "pure" conception of research or health promotion but rather to create a convergence of means and approaches. This convergence can also go as far as the very definition and purpose of research projects, as shown by the JOBS Program. This programme combines the aims of health promotion and of work promotion and offers a very good example of the collaborative approach to health in all policies. This leads to a re-questioning of the very concepts that guide research action.

The collaborative and participatory dynamic of research on the health practices of individuals requires the production of specific data collection tools. The challenge is to allow the adaptation of proven tools in context so that they can be used and make sense for the populations concerned. This meticulous process of producing a relevant data collection tool is presented step by step in the context of research on the determinants of breastfeeding in the Philippines. All the elements structuring health promotion research are confronted and reworked: reformulation of the research question and its objectives and readjustment of the means used according to the audience. The challenge is to articulate and adapt established scientific data in ways and forms that make sense in the specific context of the intervention.

Finally, the last snapshot synthesizes the dual challenge of health promotion research, which is to develop knowledge for action (transformative aim) while being guided by ethical principles (principles of equity, fight against health inequalities). This involves implementing innovative approaches, such as spatial econometrics, to identify and understand the health practices of the most vulnerable and the most at-risk communities, in this case, the low-diabetes screening communities in Mississippi (United States). The aim of the research is to improve knowledge of the health determinants of specific groups and then to share this knowledge with local stakeholders for targeted action involving community organizations.

8.2 School-Based Programmes as a Research Platform for Improving Oral Health and Reducing Malaria Morbidity

Andrew J. Macnab

Our Purpose was to develop and evaluate research-based initiatives to address two community-identified health issues affecting African children: 1) poor oral health, with associated periodontal disease and a high incidence of dental caries (Macnab, 2015), and 2) malaria, where morbidity is the principal cause of absenteeism from school, and neurological sequelae can significantly compromise a child's academic potential in the long term (Macnab, 2020).

Collaborative Development was a core element of both research initiatives. We have learned previously that community discussion is an essential first step and the foundation for acceptance of a research-based global health education intervention. Ongoing dialogue maintains the commitment needed for a programme to be sustained and enables comprehensive evaluation to be achieved (Macnab, 2013). Both the oral health and malaria initiatives required the creation of school-based teacher-driven programmes. To achieve this, our multidisciplinary research team collaborated with teachers, community leaders, parents and youths in the schools to generate additions to the existing curriculum to foster knowledge and awareness and to provide the required tools for skills training. These were in-school tooth brushing for oral health and teacher-administered rapid diagnostic testing for malaria as well as Artemisinin combination therapy for those testing positive (Macnab et al., 2016).

Intersectoral Engagement: How these activities were conceived, carried out and evaluated was fundamental to the success of both the research and the achievement of the global health education objectives. Importantly, we chose to target issues identified by teachers and parents as health problems having a high impact on children in each community. Then, the community as a whole was engaged through dialogue conducted by an intersectoral team of healthcare providers, educators and researchers to ensure that: a) leaders, parents and teachers understood that morbidity from the health issues to be addressed was preventable; b) interventions implemented were selected by community members from a short list of evidence-based strategies prepared and presented by the health and education research team (i.e. the community saw the project as both appropriate and feasible) and c) all those participating recognized that the interventions involved research that required participation in evaluation measures, including data collection involving individual children and communal feedback, in order to learn "what works and why". Teachers were involved throughout as core members of the educational and research teams. They were given a central role in the dialogue that led to the choice by the community of the research interventions introduced, the mode of delivery within the school, the data collection and evaluation components and subsequent knowledge transfer within the community and to intersectoral agencies. We also have unequivocal evidence that the inclusion of young people in our teams is beneficial. Pupil representatives ensure that concepts, approaches and language resonate with their fellow pupils. Where possible we also identified "youth champions", young people with the presence and charisma necessary to bridge the age gap between researchers, teachers and parents and the children who are the target population (Macnab & Mukisa, 2019).

Use of the World Health Organization (WHO) Health-Promoting School (HPS) Model: Our approach for engagement, delivery, support and evaluation follows the WHO guidelines for the HPS programme delivery (Macnab, 2013); WHO endorses school-based research programmes addressing specific determinants of health, in addition to strategies aimed at enhancing the whole health ethos of the school. All school-based interventions offered to the communities to select from were evidence-based, and where diagnostic testing or treatment components were involved, these were validated and/or endorsed by WHO.

Evaluation: To evaluate outcomes, we followed a hypothesis-driven approach involving pre and post hoc analyses of validated measures. Questionnaires were also developed using local idioms. Teachers translate pupils' responses to ensure accuracy. Open-ended questions yield unexpected insights. Video interviews are a valuable source of novel data. Photo documentation during all phases of the research provided a valuable image bank for intersectoral reports to the government and other agencies and for knowledge transfer through publication of photo essays.

We Have Also Learned that in addition to the outcomes achieved, the conduct of collaborative school-based programmes benefits from innovative knowledge transfer that shares how health education research activities are conducted. To achieve this, community-based group sessions sharing progress and outcome data offer a "two-way street" for feedback, which provides impetus for effective programmes to be sustained and generates novel ideas and avenues for future collaboration. Other components necessary for obtaining future research support and the adoption of validated interventions are broad disseminations across governmental and scientific agencies and the health and education sectors, complemented by peer-reviewed publications.

8.3 Conducting Participatory Action Research (PAR) in a Primary School: The Key Role Played by (Unexpected) Social Actors in the Successful Completion of a School-Based Research

Danilo Di Emidio

The Health Foundation's inquiry (2019) into young people's future health identified that UK's children are amongst the most tested students in the world, with negative impact on students' mental health and well-being, let alone the high costs of mental ill-health for the government. Children in the UK are formally tested three times by the age of 11 vs. one time in most European countries. Therefore, my research intended to explore the nature of pre-adolescent mental health within the ambivalent features of the school environment in the "exam-focused" school. Further attention was placed on the factors enhancing the researcher–user interaction, "take-up" and impact through varying degrees of service–user engagement (here, service users refer to any participants from the school and also users such as school governors who did not participate but "used" the research findings as guidance). The research, part of my master's degree, was carried out in June/July 2019 over 6 weeks in a primary school in central London (UK). It involved 8 year-6 students (10/11 years old) who had just completed the Statutory Assessment Tests (SATs), their final exam of primary education.

The school selection was part of a wider design to inform my follow-up PhD research, which would focus on the influence of the exam-focused school on pre-adult adolescent mental health – 16/18 years of age. Therefore, I selected a local primary school as part of a preparatory pilot study to gather data on the same theme from a different age group, undergoing the same "final year" exams. A number of lessons were learned about conducting participatory action research (PAR) alongside an ethnographic methodology.

First, it is essential to have a research plan to share with the school's social actors to identify commonalities of intent and expected outcomes. It initiates a working relationship rather than a formal handover of a research terrain often difficult to access. For example, once I got the head teacher on board, I was assigned a gatekeeper who was in charge of students' well-being and inclusion. The gatekeeper coordinated my day-to-day work in the school and also assigned a teaching assistant to the research, facilitating further rapport building with other school staff. This enabled smooth operations throughout the fieldwork. In short, the school wanted to have a broader, more inclusive view than the one I had planned, and my flexibility paid off.

Second, while the ongoing sharing of views/expertise with the (unexpected) social actors implied a slight reworking of the original plan (i.e. to involve only students), it also contextualized and grounded my plan in the "field". Not only was showing such flexibility useful for a richer thematic analysis but it also helped reach other key social actors (teachers, teaching assistants and parents), offering additional analytical and methodological scope that I had not contemplated before.

Building on the previous points, a third important learning curve emerged while witnessing a discrepancy between methodological theory and practice. Even though most PAR theories do not advocate fixed procedural criteria, they still invite to adhere to standard iterative procedures to ensure reliability and rigour. For example, on reflection, while I was the research facilitator who involved different social actors according to their different roles, I noticed that "varying degrees" of PAR were unfolding rather than a standard PAR cycle. Amongst the many changes of plan or adaptations, a few are worth consideration.

First, I was unexpectedly asked to wait for 2 weeks before starting to engage with the year-6 students, causing research worries about completion. However, the assigned gatekeeper took prompt action and, with the support of the teaching assistant, arranged that I worked with a group of year-5 students for a short while. It turned out to be invaluable preparatory time, to get a "feel" of the research field, experiencing the school ethos first-hand, getting to know the new staff and the school environment and testing the year-5's curiosity and anxiety about turning year 6 soon.

Second, my initial research question had to change and adapt following some of the suggestions from the head teacher. Again, such a move had further implications as I was asked to drop "mental health" from my research focus and replace it with "well-being", in line with the internal school policy to focus only on well-being; a separation that opened up to nuanced speculation on educational policies in my follow-up PhD.

Third, for a variety of reasons, the number of participants' parents (to be interviewed) went from the initially recruited 10 to 2. On this occasion, the deputy head (a new social actor appearing on the scene) reassured me that we could have reached a greater number of parents, often those hard to reach, through a survey/questionnaire. She facilitated the submission of an online questionnaire for all year-5/6 parents, adding alternative valuable data, and increased the voices to be heard to further contextualize students' perceived well-being in relation to exams/tests. Once again, this shows that the "degrees of PAR" involvement vary across the social actors involved.

In conclusion, following a rich analytical triangulation of data collection (parents, staff and students), three major findings, focusing on well-being promotion, were presented to the school governors. Surprisingly, these findings were included in the school's "improvement plan" document for the following year. Such a participatory approach blended well with a growing interest in research "use/influence", which, as Wright (2008) argues, goes further than communicating research to a limited privileged few, instead, moving towards embedding strategies of service–user engagement and seeing research as a driver of wider social change.

By keeping a flexible research mind-set, a PAR approach brings with it twists and turns, let alone new social actors, which cannot be "designed" but can surely add value to the research outcome.

8.4 Evidence-Based Health Promotion Among Unemployed People: An Example of the JOBS Program Germany

Alfons Hollederer

Mass unemployment is a social determinant of health, which stresses individuals, communities and state systems. Unemployment increases the risk of diseases, and health impairments reduce the chance of reintegration into the labour market. Health promotion among the unemployed aims to improve health and labour market integration. Health promotion measures among unemployed people were met with varying success in the past. The research shows evidence of improved mental health and employment promotion effects for established approaches like the JOBS Program in Anglo-American countries. The JOBS Program is a multimodal approach that implements not only training in applying for jobs but also various elements of social learning based on social-cognitive theories and self-efficacy. The adaptation requires confirmatory studies. The objective of a study of the University of Kassel is to investigate the effects of the JOBS Program intervention on reintegration into the labour market and on health among approximately 1400 unemployed people in Germany. This confirmatory study was designed as a randomized controlled intervention trial (RCT) with a waiting list group of over 6 months. It was part of large-scale efforts to combine employment promotion and health promotion at the community level in Germany. In addition, a first international meta-analysis is in preparation for health promotion among the unemployed.

8.4.1 Background

The ongoing global COVID-19 pandemic is a health problem, which triggered a global economic crisis and a related labour market crisis. The global economic crisis caused persistently high unemployment. Unemployment figures are rising in many industrialized countries (International Monetary Fund, 2020). The risk of becoming unemployed is not equally distributed among regions and social groups. Especially, young people and low-skilled workers were often the first to lose their jobs during the crisis. Involuntary mass unemployment is a major challenge for public health. Unemployment is one of the factors affecting the complex interrelationships of lifestyles, working and living conditions that determine population health. The Commission on Social Determinants of Health of the World Health Organization (WHO) concluded that unemployment as a social determinant of mental health constitutes both a differential exposure at the individual level and a significant socio-economic context factor (CSDH, 2008).

According to the existing research, unemployment is related to health problems. Compared to the employed population, unemployed people are characterized by a substantially worse health status. International meta-analyses consistently identified a negative impact of unemployment on morbidity (McKee-Ryan et al., 2005; Paul & Moser, 2009) and on premature mortality or suicide of exposed individuals (Roelfs et al., 2011; Milner et al., 2013). After losing their jobs, people tend to suffer from impaired mental health, whereas their mental well-being clearly improves as soon as they find their way back into employment (Paul & Moser, 2009). The causal relationship is not yet fully understood. The employed and unemployed differ substantially in terms of socio-demographic and health-related characteristics. Unemployed persons more often report worse or bad self-rated health and feel being rather or much impaired by mental health issues. Lower self-rated health is associated with a higher unemployment risk for employed people as well as a lower probability of reintegration for unemployed people.

In accordance with the EU-SILC survey, analyses show significant health disparities to the detriment of unemployed people of all European countries (database of Eurostat 2021). They also refer to a need for prevention regarding health and employment. Differential unemployment research considered not only the heterogeneous risks of becoming unemployed but also the inequality in the distribution of psychosocial and health risks among this group. Thus, such predictor variables can provide important insights for intervention approaches and the definition of target groups for health promotion efforts.

It remains an open research question as to how people can at best, and with the least damage to their health, master the involuntary loss of their jobs and their unemployment. The interactions between unemployment and health create a need for specific interventions for health promotion. A significant evolution can be observed in the quality and quantity of health promotion for the unemployed over time. An international overview by Hollederer (2019) provides information on how health promotion for the unemployed has been approached with an analysis of controlled intervention studies. The health promotion measures were generally based on individual counselling, case management, training or group services. The overview demonstrates the breadth of variation in target groups and types of measures. Their result indicators for health and integration into the labour market vary substantially, as do the employment promotion effects. However, effects are rather moderate or low in magnitude, and the effect mechanisms often remain unclear. Effects weaken over time. Success is more common in the areas of health, physical activity, nutrition and stress relief.

Intervention strategies that take account of the diversity of the unemployed and their different needs should be developed. For their further development, prevention and health promotion measures for unemployed people need better framework conditions to break or at least mitigate the vicious circle of unemployment and health. There is also a need for targeted health promotion as an integral part of a general health promotion policy, which has already been postulated by the WHO Ottawa Charter (1986) or in the Health in All Policies Approach. Health promotion interventions would help the unemployed maintain their health as well as their ability to work.

8.4.2 JOBS Program Germany for Health Promotion Among the Unemployed in the Communities and with Labour Promotion Institutions

Unemployment is a major risk factor for poverty and social exclusion. Participation in work has an important function in overall social integration. "Labour market-integrative health promotion" (Hollederer, 2021) is an approach for the target group of unemployed people. It goes beyond the prevention of illness, since it focuses on the maintenance of employability and aims at labour market integration. The approach often combines health promotion measures with employment promotion.

A systematic review by Hollederer (2019) identified 30 health interventions for the unemployed in the literature and analyzed 14 intervention studies with a controlled study design. The interventional approaches have varying degrees of success. For internationally established approaches such as the JOBS Program, there is evidence of improvement, especially in mental health among the unemployed. The intervention studies that followed the JOBS Program II have also shown positive effects on labour market integration. On average, studies with explicitly voluntary access had better effects. However, the number of randomized controlled trials is still small overall.

The JOBS Program was being transferred to Germany (study protocol by Hollederer et al., 2021). It combines job application training with various elements of social learning based on social-cognitive theories and self-efficacy (Bandura, 1977, 2004). The JOBS Program was developed on the basis of scientific findings by the Michigan Prevention Research Center (MPRC) (http://webservices.itcs.umich.edu/drupal/mprc/projects/jobs). Variants of this JOBS Program have been used in the USA, Finland, Ireland, the Netherlands, China, Korea and other countries.

The research project "JOBS Program Germany for health promotion among the unemployed in the communities and with labour promotion institutions (JobsProgramDtl)" aims to systematically improve the health of unemployed people. It is an ongoing randomized controlled trial with a 6-month follow-up. The study design follows a mixed methods research. The study targets officially registered unemployed people aged between 18 and 65 years in Germany. Regional information events on the aims, procedures and contents of the JOBS training courses will be held by the trainers. Participation is voluntary, and withdrawal is possible at any time without consequences. Unemployed people who would like to participate in the JOBS training courses after the information events can subsequently submit an expression of interest. Following expressions of interest in participating in the training courses, approximately 700 unemployed people are randomly assigned to the intervention groups and approximately 700 unemployed people to the waiting control groups. To validate the questionnaires, a pre-test was be carried out with approximately 70 unemployed people. The unemployed people are then contacted via computer-assisted telephone interviews. This involves repeated questioning of willingness to participate, randomized allocation to intervention and waiting control groups and invitation to the JOBS training for the intervention group. During the computer-assisted telephone interviews, the current employment status and biographical and socio-demographic variables of employment are collected. Target variables are mental health and well-being and labour market integration. Constructs such as self-efficacy and self-esteem are also of interest. The voluntary offer of the JOBS Program intervention is also planned for the approximately 700 unemployed in the waiting control group after the study, and the financing is already secured. This means that the control group can also benefit from the intervention later if they wish.

The JOBS Program Germany will be introduced under "real-world conditions". The research project generates hints for adaptation and results for implementation and achievement of objectives. In case of a successful implementation of the project "JOBS Program Germany", the trained trainers can continue the interventions beyond the pilot's project phase. The combination of health promotion with work promotion in Germany is a positive example of a collaborative Health in All Policies approach, which can also serve as a model for other countries.

Integrative health promotion goes beyond disease prevention and increasing health resources in the target definitions, as it also aims at improving employability and labour market integration. The implementation of the measures requires innovative strategies for addressing the vulnerable target groups and a structural interlinking of work promotion and health promotion with steering committees. The expansion of intervention research among the unemployed people represents likewise a "current challenge for public health" (Hammarström & Janlert, 2005).

The systematic review by Hollederer (2019) showed a considerable development for health promotion among the unemployed in terms of quality and quantity of intervention studies. Overall, there is little evidence on the mechanisms of action of individual components and in different social target groups. There is a need for further research on the effectiveness and the longer-lasting maintenance of the effects of the interventions. In perspective, some of the evaluated intervention approaches appear to be good to combine. The first international meta-analysis using quantitative empirical methods was conducted by Paul and Hollederer (2022) on the evidence base of health promotion among the unemployed.

8.4.3 The Research Conducted on the JOBS Program

8.4.3.1 The Specific Health Promotion Practices Investigated: Who Were the Actors? What Were They Doing? For What Purposes?

There is evidence of improved health and labour market integration for established approaches like the JOBS Program. The JOBS Program approach has been broadly adopted in Germany by the German Federal Centre for Health Education (BZgA) and is supported by the National Association of Statutory Health Insurance Funds (GKV-Spitzenverband) for 2020. It aims to implement health promotion measures within the regular structures of Jobcenters, occupational retraining organizations and employment promotion. It is part of a community-oriented initiative. The German Federal Centre for Health Education (BZgA) plays a key role in the transfer of JOBS Program activities into practice. It provides support for the locations where JOBS activities are conducted and adapts the project results for further implementation to ensure its sustainability. The German Federal Centre for Health Education (BZgA) was assigned with the implementation of the JOBS Program by the National Association of Statutory Health Insurance Funds (GKV-Spitzenverband). Established administrational structures of the "Alliance for Health" were used for implementing the JOBS Program. It is an initiative of the Statutory Health Insurance to develop and implement measures of health promotion and prevention in communal settings. To implement the JOBS Program, every location of this Alliance formed a steering committee composed of representatives from the Jobcenters and the Statutory Health Insurance as well as from several community facilities, who supported the implementation on a local level.

Training will be provided in daily sessions of 5 hours each over 1 week using the following methods:

- Training in job-search skills.
- Active teaching and learning methods.
- Qualified instructors for programme implementation.
- An active and supportive learning environment.
- Inoculation against setbacks.

The courses aim to enhance social support among group participants and to increase self-efficacy in acquiring job-search skills.

8.4.3.2 The Purpose of the Research Project or Programme: What Were the Objectives? In which Context Were They Defined? Who Participated in Their Definition? Were Values Other Than Knowledge Production Pursued Through This Research? If Yes, What Were They? Who Defined Them?

In international comparisons, the population of the unemployed in Germany is characterized by a persistent number of people with placement obstacles, such as the long-term unemployed, the unemployed of high age or with lower qualifications or health restrictions. In addition, the labour market in Germany is generally much less flexible than in other countries and offers fewer part-time jobs. The main objective of the confirmatory study is therefore to investigate whether the JOBS Program approach can be transferred to German conditions and whether the unemployed people in Germany evolve the same positive health and labour market effects examined in other international evaluations of the JOBS Program. In terms of health goals, the effectiveness of the JOBS Program on mental health was of particular interest. New scientific knowledge on health needs among the unemployed people should be generated. It is of interest to create evidence of transfer in the everyday life of vulnerable groups.

8.4.3.3 The Research Framework: Which Research Paradigm Was Framing the Research and Why? Which Theory or Theories Were Used? How Was the Theory Used?

The Michigan Prevention Research Center developed the "JOBS Program" (Caplan et al., 1989; Vinokur et al., 1995). This is a multimodal approach that incorporates not only training in applying for jobs but also various elements of social learning based on social-cognitive theories and self-efficacy (Bandura, 1977, 2004). The effects were evaluated in two intervention studies among persons who had been unemployed for 3–4 months. The studies were conducted in Michigan, with control groups and randomized access, and revealed many positive effects. In a 2-year follow-up, significant positive labour market effects and health outcomes were still found among the JOBS II intervention group, as was a decrease in depressive symptoms (Vinokur et al., 2000).

The Työhön Job Search Program is the Finnish version of the JOBS Program II approach, but, in this case, unemployed people were trained as instructors (Vuori et al., 2002). After 2 years, an intervention effect was found in depressive symptoms and self-esteem as well as in general labour market commitment (Vuori & Silvonen, 2005).

The coherences of work and health framed the implementation of the JOBS Program. The ability to work is a requirement for (re)integration into the labour market. Therefore, work-integrative health promotion activities address the capabilities and potentials of (still) healthy unemployed people to maintain or enhance their health status and by that also their ability to work. Despite that, there is a lack of prevention addressing unemployed people. Health promotion often does not apply for unemployed people because they are hard to reach by the conventional approaches. Thus, the communities and federal structures of the Statutory Health Insurance were of great importance for the implementation. They enabled an approach by regarding people's living conditions (behavioural and environmental prevention). Regarding the behavioural aspects of the programme, the theory of cognitive behaviour built the framework for the JOBS trainings, which addresses both – the convenience in having the capability to find a new job and by that stay mentally healthy with a positive attitude towards the given circumstances of unemployment.

8.4.3.4 The Relationship with Those Whose Practices Were Investigated: How Were Research Participants Involved in the Planning and Conducting of the Research? Were Research Results Shared with Non-researchers? If Yes, How and for What Purpose?

Before the main study, a qualitative pre-study will be conducted to provide access to the target group and to gather initial knowledge about their experiences, needs and demands concerning the JOBS Program. Therefore, one will attend the JOBS training to gain explorative knowledge on three levels: problem-centred interviews, focus group discussions and participating observations. Especially, the focus group, as a culturally sensitive and participative research method, offered an opportunity to involve the participants in the planning and further conduction of the JOBS Program. Unemployed people have the chance to bring their own experiences in dealing with periods of unemployment, challenges they are confronted with and their expectations on a programme like JOBS to the group. These insights will be used to reconsider and adapt the upcoming implementation of the JOBS Program. Involving the target group in this way should not only increase the acceptance of the planned intervention but also increase its success and sustainability.

8.4.3.5 The Methods Used: What Kinds of Data Were Collected? How Were they Collected and Analyzed?

The University of Kassel carried out a randomized controlled trial (RCT) with an intervention group and a waiting-list control group (Hollederer et al., 2021). Approximately 60 intervention workshops were delivered by co-trainers. The data of $N = 1400$ unemployed people is currently being collected, containing one treatment group who took part in the JOBS Program immediately and one waiting control group that took part in the intervention after 6 months. Participation was voluntary. After the JOBS coaching, the participants were interviewed by computer-assisted telephone interviews (CATIs) at three times of treatment (T0 before the intervention, T1 after the intervention). The data were evaluated by logistic regression analyses to identify the independent variables influencing the dependent variables and to determine the strength and direction of this influence.

8.4.3.6 Specific Challenges of Health Promotion Research Enlightened by the Project or Programme: How Does the Research Contribute to Advances in Health Promotion Research?

The evaluation of the JOBS Program advances health promotion research by creating highly needed evidence in the field of health promotion and prevention for unemployed people. Furthermore, it shows where the JOBS Program must be adapted to fit consistently into German labour market conditions, to the extent that at the interlinking of employment promotion and health promotion, actors like the Statutory Health Insurance and Jobcenters need more evidence-based approaches. The JOBS Program has the potential to close this gap. It is integrated into the existing municipal structures.

The research project on which this report is based was funded by the German Federal Ministry of Education and Research under the funding code 01EL2001. The author is responsible for the content of this publication. The JOBS Program Germany was launched on behalf of the funding of the German Federal Centre for Health Education (BZgA) and supported by the National Association of Statutory Health Insurance Funds (GKV-Spitzenverband).

The research contributes to the evidence base. The first international meta-analysis on health promotion among the unemployed was being prepared in parallel (Paul & Hollederer, 2022).

8.5 Employing Survey as a Research Method in Breastfeeding Health Promotion Research: A Philippine Perspective

Efrelyn A. Iellamo, Jimryan Ignatius B. Cabuslay,
Ivan Rene G. Lim, Shannen G. Felipe, and Bridget Ira C. Arante

8.5.1 *Introduction*

Data collection remains one of the vital facets of the research process. Among many research tools, a survey questionnaire is commonly used for collecting data on human behaviour by indirectly observing respondents (Jones et al., 2013). Data collected on health behaviours become an invaluable asset in health promotion as they serve as a major thrust to create programmes and interventions that promote optimal health practices.

Breastfeeding practices of mothers in developing countries have emerged as a relevant subject in health promotion research. The utilization of a survey questionnaire was demonstrated to be useful in identifying factors related to breastfeeding practices. This chapter explores how descriptive correlational survey research on breastfeeding practices utilized a questionnaire as part of a research instrument for data collection.

8.5.2 *Designing the Survey Questionnaire*

Designing a survey questionnaire entails ample amount of time for planning. Planning started during the initial step – formulation of the research question and objectives. The study aimed to answer the question, "What are the factors that affect breastfeeding practices of mothers, and how do healthcare workers affect breastfeeding practices?" The research question and objectives provided a clear direction in the research.

The theoretical and conceptual framework guided the researchers in considering variables and corresponding relationships in the study. After identifying the variables, researchers have to conduct a literature search to identify and appraise the existing instruments measuring breastfeeding knowledge, attitudes, practices and intention (Casal et al., 2017). Researchers carefully considered validity and reliability prior to the selection of an instrument. Authors of selected breastfeeding instruments granted permission for their use for research purposes. Selected breastfeeding instruments such as the IOWA Infant Feeding Attitude Scale (Mora et al., 1999) needed adaptation to the local context; hence, researchers obtained official Filipino language translation and ensured items remained appropriate for the study. The questionnaire was submitted to the Faculty of Maternal and Child Nursing of the University of the Philippines College of Nursing and underwent content and face validation to ensure that the items in the questionnaire were appropriate to the specific objectives of the study.

The researchers conducted pre-testing to evaluate how a sample of mothers would respond to the self-administered questionnaire. A sample size of 20 mothers and 10 community healthcare workers were recruited by convenience sampling for pre-testing the tools. Feedback from the respondents was noted to improve the questionnaire. Clarifications were raised on formatting and the sequence of questions, and changes were made.

8.5.3 Challenges Addressed During Data Collection

Several challenges surfaced during data collection. Some respondents had difficulty in reading the items since it was self-administered, and others were not able to follow the instructions thoroughly; hence, they needed assistance from the team. Although addressed during pre-testing, researchers recommend that immediate evaluation of the validity of the responses of the submitted questionnaires be done to prevent data encoding errors.

Data collection performed during the weekdays also posed a challenge. Since the team has to coincide data collection with well-baby clinics during weekdays at the local health centres, some working mothers were often not available to accompany their child, hence further decreasing the number of respondents available for data collection. Researchers ensured that working mothers were also covered to yield meaningful research data. Posters approved by the Research Ethics Board have been posted for recruitment.

Local health centres with higher population coverage turned out to have higher response rates when compared to those of other health centres in the same district. Researchers have to address this concern by reaching out to the urban community covered by the health centre.

An official Filipino language translation of the tools was obtained; thus, the team did not encounter difficulty in terms of the participants' comprehension regarding the questionnaire. The team accounted for any possible language barriers that could arise during data collection since the City of Manila comprises people from various regions of the country with distinct languages and from all walks of life. During instances wherein a particular item seemed to be unclear or vague for respondents, the researchers offered assistance to guide the mothers.

8.5.4 *Conclusions*

The use of a survey questionnaire significantly facilitated identifying the determinants affecting breastfeeding practices in District V, City of Manila. Breastfeeding knowledge, attitudes, practices and intention were obtained purposefully through the use of specific, valid and reliable research instruments.

A key lesson in designing and adapting a survey questionnaire is the formulation of the research question and objectives that guided the team in efficiently gathering data. A survey questionnaire should be designed with decisive consideration of the target respondent population's demographics and literacy, among other factors.

Pre-testing played a vital role in gauging the appropriateness of the questionnaire in the conduct of breastfeeding research in the local context. It revealed the possible challenges and constraints in administering the questionnaires; hence, researchers addressed these concerns immediately to ensure efficient and organized data gathering.

Survey research is among the research methods that can be utilized to yield relevant information related to health behaviour to facilitate health promotion of breastfeeding practices in the context of a developing country such as the Philippines. With increased awareness of various factors that can influence breastfeeding practices, findings of this survey research can be used as local data to explore future public programmes and interventions that can be implemented with the aim to improve the maternal breastfeeding outcomes in the country and eventually to reach the targeted breastfeeding rate in the Philippines.

8.6 Researching Practices That Promote the Population Health of Older Adults: Utilizing a Spatial Approach to Guide Diabetes Care

Andy Sharma

8.6.1 *Introduction*

Diabetes is the seventh leading cause of death in the United State (US) and is a significant health concern for older minority adults, particularly Blacks, due to higher prevalence rates (Heron, 2019). Despite ongoing initiatives to reduce the burden of diabetes in the past decade, it remains near the top of the list of public health issues. Recognizing this need, this section explains how new knowledge was generated in this area and how results from the spatial analyses were utilized by health professionals to enrich practices that promote population health. What makes this work fall into the category of health promotion research is the dynamic link between knowledge production and sharing with healthcare professionals.

8.6.2 *Generating New Knowledge by Utilizing a Spatial Approach Within a Socio-Environmental Framework*

Effective diabetes management begins with the person (i.e. unit of analysis at the individual level). However, managing diabetes can be challenging for individuals, particularly older minority adults who may also suffer from disabilities, limited economic resources and isolated family and social networks (Walker et al., 2021). In these instances, a community-based approach could be a practical health promotion strategy.[1] That is, diabetes management can be facilitated by involving community organizations/members in the treatment and care process. While such an approach has been received favourably by healthcare professionals, identifying clusters (i.e. small geographic areas) which could benefit from such an approach for older Blacks in largely rural areas had not been studied extensively (Glenn et al., 2020). As such, generating new knowledge in this area has the potential to improve the quality of life for older adults. To accomplish this, a spatial framework was constructed to identify clusters of low diabetes testing. Next, this knowledge was shared with health practitioners with the goal of devising interventions for specific areas.

In order to better understand how to incorporate space into the analysis, this study applied concepts from spatial econometrics. That is, recognizing the influence of spatial interaction and structure (i.e. spatial autocorrelation and heterogeneity). More specifically, units interact in space and are influenced by other nearby units. Due to this, observations are no longer independent of each other (violation of the Gauss–Markov assumptions). A spatial lag model is one such model that can account for this autocorrelation by adding neighbouring values as an additional independent variable based on a spatial weights matrix. Using the state of Mississippi as a case study, a spatial lag model was constructed with the county as the unit of analysis (total of 82 counties).[2] Since one objective was to identify clusters that could benefit from improved diabetes care practices, the model was formulated where testing rates for low-density lipoprotein or LDL (i.e. bad cholesterol) served as the outcome variable and the percentage of the population identifying as Black functioned as the main independent variable of interest. As stated previously, this was an advancement in health promotion research in diabetes care because earlier work focused at the individual level, whereas this framework applied a socio-environmental approach at the county level. The regression estimates revealed that counties with a higher percentage of the older Black population maintained lower LDL testing rates and both the spatial autocorrelation and clustering analyses uncovered a distinct pattern of low testing rates in (a) northwestern and (b) western Mississippi.

8.6.3 Applying New Knowledge to Inform Diabetes Care Practices

At the same time as the data collection, the knowledge transfer process was launched. The objective of this work is to equip practitioners with an understanding of the spatial patterns and then to increase awareness of the role of social determinants in diabetes management. The partners of this process were the Mississippi State Department of Health, the Office of Health Disparity Elimination and the Mississippi Diabetes Prevention and Control Program. As part of the research project, we devised a communications strategy, which involved sharing both the results and the accompanying cluster maps with the Diabetes Coalition unit and various local public health professionals. By focusing on statistically significant clusters of low levels of testing, targeted efforts could be initiated by involving community organizations when hosting health promotion efforts (particularly during holidays and special events) where multiple nearby counties could offer testing during the week. By coordinating inter-county events, a larger audience could be reached while costs related to marketing and promotion could be minimized. With this approach, the state now had another approach to identify the needs of people living with diabetes and to understand the factors influencing diabetes management.

[1]This should not be confused with community-based participatory research (CBPR), which involves shared decision-making authority by community members.

[2]Mississippi, a state in southeast US, was selected because it ranks near the top for diabetes prevalence and also has a significant older Black population.

Article for Additional Information

Sharma, A. (2014). Spatial analysis of disparities in LDL-C testing for older diabetic adults: A socio-environmental framework focusing on race, poverty, and health access in Mississippi. *Applied Geography*, *55*, 248–256. Available at: https://doi.org/10.1016/j.apgeog.2014.09.017

References

Bandura, A. (1977). Self-efficacy: Toward a unifying theory of behavioral change. *Psychological Review, 84*(2), 191–215.

Bandura, A. (2004). Health promotion by social cognitive means. *Health education & behavior: the official publication of the Society for Public Health Education, 31*(2), 143–164.

Caplan, R. D., Vinokur, A. D., Price, R. H., & van Ryn, M. (1989). Job seeking, reemployment and mental health: A randomized field experiment in coping with job loss. *Journal of Applied Psychology, 74*(5), 759–769.

Casal, C. S., Lei, A., Young, S. L., & Tuthill, E. L. (2017). A critical review of instruments measuring breastfeeding. attitudes, knowledge, and social support. *Journal of Human Lactation, 33*(1), 21–47.

CSDH. (2008). *Closing the gap in a generation: Health equity through action on the social determinants of health: Final report of the commission on social determinants of health.* World Health Organization.

Glenn, L. E., Nichols, M., Enriquez, M., & Jenkins, C. (2020). Impact of a community-based approach to patient engagement in rural, low-income adults with type 2 diabetes. *Public Health Nursing, 37*(2), 178–187.

Hammarström, A., & Janlert, U. (2005). An agenda for unemployment research: A challenge for public health. *International Journal of Health Services, 35*(4).

Heron, M. P. (2019). Deaths: leading causes for 2017. *National vital statistics reports, 68*(6), 2019–1120.

Hollederer, A. (2019). Health promotion and prevention among the unemployed: A systematic review. *Health Promotion International, 34*(6), 1078–1096.

Hollederer, A. (2021). *Gesundheitsförderung bei Arbeitslosen (health promotion among unemployed).* Fachhochschulverlag.

Hollederer, A., Jahn, H. J., & Klein, D. (2021). JOBS program Germany for health promotion among the unemployed in the community setting with institutions for employment promotion (JobsProgramDtl): Study protocol for a randomized controlled trial. *BMC Public Health, 21*(1), 261.

International Monetary Fund (Ed.) (2020). *World economic outlook.* The Great Lockdown.

Jones, T. L., Baxter, M. A., & Khanduja, V. (2013). A quick guide to survey research. *Annals of the Royal College of Surgeons of England, 95*(1), 5–7. https://doi.org/10.1308/003588413X13511609956372

Macnab, A. (2013). The Stellenbosch consensus statement on health promoting schools. *Global Health Promotion, 20*(1), 78–81.

Macnab, A. J. (2015). Children's oral health: The opportunity for improvement using the WHO health promoting school model. *Advances in Public Health, 2015.*

Macnab, A. J. (2020). School-based initiatives to reduce malaria morbidity and promote academic achievement in children. In A. J. Macnab, A. Daar, & C. Pauw (Eds.), *Health in transition: Translating DOHaD science to improve future health in Africa* (pp. 247–288). Sun Media (STIAS Book Series) Stellenbosch University Press.

Macnab, A. J., & Mukisa, R. (2019). Celebrity endorsed music videos: Innovation to foster youth health promotion. *Health Promotion International, 34*(4), 716–725.

Macnab, A. J., Mukisa, R., Mutabazi, S., & Steed, R. (2016). Malaria in Uganda: School-based rapid diagnostic testing and treatment. *International Journal of Epidemiology, 45*(6), 1759–1762.

McKee-Ryan, F. M., Song, Z., Wanberg, C. R., & Kinicki, A. J. (2005). Psychological and physical well-being during unemployment: A meta-analytic study. *The Journal of Applied Psychology, 90*(1), 53–76.

Milner, A., Page, A., & LaMontagne, A. D. (2013). Long-term unemployment and suicide: A systematic review and meta-analysis. *PloS one, 8*(1), e51333. https://doi.org/10.1371/journal.pone.0051333

Mora, A. D. L., Russell, D. W., Dungy, C. I., Losch, M., & Dusdieker, L. (1999). The Iowa infant feeding attitude. scale: analysis of reliability and validity. *Journal of Applied Social Psychology, 29*(11), 2362–2380.

Paul, K., & Hollederer, A. (2022). *The effectiveness of health-oriented interventions and health promotion for unemployed people – a meta-analysis.* (submitted)

Paul, K. I., & Moser, K. (2009). Unemployment impairs mental health: Meta-analyses. *Journal of Vocational Behavior, 74*(3), 264–282.

Roelfs, D. J., Shor, E., Davidson, K. W., & Schwartz, J. E. (2011). Losing life and livelihood. A systematic review and meta-analysis of unemployment and all-cause mortality. *Social Science & Medicine, 72*(6), 840–854. https://doi.org/10.1016/j.socscimed.2011.01.005

The Health Foundation. (2019). *Making the grade: How education shapes young people's mental health.* CentreforMH_CYPMHC_MakingTheGrade_PDF_1.pdf (centreformentalhealth.org.uk). Accessed 5th January 2021.

Vinokur, A. D., Price, R. H., & Schul, Y. (1995). Impact of the JOBS intervention on unemployed workers varying in risk for depression. *American Journal of Community Psychology, 23*(1), 39–74.

Vinokur, A. D., Schul, Y., Vuori, J., & Price, R. H. (2000). Two years after a job loss: Long-term impact of the JOBS program on reemployment and mental health. *Journal of Occupational Health Psychology, 5*(1), 32–47.

Vuori, J., & Silvonen, J. (2005). The benefits of a preventive job search program on re-employment and mental health at 2-year follow-up. Short research paper. *Journal of Occupational and Organizational Psychology, 78*(1), 43–52.

Vuori, J., Silvonen, J., Vinokur, A. D., & Price, R. H. (2002). The Työhön job search program in Finland: Benefits for the unemployed with risk of depression or discouragement. *Journal of Occupational Health Psychology, 7*(1), 5–19.

Walker, R. J., Garacci, E., Campbell, J. A., Harris, M., Mosley-Johnson, E., & Egede, L. E. (2021). Relationship between multiple measures of financial hardship and glycemic control in older adults with diabetes. *Journal of Applied Gerontology, 40*(2), 162–169.

World Health Organization, Regional Office for Europe. (1986). Ottawa charter for health promotion.

Wright, K. (2008). *Conceptualizing influence and impact in development research.* Briefing Paper for ESRC- DFID.

Part II
Researching the Practices of Professionals

Chapter 9
Fostering Cultural Safety in Health Care Through a Decolonizing Approach to Research with, for and by Indigenous Communities

Marie-Claude Tremblay and Sandro Echaquan

9.1 Introduction

On September 28, 2020, in the moments before her death at the Centre hospitalier de Lanaudière, Joyce Echaquan, an Atikamekw woman from the community of Manawan (Québec), broadcast live on social media the racist and degrading comments made towards her by the nursing staff (Kamel, 2021). This video quickly made the rounds of global media, generating shock, horror and outrage and triggering conversations about systemic racism against Indigenous peoples. The case of Joyce Echaquan is a poignant example of the racism that Indigenous peoples experience in the health system. Racism towards Indigenous peoples, whether interpersonal or systemic, is inextricably linked to colonialism, a racist ideology that presupposes the superiority of Western culture over others and permeates the structure of our public institutions (Allan & Smylie, 2015). Recently, in Canada, the Truth and Reconciliation Commission (2015), the National Inquiry into Missing and Murdered Indigenous Women and Girls (Buller et al., 2019) and the Public Inquiry Commission on relations between Indigenous peoples and certain public services (Gouvernement du Québec, 2019) have brought to light the discrimination, rights violations, trauma and harm suffered by Indigenous peoples with various institutions. These commissions have all called for actions to address the root causes of institutional violence and systemic racism through decolonization and cultural safety approaches based on respectful partnerships with Indigenous communities.

This tragic example leaves no doubt that health services are a high-level determinant of health that can increase the burdens of health inequalities for Indigenous

M.-C. Tremblay (✉)
Department of Family Medicine and Emergency Medicine, Université Laval, Québec, Canada
e-mail: Marie-Claude.Tremblay@fmed.ulaval.ca

S. Echaquan
Masko-Siwin Health Center and Mihawoso Social Pediatrics Center, Québec, Canada

L. Potvin, D. Jourdan (eds.), *Global Handbook of Health Promotion Research, Vol. 1*,
https://doi.org/10.1007/978-3-030-97212-7_9

populations and contribute to the systemic marginalization of minority groups. Health promotion, as a field of practice and research, has an important role to play to ensure equitable, anti-racist and culturally safe health care.

The purpose of the research discussed in this chapter is to contribute to reorienting health services by ensuring cultural safety in the provision of health care to Indigenous populations in the province of Québec (Canada). To do so, it aims to co-develop a new intervention model to ensure cultural safety for Atikamekw patients in the health system. The Atikamekw Nehirowsiw are a Nation that is part of the Algonquin cultural area and upholds values such as caring for extended family and community members, respect for Elders, equality between men and women and a close connection with the land (Atikamekw Sipi, 2019). Three Atikamekw communities are located in the traditional territory of Nitaskinan, in the Saint-Maurice River Valley (Québec): Manawan, Wemotaci and Opitciwan. These three communities together comprise around 7800 members, most of whom speak Atikamekw. The Atikamekw were traditionally a nomadic people, and many traditional activities such as fishing and hunting continue to be practised today. Like many Indigenous peoples, the Atikamekw have unique and specific cultural health practices, traditional knowledge and perspectives on health, which are central to their well-being but are often devalued or ignored by Western science and medicine (Tremblay et al., 2020). This research has been developed and implemented in full partnership with the Atikamekw communities of Manawan, Wemotaci and Opitciwan, as well as with the Atikamekw Nation Council (ANC), to address the concerns and needs that they have identified.

9.2 What Is Cultural Safety?

Indigenous peoples in Canada experience substantial health inequities, including shorter life expectancies, higher rates of suicide and greater prevalence of mental illness and chronic and infectious diseases (Hackett et al., 2016; Kolahdooz et al., 2015; Loppie Reading & Wien, 2009; Zambas & Wright, 2016). These inequities result from the continuing impact and lasting effects of colonialism on health determinants such as access to health services (Gao et al., 2008; Loppie Reading & Wien, 2009; Marrone, 2007; Peiris et al., 2008). Barriers to health services access include programmes and interventions inherently structured on the basis of dominant (Western) cultural values, principles and perspectives not relevant to Indigenous patients' needs (Jacklin et al., 2017; Kolahdooz et al., 2015; Tang & Browne, 2008). Health services built and managed in keeping with Western worldviews have reinforced Western cultural supremacy, making it possible to socially and politically disavow traditional Indigenous health practices and knowledge (Gouvernement du Québec, 2019). As a reflection of the structural racism embedded in social institutions, interactions between Indigenous patients and health providers are often characterized by stigmatization, discrimination and racism (Allan & Smylie, 2015; Gouvernement du Québec, 2019; Jacklin et al., 2017; Janzen et al., 2018; Loppie

Reading & Wien, 2009; Reading, 2009; Tang & Browne, 2008). Research has demonstrated that patients who experience racism and discrimination when receiving health care tend to anticipate such interactions with health professionals, under-utilize healthcare services and under-report their symptoms to health professionals (Allan & Smylie, 2015; Tang & Browne, 2008). This increases the intensity and frequency of crisis situations and delays screening and provision of care (Allan & Smylie, 2015; Gouvernement du Québec, 2019). Along with other microaggressions and environmental stressors that diminish the capacity to manage stress, experiences of racism and discrimination in health care contribute to the allostatic load of Indigenous populations, precipitating the decline of biological functions and increasing the risk of physical illnesses (Duru et al., 2012).

Many health professionals respond to the issue of racism by aiming to be socially and culturally neutral in their practice, consequently adopting a "culture-blind" approach to service delivery (i.e. asserting that race or ethnicity should not affect treatment) (Beagan & Kumas-Tan, 2009). However, this approach wrongly assumes that neutrality is possible and desirable while hindering recognition of the substantial impact of historical and socio-cultural factors on Indigenous patients' health. Health professionals who adopt a so-called "culturally neutral" practice may ignore the significant influence of generalized social patterns on Indigenous health (Beagan & Kumas-Tan, 2009), e.g. how intergenerational trauma and frequent experiences of racism impact stress, hypertension, depression or coping behaviours. Moreover, "culture blindness" in health care is a misnomer for a practice that defaults to dominant (Western) cultural beliefs and denies the existence of specific Indigenous worldviews and health perspectives (Beagan & Kumas-Tan, 2009; McKinstry, 2017).

Cultural safety is proposed as a transformative approach to health care that draws attention to the values, needs, expectations, rights and identities of Indigenous patients (Ramsden, 1990, 1992; Smye et al., 2010; Wood & Schwass, 1993). The goal of cultural safety is to support Indigenous patients by bringing attention to, and dismantling, the colonial lens of the healthcare system. The cultural safety approach emphasizes equal partnerships between professionals and patients, the commitment and active participation of patients/professionals in the provision of health care and protection of the cultural identities of Indigenous patients (Gerlach, 2012). Cultural safety offers a way to counter "culture-blind" approaches to care by bringing the cultural and social determinants of health to the forefront of care. In keeping with this perspective, the core characteristics of culturally safe care must be defined by the communities receiving the care, in accordance with their specific needs, their own values and cultural norms (Association des Médecins Indigènes du Canada and Association des facultés de médecine du Canada, 2009; Brascoupé & Waters, 2009). This shift in the power dynamics underlying current healthcare practices, structures and policies centres the historically marginalized voices, cultures and rights of Indigenous populations in the care they receive (Gerlach, 2012).

Although recognized by many actors as a promising idea with the potential to generate significant benefits for Indigenous patients (Aboriginal Nurses Association of Canada & Canadian Association of Schools of Nursing, 2009; Indigenous Physicians Association of Canada, & Association of Faculties of Medicine of

Canada, 2009), cultural safety remains a complex concept that is difficult to grasp and translate concretely into practice (Brascoupé & Waters, 2009; Gerlach, 2012). Implementation of cultural safety cannot be reduced to applying a checklist or by offering general guidelines (Gerlach, 2012). Moreover, because cultural safety is a relative concept that is both contextual and personal, there is currently no consistent way to define or assess its application (Brascoupé & Waters, 2009).

9.3 What Are the Ontological, Epistemological, Methodological and Ethical Premises of This Research Programme?

This research builds on the premise that for Indigenous needs, rights and identities to be fully taken into consideration in a Western-based healthcare system, we need corresponding research approaches that allow for the decolonization of Western science. In a decolonization approach to research, the purpose of research goes beyond producing new knowledge; it allows the research process to refocus on the specific knowledge, worldviews and methodologies of Indigenous peoples, in order to counteract the power relationships that are inherently embedded in Western knowledge production (Martin, 2012). In this research, we build on Two-Eyed Seeing, or Etuaptmumk in Mi'kmaq, a principle of research decolonization that promotes the integration of Indigenous and Western worldviews and ways of knowing (Bartlett et al., 2012; Iwama et al., 2009; Martin, 2012). Two-Eyed Seeing fosters an open and respectful dialogue between Indigenous and Western sciences (ways of knowing), including their various ontological, epistemological and methodological dimensions (Iwama et al., 2009). Building on this decolonization approach to knowledge production, this research aims to achieve a more effective way to address power differentials and colonialism in the healthcare system.

Enabling Two-Eyed Seeing first involves implementing participation and co-learning processes in which ways of knowing and worldviews from both visions (Indigenous and Western) can be brought together, discussed and integrated into relevant co-constructed solutions (Bartlett et al., 2015). This co-construction approach requires that researchers adopt a humble attitude towards co-learning, reflexively examine their beliefs, assumptions and values in the research process and welcome alternative perspectives and Indigenous spiritual wisdom (Bartlett et al., 2015). Thus, this research is ontologically rooted in a relative conception of reality, in which reality is a relational construct that can vary from different perspectives. On an epistemological level, this research builds on subjectivism, which holds that "reality" is constructed by the multiple experiences of social actors. On a methodological level, this research builds on a dialectical approach, welcoming methods established by not only Western science but also Indigenous narratives, stories, metaphors and spirituality as significant sources of knowledge informing the problems and situations at stake (Martin, 2012). For instance, in the process of creating the model, we used talking circles as a methodology to gather specific cultural significations, values and beliefs to incorporate with other types of data. In so doing, we aim to forge a unique vision that respectfully incorporates Atikamekw knowledge and ways of knowing, with the potential to better address the barriers presently faced by Atikamekw populations in the health system.

This research complies with the Chap. 9 of the Tri-Council Policy Statement principles for research involving the First Nations, Inuit and Métis peoples of Canada (Canadian Institutes of Health Research et al., 2018). This important statement formulates ethical principles such as seeking Indigenous engagement from communities, organizations and governing authorities in research; building on participatory or collaborative approaches to research; jointly defining the level of engagement of the different entities in research; considering the views of all relevant sectors (including marginalized voices) in the research process; fostering mutual benefits in research; respecting the relevant customs and codes of research that apply in specific communities; defining an engagement plan and setting out a research agreement with the involved communities (Canadian Institutes of Health Research et al., 2018).

In line with the principles of this policy statement, in this research, we sought engagement from, and developed respectful collaboration with, the Indigenous communities and organizations involved in the project. Owing to the pilot work (described below) and preliminary exploratory meetings with potential stakeholders, the research was developed based on the needs expressed by community stakeholders, thus ensuring that the research has mutual benefits. The objective of this project was identified and defined in partnership with the Atikamekw communities of Manawan, Wemotaci and Opitciwan as well as with the Atikamekw Nation Council (Conseil de la nation Atikamekw). After preliminarily defining the objective of the project with the Indigenous partners, we also established collaborations with actors of the health system (i.e. local health and social service authorities). We wanted to give priority to Indigenous voices to discuss the problems at hand before reaching out to stakeholders in the health system.

A participatory approach is considered a gold standard in health promotion research (Tremblay & Richard, 2014), but, for this research, meaningfully involving Indigenous stakeholders was considered a moral and political imperative. In practice, adopting a participatory approach helps safeguard the political, moral and ethical principles that fight oppression and allows a repositioning of the unique knowledge, beliefs and values of Indigenous peoples in research and various social institutions of society (Martin, 2012; Bartlett et al., 2012; Iwama et al., 2009; Bartlett et al., 2015; Canadian Institutes of Health Research et al., 2018; Tremblay & Richard, 2014; Assemblée des Premières Nations du Québec et du Labrador, 2014). Such an approach ensures the self-determination and capacity building of the stakeholders and actors involved in the process, facilitates the transfer of knowledge and its application in practice and promises significant and lasting effects for the parties involved (Baum et al., 2006; Cargo & Mercer, 2008). On initiation of this research, we approached the community councils that act as the authority for each community. The research project was presented to each of these community governance bodies and agreed upon through formal collaboration agreements. In addition, this research respects and upholds the principles established by the Assembly of First Nations, which are principles accepted by the community partners. This protocol stipulates specific principles regarding the ownership, control, access and possession of data and research results by the community partners. Based on these principles, each step of the research is based on a transparent process with the partners and the communities involved. It implies that the First Nations control data collection processes in their communities and that they own, protect and control how their information is used (Cargo & Mercer, 2008; Assemblée des Premières Nations du Québec et du Labrador, 2014).

9.3.1 How Was This Research Developed?

The research was designed to build on the results of a pilot community-based participatory study. The goal of the pilot study was to identify the potential barriers to and enablers of cultural safety in the provision of health care to Atikamekw populations in the province of Québec (Canada) (Tremblay et al., 2020). The pilot study was built on a qualitative descriptive design and involved conducting talking circles with different actors (Atikamekw patients and health professionals) to seek insights into the struggles that Indigenous patients face when interacting with health organizations and to generate ideas for practical solutions that could enhance cultural safety within clinical encounters and health organizations.

The study's most important finding was that racism is a major barrier to healthcare access for Indigenous populations, with many participants reporting having directly experienced or heard other Indigenous peoples describe receiving differential treatment due to their Indigenous status, not being taken seriously by health professionals or being treated disrespectfully (Tremblay et al., 2020). In addition, the current organization of health services was pinpointed as being ill-adapted to the social organization and values of the Atikamekw culture, by discouraging community social support and the involvement of the extended family in healthcare decisions. In contrast, health professional participants underlined the fact that congestion in the healthcare system and busy schedules make it hard to implement a patient-centred approach, which takes time but would allow better consideration of the cultural diversity of the clientele. Other important barriers to culturally safe healthcare access were related to language and communication. These barriers concern the fact that many Atikamekw are unable to obtain services in their own language (i.e. Atikamekw) if consulting outside their community. In addition, the medical jargon used by health professionals further exacerbates this issue, hindering mutual understanding and trust even when patients speak French. Finally, healthcare professionals' ignorance of Atikamekw traditional practices and cultural perspectives on health was underlined as an important obstacle to culturally safe care. Health professionals expressed their desire to know more but were unsure about where to start and how to apply this knowledge in practice (Tremblay et al., 2020).

Following the pilot study, a deliberative dialogue workshop (Lavis, 2010) was organized with all stakeholders of the project to discuss the results and prioritize potential solutions to improving cultural safety. A total of 21 people attended the event, including Atikamekw patients, representatives of the Atikamekw Council of Manawan, professionals from the Native Friendship Centre, health professionals and healthcare decision-makers from the local hospital and regional health and social service authority. Before the workshop, all participants received a summary of the results in an accessible language. Through small groups and plenary discussions, participants were invited to identify and prioritize potential solutions for improving the cultural safety of care. The proposed solution consisted of developing and implementing an intervention involving a new professional role dedicated to cultural safety in healthcare organizations. Participants of the workshop suggested involving the two other Atikamekw communities (Wemotaci and Opitciwan) in future research activities. Following this workshop, the research began to take form in close partnership with these three Indigenous partners as well as with the Atikamekw Nation Council. As we wanted to prioritize Indigenous voices and concerns in the project, the roles and nature of collaboration with regional health and social service authorities (in the three involved regions) were defined a little later in the project. Formal agreements were defined with these organizations, following the submission of a new grant application for this project. A representative from each regional authority was then delegated to take part in the project research team and serve as the contact person in the project.

9.3.2 The Research Governance

This research involves partnerships with academic, Indigenous and health service actors. We decided to adopt a ternary structure of governance inside the project to facilitate dialogue between the three entities embodied by the research team, the advisory committee and the regional health and social service authorities, respectively (Fig. 19.1). Each of these distinct partners brings crucial and specific expertise to the research: scientific expertise related to cultural safety and the organization of care; lived experience of the Atikamekw culture and concepts of health; and practical experience of the particular organizational contexts and related administrative or implementation constraints of the healthcare system. To foster cultural safety in the model being developed as well as in the research approach, we have put in place an advisory committee with representation from the three Atikamekw communities in Québec and a representative of the Atikamekw Nation Council. Composed of Atikamekw health professionals and community leaders, this advisory committee oversees and takes an active role in all steps of the project, meeting once every 6 weeks. It is responsible for providing work directions for development of the model, as well as for the project more generally, and for acting as a link between the research team and the communities. The research team is responsible for liaising with the participating regional health and social service authorities to

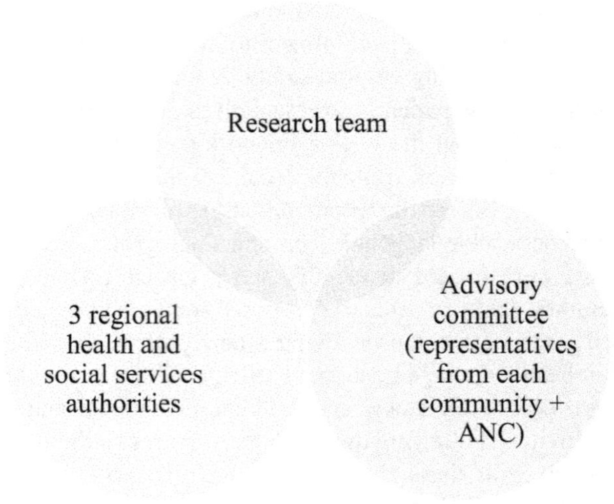

Fig. 19.1 Governance structure of the project

report on project progress, to mutually share information and to incorporate their comments, reactions and suggestions into the model. Representatives from these organizations will be invited to attend some of the advisory committee meetings, to take part in the crucial steps of the model's development and to contribute their practical knowledge of the healthcare system context. At the end of the initial development phase (1 year), a community forum will be organized to gather the perspectives of a broad base of actors from the three communities and the healthcare system sector.

For this research, we relied on different mechanisms to respectfully and meaningfully integrate Indigenous and Western ways of knowing and worldviews, following a Two-Eyed Seeing approach. These mechanisms include implementing strong, trusting relationships and formal processes of participation with Indigenous partners. This has been achieved through the engagement of the community partners since the beginning of the project and through the advisory committee. In addition, at the beginning of the project, a gathering including ceremonies was organized with all project partners and research team members, with the desire to build the communion required for this project to be successful. This gathering was supposed to be held in 2020 on the traditional lands of the Atikamekw but was finally held in 2021 due to the pandemic context. To develop a model that would weave together Indigenous and Western worldviews, we relied on different methodological traditions, such as a rapid literature reviews, to identify the fundamental components of cultural safety interventions in health care, as well as talking circles with Atikamekw Elders, healers and health professionals to identify the essential cultural elements that would inform the model (e.g. stories, narratives, values, meanings and perspectives of health). Building on all these sources of knowledge, the intervention model is being developed in full partnership with the advisory committee by weaving together Indigenous and Western perspectives and ways of knowing. A final important element to point out is the fact that many members of the advisory committee are Atikamekw health professionals and thus can more easily integrate the different forms of knowledge. Their cultural background coupled with their professional expertise nurtures rich and relevant perspectives that facilitate the articulation of diverse forms of knowledge within the model's development. So far, the main ideas for the intervention model include facilitation of bidirectional changes in healthcare organizations, i.e. changes at the interface of care that allow Indigenous patients and their families to better navigate the existing services and changes in professional and organizational practices that allow for greater openness to and consideration of Indigenous realities, value systems and practices in the healthcare system. The preliminary results of the project's development phase identified certain key elements to consider in the construction of the model, e.g. placing Indigenous staff at the centre of the intervention, supporting interprofessional collaboration within the care team and allowing the involvement of family in interventions. In addition to the community forum, later phases of the project will involve co-developing concrete modalities for intervention implementation with the advisory committee and partners.

One of the key challenges that we face in this project relates to the volatile and action-oriented nature of the health system context, especially in the aftermath of the death of Joyce Echaquan. Although this tragic event has brought public and political attention to the issue of racism against Indigenous peoples and has highlighted the need to rethink current healthcare practices, it has also meant a quickly evolving context for this project, one that requires constant adaptation to rapid changes in the political and institutional environments. At the end of 2020 and the beginning of 2021, for example, the federal (Gouvernement du Canada, 2021) and provincial governments (Gouvernement du Québec, 2020) allocated new funds to regional authorities and to the community of Manawan to foster cultural safety through training and new models of health care such as patient navigators. At around the same time, the Council of Manawan began a political process aiming to eradicate systemic racism in public institutions (see Joyce's Principle – Conseil des Atikamekw de Manawan and Conseil de la Nation Atikamekw, 2020). Although our team took part in the consultation for this brief, this was a political process carried out by the community of Manawan and the Atikamekw Nation Council. These sudden contextual transformations pose specific challenges related to adaptability as well as our position as a research team. Being a research team external to the health system, we must remain up to date and engaged in the ongoing transformations of the healthcare system via the three regional health and social service authorities participating in this project. To do so, we try to engage with high-level leadership within the different organizations as well as frequently mobilize our contact people in each organization. At the same time, to keep the trust of our Indigenous partners, it is important that we respect the inner pace and initial vision of the project by not rushing the model's development in response to external pressures or political agendas.

9.4 Conclusions

Health services are a determinant of health that play a role in increasing social health inequities and systemic marginalization of minorities such as Indigenous peoples (Allan & Smylie, 2015; Peiris et al., 2008; Tang & Browne, 2008). As such, health professionals and health organizations must be considered as key actors in the field of health promotion. This research, working at the intersection of public health and healthcare research, aims to contribute to the reorientation of health services towards ensuring culturally safe care, by building on respectful, reciprocal and equitable partnerships with Indigenous partners. To this effect, it builds on a decolonizing approach to research based on the principle of Two-Eyed Seeing, which promotes the respectful integration of Indigenous and Western knowledge and science in research. In so doing, this research centres the expertise of Indigenous communities in the development of solutions relevant to their needs and aims to elevate and integrate Indigenous conceptions of health, values and cultural practices into Canadian (Western-based) health and research systems. This research's approach and process propose useful research strategies for enacting the established values of health promotion such as participation, empowerment, social justice and equity. The major contributions of this research include advancement of the application of the principle of Two-Eyed Seeing, which is still little formalized or exemplified in the scientific literature, as well as proposing an approach to operationalize the concept of cultural safety in practice, in full partnership with local communities and healthcare stakeholders.

References

Allan, B., & Smylie, J. (2015). *First peoples, second class treatment: The role of racism in the health and well-being of indigenous peoples in Canada*. The Wellesley Institute: Toronto. 17 pages.

Assemblée des Premières Nations du Québec et du Labrador. (2014). *Protocole de recherche des Premières Nations au Québec et au Labrador*. APNQL, Wendake, 98 pages.

Aboriginal Nurses Association of Canada & Canadian Association of Schools of Nursing. (2009). *Cultural competency and cultural safety in nursing education. A framework for First Nations, Inuit and Métis nursing*. ANAC, Ottawa, 15 pages.

Indigenous Physicians Association of Canada, & Association of Faculties of Medicine of Canada. (2009). *First Nations, Inuit, Métis Health Core Competencies*. IPAC and AFMC, Ottawa, 7 pages.

Atikamekw Sipi. (2019). Atikamekw Sipi. https://www.atikamekwsipi.com/

Bartlett, C., Marshall, M., & Marshall, A. (2012). Two-eyed seeing and other lessons learned within a co-learning journey of bringing together indigenous and mainstream knowledges and ways of knowing. *Journal of Environmental Studies and Sciences, 2*(4), 331–340. https://doi.org/10.1007/s13412-012-0086-8

Bartlett, C., Marshall, M., Marshall, A., & Iwama, A. (2015). Integrative science and two-eyed seeing: Enriching the discussion framework for healthy communities. In *Ecosystems, society and health: Pathways through diversity, convergence and integration* (pp. 280–326). McGill-Queen's University Press.

Baum, F., MacDougall, C., & Smith, D. (2006). Participatory action research. *Journal of Epidemiology and Community Health, 60*(10), 854–857. https://doi.org/10.1136/jech.2004.028662

Beagan, B. L., & Kumas-Tan, Z. (2009). Approaches to diversity in family medicine: "I have always tried to be colour blind". *Canadian family physician Medecin de famille canadien, 55*(8), 21–28.

Brascoupé, S., & Waters, C. (2009). Cultural safety exploring the applicability of the concept of cultural safety to aboriginal health and community wellness. *Journal of Aboriginal Health, 5*(2), 6–41.

Buller, M., Audette, M., Robinson, Q., & Eyolfson, B. (2019). *Réclamer notre pouvoir et notre place: le rapport final de l'Enquête nationale sur les femmes et les filles autochtones disparues et assassinées*. Bureau du Conseil privé.

Canadian Institutes of Health Research, Natural Sciences and Engineering Research Council of Canada, and Social Sciences and Humanities Research Council. (2018) *Tri-Council Policy Statement: Ethical Conduct for Research Involving Humans.* TCPS, Ottawa, 23 pages.

Cargo, M., & Mercer, S. L. (2008). The value and challenges of participatory research: Strengthening its practice. *Annual Review of Public Health, 29*, 325–350. https://doi.org/10.1146/annurev.publhealth.29.091307.083824

Conseil des Atikamekw de Manawan, & Conseil de la Nation Atikamekw. (2020). Principe de Joyce: Mémoire présenté par le Conseil des Atikamekw de Manawan et le Conseil de la Nation Atikamekw. https://www.atikamekwsipi.com/public/images/wbr/uploads/telechargement/Doc_Principe-de-Joyce.pdf

Duru, O. K., Harawa, N. T., Kermah, D., & Norris, K. C. (2012). Allostatic load burden and racial disparities in mortality. *Journal of the National Medical Association, 104*(1–2), 89–95. https://doi.org/10.1016/s0027-9684(15)30120-6

Gao, S., Manns, B. J., Culleton, B. F., Tonelli, M., Quan, H., Crowshoe, L., et al. (2008). Access to health care among status aboriginal people with chronic kidney disease. *Canadian Medical Association Journal, 179*(10), 1007–1012. https://doi.org/10.1503/cmaj.080063

Gerlach, A. J. (2012). A critical reflection on the concept of cultural safety. *Canadian Journal of Occupational Therapy, 79*(3), 151–158. https://doi.org/10.2182/cjot.2012.79.3.4

Gouvernement du Canada. (2021, February 10). *Le gouvernement du Canada accorde deux millions de dollars au Conseil des Atikamekw de Manawan et au Conseil de la Nation Atikamekw pour soutenir le Principe de Joyce*. Gouvernement du Canada [Press release]. https://www.canada.ca/fr/services-autochtones-canada/nouvelles/2021/02/le-gouvernement-du-canada-accorde-deux-millions-de-dollars-au-conseil-des-atikamekw-de-manawan-et-au-conseil-de-la-nation-atikamekw-pour-soutenir-l.html

Gouvernement du Québec. (2019). *Commission d'enquête sur les relations entre les Autochtones et certains services publics: écoute, réconciliation et progrès* (Rapport final). Commission d'enquête sur les relations entre les Autochtones et certains services publics. https://www.cerp.gouv.qc.ca/fileadmin/Fichiers_clients/Rapport/Rapport_final.pdf

Gouvernement du Québec. (2020, November 6). Investissement de 15 M$ pour la sécurisation culturelle auprès des membres des Premières Nations et des Inuits dans le réseau de la santé et des services sociaux Québec [Press release]. https://www.msss.gouv.qc.ca/ministere/salle-de-presse/communique-2427/

Hackett, F. J., Abonyi, S., & Dyck, R. F. (2016). Anthropometric indices of First Nations children and youth on first entry to Manitoba/Saskatchewan residential schools-1919 to 1953. *International Journal of Circumpolar Health, 75*, 30734. https://doi.org/10.3402/ijch.v75.30734

Iwama, M., Marshall, M., Marshall, A., & Bartlett, C. (2009). Two-eyed seeing and the language of healing in community-based research. *Canadian Journal of Native Education, 32*, 3–23.

Jacklin, K. M., Henderson, R. I., Green, M. E., Walker, L. M., Calam, B., & Crowshoe, L. J. (2017). Health care experiences of Indigenous people living with type 2 diabetes in Canada. *Canadian Medical Association Journal, 189*(3), E106–E112. https://doi.org/10.1503/cmaj.161098

Janzen, B., Karunanayake, C., Rennie, D., Katapally, T., Dyck, R., McMullin, K., et al. (2018). Racial discrimination and depression among on-reserve First Nations people in rural Saskatchewan. *Canadian Journal of Public Health, 108*(5–6), e482–e487. https://doi.org/10.17269/cjph.108.6151

Kolahdooz, F., Nader, F., Kyoung, J. Y., & Sharma, S. (2015). Understanding the social determinants of health among Indigenous Canadians: Priorities for health promotion policies and actions. *Global Health Action, 8*(0), 1–16. https://doi.org/10.3402/gha.v8.27968

Lavis, J. (2010). *Organizing and evaluating deliberative dialogues in Canada and elsewhere*. 13es Journées annuelles de santé publique, Montreal. https://www.ncchpp.ca/docs/DeliberationJASP2010_LAVIS_EN.pdf

Kamel, G. (2021). Rapport d'enquête concernant le décès de Joyce Echaquan. Québec, CA: Bureau du coroner. https://www.coroner.gouv.qc.ca/fileadmin/Enquetes_publiques/2020-EP00275-9.pdf

Loppie Reading, C., & Wien, F. (2009). *Inégalités en matière de santé et déterminants sociaux de la santé des peuples autochtones* (Centre de collaboration national de la santé autochtone (Ed.)). Prince George

Marrone, S. (2007). Understanding barriers to health care: A review of disparities in health care services among indigenous populations. *International Journal of Circumpolar Health, 66*(3), 188–198. https://doi.org/10.3402/ijch.v66i3.18254

Martin, D. H. (2012). Two-eyed seeing: A framework for understanding indigenous and non-indigenous approaches to indigenous health research. *The Canadian Journal of Nursing Research, 44*(2), 20–42.

McKinstry, S. (2017). Indigenous oral health inequity: An indigenous provider perspective. *Canadian Journal of Public Health, 108*(3), e221–e223. https://doi.org/10.17269/CJPH.108.6243

Peiris, D., Brown, A., & Cass, A. (2008). Addressing inequities in access to quality health care for indigenous people. *CMAJ, 179*(10), 985–986. https://doi.org/10.1503/cmaj.081445

Ramsden, I. (1990). Cultural safety. *The New Zealand Nursing Journal Kai Tiaki, 83*(11), 18–19.

Ramsden, I. (1992). Teaching cultural safety. *The New Zealand Nursing Journal, 85*(5), 21–23.

Reading, J. (2009). *Les déterminants sociaux de la santé chez les Autochtones : Approche fondée sur le parcours de vie.* Ottawa: Sous-comité sénatorial sur la santé de la population. 164 pages.

Smye, V., Josewski, V., & Kendall, E. (2010). *Cultural safety: An overview.* Mental Health Commission of Canada Canada, First Nations, Inuit and Métis Advisory Committee. https://www.troubleshumeur.ca/documents/Publications/CULTURAL%20SAFETY%20AN%20OVERVIEW%20(draft%20mar%202010).pdf

Tang, S. Y., & Browne, A. J. (2008). 'Race' matters: Racialization and egalitarian discourses involving aboriginal people in the Canadian health care context. *Ethnicity & Health, 13*(2), 109–127. https://doi.org/10.1080/13557850701830307

Tremblay, M. C., & Richard, L. (2014). Complexity: A potential paradigm for a health promotion discipline. *Health Promotion International, 29*(2), 378–388. https://doi.org/10.1093/heapro/dar054

Tremblay, M. C., Bradette-Laplante, M., Witteman, H. O., Dogba, M. J., Breault, P., Paquette, J. S., et al. (2020). Providing culturally safe care to indigenous people living with diabetes: Identifying barriers and enablers from different perspectives. *Health Expectations*. https://doi.org/10.1111/hex.13168

Truth and Reconciliation Commission of Canada. (2015). *Truth and Reconciliation Commission of Canada: Calls to action.* https://www2.gov.bc.ca/assets/gov/british-columbians-our-governments/indigenous-people/aboriginal-peoples-documents/calls_to_action_english2.pdf

Wood, P. J., & Schwass, M. (1993). Cultural safety: A framework for changing attitudes. *Nursing Praxis in New Zealand, 8*(1), 4–15.

Zambas, S. I., & Wright, J. (2016). Impact of colonialism on Maori and aboriginal healthcare access: A discussion paper. *Contemporary Nurse, 52*(4), 398–409. https://doi.org/10.1080/10376178.2016.1195238

Chapter 10
Conducting Research with People: Hepatitis C and Intensive Engagement with High-Risk Occupational Groups in Karachi, Pakistan

Tassawar Ali and Nance Cunningham

10.1 Introduction

This chapter describes the research approach implemented with the aim of developing a population's capacity to fight against the neglect and spread of hepatitis C virus (HCV). The intervention, aiming to promote the engagement of hepatitis C diagnosis and treatment in high-risk occupational groups of hepatitis C in urban Pakistan, falls under the heading of health promotion because it goes beyond simply informing the public to invoke various determinants of community engagement against hepatitis C and builds awareness and creates interest among the inhabitants to respond to this silent epidemic. In this chapter, we will look at the role of research and health promotion in a project for intensive engagement of hepatitis C diagnosis and treatment in high-risk occupational groups of hepatitis C in urban Pakistan. We begin with a background of HCV and the HCV epidemic in Pakistan. After noting the characteristics of HCV and Machar Colony, which makes for an appropriate site for a health promotion intervention, we describe in detail the health promotion implementation research.

T. Ali (✉)
Médecins Sans Frontières/Doctors Without Borders, Karachi West, Pakistan
e-mail: tassawara83@gmail.com

N. Cunningham
University of British Columbia, Vancouver, BC, Canada

British Columbia Centre for Excellence in HIV/AIDS, Vancouver, BC, Canada

L. Potvin, D. Jourdan (eds.), *Global Handbook of Health Promotion Research, Vol. 1*,
https://doi.org/10.1007/978-3-030-97212-7_10

10.2 HCV Background

HCV causes great loss of life around the world and in Pakistan (Thrift et al., 2017; Hafez, 2018) Details of historical spread are speculative, as there was no test for the virus until 1989, but, by the early twenty-first century, more than 1 in 100 people worldwide had been exposed to HCV, and infection persisted in about 7 out of 10 (Noor-Ul-Huda et al., 2016; Blach et al., 2017). If HCV infection is not cleared by the immune system within 6 months or treated, it typically becomes a lifelong infection, and a significant proportion of people with chronic infection will suffer liver damage (Seeff, 2009). Although HCV can cause liver damage within a few years, more typically liver cirrhosis, cancer or other irreversible damage does not begin for a decade or longer (Kanwal et al., 2014).

In Pakistan, at the time of a 2007 survey, nearly 5% of the population had been exposed to HCV (Qureshi et al., 2010). At the time of the 2007 national survey, HCV antibody prevalence in the Sindh province, where Karachi is located, was estimated at 5.0%; in a 2019 estimate, the prevalence in Sindh had climbed to 7% (Mahmud et al., 2019). HCV has only humans as a reservoir (Pfaender et al., 2014). It is mainly spread through blood contact and probably initially spread widely through transfusions and contaminated shared medical equipment (Thrift et al., 2017). Even after HCV tests became available, blood, plasma and other blood products have not always been universally tested (Luby et al., 1997; Safe Blood Transfusion Programme, 2013; Alaei et al., 2018) Although sterilization of medical and other skin-piercing equipment improved after the implementation of universal precautions spurred by HIV-related policies, medical and dental equipment are still a source of HCV transmission where there are lapses in sterilization. HCV is believed to spread mainly outside formal medical facilities in Pakistan, but, aside from a few outbreaks, the extent of transmission from different sources is unknown (Khan et al., 2020). HCV can remain infective for days or weeks on contaminated equipment and could be transmitted via shared hookah and pipe stems, razors, ear-piercing needles, suturing needles, syringes, tattooing equipment, equipment for other treatments such as cupping and acupuncture and any shared sharps, including for substance use (Safi et al., 2012; Waheed et al., 2009; Paintsil et al., 2014).

Treatment for HCV with direct-acting antiviral agents (DAAs) is effective during the acute and chronic phases of infection (Abozeid et al., 2018; Capileno et al., 2017). There is no vaccine for HCV, and immunity is weak, causing most reinfections to result in chronic infection (Hajarizadeh et al., 2020; Martinello et al., 2019). Even though HCV may not have an impact on health immediately, people with HCV should be treated early in their infection. Early treatment minimizes the chance of transmission to others and maximizes the chance of a cure with DAAs (Nahon et al., 2017).

10.3 The Determinants of HCV Transmission in the Population

HCV is an excellent target for health promotion intervention, as it is a virus with no animal reservoir, causing great human and economic burdens, with known and controllable transmission pathways and with a cure (Hajarizadeh et al., 2016; Martinello et al., 2019). Accurate and affordable tests can detect it, and 95% of cases can be cured within 6 months by a drug with few adverse effects. Most HCV transmissions can be interrupted when institutions follow the existing regulations for testing and sterilization and by motivated individual actions, which are neither difficult nor expensive. However, in practice, a pattern of frequent low-risk exposures over the course of years makes it difficult to prevent transmission in the general public in Pakistan. The behaviours that spread it are different in different populations and places, as are the ways to interrupt transmission. The risks also change over time. Surveys of HCV prevalence and risk behaviours reflect the lifetime risk of those behaviours, not the current risk of the same behaviours. History of blood transfusion was a risk factor, but blood transfusions were far more risky in the twentieth century, before testing of donated blood became widespread. The average number of injections per year was also seen as a significant risk factor in national surveys in Pakistan. However, single-use needles have come down in price and in the late 2010s are much more common than any time earlier. The current major risks were not known with confidence. Health promotion research can identify the most likely transmission routes in a context, allowing prevention efforts to focus on the highest risk behaviours while continuing general health education.

10.4 The Context: Machar Colony in Karachi

Karachi is Pakistan's largest city, with a population of about 20 million, approximately 10% of the total population of Pakistan. Machar Colony, also called Muhammadi Colony, is one of the largest unplanned, informal settlements of Karachi. Machar Colony comprises 4.5 km^2 and is bordered by the Port of Karachi in the south, a mangrove forest in the west, a shoreline in the north and a railway line in the east. The population is estimated to be 120,000. Machar Colony is home to people of a variety of ethnicities, including Bengalis, Burmis, Sindhis, Pashtuns, Punjabis and other smaller communities. The population has a steady natural growth, but there is little movement into the area. According to project research, most resident families have been living in the Machar Colony for at least 20 years.

There are large economic and cultural differences in Machar Colony. The communities tend to live and work separately. The large businesses are mainly in the fishing industry. The Bengali and Burmi communities mainly live near the port in the southern part of Machar Colony, where most families are supported by work in fisheries in one way or another. Common work includes catching fish or shrimp, whether on boats that go out daily or for weeks or months at a time, cleaning fish, peeling shrimp, packing the processed seafood and building or breaking fishing ships. There are many small businesses and market stalls as well. In Bengali and Burmi families, many of the women are employed in the fishing industry. More of the Pashtu population lives in the northern part of Machar, and many of the men work in transport. In the Pashtu community, women are much less likely to work outside the home, and, in many families, women have limited access to education and have low health autonomy. The common language in Pakistan generally is Urdu, but, in Machar Colony, many of the adults do not understand Urdu. Many Machar residents speak only their mother tongue, some with additional languages other than Urdu. Literacy in any language is also low. Not all Machar Colony community members are legally registered with the government, and those without government identification cards have restricted opportunities to access employment and education. A national identification card is necessary to receive hepatitis C treatment from the government health service.

10.5 Health Promotion Actors and Activities

The prominent social actors in Machar Colony included imams and other religious leaders, large business owners and community leaders from the various ethnic communities. Health care was provided by one government health clinic, a handful of free clinics operated by not-for-profit organizations and numerous unlicensed health practitioners of various levels of skills and knowledge. The majority of healthcare service was from unlicensed practitioners, who ranged from trained nurses and pharmacists to people with no formal education. Demand for their services was high, as they provided quick and inexpensive relief, in most cases by injection.

Médecins Sans Frontières (MSF), a medical humanitarian organization, began working in Machar Colony in 2012, building on a history of working in Pakistan since 1986. MSF had collaborated with health authorities in various parts of the country. From 2012, MSF supported and expanded the work of a Sina Health, Education and Welfare Trust clinic. Sina is a community service not-for-profit organization working since 1998. Sina and MSF operated a primary healthcare clinic (PHC) in Machar Colony on an open-door model, offering outpatient care free of cost to all who arrived at their facility. In addition to typical primary health care, the Machar Colony PHC provided emergency services, transfer to hospital, hepatitis C care and health promotion (HP) activities. The nine-member HP team included seven health promoters. Among their HP activities, they verbally screened people waiting in the PHC clinic for HCV risk factors and offered HCV testing if any results were positive. For those who tested positive, further laboratory tests needed for diagnosis and HCV treatment were offered.

At the time, most hepatitis care in Pakistan was offered out of tertiary care hospitals. Operational research carried out at the Machar Colony clinic demonstrated the effectiveness of MSF's decentralized model of care (Capileno et al., 2017;

Khalid et al., 2018). The decentralized care brought highly effective HCV treatment for uncomplicated cases to the PHC level but still relied on patients seeking health care at the clinic.

In 2019, the clinic building was slated for demolition. Sina put their resources into their other clinics. MSF converted their project to a dedicated clinic for screening and treating HCV and developed further collaborations with local health partners in Machar Colony. The HP component and its expanded community-based approach were crucial for the project to achieve its objective of a high standard of care reaching the segments of the population with the poorest access to health care. The health promotion team had already carried out community-based health education work in the PHC phase of the project. In the HCV-clinic phase, work in the community intensified as new core objectives of the health promotion programme were developed.

The health promotion team's five major roles in the project's 2019 strategy reflected a socio-ecological theoretical model, which seeks to understand and support a community as a set of interacting systems. In this case, the systems ranged from the individual, household and close-knit cultural communities through outer systems of employment and informal and formal health care. The roles were: (1) active case finding focusing on the key populations in the community, (2) collaboration with local health partners, (3) household treatment, including supporting individual patient adherence and tracing, (4) specialized prevention activities for those who pose a transmission hazard to others and (5) community sensitization for the general public. The monitoring and evaluation was designed to increase the project's efficiency and provide an understanding of Machar Colony's population dynamics and occupational issues related to HCV.

10.6 Producing Knowledge with the Communities in Machar Colony

Community leaders in Machar Colony were supportive of MSF's presence and services. As is typical of a silent epidemic, despite its high prevalence, HCV was not well known among leaders or community members before MSF began providing testing and treatment in 2012. By the time MSF opened the dedicated HCV clinic in 2019, community leaders had a good understanding of HCV, and some had been treated for it.

Community support was key to reaching the different communities in Machar Colony, but more information was needed to provide testing and treatment to people who needed them most. It was clear that relying on the passive case finding of the open-door model would not reach them. To make the greatest, fastest and longest lasting reduction in HCV prevalence and transmission, the project needed the HP team to understand more about the communities in Machar Colony. Little reliable data were available about Machar Colony's demographics, social and economic factors, health status, health-related infrastructure or HCV prevalence at the start of the project. The lack of data made planning for a health promotion approach difficult. In order to better serve the community, the HP team expanded screening questions to include information about occupations, household size, mobility, language proficiency, health information preferences, health-seeking behaviour and HCV knowledge.

This research enabled the HP team to better match its resources to the community needs. It showed how the community interacted with the health service systems. It also allowed the team to adapt health messages to community knowledge and beliefs and to find segments of the community with the least knowledge of HCV. Questions about people's sources for health information revealed the preferences of different linguistic and demographic communities, allowing for more efficient communication. Open-answer questions about HCV showed what was generally known about HCV and what misunderstandings prevailed. This allowed the HP team to monitor how health education messages about HCV were received by the population and to adapt the health education talks to address rumours or other issues as they arose. Incorporating the additional questions into the screening allowed the HP team to show that many of those who tested positive worked in the fishing industry and were monolingual Bengali or Burmi.

The next step for the HP team was to act on the information emerging from this research and invoke connections with community leaders to arrange for testing of fisheries workers. Factory owners were supportive and allowed the HP team to provide health education to all the workers at each worksite, during workday hours. The MSF team offered individual pre-test counselling in all languages spoken. The uptake of the screening test was extremely high. All received post-test counselling in their preferred language, and those who tested antibody positive were linked to care. The HP team developed a typology of factories as more were tested, allowing outreach and community work to focus on the type likely to have the highest prevalence of HCV. At various workplaces, generally with 100–200 employees tested, 15%–35% of fisheries workers tested positive for antibodies to HCV.

All people who tested antibody positive, and who did not live alone, were counselled to have household members tested. More HCV-positive persons were found in the households. Those who were under working age, housebound or others who otherwise would be unlikely to receive testing could receive testing services in this way. MSF continued to gather data during the screening processes, accumulating evidence to allow for better estimates of HCV health needs and to allow for planning to match the number of patients with the treatment capacity of the clinic.

10.7 Gathering Data and Risk Mapping for Further Steps

Based on the outreach testing, it appeared that fish packing was one high-risk occupation for HCV. The basis of the risk was working with sharps and contact with surfaces handled by other workers. The HP team's mapping of potential transmission risks in Machar Colony had provided a basis for further contact with other high-risk groups as well. Traditional birth attendants also worked with sharps and encountered blood. Beauticians and barbers used razors on many customers and may encounter traces of blood. Unlicensed local health practitioners handled minor injuries and illnesses and gave injections to about 95% of their customers. Truck drivers visited such local practitioners in many different places along their driving routes, and some were at higher risk of sexual transmission. Each of these occupational groups had formal or informal leading bodies, with which the HP team was in contact. The HP team was able to work with these bodies to contact participants for further research and analysis.

The HP team held focus group discussions with members of each of these occupational groups. In the focus group discussions, participants shared their concerns, revealed their HCV-related knowledge and gave detailed information about practices with a potential to transmit HCV. The goal of the HP team was to understand both the participants' concerns about and risk of acquiring HCV when practicing as usual and the risk of transmitting HCV to clients, co-workers or other contacts. This allowed the HP team to respond to occupation-specific concerns and offer the most relevant information and support to each group. In some cases, the HP team was able to offer participants HCV testing and priority for initiating HCV treatment in the MSF clinic. Once the HP team had data, allowing a better understanding of the typical risks of each occupation and some indication of the prevalence of HCV as well, the team could establish priorities for interventions in partnership with members of these communities.

The results of testing of high-risk occupational groups other than fish factory workers ranged from no positives (among 5 beauticians) to 57% positive (8 of 14 traditional birth attendants). While the total number tested was small (121 potential high-risk occupation workers were tested outside the fish factories), overall, 17% tested antibody positive, 2.4 times the provincial average, and all 21 were diagnosed with active HCV infection, raising the ratio to about 2.7 times the provincial average.

Most concerning was the HCV prevalence among 58 members of groups, which could spread HCV to many others through networks, namely, local health practitioners, barbers, beauticians and traditional birth attendants. Testing of a total of 58 persons revealed a prevalence of chronic HCV infection of 28%, more than 4.5 times the provincial average. These findings were only provisional, as they were from a convenience sample of a small number of persons. Nevertheless, the results were indicative of a need for further attention. The plausibility of high prevalence was sufficient justification for planning further activities with these groups. However, prevalence findings could not be shared with the groups because of medical confidentiality concerns.

Transport workers did not have the same potential to transmit HCV through a well-defined client network. Nevertheless, they were of particular interest, as people who may have elevated risk while on the road, and 63 were tested. Prevalence in the sample was at 8%, slightly above the estimated provincial average. This was a small convenience sample which cannot be generalized to all drivers or other transport workers. However, drivers were of epidemiological concern as they are some of the few Machar Colony residents who regularly travel in and out of the community. They would need special attention in future comprehensive prevention efforts aimed at eliminating HCV in Machar Colony. For example, transport workers could be among the groups that are offered annual testing.

This work, carried out not on the populations but with them, makes it possible to help them understand silent risk, react to their most urgent concerns, prioritize risks and activities according to community values, give meaning to the data collected and organize the activities for safer occupational practice with the trust and support of the community.

10.8 Conclusions

Ideally, all health promotion projects would take place after thorough community consultation and a comprehensive needs assessment. In practice, many projects are subjected to severe constraints in terms of human resources, time pressures, changing circumstances and scant data. Some health issues, including HCV, are not apparent to the communities that they affect. This highly successful health promotion programme is an example of one built on the known strengths of health promotion, including hiring from the communities and consultation with a variety of community stakeholders. As the project progressed, the HP team was able to gather data to increase its understanding of and connections with the key populations in the community. Community leaders, including religious leaders who were highly prominent, and also business leaders, occupational bodies and influential community members became more knowledgeable and concerned about HCV as they became aware of its extent and effects in their communities.

As a primary healthcare clinic transformed into a dedicated hepatitis C clinic, the HP department collected specific data while carrying out its usual activities, which enabled recognition of previously unidentified priority areas and populations. This allowed the project to allocate resources to where they were most needed. The HP team reached high-prevalence populations and established a strong basis for community-based prevention activities in high-risk occupations. In doing so, they deepened their connections with the community, allowing communities to address the risks in their practices as the team learned about sensitive issues, such as lack of instrument sterilization and sexual behaviours, which put participants at higher risk of HCV transmission. Research was tightly integrated into health promotion activities, and all team members were encouraged to contribute knowledge and ideas for next steps. The results were shared with other departments and helped guide the priorities of the project. Findings were also shared with the population through key stakeholders and through direct community connections and contacts, which facilitated knowledge exchange and relationships of mutual respect.

References

Abozeid, M., Alsebaey, A., Abdelsameea, E., Othman, W., Elhelbawy, M., Rgab, A., et al. (2018). High efficacy of generic and brand direct acting antivirals in treatment of chronic hepatitis C. *International Journal of Infectious Diseases, 75*, 109–114. https://doi.org/10.1016/j.ijid.2018.07.025

Alaei, K., Sarwar, M., & Alaei, A. (2018). The urgency to mitigate the spread of hepatitis C in Pakistan through blood transfusion reform [Report]. *International Journal of Health Policy and Management, 7*, 207–209. https://doi.org/10.15171/ijhpm.2017.120

Blach, S., Zeuzem, S., Manns, M., Altraif, I., Duberg, A. S., Muljono, D. H., et al. (2017). Global prevalence and genotype distribution of hepatitis C virus infection in 2015: A modelling study. *The Lancet Gastroenterology and Hepatology, 2*(3), 161-176, doi: https://doi.org/https://doi.org/10.1016/S2468-1253(16)30181-9.

Capileno, Y. A., Van Den Bergh, R., Donchunk, D., Hinderaker, S. G., Hamid, S., Auat, R., et al. (2017). Management of chronic hepatitis C at a primary health clinic in the high-burden context of Karachi, Pakistan. *PLoS ONE, 12*(4). https://doi.org/10.1371/journal.pone.0175562

Hafez, T. A. (2018). Public health and economic burden of Hepatitis C infection in developing countries. In S. M. Kamal (Ed.), *Hepatitis C in developing countries: Current and future challenges* (pp. 25–32). Academic Press.

Hajarizadeh, B., Grebely, J., Martinello, M., Matthews, G. V., Lloyd, A. R., & Dore, G. J. (2016). *Hepatitis C treatment as prevention: evidence, feasibility, and challenges* (Vol. 1, pp. 317–327). Elsevier Ltd.

Hajarizadeh, B., Cunningham, E. B., Valerio, H., Martinello, M., Law, M., Janjua, N. Z., et al. (2020). Hepatitis C reinfection after successful antiviral treatment among people who inject drugs: A meta-analysis. *J Hepatol, 72*(4), 643–657. https://doi.org/10.1016/j.jhep.2019.11.012

Kanwal, F., Kramer, J. R., Ilyas, J., Duan, Z., & El-Serag, H. B. (2014). HCV genotype 3 is associated with an increased risk of cirrhosis and hepatocellular cancer in a national sample of U.S. Veterans with HCV, Hepatology (Baltimore, MD), *60*(1), 98-105, doi:https://doi.org/https://doi.org/10.1002/hep.27095.

Khalid, G. G., Kyaw, K. W. Y., Bousquet, C., Auat, R., Donchuk, D., Trickey, A., et al. (2018). From risk to care: the hepatitis C screening and diagnostic cascade in a primary health care clinic in Karachi, Pakistan—a cohort study. *International Health*. https://doi.org/10.1093/inthealth/ihy096

Khan, A., Altaf, A., Qureshi, H., Orakzai, M., & Khan, A. (2020). Reuse of syringes for therapeutic injections in Pakistan: Rethinking determinants. *Eastern Mediterranean Health Journal, 26*(3), 283–289. https://doi.org/10.26719/emhj.19.028

Luby, S. P., Qamruddin, K., Shah, A. A., Omair, A., Pahsa, O., Khan, A. J., et al. (1997). The relationship between therapeutic injections and high prevalence of hepatitis C infection in Hafizabad, Pakistan. *Epidemiology and Infection, 119*(3), 349–356. https://doi.org/10.1017/s0950268897007899

Mahmud, S., Al Kanaani, Z., & Abu-Raddad, L. J. (2019). Characterization of the hepatitis C virus epidemic in Pakistan. *BMC Infectious Diseases, 19*(1), 809. https://doi.org/10.1186/s12879-019-4403-7

Martinello, M., Hajarizadeh, B., Grebely, J., Matthews, G. V., & Dore, G. J. (2019). Cure and control: What will it take to eliminate HCV? In M. J. Sofia (Ed.), *HCV: The journey from discovery to a cure* (Vol. II, pp. 447–490, Current topics in medicinal chemistry, Vol. 32). Springer Nature.

Nahon, P., Bourcier, V., Layese, R., Audureau, E., Cagnot, C., Marcellin, P., et al. (2017). Eradication of hepatitis C virus infection in patients with cirrhosis reduces risk of liver and non-liver complications. *Gastroenterology, 152*(1), 142-156 e142. https://doi.org/10.1053/j.gastro.2016.09.009

Noor-Ul-Huda, G., Shafique, A., Muhammad Qasim, H., & Anjum, S. (2016). The phylogeographic and spatiotemporal spread of HCV in Pakistani population. *PLoS ONE, 11*(10). https://doi.org/10.1371/journal.pone.0164265

Paintsil, E., Binka, M., Patel, A., Lindenbach, B. D., & Heimer, R. (2014). Hepatitis C virus maintains infectivity for weeks after drying on inanimate surfaces at room temperature: Implications for risks of transmission. *The Journal of Infectious Diseases, 209*(8), 1205–1211. https://doi.org/10.1093/infdis/jit648

Pfaender, S., Brown, R. J., Pietschmann, T., & Steinmann, E. (2014). Natural reservoirs for homologs of hepatitis C virus. *Emerging Microbes & Infections, 3*(3), e21–e21. https://doi.org/10.1038/emi.2014.19

Qureshi, H., Bile, K. M., Jooma, R., Alam, S. E., & Afridi, H. U. R. (2010). Prevalence of hepatitis B and C viral infections in Pakistan: Findings of a national survey appealing for effective prevention and control measures. *Eastern Mediterranean Health Journal, 16*, S15–S23. https://doi.org/10.26719/2010.16.Supp.15

Safe Blood Transfusion Programme. (2013). *National baseline survey based on WHO evaluation framework/tool for assessment, monitoring and evaluation of blood screening systems in Pakistan.* https://www.who.int/bloodsafety/transfusion_services/PakistanMonitoringEvaluationBloodScreeningSystems.pdf. Accessed 19 Sept 2020.

Safi, A. Z., Waheed, Y., Sadat, J., Solat Ul, I., Salahuddin, S., Saeed, U., et al. (2012). Molecular study of HCV detection, genotypes and their routes of transmission in North West Frontier Province, Pakistan. *Asian Pacific Journal of Tropical Biomedicine, 2*(7), 532–536. https://doi.org/10.1016/s2221-1691(12)60091-4

Seeff, L. B. (2009). The history of the "natural history" of hepatitis C (1968–2009). *Liver International, 29*, 89–99. https://doi.org/10.1111/j.1478-3231.2008.01927.x

Thrift, A. P., El-Serag, H. B., & Kanwal, F. (2017). Global epidemiology and burden of HCV infection and HCV-related disease [Report]. *Nature Reviews Gastroenterology & Hepatology, 14*, 122–132.

Waheed, Y., Shafi, T., Safi, S. Z., & Qadri, I. (2009). Hepatitis C virus in Pakistan: A systematic review of prevalence, genotypes and risk factors. *World Journal of Gastroenterology, 15*(45), 5647–5653. https://doi.org/10.3748/wjg.15.5647

Chapter 11
Respectful Maternity Care: A Methodological Journey from Research to Policy and Action

Manmeet Kaur

11.1 Introduction

Health promotion relates to behaviours within social and physical environments. However, human behaviour has been mostly linked to biological and psychological traits, and the role that society plays in shaping the behaviours has largely been ignored (Cacioppo et al., 2000). Psychological theories have predominated in explaining human behaviours, but power relations in society cannot be ignored as determinants of behaviour (Guinote, 2007). Power does not necessarily come from personality, but from knowledge and skills, broadly in line with an individual's socio-economic standing in society (Gaventa & Cornwall, 2008).

Power relations also play an important role in the healthcare system, irrespective of the clamour for ethics and rights (Nimmon & Stenfors-Hayes, 2016; Miller & Lalonde, 2015). Often, although health service providers use the power of knowledge, they fail to provide the space for health service users to express their needs. Power relations are also visible in the maternity care provided to women in a healthcare facility setting where disrespect and abuse are prevalent across the globe (Miller & Lalonde, 2015). According to World Health Organization, Respectful Maternity Care (RMC) means "care organized for and provided to all women in a manner that maintains their dignity, privacy and confidentiality, ensures freedom from harm and mistreatment, and enables informed choice and continuous support during labour" (WHO, 2018). It indicates that respect in maternity care is the responsibility of the service provider.

As a result, the RMC research was envisaged to help understand the behaviours of service providers, advocate with policymakers to review and revise policies and

M. Kaur (✉)
School of Public Health, Post Graduate Institute of Medical Education and Research, Chandigarh, India
e-mail: kaur.manmeet@pgimer.edu.in

L. Potvin, D. Jourdan (eds.), *Global Handbook of Health Promotion Research, Vol. 1*,
https://doi.org/10.1007/978-3-030-97212-7_11

programmes and engage with service providers for participatory action for RMC in a tertiary care hospital in North India. Several theoretical and methodological issues were encountered during the conceptualization and implementation phases of this project, particularly while linking the research to advocacy, a process that is at the heart of health promotion.

11.2 The Context

In India, many women die while giving birth. Birthing at home was a common practice in India until recently, but, by 2015, 70% of women were presenting themselves for childbirth at health institutions (MoH&FW, 2017a). Birthing at a health facility has been considered a key intervention to save mothers and newborns in India where the maternal mortality ratio per 100,000 live births is still 113. However, the increase in the institutional delivery rate has not led to the expected decline in maternal and newborn mortality. Both policymakers and researchers have raised concerns about the "quality of care" available to women birthing in public health facilities. Some of the observed disrespect and violence to which women were subjected during delivery at such facilities was considered to be a factor that discouraged women from approaching health institutions for birthing, even when facing complications or needing specialized care.

As the Government of India had already initiated a programme for improving the quality of maternity care by improving the hospital infrastructure and technical capacities of health service providers, we initiated a project on respectful maternity care with financial support from the MacArthur Foundation, the Centre for Catalyzing Change (C3) and the White Ribbon Alliance.

11.3 Project Conceptualization

The fundamental question we needed to answer was how disrespect has emerged between the service user and service provider, and, so, the first call was to understand the unequal relationship between service providers and service users. The scientific literature on this question was scanty. We reviewed the history of medicine and public health and realized that the balance in power relations between a service user and a service provider has been contextual, i.e. different in different political and economic structures (Addicott & Ferlie, 2007).

In the Indian context, incidents of violence were reported in healthcare institutions. Although the vast majority of incidents involved disrespect or abuse of patients by service providers, it should be noted that there have also been cases of service users using violence against service providers who were perceived to be providing low-quality services or were perceived to be negligent (Kumar et al.,

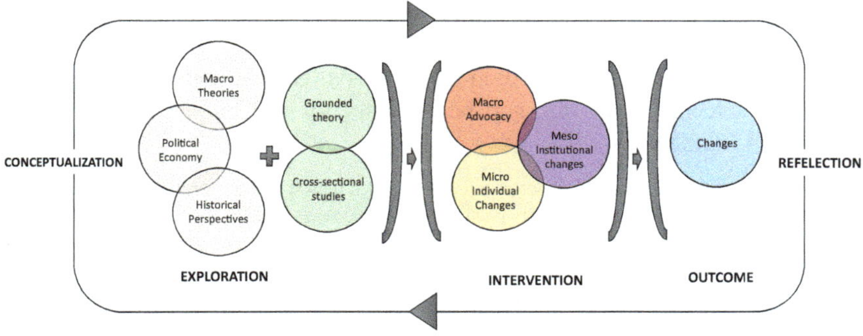

Fig. 11.1 RMC: paradigms of change

2016). This indicated that the power of knowledge (of service providers) can be challenged by those who are most vulnerable (the users of service).

It was expected that understanding the drivers of disrespect and abuse, as well as changing behaviours and advocating for the rights of women seeking maternity care, might be another phase in the history of medicine and public health, and a multidisciplinary approach would be required to understand the phenomenon of power relations in a medical setting. Therefore, a team comprising an epidemiologist, a sociologist, a social psychologist, an anthropologist, a gynaecologist and a lawyer was put together to work on the RMC project, for providing both theoretical and methodological inputs. According to Davies, "a discipline needs the ability to attract like-minded individuals and groups with similar beliefs, goals and vision" (Davies, 2013). Hence, the RMC project adopted a multidisciplinary approach.

After extensive deliberations, a novel approach of linking research to policy and action was agreed. It differed from most of the earlier approaches, which focused on individual behaviour change and usually ignored organizational and social changes (Baum & Fisher, 2014). After considering the chaos theory (Gleick, 1987), the use of social structural theories was considered to be apt for the RMC project. A critical realist approach advocated by Bhaskar (Bhaskar, 1975), in which there is space for being critical, was used to help understand the whole of society in the context of its history. This was useful in planning the paradigms of change for the RMC project from exploration to intervention and outcome (Fig. 11.1). The intervention strategy was kept flexible for policy, institutional and individual contexts.

11.4 Research Strategy

In scientific disciplines, a conventionally positivist approach is used to provide evidence that is based on experiments, e.g. randomized controlled trials (RCTs). However, science is a product of historical development. The constructivist approach has broken the boundaries and limits of the rules on what evidence means. Therefore, in the RMC study, we carefully followed both positivist and constructivist approaches in the various phases of the project.

The RMC project was carried out in three phases. The methods used in all three phases were selected to fill the gap between theory and empirical learning, as according to Charmaz:

> neither data nor theories are discovered but are constructed by the researcher as a result of their interactions with the field and its participants (Charmaz, 2000).

We ensured that each phase had its own specific methodology and that a separate protocol was submitted for financial support and ethical approval for each phase. However, each phase is linked with other phases starting from the conceptualization through to outcomes and reflections on changes made in policies and practices.

11.4.1 Phase I: Evidence for Advocacy

The aim in the first phase of the RMC study was to provide evidence on the extent and pattern of disrespectful behaviours (if any), to identify drivers of disrespect and draw lessons for policy changes and actions to be implemented in the programme. The research questions were: 1) What are the perceptions of service providers on RMC and the rights of women in the antenatal, natal and postnatal phases? 2) What are the gaps in the perceptions of service providers and users about RMC? 3) What are women's experiences of RMC? 4) What are the drivers of disrespect in care?

The specific objectives were to measure the prevalence of RMC and identify the factors leading to disrespect during the antenatal, natal and postnatal periods.

In this phase, a concurrent exploratory mixed methods (Creswell et al., 2003) study design was used. Random sampling strategy to collect quantitative data and purposive sampling to collect qualitative data from different levels of health institutions were harnessed. The data were collected using a structured questionnaire for the quantitative component, a topic guide for in-depth interviews and focus group discussions (FGDs) and a checklist for non-participatory observations. While observations and in-depth interviews with mothers and service providers were conducted in health institutions, in-depth interviews with postnatal mothers and FGDs with community members were held in a community setting. Health care providers working at different levels of public health facilities (primary, secondary and tertiary) were interviewed and observed in their own settings.

Descriptive analyses were carried out to find the prevalence of disrespect and to identify the factors involved. Thematic analyses of qualitative data were carried out manually as the team wanted to make a continuous comparison of data to find the links between themes. Grounded theory (Glaser & Strauss, 1967), in which a constant comparison within the data was applied to identify themes and defining categories, was used for the analyses. The QUAN and QUAL data were triangulated at the time of analyses, and QUAL findings were used to explain the reasons for disrespect (Fig. 11.2).

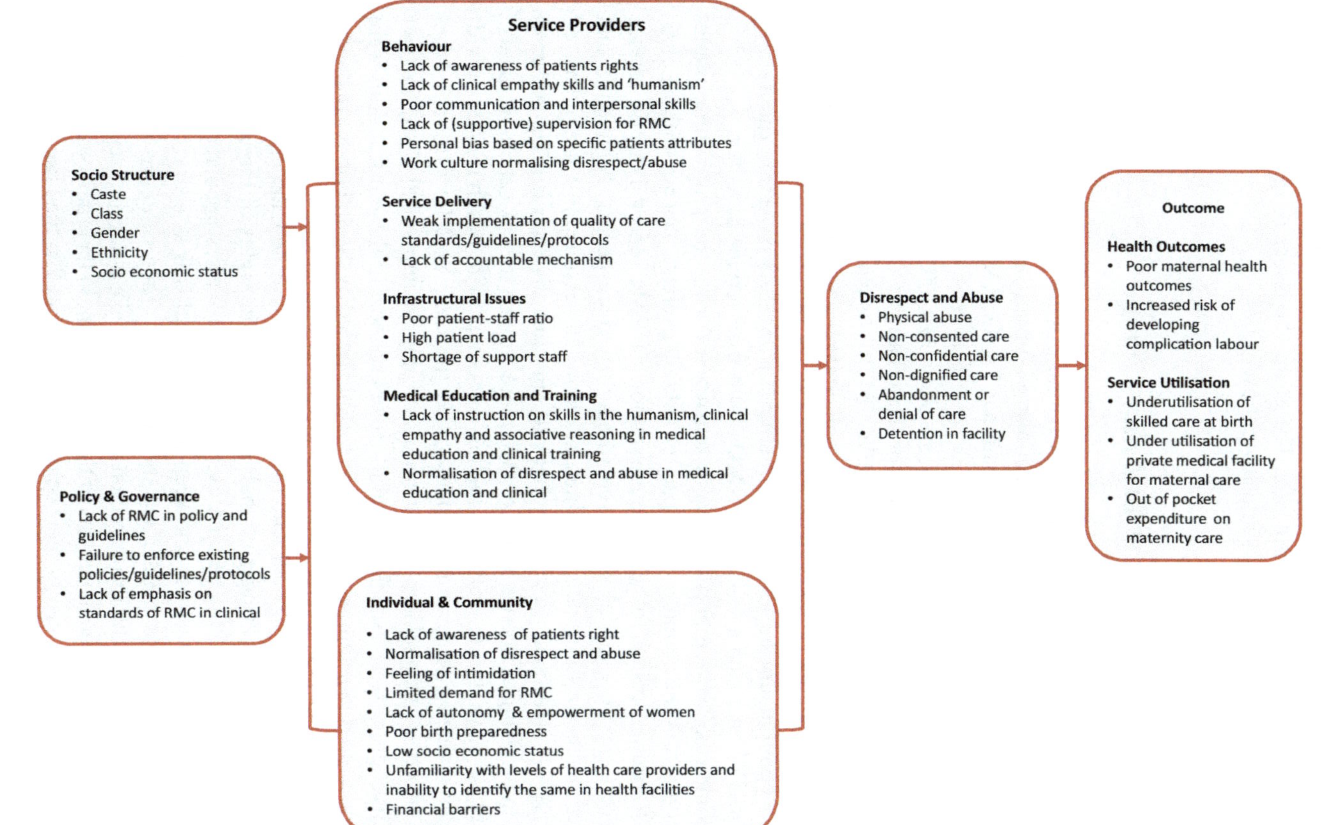

Fig. 11.2 Contributors to disrespect and abuse: findings from the RMC study

The interactions with service providers and service users at different levels of service delivery made it extremely clear that the medical education system has made service delivery more outcome-oriented, and this has led to the "normalization" of disrespect while providing care. Therefore, the issues of inequality within the health system must be addressed using policy spaces.

11.4.2 Phase II: Advocacy for Policy Change

The advocacy strategy included coalition building with allies, public awareness campaigns through mass media and meetings with policymakers. For agenda setting, a short documentary was aired on national TV (Deb, 2018), and several meetings were held with stakeholders.

A window of opportunity to communicate our work on RMC that emerged as the National Program on Quality of Care for Maternal and Child Health was to be launched on 11 December 2017 (MoH&FW, 2017b). As part of this event, we were able to share the findings of phase I with policymakers and programme managers. Based on these findings, RMC was included as an important component of the Labour Room Quality Improvement Initiative (LaQSHYA) program. The training for LaQSHYA included a session on RMC to sensitize service providers.

Although the service providers were sensitized during the programme implementation across the country, this capacity-building exercise was not without challenges. Resource persons for sensitization sessions on RMC reported that the service providers were in a denial mode regarding their disrespectful behaviours and remained defensive for quite some time. In the initial sessions, it was emphasized that though obstetricians save many lives despite this disrespectful behaviour, it needed to be changed in order to encourage more women to seek care in hospitals.

Advocacy with stakeholders and training workshops with health service providers helped in finding programme partners to take the RMC work forward. The experiences of other stakeholders who were also trying to implement RMC in their health institutions were especially useful. However, most of these institutions were following a top-down approach, i.e. change would be led by the authorities in power.

It was apparent that service providers themselves are bound by hierarchies in society and in the health system, and they automatically follow the instructions of the authorities without considering their own rights, the rights of the women they care for or the needs of the service users. Service providers appeared to remain distant from their own realities and keep their minds closed as everyone followed the existing routines and maintained the status quo. They often do not ask for improvements in the health infrastructure but rather make compromises on quality. There is no space for critical analysis of the environment in their personal or professional lives. The experts justify their behaviour by saying that they use their expertise to save mothers and babies, offering this as a rationale for not changing disrespectful behaviours.

11.4.3 Phase III: Participatory Action

Experiences from the training workshops and from other organizations, with both positive and not so positive outcomes, indicated that a top-down approach may not be sustainable. The research team also admitted bringing about changes in practice at tertiary care hospitals, where experts are recognized for their knowledge and skills, is a big challenge. Therefore, we decided to use a participatory action approach (Lewin, 1946) to change the behaviours of health service providers and to draw lessons for future health promotion research.

The purpose of the intervention in this phase was to learn and change together to realize the rights of childbearing women. The intervention was designed, implemented and evaluated by the study participants, i.e. the service providers; the research team only facilitated the processes.

The intervention was initiated in December 2018 in a tertiary care hospital. As there is no midwifery practice in India, women receive antenatal care at the primary care level, but, for birthing, they approach secondary or tertiary care facilities.

Participatory action is a continuous process, and spirals of change are followed. In the RMC programme, most of the planning and implementation of activities for change shifted from the facilitator of change, the researcher, to the service providers themselves. The service providers, particularly the residents and consultants, were able to change the hospital infrastructure and the behaviours by involving partners including institutional authorities, funding agencies and government representatives. They started to provide respectful services to pregnant and birthing women using their own innovations (such as drawing up a chart to observe their own behaviour and identifying what they could do differently, even during the COVID-19 crisis and periods of lockdown.

However, involvement of the service providers in the RMC programme implementation was quite complex. Deciding on the level of support required by the research participants, especially the senior obstetricians, was the biggest challenge. Achieving the dynamism and flexibility required in the use of research methods for data collection, intervention implementation and evaluation at different levels and integrating the qualitative findings and outcomes appropriately at different points in time without losing focus on the participants' needs sometimes presented difficulties for the team.

11.5 Methodological Rationale and Challenges

The following theoretical and methodological challenges had to be addressed while conducting the RMC project, especially linking the research evidence to advocacy and policy action.

11.5.1 Use of Theories and Models

Identifying and appropriately using theories and models for understanding the behaviours and environments of a variety of stakeholders, including pregnant women, service providers and political leaders, was a challenge. Health promotion has about 89 meso- and micro-level theories and models that explain how behaviours can be changed (Michie et al., 2014). The theory of change and the behaviour change wheel were both explored and the principles of both were applied, but, following the theory of critical realism, a concurrent mixed methods design (Michie et al., 2011) was used in the first phase. The capacity, opportunity and motivation (COM-B) part of the behaviour change wheel helped in understanding the capacity of participants. A trans-theoretical model was used to understand the stage of change of the study participants before starting with participatory actions, and, to find the drivers of mistreatment during childbirth, we used the conceptual framework of Bowser and Hill (Bowser & Hill, 2010; WHO, 2014).

There was a dilemma as to whether structural (Foucault, 1970; Althusser, 2009) or functional theories (Malinowski, 1944) should be used to help study participants understand how all relations are bound by power hierarchies. Structuralists are often critical of power and are in favour of change in power to bring about equality, whereas functionalists support maintaining the status quo by respecting the hierarchies and power. These theories help in understanding how domination by one class or social group provides space and opportunities for disrespectful behaviours to persist while the status quo is maintained. A review of the political economy of different countries indicates that inequities and power relations within systems are bound by political and economic structures, which also define the relationship between a health service provider and a user (Stuckler et al., 2010).

The use of social theories in deciding which research methods and intervention implementations are more effective and sustainable is now well established. There has been good use of theories in the health promotion research, but researchers mostly apply meso-level theories (Sabatier, 1988) for understanding or changing behaviours. Human behaviours are complex and dynamic; therefore, one theory or a set of theories cannot be advocated, and the choice of theories must be determined by the researcher's own philosophical underpinning, ideology and, at times, the need to be pragmatic according to the requirements of the setting in which they work.

11.5.2 Settings and Methods

The project was carried out in both community (phase I) and hospital (phase III) settings. Advocacy sessions, workshops and meetings were held with the policymakers and experts in an office setting (phase II). The intervention has currently only been implemented in a hospital setting, but, to change the behaviours of a community, there is also a need to develop interventions in that community after careful consideration of the community context. Working in multiple settings is a challenge; however, the use of phasing helps.

Presently, the focus is more on changing the behaviours of service providers. There is also a need to change the behaviour of pregnant women who are vulnerable to abuse or violence as they are never made aware of their rights, knowledge that is essential when approaching a health institution to seek care. An intervention to change the behaviour of pregnant women should also be designed and implemented.

Appropriate choice of research design, sampling strategy and methods of data collection were difficult in the RMC study as it involved several phases with specific purposes. Research methods were borrowed from social science and epidemiology. The policy intervention development and implementation were also not easy; hence, it was necessary to maintain flexibility of approach during the different stages.

While deciding on which methods to consider for a specific setting for both data collection and intervention, it is important to recognize that health promotion research is complex and requires more than one method. Cross-sectional design can be used for measuring the prevalence of behaviours quantitatively. However, it should not be considered a complete method until it is supplemented by qualitative methods to identify the root causes of behaviours, which is essential when advocating for change. Therefore, a mixed methods design is appropriate, even for short or smaller health promotion studies.

11.5.3 Evidence for Advocacy

In the absence of local evidence on RMC, advocacy with the policymakers was difficult. Hence, the first phase was planned to provide data on actual behaviours performed at a given point in time and within the given context. Without understanding the drivers of the behaviours, the application of behaviour change models would not have been effective. Therefore, an exploratory concurrent mixed methods design was used for simultaneous collection and analysis of quantitative and qualitative methods. The learnings from thematic analyses of qualitative research provided information on not only the reasons for disrespect but also the circumstances under which disrespect occurs and on the kind of relationship that exists between service users and providers.

Asymmetry in knowledge between the service user and provider was one of the major reasons for unequal relationships and subsequent abuse and disrespect during the provision of services. Most women acknowledged the occurrence of violence but always referred to other women who had experienced it. None of the women shared their own experience of violence that they might have encountered. It is possible that the women perceived a loss of dignity or a sense of shame in experiencing physical or verbal abuse.

Almost all the service providers acknowledged that violence has become a part of their care routines and it has been "normalized", though it is not considered to be desirable. They admitted that they do not approach the powers that be in the health system for an increase in resources but rather abuse the women who come to them in large numbers for availing themselves of services in resource-constrained situations. The insights gained from the multiphase mixed methods research were substantially effective in advocating for RMC. Therefore, while planning for health promotion, the research focus should be on generating evidence for advocacy for policy change interventions.

11.5.4 Intervention Development

Intervention research has been conceptualized by Rothman and Thomas (1994). It uses three facets: knowledge development, knowledge use and design and development (Rothman & Thomas, 1994). In the RMC research project, knowledge was generated in phase I; this was used for advocacy with the policymakers in phase II as well as for designing intervention for changing behaviours of service providers in phase III.

Advocacy, after the first phase, was intended to bring policy and programme-level changes. However, as the top-down approach was not found to be adequate, it was decided that the bottom-up approach would be used for co-development of the intervention, following the principles of participatory action research, i.e. the spiral approach of planning, action and evaluation.

It was considered beneficial to use a self-reflective approach with the practitioners who are experts in their own fields. Bogdan and Biklen have noted "practitioners marshal evidence or data to expose unjust practices or environmental dangers and recommend actions for change" (Bogdan & Biklen, 1992).

Therefore, practitioners were actively involved in the cause for which the research was being conducted. For others, such commitment is a necessary part of being a practitioner or a member of a community of practice. Thus, various projects designed to enhance practice could be referred to as "action research" (Goetschius et al., 1967).

The RMC project can be considered as action research, bringing need-based change in individuals, systems, organizations, communities and in the policies for changing structures. Thomas recognizes that the central idea is for "problem-solving in whatever way it is appropriate" (Thomas, 2007).

Whereas McNiff (2016) argues that it cannot be considered as a technique but should be viewed as a kind of conversation (McNiff, 2016). According to Thomas, action research is all about people:

> thinking for themselves and making their own choices, asking themselves what they should do and accepting the consequences of their own actions (Thomas, 2007).

11.5.5 Intervention Implementation

Implementation of action research in a tertiary care hospital is difficult as this hospital is a centre of excellence that provides care for women with complications of pregnancy and childbirth and has a load of 6,000–7,000 births per year; approximately 40% of these are caesarean section cases.

Disrespect towards pregnant and birthing women was found to be a "normalized" behaviour. Changing such behaviours has been a challenge. It calls for more than the issuing of guidelines and orders from the top authorities. Discriminatory and disrespectful behaviour was not only acceptable but also encouraged at times under the guise of saving the life of the mother and child. Discussions at all levels, during advocacy, raised questions in the minds of participants and provided opportunities for the researcher to understand how some behaviours in certain professions become normal when linked to service delivery outcomes or to targets for the reduction of maternal and newborn mortality.

The first demand that was raised by service providers during the advocacy session was that of hospital infrastructural development, e.g. one of the domains of respectful maternity care is privacy and access to the delivery room for a birth companion from the family. Service providers argued that this was not possible due to poor infrastructure. Lack of infrastructure or lack of resources was cited by service providers as a reason to avoid behaviour change, which provided another important lesson for the design of the intervention.

Health promotion also relates to "providing environment for change". Infrastructure is an environmental issue, and, many a time, it is beyond the control of the service provider. There is always a cultural lag between material and non-material culture (Ogburn, 1922). In individual and family lives, material culture grows faster than non-material culture as it is based on technology and the marketing of products. In health systems, the indicators of performance are based either on service coverage or on lives saved in low-resource countries (WHO, 2000), and these do not have much impact on the environment. It raises another question: Does it mean that work be done on other behavioural issues until there is a conducive environment?

Although environmental requirements were discussed, the communications during the workshops and meetings led to the understanding that power relations are deeply rooted in society and in social systems such as the health system. It became clear that it is not only the physical infrastructure that needs to be changed but also the social and economic structure calls for bigger changes to address RMC and the larger issue of health inequity.

Several meetings, workshops and visits by the facilitator in the labour room had to be carried out. The facilitator helped the service providers understand the issues around disrespect and how to resolve them while being respectful. Initially, there was denial that there was a problem of disrespect and significant resistance to change from the service providers' side.

11.5.6 Measuring the Impact

Health promotion research need not always have a control group to test the hypothesis as in RCTs, but it can follow the spirals of change of action research. Evaluation of the change in action research is quite challenging, but the qualitative reflections of the stakeholders can reveal whether it leads to policy change and desired actions at both the institutional and individual levels. For example, evidence-based advocacy helped in providing a platform for following the RMC approach for pregnant women and newborns at the national level, and qualitative observation led to the discovery that there were some institutions where the change towards RMC was becoming visible. The change in the public sector institutions was found to depend on the leadership of the higher authorities as staff in subordinate roles often follow the guidelines provided for the change. This top-down approach led to some changes taking place without the service providers even realizing that there had been a change, what the change had been or who gained and who lost after the change. It was clear that imitation of the behaviour of others played a large part in the process of change, but it is important to recognize that evidence-based advocacy did lead to questioning the status quo.

In the second spiral of change, after 3 months, the obstetricians and resident doctors started to acknowledge the existence of disrespect and reflect on their behaviour. By the end of 1 year, they had started to address this issue on their own. They had begun to identify the issues, plan the steps needed to address them and present their plans during the workshops. This process is being followed more closely and more often by nurses and medical doctors rather than by other categories of staff.

The role of a facilitator was reduced as some service providers stepped into that role. The measurement of outcome was not how much change had happened quantitatively, as is the case for RCTs, but the qualitative measure that explains the extent and type of change and its effect on the well-being of service providers and users.

11.6 Conclusions

In the RMC project, the individual behaviour change concept had to be stretched to a wide range of social and environmental changes. Since a great deal of time had to be spent building the recognition, even among the research team, it is necessary to understand the social contexts and the root causes of the behaviours of both the service providers and the users so as to advocate for respectful maternity care service. It is imperative for health promotion researchers to recognize their own philosophical outlook before starting the research work. Critical realism, as well as historical and theoretical perspectives on the relationship between a health service provider and a user, was useful for designing a complex health promotion research project.

Field observations, along with in-depth interviews, helped in advocating and in negotiating with the political system to create a policy space for RMC. Various theories were used within the given context to understand the behaviours and to initiate change. The service providers were involved from the planning stage to implementation, evaluation and re-planning cycles to ensure continuity while making conscious efforts to improve quality of care. The RMC research experience suggests that change can be more acceptable, practicable and sustainable if the actors of change have been engaged in recognizing their beliefs and current behaviours. People themselves need to test and learn from their own change process; control of change needs to be in the hands of the people who are changing themselves. The researcher needs to be a facilitator. The journey of RMC is continuing, and change has become an internal rather than an external process.

RMC has emerged as a social phenomenon, which also has physical and psychological aspects. The RMC journey reveals that individual change needs to be understood within environmental changes and that change is a process. Hence, there is a need for a paradigm shift. Health promotion needs to be rooted in social science, socio-political and cultural contexts and systems. The core of health promotion lies in "change". The existing macro-, meso- and micro-level theories of change are relevant, but health promotion scientists need to be more realistic and at the same time more critical to bring about change not only in behaviours or systems but also in structures.

References

Addicott, R., & Ferlie, E. (2007). Understanding power relationships in health care networks. *Journal of Health Organization and Management, 21*, 393–405. https://doi.org/10.1108/14777260710778925

Althusser, L. (2009). Stanford encyclopedia of philosophy (Fri Oct 16). https://plato.stanford.edu/entries/althusser/

Baum, F., & Fisher, M. (2014). Why behavioural health promotion endures despite its failure to reduce health inequities. *Sociology of Health & Illness, 36*(2), 213–225. https://doi.org/10.1111/1467-9566.12112

Bhaskar, R. (1975). *A realist theory of science*. Routledge, Taylor & Francis Group.

Bogdan, R., & Biklen, S. (1992). *Qualitative research for education: An introduction to theory and methods*. Allyn and Bacon.

Bowser, D., & Hill, K. (2010). *Exploring evidence for disrespect and abuse in facility-based childbirth*. USAID-TRAction Project, Harvard School of Public Health.

Cacioppo, J. T., Berntson, G. G., Sheridan, J. F., & McClintock, M. K. (2000). Multilevel integrative analyses of human behavior: Social neuroscience and the complementing nature of social and biological approaches. *Psychological Bulletin, 126*(6), 829.

Charmaz, K. (2000). Grounded theory: Objectivist and constructivist methods. *Handbook of Qualitative Research, 2*, 509–535.

Creswell, J. W., Plano Clark, V., Gutmann, M. L., & Hanson, W. E. (2003). Handbook of mixed methods in social and behavioral research. *Advanced mixed methods research designs* (p. 209).

Davies, J. (2013). Health promotion: A unique discipline? In *Health promotion forum of New Zealand.*

Deb, S. (2018). India matters: Respectful maternity care. *India Matters* (pp. 20 Min, 38 Sec). NDTV, India.
Foucault, M. (1970). *The order of things: An archaeology of the human sciences* (A. Sheridan, Tran.). Tavistock).
Gaventa, J., & Cornwall, A. (2008). Power and knowledge. *The Sage handbook of action research: Participative inquiry and practice* (Vol. 2, pp. 172–189).
Glaser, B., & Strauss, A. (1967). *The discovery of grounded theory* (pp. 1–19). Weidenfield & Nicolson.
Gleick, J. (1987). *Chaos: Making a new science*. Viking Penguin Inc.
Goetschius, G. W., Tash, M. J., Association, L. Y. W. s. C., & London, Y. W. s. C. A. (1967). *Working with unattached youth: problem, approach, method: The Report of an enquiry into the ways and means of contacting and working with unattached young people in an inner London borough*. Routledge & K. Paul.
Guinote, A. (2007). Behaviour variability and the situated focus theory of power. *European Review of Social Psychology, 18*(1), 256–295. https://doi.org/10.1080/10463280701692813
Kumar, M., Verma, M., Das, T., Pardeshi, G., Kishore, J., & Padmanandan, A. (2016). A study of workplace violence experienced by doctors and associated risk factors in a tertiary care hospital of South Delhi, India. *Journal of Clinical and Diagnostic Research: JCDR, 10*(11), LC06.
Lewin, K. (1946). Action research and minority problems. *Journal of Social Issues, 2*(4), 34–46.
Malinowski, B. (1944). The functional theory. *A Scientific Theory of Culture*, 145–176.
McNiff, J. (2016). *You and your action research project*. Routledge.
Michie, S., van Stralen, M., & West, R. (2011). The behaviour change wheel: A new method for characterising and designing behaviour change interventions. *Implementation Science: IS, 6*, 42. https://doi.org/10.1186/1748-5908-6-42
Michie, S., West, R., Campbell, R., Brown, J., & Gainforth, H. (2014). *ABC of behaviour change theories*. Silverback Publishing.
Miller, S., & Lalonde, A. (2015). The global epidemic of abuse and disrespect during childbirth: History, evidence, interventions, and FIGO's mother– Baby friendly birthing facilities initiative. *International Journal of Gynecology & Obstetrics, 131*, S49–S52.
Ministry of Health & Family Welfare. (2017a). *National family health survey* (NFHS-4, 2015-16). International Institute for Population Sciences (IIPS).
Ministry of Health & Family Welfare. (2017b). Labour Room Quality Improvement Initiative (LAQSHYA). In N. H. M. (NHM) (Ed.), (p. 144). Government of India.
Nimmon, L., & Stenfors-Hayes, T. (2016). The "Handling" of power in the physician-patient encounter: Perceptions from experienced physicians. *BMC Medical Education, 16*(1), 1–9.
Ogburn, W. F. (1922). *Social change with respect to culture and original nature*. BW Huebsch Incorporated.
Rothman, J., & Thomas, E. J. (1994). *Intervention research: Design and development for the human service*. Psychology Press.
Sabatier, P. A. (1988). An advocacy coalition framework of policy change and the role of policy-oriented learning therein. *Policy Sciences, 21*(2/3), 129–168.
Stuckler, D., Feigl, A., Basu, S., & McKee, M. (2010). *The political economy of universal health coverage*. Background paper for the global symposium on health systems research.
Thomas, G. (2007). *Education and theory: Strangers in paradigms*. McGraw-Hill Education (UK).
WHO. (2000). *The world health report 2000: Health systems: Improving performance*. World Health Organization.
WHO. (2014). *WHO statement: The prevention and elimination of disrespect and abuse during facility-based childbirth*. WHO.
WHO. (2018). *WHO recommendations: Intrapartum care for a positive childbirth experience*. WHO.

Chapter 12
Valuing Indigenous Health Promotion Knowledge and Practices: The Local Dialogue Workshop as a Method to Engage and Empower Matrons and Other Traditional Healers in Haiti

Obrillant Damus, Maude Vézina, and Nicola J. Gray

12.1 Introduction

In Haiti, institutional resources and the welfare state are weak. Within rural communities, people have developed local knowledge, ways of thinking and action in order to address their ontological vulnerability[1] (Damus, 2016; Boublil, 2018) and their economic poverty. Much of the local and ancestral knowledge is associated with the conservation and sustainable use of biodiversity and ecosystems[2] and holds various benefits for communities, allowing them not only to survive in adverse conditions but also to maintain a certain balance with environmental considerations

[1]This expression refers to the faculty of being "affected", which characterizes each of us living creatures. It not only refers to the human condition but also to those of non-humans (animals and plants), especially at the physical level. The distinction is that unlike animals and plants, we, humans, experience vulnerability on all levels: physical, psychological and moral. Unfortunately, according to a common and false belief, pregnant women, the so-called disabled, children and the elderly are the only ones who are vulnerable.

[2]This term refers to the ecological unity or interdependence between humans and non-humans.

O. Damus (✉)
Institut Supérieur d'Études et de Recherches Africaines d'Haïti, State University of Haiti, Port-au-Prince, Haiti
e-mail: oobrillant@yahoo.fr

M. Vézina
Interdisciplinary School of Health Sciences, University of Ottawa, Ottawa, Canada

SPOT-CCSE Health Clinic, Québec, QC, Canada

N. J. Gray
'Global Health and Education' Research Group, Clermont Ferrand, France

University of Huddersfield, Huddersfield, West Yorkshire, England, UK

L. Potvin, D. Jourdan (eds.), *Global Handbook of Health Promotion Research, Vol. 1*,
https://doi.org/10.1007/978-3-030-97212-7_12

through respect for biodiversity. Such knowledge that serves health promotion objectives, well-being and community survival allows rural dwellers, to a certain extent, to cope with the weakness of the modern medical sector and the virtual absence of industrial agricultural practices. Rural dwellers who are equipped with ancestral and local knowledge contribute – to a large extent – to the resilience of their communities.

The setting for the study was Jean-Rabel, a rural commune in northwest Haiti. Jean-Rabel was chosen as the focus not only for the richness of its biodiversity and its ecosystem value but also for its age as it was founded in 1743. The commune consists of a large town and seven villages. These are divided into hamlets, which are further subdivided into localities. The commune is located about 250 km from Port-au-Prince, the capital city of Haiti, and 95% of its population lives on agriculture and animal husbandry (Jean-Gilles, 2004). In the rural communes, dwellings and villages of Jean-Rabel where they live, there are no hospitals. The nearest town has only one hospital (Notre-Dame de la Paix Hospital), which is unable to meet the needs of local populations. In the absence of modern medical care, these local populations turn to the local and Indigenous knowledge of the matrons, leaf doctors, mambos, houngans, etc., regarding the management of health and illness.

These rural healers are consulted for cultural, social and economic reasons. Healers and the people who consult them share the same beliefs, the same visions of the world and the same lifestyles, and many traditional healers provide care almost free of charge. Their profession is accessible to all social classes, and the perception of personal and professional effectiveness of healers is linked to the number of years for which they have practised their profession. They are consulted not only by rural people but also by urban dwellers. Many women of rural origin living in urban areas prefer to travel to the countryside to give birth instead of suffering psychological, moral and obstetric challenges in a poorly equipped hospital centre. Moreover, local healers' knowledge saves lives. Contrary to what the medical community might think, the maternal mortality rate would be higher in Haiti – according to WHO (World Health Organization) estimates (2019), there were, in this country, 480 maternal deaths in 2017 – if the matrons did not attend to poor women, particularly those living in rural areas where health and road infrastructures are absent. In 2013, matrons performed 97.10% of home births, according to a report from the Haiti Ministry of Public Health and Population (2014).

When living in techno-medically and materially deprived environments, knowledge of health, spirituality, biodiversity and ecosystems is essential for human orientation. The specific health promotion practices studied in the research project concerned sustainable development actions and good eating and agricultural habits, which allow farmers to manage their health and the health of their relatives in those communities. Thus, the questions asked were as follows:

- What characterizes rural dwellers' knowledge relating to the management of both community health and sustainable development?
- To what extent do the local and Indigenous knowledge and the resulting practices of the participants in our intra-cultural dialogue on health promotion contribute to the management of community health, biodiversity and ecosystems?

Most of the data collected during the dialogue workshop concerned phytotherapy. Plants play a fundamental role in the treatment of natural (medicinal plants) and supernatural (magical plants) diseases. Holders of local and Indigenous knowledge use and protect plants for therapeutic, magical and symbolic purposes. In fact, the medical, the magical and the religious are inseparable, which adds complexity to health-promoting practices. The survival and quality of life of rural populations are intimately linked to the natural resources provided by biodiversity and ecosystems. Rural populations consume traditional herbal medicines, which they assert, according to the data collected, have no side effects. They do not use chemicals in their farming practices or for the storage of grains. They prefer food products obtained from their organic farming to those imported from other places in order to prevent diseases. Traditional zoo medicines (prepared with animal substances) play a secondary role in their lives; animal parts are rarely consumed for therapeutic purposes. Nature is a complete natural "pharmacy" to which they can turn in order to seek a remedy for their health problems.

The participants of the dialogue workshop explore and manage the ecosystems of the Jean-Rabel region to ensure their survival. Their health depends on the management and sustainable use of plants, animals (biotic elements) and water (abiotic element). They plant trees in the proximity of springs to prevent them from drying up. Therefore, they know that there is an insufficient local supply of fresh water and that one of the specific factors linked to their survival is water security. Animals, plants and humans need it. The holders of local and Indigenous knowledge use water to prepare their natural medicines (infusions and decoctions of leaves, roots and peels). Living in rural areas, where synthetic drugs and modern care are practically non-existent, they have no choice but to turn to traditional medicines by exploring the local flora and fauna.

We heard evidence of values of confidence and courage from the words gathered during the local dialogue workshop: the solidarity practices praised by participants during the workshop allowed us to deduce that they are driven by a sense of common destiny. Participants show this by taking care of their health and that of others (see Table 12.1).

Table 12.1 Defining the characteristics of different types of traditional healers (table constructed from data collected during local dialogue workshops)

	Traditional healer	Uses plants and loa (voodoo spirits) to heal	Only uses plants (and/or prayers) to heal
Mambo	+	+	–
Houngan	+	+	–
Leaf doctor	+	–	+
Matron	+	–	+
Matron–mambo	+	+	–

12.2 Research to Elicit Health Promotion Knowledge in Rural Dwellers in Haiti: Features of the Dialogue Workshop Method

This research was based on a community-based participatory research (CBPR) approach (Wallerstein & Duran, 2006). This approach has emerged in recent decades as an alternative paradigm for achieving health promotion research objectives and is particularly used for research aiming at reducing health inequities (Wallerstein & Duran, 2006). The CBPR approach is rooted in four central foundations, which are: (1) the establishment of academic and community co-learning partnerships alongside the research activities, (2) inclusion of capacity building in the research efforts, (3) the results must benefit all partners and (4) the participatory research must involve long-term commitments (Wallerstein & Duran, 2006). That said, CBPR aims not only at defining objectives based on the needs expressed by community members but also at generating knowledge *with* and *for* communities (e.g. Potvin et al., 2003). Although the field of health promotion has encountered difficulties relating to the sometimes challenging compatibility of a participatory approach with biomedical research guidelines (Koelen et al., 2001), a CBPR approach remains an essential tool and method for strengthening the connection between communities and the development of health-related knowledge.

In order to develop the objectives with local participants, and to answer the research questions, a 2-day workshop was organized in Jean-Rabel on November 26 and 27, 2016. The workshop participants came from a number of rural communities administratively attached to Jean-Rabel: Morne-Pasteur, Bois-Changé, Nan Ogé, Ruelle Rivière, Belle Dorée, Porrier, Lalande, Grande-Source, Galata, etc. The life history of the participants, as well as their socio-demographic and socio-economic descriptions of their communities, was the focus of interest. Prof. Damus first met some of the matrons in Jean-Rabel in 2012. When the researchers returned in 2016, these matrons acted as gatekeepers to bring other holders of knowledge to the local workshop. The research team asked community representatives to inform other rural actors of their arrival at Jean-Rabel, and these matrons were paid to circulate the topics for discussion to local families.

The objectives of the local dialogue workshop – examining both conscious and unconscious health promotion practices – were to: (1) identify strategies for health promotion as well as management and sustainable use of biodiversity and ecosystems; (2) describe the ways of thinking and actions of rural dwellers who promote an osmotic relationship between health promotion and management and sustainable use of biodiversity and ecosystems; (3) describe the capacity of male and female rural dwellers to explore the resources offered by nature to promote health and (4) describe the eating habits and agricultural actions that serve individual, family and community health. The two main values pursued by the project were solidarity, by sharing knowledge related to health promotion, and promoting sustainable development in rural communities. These objectives and values were defined collectively during the dialogue workshop.

The workshop was organized around the following themes: biodiversity and ecosystem management techniques; biodiversity, health and spirituality; food sovereignty (organic, family, peasant and food-producing farming) and biodiversity; breastfeeding and nature and methods of transmitting local and Indigenous knowledge. Examples of questions asked in the workshop, generated as the discussions took place and noted in situ to show the dynamism of the dialogue, can be found in the Appendix.

The workshop was held over 2 days, running from 7 a.m. to 4 p.m. each day. Breakfast and lunch were offered free of charge to participants. After having breakfast together on the first day, the researchers said to participants,

> You are our teachers. We came here to learn. You are all holders of knowledge. When a person speaks, she should not be corrected. You have to let her speak. Everyone has their own practices or experiences. All the experiences can be considered. You can add to what a participant has to say if the person has a memory lapse. As soon as she finishes her testimony, you can criticize her in order to energize the dialogue workshop. (English translation from the original Creole version.)

The objective was to have them reflect on their professional experiences. Each of the participants was asked to introduce themselves in Creole, first stating their name, profession and socio-geographic origin (including the name of the rural commune to which they belonged). Questions were asked about each of the workshop themes, which were also discussed over lunch. The researchers kept encouraging participants to respect the lived experience of their fellow human beings. The participants challenged and corrected each other while following the dialogue workshop facilitator's instructions.

The researchers avoided presenting a judgmental attitude towards the participants. For the first time in their lives, they were treated as holders of valuable knowledge and not as ignorant people who had to be taught about proper health promotion practices. In effect, researchers took on the role of ignorant people who went to *their* school. Eating the midday meal did not interrupt the flow of the dialogue workshop. A few participants used this convivial moment to share knowledge with the team; they asked questions, including whether the researchers might dedicate the second day of the dialogue workshop to a training seminar for them. The chosen approach – encouraging them to recognize their own health promotion knowledge – did not allow the team to do this. Instead, part of the afternoon of the second day was dedicated to the collective promotion of behaviours supporting not only the conservation and improvement of health but also environmental sustainability, through a presentation in Creole of a section of the results obtained through preliminary analysis of the data already collected.

The researchers carried out 40 individual and 4 group interviews during the dialogue workshop with the holders of local and ancestral knowledge: 23 matrons, 7 leaf doctors, 5 houngans and 5 mambos. They conducted structured, unstructured and semi-structured interviews, which were transcribed verbatim. The combination of individual and group interviews allowed the team to address the complexity of local and Indigenous knowledge about health promotion, biodiversity and ecosystem management. In addition to taking notes, they made audio and video recordings. Quantitative data about biodiversity and ecosystem management strategies, and their sustainable use, were also collected during the dialogue workshop. These quantitative data included the number of medicinal plants used in order to treat health problems, the number of leaves used in the preparation of a decoction/infusion and the number of trees planted each year. As most of the knowledge generated related to plants and farming, nature walks were conducted with participants after the workshops each day to confront their knowledge and the researchers' own assumptions of reality.

Content analysis techniques (Bardin, 1993; L'Écuyer, 1987) were used for the interviews according to the classical inductive methods of comprehensive sociology (Glaser & Strauss, 1967) to elicit themes within local and Indigenous knowledge associated with health promotion, biodiversity and ecosystems. As there is no sociology without induction, the double phenotypic (manifest meaning, explicit meaning, *said*) and genotypic (implicit meaning, *unsaid*) dimensions of the empirical material were both taken into account. The data analysis process consisted of identifying themes and sub-themes in the data, through both the breakdown (identification and coding of the units of meaning) and the categorization (grouping semantic units within various categories) of this material. Since the subject–object and the researcher both participate in the construction of reality, its meaning results from the fruitful conjunction of *emic* constructs (descriptions and interpretation suggested by the holder of local and Indigenous knowledge) and *etic* constructs (descriptions and attempts at objectifying interpretation from the researcher).

Perfect mastery of Creole, the mother tongue of the participants, allowed researchers to grasp the hidden (implicit) meaning of their discourse and the deep meaning that they brought to their own experiences. This complex experiential teaching was based on the pedagogy of the oppressed (Freire, 1980). In order to describe in detail the local and ancestral knowledge and practices recorded during the dialogue workshop, researchers turned to the following disciplines, wishing to address the complexity of the factual elements collected: natural sciences, ethnomedicine, sociology, anthropology, etc. The objective was to "bring together unrelated knowledge into relevant knowledge" in a health promotion perspective, resulting in a "transparadigmatological"[3] (Damus, 2016) posture.

Given the inevitable influence of the context of enunciation on both the form and content of the speech of the people who participated in the local workshop, it is useful to make a distinction here between the words "text" and "speech". When an interview is transcribed, it should be considered as a text. However, a text is an "empirical object considered independently from its production conditions". Even if certain elements of empiricism can be analyzed independently from their context (universalist posture), our principle of analysis and interpretation is based on the fact that the meaning of empirical material is intimately linked to its context of production (contextualist posture). In this case, it thus seems more relevant to prefer the notion of "discourse", which is defined as an "empirical object with its production

[3] Used in this context, this concept refers to the process of transcending disciplinary frontiers.

conditions", rather than the word "text". The conscious knowing of the existence of a spatio-temporal bias inherent to the collection of empirical data allowed the team, during the analysis process, to benefit from this trilogy: discursive material, socio-anthropological questions and the empirical context.

Beyond qualitative analysis, the adoption of a transparadigmatic posture enabled the researchers to apply theoretical reasoning to their conceptualization of the rich data. The ways of thinking and acting of the holders of local knowledge, on the one hand, and the symbiosynergic[4] paradigm, on the other, characterize their profession and allow the conservation of the environment. There is no separation between their professional practices and the latter. Traditional childbirth, for example, is based on cultural factors (myths, taboos, symbols, values, cosmovisions,[5] etc.), which promote the conservation of biodiversity and ecosystems.

To cope with the complexity of life, matrons, leaf doctors, mambos and houngans have developed for centuries a way of thinking with multiple dimensions and at the service of ritual actions: magical, symbolic, mythological, empirical, technical and rational. This organic or holistic thinking is linked to global determinism or to the multi-determined nature of social and cultural facts. It generates cognitive categories, which are part of the fight against ontological vulnerability and which constitute an invaluable patrimonial (or matrimonial) wealth. These cognitive categories are based on the non-separation of body and mind, reality and imagination and culture and nature. *Volens nolens*[6] means that they are part of the intangible heritage of humanity.

Participants in the local dialogue workshop hold complex knowledge regarding the management and sustainable use of biodiversity and ecosystems. Most of their knowledge and beliefs are at the service of community, animal and plant health (human and environmental sustainability).

12.3 Critical Review of Methodological Successes and Challenges

The data collected during the workshop allowed us to make several major observations: (1) The participants hold knowledge expressed through multiple dimensions, which serve both human and ecological health. (2) The holders of local and Indigenous knowledge protect the sacred trees as well as the plants and animals they use. (3) These people are specialists in Creole medicine (this type of medicine is "ecocentric" as its practitioners must, within the framework of their healthcare

[4]The symbiosynergic paradigm (from the Greek sumbiôsis, communal life/from the Greek Sunergia, cooperation; from 'sun' = with and ergon = work) is defined by three interrelated elements: the person, the sociolinguistic–epistemic community and nature.

[5]Refers to visions of the world and the universe.

[6]Refers to a Latin expression meaning "whether we want it or not".

practices, explore and use the resources of nature in a sustainable way – it does not separate man from his environment). (4) Synergy was noted between the traditional medical knowledge of the participants, who are at the service of biodiversity and ecosystems, and their traditional agricultural knowledge.

One of the implicitly formulated objectives was to encourage rural actors to become aware of the role of their "unsuspected" knowledge in health management and to develop a certain "*libido sciendi*" (passion for knowledge, desire to learn) by allowing them to enrich their cognitive resources. We were hoping to develop, *with* them and not *for* them (Freire, 1975), knowledge related to health promotion by asking them to talk, without inhibition, about their social and cultural practices (using the logic of cognitive co-production). A climate of mutual trust had to be developed. The many questions that were asked during the local dialogue workshop made them aware of a certain amount of knowledge that they already possessed related to health promotion. The knowledge shared during the dialogue workshop helped strengthen their sense of empowerment. Each participant was able to benefit from the experiential knowledge of others. "We, the matrons, take care of the development of our communities", was said during the dialogue workshop. They were not considered as anonymous participants but as traditional health promoters.

During the dialogue workshop, the researchers tried to get the participants to articulate knowledge and beliefs that usually belong to a non-verbal approach of practice. As the participants knew each other, they were used to sharing knowledge in informal communication situations. There will remain, undoubtedly, experiential knowledge that they did not share. The dialogue workshop only allowed the team to access an emerging tip of the iceberg of knowledge related to the promotion of human and ecological health.

One of the challenges of the dialogue workshop was to strengthen the participants' self-confidence, self-esteem and sense of competence and personal efficacy (Bandura, 2003) in order to have them define themselves as subjects capable of exploring the thematic universe relating to the promotion of intra- and inter-community health. Given the fact that the holders of this traditional knowledge have always been treated as subordinates or ignorant by the holders of the so-called scientific and technical knowledge, they were hesitant to speak up to share their knowledge. Despite strategies to encourage knowledge sharing, some of them never spoke during the workshops. They convinced themselves that they were attending a training seminar. Indeed, they had asked for a training seminar during their first meeting. As most of the participants were used to participating in biomedically oriented didactic training on disease prevention and health promotion, it was difficult to convince them to share their experiential knowledge because it has never been valued among official health promotion practices. The relationship of subordination that they maintain with holders of universal knowledge about health nourishes their feeling of inferiority, which constitutes an obstacle to speaking in public and sharing what they know. They identified the team with holders of non-erroneous or correct knowledge. They were afraid of being criticized or of being considered ignorant.

12.4 Contribution to the Progress and Structuring of Health Promotion Research

How are these research objects distinctive of health promotion? The team chose not to burden themselves with predetermined objectives until they went into the field. In general, in the domain of health promotion, local populations do not participate in the development of cognitive research objectives (co-reflections on health practices; transmission of knowledge with complex dimensions) and discussion topics. The "dialogical" dimension (Freire, 1980) of this research is nonetheless intrinsically linked to the fact that the objectives and reflexive themes were developed jointly with the participants of the dialogue workshop.

The success of this local dialogue workshop around the role of the rural dwellers' knowledge in promoting health in communities shows that, unlike what we are used to thinking, the poverty of income is not linked to a poverty of thought and knowledge. The holders of local knowledge in Jean-Rabel are co-authors of the work that resulted from the dialogue workshop. After inducing their cognitive pregnancy, the team accompanied them in the delivery of sincere and authentic health-related interviews. Since the most vulnerable people should not be seen as blank pages to be printed on, there is a need to help them assess their experiences with health promotion before trying to force any knowledge on them or before asking them to participate in any health education programme.

This methodological approach differs from classical health promotion research mainly because it is primarily aimed at *strengthening behaviours* favourable to both human and ecological health among the holders of local and Indigenous knowledge – rather than teaching them, unilaterally, things that perhaps do not make sense to them. It allowed us to realize that health promotion is a complex phenomenon which grows outside the rules of linear causality and which is anchored in a multi-dimensional thought process (symbolic, magical, mythological, technical, rational, religious, etc.). Finally, unlike classical health promotion research, which is essentially based on the "rational paradigm or the Man as he should be" (Jourdan, 2010), this approach is not rooted in the dichotomy between *knowing* and *non-knowing* or between *savants* and *believers*. It is not characterized by socio-epistemic separation of professionals and lay people but rather by the epistemological mutual aid necessary for the survival of local populations abandoned by the state. Unsustainable dichotomies (man/nature; us/them; nature/culture; rational/irrational, etc.), on human and ecological levels, do not characterize this methodological approach.

We will see that cultural and social practices that seem irrational or residual are put at the service of health promotion in the broadest sense if we take a look at them from that angle. It should be noted that the mastery of Creole, which is the prism used by the participants to comprehend the world around them, allowed the researchers to understand the complexity of the data collected; the first interpretation of the data was suggested collectively by the participants.

> Nothing can be understood, we have to be convinced, that has not been reduced to language. As a result, language is necessarily the instrument suitable for discovering, conceptualizing

> and interpreting both nature and experience, therefore this compound of nature and experience which is called society. (English translation from the original version.) (Benveniste, 1974, p. 97)

When the participants and the facilitator do not speak the same language, or when the latter pretends not to be able to express himself/herself correctly (linguistic gibberish) in the local language, this constitutes an obstacle to real cultural immersion. The use of French or *Franci-Creole* (linguistic gibberish made up by people who can read and write) in health promotion research with unilingual Creole speakers reinforces the abyssal line that exists between those two groups. In this workshop, the cultural invasion, which characterizes classical research in health promotion (a heuristic and pragmatic perspective), gave way to the cognitive co-construction respectful of language, cosmovisions, culture and logics of action of traditional health promoters. This local dialogue workshop was a serendipitous process insofar as the knowledge gathered was not anticipated.

The collective assessment of local knowledge relating to health promotion increased the participants' desire to learn; they kept telling the team during the dialogue workshop: "We are passing on our knowledge to you. You have to give us yours in return." This statement indicates that health promotion research must be located at the crossroads of knowledge from the south and knowledge from the north (by calling ourselves doctors, we have been seen as northern holders of knowledge). Health promotion should be rooted in the Freirian principle (1998) that "No one knows it all; no one is ignorant of everything." Whatever the country in which one is located, it is necessary to consider the mother tongue, the level of education, the culture and the ways of thinking of the local populations in any implementation of action to promote health, including health promotion research. If the most vulnerable people should participate in the design and implementation of health promotion objectives, it is because they are able to think about and manage their own health.

The diversity of local knowledge collected during the dialogue workshop was nothing but proof that health promotion research practices should not be kept prisoners of a net belonging to a single discipline but should rather be approached from an interdisciplinary perspective. Holistic and participatory health promotion actions should not be confused with current prevention practices that are essentially focused on a risk management model with limited scope. The conscious and unconscious health promotion practices shared with us by the dialogue workshop participants are rooted in multidimensional thinking and in a paradigm of conjunction, whereby human and natural elements are mutually dependent.

Anchored in the humanist paradigm (Jourdan, 2010), the technique of the dialogue workshop – which we believe should be the keystone of the future of health promotion (employing a pragmatic perspective) across northern and southern countries – allows us to describe three processes concerning the destruction of local knowledge:

1. *Self-epistemicide*: This refers to local knowledge disappearing on its own due to a lack of valorization and utilization by actors, especially young people. This

process of destruction of knowledge can be explained by factors such as rural exodus, the pursuit of primary, secondary and university studies by young people in cities, climatic migrations, etc. The absence of young people, or the lack of interactions between them and their parents in rural communities, weakens the process of transmission of traditional knowledge involved in the management of health and biodiversity.
2. *Endo-epistemicide*: Custodians of ancestral knowledge, such as the matrons of Haiti, cease to use certain types of local knowledge, which were until then effective, because of the training seminars unilaterally led by holders of biomedical knowledge employed by the Ministry of Public Health and Population or by a local or Western non-governmental organization (NGO) specializing in the field of health.
3. *Exo-epistemicide*: This refers to Western-centred interventions encouraging the disappearance of much of the local knowledge and "know-how" that were considered effective until that intervention point. Western-centred interventions consciously and unconsciously remove local knowledge and skills that were previously effective at high speed. For example, Western-centred trainers have asked matrons to abandon steam baths and *lòk* (a centuries-old traditional remedy that allows the baby to get rid of meconium), administered to the mother and her baby, respectively. Moreover, it should be noted that, unlike that of voodoo, the Catholic/Protestant spirituality encourages many matrons and parents to give up an ecological practice, which consists of planting the baby's umbilical cord with a fruit tree.

The local dialogue workshop is a method used in this research to collect information related to conscious and unconscious health promotion practices in the rural communities of Jean-Rabel in Haiti. Unlike biomedically oriented and "rigid" data collection techniques, this method is not characterized by predetermined categories but mostly by an open epistemological posture and by the prominence given to serendipity (that is, the discovery of unforeseen facts). Indeed, the objectives and themes of the research were discussed during the first meeting with the holders of local and ancestral knowledge, at the beginning of the first workshop discussion. Many questions were suggested by the participants, both consciously and unconsciously. The dialogue workshop, as facilitated here, is a technique of knowledge sharing in which the anti-epistemological dichotomy of knowing/ignorance is brought under control. Owing to the reversal of the usual roles (the workshop leader, being a holder of scholarly knowledge, behaved like a curious student and the participants were encouraged to behave like teachers), the majority of participants in the dialogue workshop realized that they represented multidimensional knowledge guardians.

In line with the dual objectives to learn more about the practices of traditional healers in this rural setting, and in parallel to raise their consciousness of their role within their community, participants gave descriptions of their health- and sustainability-related practices overlaid by a greater understanding of their sense of self and their local mission. We believe that health promotion research should explicitly explore these aspects of the work of actors in health in any community of the world. We have described the different types of interconnected knowledge realized through this project and propose them as learning points for the development of health promotion research in general. That is, to consider: information about the actors; information about their health promotion practices; connections between health promotion and the wider context and applying theoretical principles to extend the meaning of the research findings.

12.5 Conclusions

The use of the local dialogue workshop method in the field of health promotion research allowed the prevention of qualitative limitations of this field, the reinforcement of the participants' empowerment and the stimulation of practices of solidarity in communities isolated from official public health promotion policies. The implementation of this qualitative data collection technique requires us to adopt an unconditionally positive view about the participants with whom we must develop substantial cultural proximity. The local dialogue workshop allowed us to understand that the relationship between rural dwellers' knowledge and health promotion focuses on a cosmocentric orientation, which is characterized by the non-separation between man, the world below and the world above, or by complex sustainability (mutual dependence between humans, non-humans and natural and sacred forces). Alternative ways of thinking and acting in health promotion encourage us to question the one-dimensional anthropocentric thinking that essentially constitutes the phreatic zone of conventional research in health promotion. The ecology of the ways of thinking and acting should be the cornerstone of the future of health promotion. The contribution of our research to the advancement of health promotion knowledge also lies in our understanding that health promotion will not be useful if it is not based on beneficial solidarity, otherness, the feeling of common destiny, trust in others and the courage to act with and for others and if it does not try to strengthen the actors' own sense of empowerment.

Appendix: Examples of Questions Asked of the Participants During the Dialogue Workshop (99 in Total) (Original Creole Version, with Examples Translated into English)

(a) **Techniques of biodiversity use and management (49 questions)**

1. Ki plant ou itilize lè akouchman frèt? *(Which plants do you use to accelerate childbirth?)*

2. Kijan ou prepare remèd sa yo pou fanm ki ap akouche a? *(How do you prepare the plant remedies that you give to the woman who is giving birth?)*
3. Ki kote ou jwenn plant sa yo? *(Where do you collect these plants?)*

(b) **Use and management of animal biodiversity (22 questions)**

1. Kijan nou jere bèt ki nan dlo yo? Nan bwa yo? Kijan bèt sa yo rele? *(How do you manage animals living in the water and in the woods? What are their names?)*
2. Èske gen anpil bèt nan forè yo? Bay non yo. *(Are there many animals in the forests? Give me their names.)*
3. Ki zwazo ak lòt bèt nou konnen? *(What birds and other animals do you know?)*

(c) **Agrobiodiversity/food sovereignty (28 questions)**

1. Kisa nou kiltive pou nou manje? Kòman nou plante yo? Ki kote nou plante? *(What food plants do you cultivate? How do you cultivate them? Where do you grow them?)*
2. Kisa nou fè ak rekòlt yo? (*What do you do with the crops?)*
3. Èske nou koupye pyebwa avan nou plante? (*Do you cut down trees before seeding?)*

References

Bandura, A. (2003). *Auto-efficacité: Le sentiment d'efficacité personnelle*. De Boeck.

Bardin, L. (1993). *L'analyse de contenu*. PUF.

Benveniste, É. (1974). *Problèmes de linguistique générale, t. 2*. Gallimard.

Boublil, E. (2018). The ethics of vulnerability and the phenomenology of interdependency. *Journal of the British Society for Phenomenology, 49*(3), 183–192.

Damus, O. (2016). *Homo vulnerabilis. Repenser la condition humaine*. Publibook.

Freire, P. (1975). *Conscientisation*. Conseil œcuménique des églises.

Freire, P. (1980). *Pédagogie des opprimés*. La découverte.

Freire, P. (1998). *Teachers as cultural workers: Letters to those who dare teach* (pp. 39–45). Westview Press. Fourth Letter.

Glaser, B. G., & Strauss, A. L. (1967). *The discovery of grounded theory: Strategies for qualitative research*. Aldine.

Jean-Gilles, G. (2004). *À la recherche de Jean-Rabel*. Éditions CIDIHCA.

Jourdan, D. (2010). *Éducation à la santé. Quelle formation pour les enseignants?* Inpes.

Koelen, M. A., Vaandrager, L., & Colomér, C. (2001). Health promotion research: Dilemmas and challenges. *Journal of Epidemiology & Community Health, 55*(4), 257–262.

L'Écuyer, R. (1987). L'analyse de contenu: notion et étapes. In D. J. P. Deslauriers (Ed.), *Les Méthodes de la recherche qualitative* (pp. 49–65). Presses de l'Université du Québec.

Ministère de la Santé Publique et de la Population. (2014). *Haiti Ministry of Public Health and Population annual report 2013*. Ministry of Public Health and Population (Haiti).

Potvin, L., Cargo, M., McComber, A. M., Delormier, T., & Macaulay, A. C. (2003). Implementing participatory intervention and research in communities: Lessons from the Kahnawake Schools Diabetes Prevention Project in Canada. *Social Science & Medicine, 56*(6), 1295–1305.

Wallerstein, N. B., & Duran, B. (2006). Using community-based participatory research to address health disparities. *Health Promotion Practice, 7*(3), 312–323.

World Health Organization, UNICEF, UNFPA, World Bank Group, United Nations. (2019). *Trends in maternal mortality 2000 to 2017: estimates by WHO, UNICEF, UNFPA, World Bank Group and the United Nations Population Division*. World Health Organization. https://www.who.int/reproductivehealth/publications/maternal-mortality-2000-2017/en/. Accessed 24 Sept 2020

Chapter 13
Aligning Research Practices with Health Promotion Values: Ethical Considerations from the Community Health Worker Common Indicators Project

Noelle Wiggins, Kenneth Maes, Leticia Rodriguez Avila, Keara Rodela, and Edith Kieffer

13.1 Introduction

Recent studies have pointed to a burgeoning community of health promotion researchers and significant new networks while at the same time identifying a need to better organize and mobilize the field (Potvin et al., 2013), crystallize a set of health promotion research principles (Woodall et al., 2018), integrate new theories and take a more transdisciplinary approach (Wingood & DiClemente, 2019). Health promotion research is recognized as "critical for identifying new and innovative strategies to improve [health]" (Wingood & DiClemente, 2019, p. S116) yet

Funding and Disclaimer: The CHW Common Indicators Project is partially supported by the Federal Award Number 5-NU38OT000286–02 and the CFDA Number 93.421, from the Centers for Disease Control and Prevention, via the National Association of Chronic Disease Directors. The observations and recommendations in this chapter reflect the opinions and findings of the authors and do not necessarily represent the views or official position of the US Department of Health and Human Services or the Centers for Disease Control and Prevention (CDC).

N. Wiggins (✉)
Wiggins Health Consulting, LLC, Portland, OR, USA
e-mail: chwcommonindicators@gmail.com

K. Maes
Oregon State University, Corvallis, OR, USA

L. Rodriguez Avila
Los Angeles County Dept. of Health Services, Los Angeles, CA, USA

K. Rodela
Immigrant and Refugee Community Organization, Portland, OR, USA

E. Kieffer
University of Michigan, Ann Arbor, MI, USA

L. Potvin, D. Jourdan (eds.), *Global Handbook of Health Promotion Research, Vol. 1*,
https://doi.org/10.1007/978-3-030-97212-7_13

needing to grow and develop to meet increasingly complicated public health threats. These words have never seemed more urgent, given the global COVID-19 pandemic, a worldwide uprising against racism and white supremacy and the increasing and unavoidable urgency of the climate crisis.

Often, when a field needs new theories and approaches, benefit can be derived from looking within that field for models that may have long existed yet have been overlooked by dominant cultures and systems. Looking to practice seems especially appropriate for the field of health promotion, which has been described as "essentially … action-oriented" (Potvin et al., 2013). In the case of health promotion, much can be learned by focusing on research with and about a group of health promotion practitioners who are emblematic of the field yet largely unknown and undervalued for their contributions.

A substantial and rapidly growing body of international research documents the unique contributions of community health workers (CHWs) as a professional group (Campbell et al., 2015; Kane et al., 2020; Kangovi et al., 2020; Kieffer et al., 2013, 2014; Maes, 2015; Morgan et al., 2016; Spencer et al., 2018). Yet, some of the same challenges that plague health promotion research generally also apply to research with and about this group of health promotion practitioners. Variation in the field makes it hard to identify a set of standardized process and outcome measures. The time horizons needed to measure outcomes of CHW interventions are often much longer than the funding periods for CHW programmes. Lack of interest in and attention to the processes by which CHWs achieve outcomes make it difficult to demonstrate the importance of particular CHW roles, skills and characteristics. A tendency to act *on* rather than *with* CHWs deprives the field of the wisdom they have to offer.

Responding to these challenges, in 2015, CHWs and researchers from around the US formed the national CHW Common Indicators (CI) Project (Rodela et al., 2021; Wiggins et al., 2021). The CI Project now comprises more than 220 people in over 35 states. The purpose of the CI Project is to contribute to the integrity, sustainability and viability of CHW programmes through the collaborative development and adoption of a set of common process and outcome constructs and indicators for programmes that employ CHWs in a variety of settings. Crucially, the CI Project is committed to lifting up and practicing a participatory epistemology that has been characteristic of the CHW profession since its inception. CHWs are well known for taking a co-learning and non-hierarchical approach with community members; the CI Project seeks to model this relationship in its work with CHWs and other stakeholders principally through the use of popular (people's) education, a liberatory philosophy and methodology that has been successfully used around the world to promote health and decrease inequities (Wiggins, 2012).

In this chapter, we reflect on how we have used this participatory approach to identify constructs and indicators for the practices, workforce conditions and outcomes of CHWs. In so doing, we suggest how wider use of this approach can support and further the deeply held values and goals of the field of health promotion.

This chapter has been organized to provide answers to the following questions:

- How do CHWs embody the emblematic traits of health promotion practitioners?
- What frameworks and approaches is the CI Project using to conduct research *with* CHWs and to understand the mechanisms that promote health at a community level, and how are these emblematic of health promotion research?
- What are the outcomes – in terms of both findings and actions taken based on findings – of the CI Project, and how are those distinctive of health promotion research?
- How is the CI Project contributing to advancing and structuring health promotion research?
- What can the CI Project teach the field about health promotion research?

13.2 CHWs as Health Promotion Practitioners

CHWs are trusted community members who promote health in their own communities through a variety of strategies (Rosenthal et al., 2011). Around the world, CHWs go by multiple titles, including health extension workers (in Ethiopia), village health workers (in Tanzania and Zimbabwe) and lady health workers (in Pakistan). In the United States (US), common titles include community health representatives (in Native/American Indian communities) and promotores(as) de salud (in Spanish-speaking communities).

According to Coulter et al. (2020), "Using the community health worker (CHW) workforce in health promotion programs to reach vulnerable and marginalized populations has become a best practice in addressing health disparities" (p. 1). Historically, a hallmark of CHW practice and a key reason for its effectiveness has been its flexibility, with CHWs taking on multiple different roles depending on the situation. Although essential, this flexibility has made it difficult to delineate a scope of practice of CHWs similar to those used in other professions (Wiggins & Rodela, 2021). However, several consecutive participatory studies in the US have identified a set of 10 core roles, which range from connecting individuals to existing services to sharing culturally centred health information with groups and to organizing whole communities to address the underlying causes of ill health and health inequities (Wiggins & Borbón, 1998; Rosenthal et al., 2018).

CHWs are, in many ways, quintessential health promotion practitioners. They seek to address the root causes of problems, often work in ways that are invisible to the larger system (Hawe et al., 1998) and seek to create conditions in which people can be healthy rather than primarily providing curative care or ameliorating problems that already exist. CHWs also operate at multiple levels of the socio-ecological model and routinely build partnerships and work in a transdisciplinary way. They seek to address all five areas of practice identified in the Ottawa Charter for Health Promotion (WHO, 1986) and reaffirmed in the Jakarta Declaration (WHO, 1997).

The roots of the CHW profession go back to natural helping and healing systems that became formalized in areas where large sectors of the population had been denied health care and conditions necessary for good health, with the intent of increasing health and social justice (Wiggins & Borbón, 1998). Arguably, CHWs' most important objective is supporting individual and community empowerment (Wiggins et al., 2014).

Formal CHW programmes in the USA have existed since the 1960s, and, despite unstable funding and fluctuating policy support, the number of CHW programmes in the USA has risen steadily since the 1980s (Viswanathan et al., 2009). CHWs were highlighted in the 2010 Patient Protection and Affordable Care Act, leading to greater recognition of CHWs and producing state-level policies for training and certification, efforts towards sustainable financing and founding of a national CHW association (Association of State and Territorial Health Officials, 2020; National Association of Community Health Workers 2020). Several notable efforts to advance the CHW model within bureaucracies and health systems have been advanced (Centers for Disease Control and Prevention 2020).

Related efforts to structure and systematize the field at the international level have included the recent WHO guidelines on health policy and system support to optimize community health worker programmes (WHO, 2018) and work being conducted by the Community Health Impact Coalition (Community Health Impact Coalition 2020) and the Population Council (Agarwal et al., 2019a, b). The COVID-19 pandemic has underlined the need for systemic support for CHWs, who can conduct outreach, share health education, provide support for marginalized individuals and communities and address the social and structural factors (particularly, systemic racism and white supremacy) that put individuals and communities at increased risk (Mayfield-Johnson et al., 2020; Rosenthal et al., 2020).

13.3 CHWs in Health Promotion Research

According to Potvin et al. (2013):

> Recent evolution in the field of health science has shown that a key element for a system's capacity is a thriving research community, enjoying a sufficient level of resources and funding for the conduct of relevant studies that inform the definition of critical problems and systems' responses to those problems. (p. 3)

A large and growing research community has documented the unique contributions of CHWs to a wide range of desirable outcomes including improved health, disease prevention and management and quality of care; better utilization of health services and reduced cost; strengthened local economies and families and increased community capacity (Campbell et al., 2015; Fedder et al., 2003; Kangovi et al., 2020; Kieffer et al., 2013, 2014; Levine et al., 2003; Morgan et al., 2016; Shah et al., 2013; Spencer et al., 2018; Witmer et al., 1995). Ethnographers have studied CHWs' working conditions and advocated for greater respect and higher pay (Maes, 2017; Maes et al., 2014).

Despite these impressive outcomes, the lack of standardized measures to assess CHW practice has made it impossible to aggregate data across programmes and regions, impeding commitment to sustainable, long-term financing for CHW programmes. Lack of easy-to-use indicators has made it difficult for grassroots programmes to report outcomes to funders and their constituencies (Wiggins et al., 2021). These reasons, among others, led to the founding of the CHW CI Project. Similar efforts are underway in low- and middle-income countries (Agarwal et al., 2019a).

A variety of studies going back more than 20 years have addressed CHWs' roles in health promotion research. Commonly, CHWs were positioned (and shown to be effective) in research as interviewers and interventionists (Allen et al., 2002; Hill et al., 1996, 1999; Levine et al., 2003). Some earlier studies (Terpstra et al., 2011) focused the "researcher gaze" upon CHWs in an effort to identify problems and limitations associated with their engagement in research. Even in this earlier period, some studies did include CHWs as co-researchers and co-creators of knowledge and identified the benefits associated with their involvement (Farquhar et al., 2008).

A recent scoping review of the positionality of CHWs on research teams (Coulter et al., 2020) has found that although CHWs are increasingly involved as members of research teams, their level of involvement and the roles they play continue to vary widely. Not surprisingly, CHWs tend to play the widest range of roles in studies using a community-based participatory research (CBPR) approach. The scoping review identified 12 benefits associated with CHW involvement in research, including increasing the research team's awareness of the broader community context, contributing to community acceptability of interventions, negotiating the inclusion of structurally vulnerable communities in research, bringing community voices to research and encouraging advocacy to sustain health-promoting individual- and system-level changes. The correspondence between these outcomes and the most cherished outcomes of health promotion is notable. In a related development, the 2018 final report of the CHW Core Consensus Project (Rosenthal et al., 2018) updated the 1998 list of CHW core roles (Wiggins & Borbón, 1998) to include "participating in evaluation and research".

13.4 The CHW Common Indicators Project as Health Promotion Research

To help fill the evaluation knowledge gap in the CHW field, in 2014, the Michigan Community Health Worker Alliance (MiCHWA) launched the CHW Evaluation Common Indicators Project (Kieffer et al., 2015). The goal was to create a common set of evaluation indicators and measures to articulate the unique contributions of CHWs to successful programme outcomes and their added value to healthcare and human service systems. Building on the work conducted by MiCHWA, in 2015, members of the Oregon CHW Consortium organized a 2-day summit, which intentionally brought together 16 CHWs, CHW programme managers and CHW programme evaluators from the academic field, health system, public health and other organizations from 5 states, all of whom had an interest in CHW evaluation. The outcomes of the Summit included a preliminary consensus list of process and outcome constructs and the founding of the national CHW CI Project. Since the initial Summit, the Project has engaged over 220 people from more than 35 states (Rodela et al., 2021; Wiggins et al., 2021).

The ultimate purpose of the CI Project is to assure that CHWs can make an optimum contribution to promoting health and eliminating inequities, by assuring that the workforce is understood, appreciated and sustainably supported. To achieve this long-term goal, the short- and medium-term objectives of the Project are:

1. To identify a relatively brief set of specific process and outcome *indicators* that can be used across CHW programmes, regardless of setting and community and
2. To identify a larger set of process and outcome *constructs* that can be recommended for CHW research and evaluation nationally but which cannot be collected uniformly in all settings.

These objectives were defined over the course of a series of participatory activities including in-person and virtual summits, meetings and presentations at state and national conferences and regular conference calls.

The research objects of the CI Project are the processes CHWs use, the workforce conditions they need and the outcomes they achieve (for a full list of constructs, see Rodela et al., 2021). The processes are distinctive of health promotion, in that they focus on relationship building and trust, are wide-ranging and adapt to the unique needs of unique communities. The outcomes are distinctive of health promotion because they focus on outcomes such as community empowerment and social support, along with more traditional health outcomes such as improved health and reduced disparities.

The CI Project addresses all five of the action areas identified in the Ottawa Charter:

1. *Supportive environments*: The constructs include the workplace conditions that CHWs need (such as compensation and advancement) to make an optimum contribution to community health.
2. *Personal skills*: Through its methodology, the CI Project increases personal skills among all members of the team. In line with the dictum from the Jakarta Declaration (WHO, 1997) that "access to education and information is essential to achieving effective participation and the empowerment of people and communities", all stakeholders in the Project are provided with the education and information they need to be able to participate meaningfully.
3. *Healthy public policy*: The CI Project works with governmental entities like the Centers for Disease Control and Prevention (CDC) that have the influence to encourage states and programmes to adopt indicators that are in line with the

historic CHW practice and support the integrity of the profession. The Project is currently in its third year of CDC funding.

4. *Community action*: By conducting the CI Project, which to date has engaged more than 220 CHWs and others in a variety of knowledge-building and organizing activities, we are engaging in community action. The knowledge produced in the Project will also be a support to further community action, as CHWs and others use the indicators to advocate for the importance of playing a full range of roles, receiving a living wage with opportunities for advancement and working in ways that increase empowerment and social support among communities and community members.
5. *Reorient health services*: There is a constant danger that health systems will reduce the roles of CHWs to those that can be most easily quantified and reimbursed, not realizing that in so doing, they are actually reducing the effectiveness of CHWs. While not discounting the importance of indicators like healthcare utilization and cost in settings where they can be collected appropriately and well, the CI Project also seeks to motivate health systems to collect process data about workforce conditions and CHW activities and outcome data like changes in empowerment and social support. These health promotion outcomes would likely not be measured in clinical settings without the support and encouragement of an outside project.

13.5 The Research Paradigm and Design of the CI Project

According to Woodall et al. (2018), paradigmatic flexibility is both characteristic of and beneficial for health promotion research. Appropriately, then, the CHW CI Project is influenced by several research paradigms including critical theory, naturalism, the participatory paradigm and pragmatism. Critical theory supports the idea, basic to popular education, that the current distribution of the world's resources, including power, is unjust and that change is possible (Kincheloe, 2005). In stressing that there is no *one right way*, naturalism supports the multiplicity of culturally centred approaches used by CHWs (Lincoln & Guba, 1985). The participatory paradigm contributes the insight, also at the heart of both the CHW model and popular education, that everyone in the community has something unique and valuable to contribute and that we need everyone's contribution to create a more just and equitable world (Koelen et al., 2001). Finally, pragmatism encourages drawing from and building on approaches that have worked in practice in multiple different communities and settings (Morgan, 2007). In terms of its design, the CI Project is most aptly described as a distinctive form of research that involves the identification, development and standardization of measures to help describe, structure and sustain the integrity of a field and/or a profession. It is exploratory and primarily qualitative, though the indicators it seeks to develop and build consensus around are quantitative.

13.6 The Research Approach and Methods of the CI Project

The research approach and methods of the CI Project are based on two primary theoretical frameworks: popular education and participatory research. These frameworks have roots in the theories and practices of the Brazilian educator and political theorist Paulo Freire and others working within a post-colonialist context during the mid to late twentieth century (Wallerstein & Duran, 2003; Wiggins et al., 2017). Drawing on these roots, popular education and participatory research derive a similar epistemology, similar sets of principles and similar practices, all of which are also quite consistent with the CHW model and progressive health promotion.

13.6.1 *Popular Education in the CI Project*

Also referred to as "people's education", popular education (PE) creates settings in which people most affected by inequities can share what they know, learn from others in their community and use their knowledge to create a more just and equitable society. The two key ideas shared between PE and the CHW model are that people most affected by inequity are the experts of their own lives and that experiential knowledge is just as important as academic knowledge (Wiggins et al., 2014).

Most closely associated with Latin American struggles for social justice, forms of PE have arisen in almost all human communities as a response to systematic oppression and a mechanism to bring about change. Strands of PE can be found in Indigenous ways of knowing around the world, in newspapers and clandestine schools meant to uplift and empower US Black communities from the seventieth century to the present, in the practices of Latin American educators and revolutionaries who sought to use education as a foundation for liberation and in many other times and places. Similarities in methodology across diverse PE settings suggest that educators seeking to undo social inequity and build critical thinking skills come organically to similar strategies (Wiggins & Pérez, 2016).

PE has demonstrated great promise as a philosophy and methodology that communities and public health practitioners can use to address the underlying social and structural determinants of health and to decrease health inequities (Wallerstein & Bernstein, 1988; Wallerstein et al., 1999). A growing number of studies have suggested that the use of PE for health promotion is associated with improved outcomes, both health-related and empowerment-related (Wallerstein & Wiggins, 2018; Wiggins, 2012). A 2016 study of the use of PE with health promotion students suggested that PE is "a valid alternative to conventional pedagogy and a useful complement to liberatory pedagogies more common in university classrooms" (Wiggins & Pérez, 2016, p. 1).

Using PE in CI Project activities means that facilitators work to create an atmosphere of trust where participants co-create goals and agendas, balance participation and power and actively elicit all voices. To achieve these goals, facilitators use techniques such as *dinámicas* (social learning games); a variety of dramatic techniques including *sociodramas*, talk shows and radio plays; cooperative learning activities; negotiation of group agreements; group evaluations and shared meals.

13.6.2 Participatory Research in the CI Project

Woodall et al. (2018) identify four characteristics of health promotion research:

1. Application to real-world contexts
2. Application of health promotion values to the research process
3. Researchers as co-researchers with the participants in knowledge production
4. Expansive methodological toolkit of health promotion research

As these authors and others point out (Koelen et al., 2001), health promotion research and a range of participatory approaches to research bear much in common, including this set of characteristics. Our commitment to participatory research in the CI Project means that we seek to embody all four of these characteristics, as we will explain, taking the characteristics in a slightly different order.

The CI Project positions community members as *co-researchers and co-participants in the production of knowledge*. In the CI Project, "community" is defined primarily as members of the CHW profession, most of whom are also members of communities most affected by inequities based on race/ethnicity, immigrant status, LGBTQ2I+ status and other marginalized identities. CHWs have been central to the CI Project since its inception. Five of 16 participants in the organizing Summit were CHWs and three acted as co-facilitators. At this Summit, the original list of process and outcome constructs was identified based on what CHWs believe they most need to be effective in their work, the processes they identify as most characteristic of their work and the outcomes they feel most uniquely capable of achieving. CHWs have been deeply involved in facilitating regular virtual meetings of the Project Advisory Group and presenting at conferences and workshops; through both activities, the list of constructs has been further refined with input from CHWs. Publications about the Project have included CHWs as co-authors. Recognizing a need to increase the number of CHWs involved in project leadership, in 2020, more CHWs joined the Project Leadership Team and a four-person CHW Council was created.

We have sought to live out our *health promotion values in the research process*. For us, these values include shared leadership and decision-making and commitment to racial equity and social justice. The structure of the Project is intended to promote shared leadership. It includes a six-person Leadership Team (LT), the previously mentioned CHW Council and an Advisory Group, which comprises more than 220 people and which meets every other month for 1.5 hours. Two members of the LT act as co-coordinators, dealing with administrative tasks and triaging correspondence with Project partners. All substantive decisions are made by consensus of the LT. In our processes, we seek to err on the side of inclusion. This means copying all LT members on most emails, jointly developing meeting agendas, sharing facilitation responsibilities during meetings and making regular time to reflect together on various actions taken by the Project. The CHW Council, which is composed of experienced CHWs, some of whom are now supervisors and trainers, serves to amplify CHW voice in the Project; members will also co-facilitate presentations and meetings and co-author publications. The Advisory Group provides advice and consent to the Project, and many members participate from time to time in more intensive interactions, such as the second Summit held via Zoom in May of 2020. At this Summit, a proposed set of 10 priority indicators was discussed and an initial plan for piloting the indicators was created. With all these actions, we hope to provide a "reliable access to the decision-making process and the skills and knowledge essential to effect change", which the Jakarta Charter (WHO, 1997) says is crucial for empowerment.

In May of 2020, following the police killings of George Floyd and Breonna Taylor, the LT decided to make explicit a previously implicit commitment to racial justice. As the first action, LT members jointly developed a statement of solidarity and commitment, which was shared with the Advisory Group. Adding more people to the LT and creating the CHW Council are further outcomes of that commitment, as all new members of both teams are Black, Indigenous and people of colour. In the subsequent year, we have adopted a racial equity lens and are applying it to actions of the Project.

The CI Project both uses and recommends an *expansive combination of methods*. Methods used to gain input from stakeholders include focus groups, individual interviews, convenings and participatory presentations. In terms of the indicators that we are recommending, they are quantitative, primarily because those indicators will be easier to apply in a consistent way with minimal expense. However, we will also develop a toolkit or implementation guide that provides background about the indicators so that CHWs can explain them in a way that is culturally centred. Furthermore, we recommend using the quantitative indicators in tandem with qualitative methods that are centred in the community and culture.

Finally, we seek to work in such a way that *knowledge is immediately applicable to practice*. Implicit in our use of popular education is adherence to a praxis model that starts with the current experience of CHWs and allies who participate in our project. The Project creates opportunities to pool this knowledge and reflect on it through a variety of modalities. Some outcomes of reflection, in the form of lists, categories and visuals, are immediately presented back to participants in our meetings, workshops and Summits. In other cases, participants can go back to their communities and immediately test ideas produced by the Project. The most substantive example of a real-world application of our ideas has come as we have begun to pilot the indicators that have been developed in previous phases of the Project. Piloting will lead to further refinement of the indicators in an iterative process that will go on for the entire length of the Project.

13.7 The Outcomes and Contributions of the CI Project

The CI Project is already generating knowledge about the barriers and solutions to fully and meaningfully engage a set of undervalued health promotion practitioners in the creation of process and outcome measures for their own field. As they are generally located at the bottom of the health system's hierarchy, CHWs often face barriers to being involved in research, even research about their own profession. These barriers include lack of support from employers to engage in research projects on work time and lack of support staff to facilitate their involvement.

Obtaining meaningful input from a diverse group of stakeholders about a project primarily concerned with measurement and evaluation presents additional challenges. During stakeholder focus groups, for example, LT members found that many stakeholders who are not trained as evaluators were commenting not on how to *measure* concepts like social support but rather on how to *increase* social support among programme participants and what they need to be successful in their work. Making the distinction between *doing the work* and *measuring the work* was challenging for focus group facilitators who were not members of the LT. This was partly because most CHW programme staff are focused on doing, not measuring, their work and because CHWs remain largely marginalized from evaluation and research processes (Rodela et al., 2021).

Despite these barriers, through the thoughtful and consistent use of popular education, the CI Project has succeeded in bringing together more than 220 stakeholders interested in identifying and using common process and outcome indicators; identifying a set of 20 process and outcome constructs that can be recommended for CHW research and evaluation nationally; identifying, modifying and developing specific indicators for 11 priority constructs; publishing about the Project in peer-reviewed journals and blogs and presenting at state and national conferences and garnering funding from the premier governmental entity for health promotion in the USA. All of this has been done in a participatory way that increases the likelihood of the indicators being adopted and used.

When fully implemented, the CHW CI Project will generate knowledge about the ways CHWs work (their processes), the conditions they need to be effective and the outcomes they achieve. In terms of processes, our research will generate knowledge about the range of roles CHWs play (with reference to a formulation of 10 core roles identified in previous research), how CHWs go about connecting participants to needed resources and the degree to which CHWs are involved in shaping and influencing health policy. We will generate knowledge about conditions needed for success including compensation and benefits, the extent to which CHWs are integrated into teams and/or to what degree they are respected and treated as equals in their workplaces and the presence or absence of a constellation of policy and system conditions that promote CHW sustainability. Finally, we will generate outcome knowledge about the degree to which CHW programmes improve self-reported health status, community empowerment and social support and increase access to health and social services.

13.8 Conclusions

In summary, our research contributes to advancing and structuring the field of health promotion research, in that we are pioneering technologies and methods to gain meaningful input from, and effectively measure the contributions of, a group of practitioners who are crucial to the health promotion enterprise but who have often been overlooked and/or devalued. As CHWs are some of the oldest and most effective health promotion practitioners, it is essential to better understand their practice so that CHW programmes can be expanded and other health promotion professionals can learn from their approach. Similarly, it is important to understand the unique contributions of CHWs to developing conditions in which communities can achieve optimum health. It is necessary to do all this using a participatory approach, since by so doing we reinforce the values and processes at the heart of the CHW model.

Acknowledgements The Leadership Team of the CHW Common Indicators Project thanks Ms. Gloria Palmisano (emerita member of our Leadership Team), the members of the CHW Council and Advisory Group, the attendees at the 2015 and 2020 Common Indicators Summits, the participants in two pre-conference workshops held in 2016 and 2019 in conjunction with the Annual Meeting of the American Public Health Association, the members of the Centers for Disease Control and Prevention (CDC) CHW Workgroup, the staff at the National Association of Chronic Disease Directors and the participants in focus groups and interviews for generously sharing their time, experience and wisdom.

References

Agarwal, S., Kirk, K., Sripad, P., Bellows, B., Abuya, T., & Warren, C. (2019a). Setting the global research agenda for community health systems: Literature and consultative review. *Human Resources for Health, 17*(86), 1–20. https://doi.org/10.1186/s12960-019-0362-8

Agarwal, S., Sripad, P., Johnson, C., Kirk, K., Bellows, B., Ana, J., et al. (2019b). A conceptual framework for measuring community health workforce performance within primary health care systems. *Human Resources for Health, 17*(86). https://doi.org/10.1186/s12960-019-0422-0

Allen, J. K., Blumenthal, R. S., Margolis, S., Young, D. R., Miller, E. R., & Kelly, K. (2002). Nurse case management of hypercholesterolemia in patients with coronary heart disease: Results of a randomized clinical trial. *American Heart Journal, 144*, 678–686.

Association of State and Territorial Health Officials. (2020). *Clinical to community connections.* https://www.astho.org/Community-Health-Workers/. Accessed 25 Feb 2020.

Campbell, J. D., Brooks, M., Hosokawa, P., Robinson, J., Song, L., & Krieger, J. (2015). Community health worker home visits for Medicaid-enrolled children with asthma: Effects on asthma outcomes and costs. *American Journal of Public Health, 105*, 2366–2372.

Centers for Disease Control and Prevention. (2020). *Promoting policy and systems change to expand employment of community health workers (CHWs).* https://www.cdc.gov/dhdsp/chw_elearning/index.html. Accessed 13 Mar 2021.

Community Health Impact Coalition. (2020). https://chwimpact.org/. Accessed 20 Oct 2020.

Coulter, K., Ingram, M., McClelland, D. J., & Lohr, A. (2020). Positionality of community health workers on health intervention research teams: A scoping review. *Frontiers in Public Health.* https://doi.org/10.3389/fpubh.2020.00208

Farquhar, S. A., Wiggins, N., Michael, Y. L., Luhr, G., Jordan, J., & Lopez, A. (2008). "Sitting in different chairs:" Roles of the community health workers in the *Poder es Salud*/Power for Health Project. *Education for Health*. http://www.educationforhealth.net/articles/subviewnew.asp?ArticleID=39

Fedder, D. O., Chang, R. J., Curry, S., & Nichols, G. (2003). The effectiveness of a community health worker outreach program on healthcare utilization of west Baltimore City Medicaid patients with diabetes, with or without hypertension. *Ethnicity & Disease, 13*, 22–27.

Hawe, P., King, L., Noort, M., Gifford, S. M., & Lloyd, B. (1998). Working invisibly: Health workers talk about capacity-building in health promotion. *Health Promotion International, 13*(4), 285–295.

Hill, M. N., Bone, L. R., & Butz, A. M. (1996). Enhancing the role of community-health workers in research. *Journal of Nursing Scholarship, 28*, 221–226.

Hill, M. N., Bone, L. R., Hilton, S. C., Roary, M. C., Kelen, G. D., & Levine, D. M. (1999). A clinical trial to improve high blood pressure care in young urban black men: Recruitment, followup, and outcomes. *American Journal of Hypertension, 12*, 548–554.

Kane, S., Radkar, A., Gadgil, M., & McPake, B. (2020). Community health workers as influential health system actors and not "just another pair of hands". *International Journal of Health Policy and Management*. https://doi.org/10.34172/ijhpm.2020.58

Kangovi, S., Mitra, N., Grande, D., Long, J., & Asch, D. (2020). Evidence-based community health worker program addresses unmet social needs and generates positive return on investment. *Health Affairs, 39*(2), 207–213.

Kieffer, E., Caldwell, C., Welmerink, D., Welch, K., Sinco, B., & Guzman, J. R. (2013). Effect of the healthy MOMs lifestyle intervention on reducing depressive symptoms among pregnant Latinas. *American Journal of Community Psychology, 51*(1–2), 76–89. https://doi.org/10.1007/s10464-012-9523-9

Kieffer, E., Welmerink, D., Welch, K., Sinco, B., Rees Clayton, E., Schumann, C., et al. (2014). Dietary outcomes of a Spanish-language randomized controlled diabetes prevention trial with pregnant Latinas. *American Journal of Public Health, 104*(3):526–533. https://doi.org/10.2105/AJPH.2012.301122. Epub 13 June 2013.

Kieffer, E., Yankey, N., Mitchell, K., Allen, C. G., Janevic, M. R., Thomas, C., et al. (2015). The role of evaluation in developing and sustaining community health worker coalitions: The example of the Michigan Community Health Worker Alliance. *Journal of Ambulatory Care Management, 38*(4), 283–296.

Kincheloe, J. (2005). *Critical pedagogy primer*. Peter Lang.

Koelen, M. A., Vaandrager, L., & Colomér, C. (2001). Health promotion research: Dilemmas and challenges. *Journal of Epidemiology and Community Health, 55*(4), 257–262. https://doi.org/10.1136/jech.55.4.257

Levine, D. M., Bone, L. R., Hill, M. N., Stallings, R., Gelber, A. C., Barker, A., et al. (2003). The effectiveness of a community/academic health center partnership in decreasing the level of blood pressure in an urban African-American population. *Ethnicity Disease, 13*, 354–361.

Lincoln, Y. S., & Guba, E. G. (1985). *Naturalistic inquiry*. Sage Publications.

Maes, K. (2015). "Volunteers are not paid because they are priceless": Community health worker capacities and values in an AIDS treatment intervention in urban Ethiopia: Community health worker capacities. *Medical Anthropology Quarterly, 29*, 97–115.

Maes, K. (2017). *The lives of community health workers: Local labor and global health in urban Ethiopia*. Routledge.

Maes, K., Closser, S., & Kalofonos, I. (2014). Listening to community health workers: How ethnographic research can inform positive relationships among community health workers, health institutions, and communities. *American Journal of Public Health, 104*(5), e1-5.

Mayfield-Johnson, S., Smith, D. O., Crosby, S. A., Haywood, C. G., Castillo, J., Bryant-Williams, D., et al. (2020). Insights on COVID-19 from community health worker state leaders. *Journal of Ambulatory Care Management, 43*(4), 268–277.

Morgan, A. U., Grande, D. T., Carter, T., Long, J. A., & Kangovi, S. (2016). Penn Center for Community Health Workers: Step-by-step approach to sustain an evidence-based community health worker intervention at an academic medical center. *American Journal of Public Health, 106*, 1958–1960.

Morgan, D. L. (2007). Paradigms lost and pragmatism regained: Methodological implications of combining qualitative and quantitative methods. *Journal of Mixed Methods Research, 1*(1), 48–76.

National Association of Community Health Workers. (2020). https://nachw.org/. Accessed 20 Oct 2020.

Patient Protection and Affordable Care Act of 2010, Pub. L. No. 111-148, sec 5101, 5102, 5313, 5403, and 3509 (2010).

Potvin, L., McQueen, D. V., de Leeuw, E., Mendes, R., Abel, T., & Larouche, A. (2013). Fostering innovation in health promotion research: The critical role of the IUHPE. *Global Health Promotion, 20*(2), 3–4. https://doi.org/10.1177/1757975913491887

Rodela, K., Wiggins, N., Maes, K., Campos Dominguez, T., Adewumi, V., Jewell, P., et al. (2021). The Community Health Worker (CHW) Common Indicators Project: Engaging CHWs in measurement to sustain the profession. *Frontiers in Public Health, 9*, 1–12. https://doi.org/10.3389/fpubh.2021.674858

Rosenthal, E. L. Menking, P., & St. John, J. (2018). *The Community Health Worker Core Consensus (C3) Project: A report of the C3 project phase 1 and 2, together leaning toward the sky.* A National Project to Inform CHW Policy and Practice. Texas Tech University Health Sciences Center.

Rosenthal, E. L., Menking, P., & Begay, M. G. (2020). Fighting the COVID-19 merciless monster: Lives on the line-community health representatives' roles in the pandemic battle on the Navajo Nation. *Journal of Ambulatory Care Management, 43*(4), 301–305. https://doi.org/10.1097/JAC.0000000000000354. PMID: 32858729.

Rosenthal, E. L., Wiggins, N., Ingram, M., Mayfield-Johnson, S., & De Zapien, J. G. (2011). Community health workers then and now: An overview of national studies aimed at defining the field. *Journal of Ambulatory Care Management, 34*, 247–259.

Shah, M., Kaselitz, E., & Heisler, M. (2013). The role of community health workers in diabetes: Update on current literature. *Current Diabetes Reports, 13*(2), 163–171.

Spencer, M., Kieffer, E. C., Sinco, B., Piatt, G., Palmisano, G., Hawkins, J., et al. (2018). Outcomes at 18 months from a community health worker and peer leader diabetes self-management program for Latino adults. *Diabetes Care, 41*(7), 1414–1422.

Terpstra, J., Coleman, K. J., Simon, G., & Nebeker, C. (2011). The role of community health workers (CHWs) in health promotion research: Ethical challenges and practical solutions. *Health Promotion Practice, 12*(1), 86–93. https://doi.org/10.1177/1524839908330809

Viswanathan, M., Kraschnewski, J., Nishikawa, B., Morgan, L. C., Thieda, P., Honeycutt, A., et al. (2009). *Outcomes of community health worker interventions* (Evidence Report/Technology Assessment No. 181. AHRQ Publication No. 09-E014). Agency for Healthcare Research and Quality.

Wallerstein, N., & Bernstein, E. (1988). Empowerment education: Freire's ideas adapted to health education. *Health Education Quarterly, 15*(4), 379–394.

Wallerstein, N., & Duran, B. (2003). The conceptual, historical, and practice roots of community based participatory research and related participatory traditions. In M. Minkler & N. Wallerstein (Eds.), *Community based participatory research for health* (pp. 27–52). Jossey-Bass.

Wallerstein, N., Sanchez-Merki, V., & Dow, L. (1999). Freirian praxis in health education and community organizing: A case study of an adolescent prevention program. In M. Minkler (Ed.), *Community organizing and community building for health* (pp. 195–211). Rutgers University Press.

Wallerstein, N., & Wiggins, N. (2018). L'empowerment améliore l'état de santé de la population: Nina Wallerstein et Noelle Wiggins ont mesuré l'impact de l'empowerment sur la santé des populations. *La Santé en Action, 446*, 10–14.

Wiggins, N. (2012). Popular education for health promotion and community empowerment: A review of the literature. *Health Promotion International, 27*, 356–371. https://doi.org/10.1093/heapro/dar046

Wiggins, N., & Borbón, A. (1998). Core roles and competencies of community health workers. In E. L. Rosenthal, N. Wiggins, N. Brownstein, S. Johnson, et al. (Eds.), *Final report of the national community health advisor study*. Annie E. Casey Foundation.

Wiggins, N., Hughes, A., Rios-Campos, T., Rodriguez, A., & Potter, C. (2014). *La palabra es Salud* (The word is health): Combining mixed methods and CBPR to understand the comparative effectiveness of popular and conventional education. *Journal of Mixed Methods Research, 8*, 278–298. https://doi.org/10.1177/1558689813510785

Wiggins, N., Maes, K., Palmisano, G., Rodela, K., Rodriguez Avila, L., & Kieffer, E. (2021). A community participatory approach to identify common evaluation indicators for community health worker practice. *Progress in Community Health Partnerships, 15*(2), 217–224.

Wiggins, N., Parajón, L. C., Coombe, C., Duldulao, A., Rodriguez-Garcia, L., & Wang, P. (2017). Participatory evaluation as a process of empowerment: Experiences with community health workers in the US and Latin America. In N. Wallerstein, B. Durán, J. Oetzel, & M. Minkler (Eds.), *Community-based participatory research for health* (4th ed.). Jossey-Bass.

Wiggins, N., & Pérez, A. (2016). Using popular education with health promotion students in the USA. *Health Promotion International*. https://doi.org/10.1093/heapro/dav121

Wiggins, N., & Rodela, D. K. (2021). Roles and competencies of community health workers. In J. St. John, S. Mayfield-Johnson, & W. Hernandez (Eds.), *Promoting the health of the community – Community health workers describing their roles, competencies, and practice*. Springer.

Wingood, G. M., & DiClemente, R. J. (2019). Accelerating the evolution of health promotion research: Broadening boundaries and improving impact. *American Journal of Public Health, 109*(S2), S116. https://doi.org/10.2105/AJPH.2019.304991

Witmer, A., Seifer, S. D., Finocchio, L., Leslie, J., & O'Neil, E. H. (1995). Community health workers: Integral members of the health care work force. *American Journal of Public Health, 85*, 1055–1058.

Woodall, J., Warwick-Booth, L., South, J., & Cross, R. (2018). What makes health promotion research distinct? *Scandinavian Journal of Public Health, 46*, 118–122. https://doi-org.proxy.lib.pdx.edu/10.1177/1403494817744130

World Health Organization. (1986). *The Ottawa charter for health promotion*. World Health Organization. http://www.who.int/healthpromotion/conferences/previous/ottawa/en/. Accessed 9 Jan 2016

World Health Organization. (1997). *Jakarta Declaration on Leading Health Promotion into the 21st Century*. https://www.who.int/healthpromotion/conferences/previous/jakarta/declaration/en/index1.html. Accessed 20 Oct 2020.

World Health Organization. (2018). *WHO launches new guideline on health policy and system support to optimize community health worker programmes*. https://www.who.int/hrh/community/guideline-health-support-optimize-hw-programmes/en/. Accessed 20 Oct 2020.

Chapter 14
Investing in Health Promotion Research Among Community Health Workers in Semi-rural Uganda Using a Partnership Approach

Linda Gibson, Deborah Ikhile, Mathew Nyashanu, and David Musoke

14.1 Introduction

This chapter explores a partnership approach to undertaking research in Uganda that has been informed by key health promotion principles that we argue inform our practice and can add to emerging debates about what makes health promotion research distinctive. The research that we outline in this chapter was conducted within a 10-year partnership between Nottingham Trent University in the UK and Makerere University in Uganda. Despite the obvious differences in geoeconomic contexts including access to research resources, notably the funding between the UK and Uganda, what enabled our research approach is a set of values drawn from the different yet similar backgrounds of interdisciplinary social sciences, public health and environmental health. The nomenclatures of departments and programmes are both historical and political within institutions and professions, but, in both our respective areas, disciplinary practices are informed by values of social justice and inclusion, enabling and empowering communities and core health promotion values as articulated in the Ottawa Charter. Makerere University has a long history of investing in environmental and health promotion and education programmes through grassroots community-based approaches. Public health at

L. Gibson (✉) · M. Nyashanu
Institute of Health and Allied Professions, Nottingham Trent University, Nottingham, England, UK
e-mail: Linda.gibson@ntu.ac.uk

D. Ikhile
Institute of Health and Allied Professions, Nottingham Trent University, Nottingham, England, UK

Brighton and Sussex Medical School, University of Sussex, Brighton, England, UK

D. Musoke
School of Public Health, Makerere University, Kampala, Uganda

L. Potvin, D. Jourdan (eds.), *Global Handbook of Health Promotion Research, Vol. 1*,
https://doi.org/10.1007/978-3-030-97212-7_14

Nottingham Trent University is informed by health promotion approaches and the social model of health, particularly the need to recognize the broader determinants of health. These values informed our research practice in the way we engaged with our target communities and the methodologies we used. This approach enabled us to undertake research that has "real-world" impact on those communities.

The World Health Organization recognizes community health workers (CHWs) as central to successful national health plans in low- and middle-income countries (LMICs). In 2001, Uganda established a CHW programme as reflected in the National Health Policy (1999) as part of the Uganda National Minimum Healthcare Package. This strategy aimed to ensure that all villages in Uganda could mobilize individuals and households for improved health outcomes. Uganda had good success in delivering an HIV/AIDs response strategy during the 1990s and early 2000s, which was globally recognized for its innovation. CHWs are a critical but undervalued workforce in delivering comprehensive primary health care (PHC) to address the multiple environmental and health challenges in current times.

Our initial baseline research identified a gap in the delivery of the training programme for CHWs, which was impacting the effective implementation of health promotion and education initiatives, thus leading to low morale. Our subsequent research focused on investing in and building the capacity of this essential health workforce. We discuss the methodological considerations and the multiple methods used, present a synthesis of our research findings and discuss the challenges that structure conducting research in this field. This chapter also includes how our research has contributed to capacity-building initiatives among CHWs in Uganda.

14.2 Methodology

The health promotion research activities we conducted among CHWs in Uganda from 2012 to 2020 included externally funded studies and student-led projects as part of their master's and doctoral programmes. Our research aims (summarized in Table 14.1) ranged from assessing the contributions of CHWs in specific health issues, such as breast cancer, general non-communicable diseases (NCDs) and antimicrobial resistance, to broader topics, such as assessing their performance in PHC delivery. The CHWs are involved in health promotion on these health issues in their communities as part of their work.

14.2.1 Research Site

Our health promotion research among CHWs in Uganda was conducted in Wakiso District. The district is peri-urban and neighbours the capital city, Kampala. The district is the most populous in the country with an approximate population of two million people according to the 2014 national census (Uganda Bureau of Statistics,

Table 14.1 Overview of the health promotion research aims and methods from 2012 to 2020

Year of research	Study reference	Research aims	Data collection methods and sample size
2012	Musoke et al. (2016)	To determine the status of the CHW programme	Key informant interviews: 10 (3 health assistants, 3 CHW supervisors and 4 local leaders) Focus group discussions with CHWs: 9
2015	Ilaboya et al. (2018)	To examine the perceived barriers to early detection of breast cancer using a socio-ecological model	Semi-structured interviews with women: 5 Key informant interviews: 7 (1 health practitioner, 2 cancer organization representatives, 1 policymaker and 3 public health researchers) Focus group discussions: 2 (1 with CHWs and 1 with a women's group)
2016	Nchafack (2016)	To explore CHWs' perspectives on the use of mobile phones to improve access to information on maternal and child health	Key informant interviews: 3 (2 health practitioners and 1 policymaker) Focus group discussions: 3 (1 with pregnant women, 1 with new mothers and 1 with female CHWs)
2016	Musoke et al. (2019a)	To assess CHWs' competence, motivation and level of support received from their coordinators	Questionnaire: 301 CHWs Focus group discussions: 6 (2 with CHWs, 3 with community members and 1 with CHW coordinators) Key informant interviews: 6 (with health practitioners, district health officials and local leaders)
2016	Musoke et al. (2019b)	To assess the performance of CHWs and associated factors	Questionnaire: 201 CHWs
2017	Marufu et al. (2017)	To explore the views, opinions and feelings of female CHWs on their performance	Focus group discussions with female CHWs: 3 Key informant interviews: 5 (3 with CHW coordinators and 2 with CHW focal persons based at the local health centres)
2018–2019	Musoke et al. (2021)	To assess involvement of CHWs in the prevention and control of NCDs	Questionnaire: 485 CHWs Focus group discussions with community members: 6
2019–2020	Musoke et al. (2020a)	To evaluate access and use of antimicrobials in the community	Questionnaire: 226 CHWs

2016). The district is characterized by a mix of urban and rural dwellers. The 2014 census showed that 59.2% of the Wakiso District population resided in urban settings (Uganda Bureau of Statistics, 2016). Our research predominantly focused on the rural population in this district due to the difficulties they face with regard to poverty and accessing health and other social services.

14.2.2 Research Methods

We used both quantitative and qualitative methods in our research with CHWs. These data collection methods generated evidence to build the capacities of the CHWs, evaluate CHW performance and improve health promotion/PHC delivery in the local communities in the area. For quantitative data collection, we used questionnaires comprising open and close-ended questions. We employed multiple methods for qualitative data collection, including semi-structured interviews, key informant interviews, focus group discussions and stakeholder workshops. Quantitative data underwent univariate, bivariate and multivariate analyses, whereas qualitative data were analyzed thematically drawing on both semantic and latent themes. The sample size of the CHWs involved in our research varied depending on the research objectives and study design. Many of our quantitative studies involved all CHWs in the area, while purposive sampling was used for qualitative studies based on their experience with PHC delivery. A summary of our health promotion research aims and methods used is presented in Table 14.1.

14.2.3 Methodological Considerations

Key methodological considerations that influenced how we conducted research with CHWs included use of the local language, involving other participants beyond CHWs and access to the research site. Our research with CHWs considered the need to collect data predominantly in *Luganda*, the local language mainly used in the area. This necessitated the use of research assistants who knew the local language to collect data or support the UK researchers in translation during interviews and group discussions. In other cases, CHWs fluent in English were purposively selected to enable UK research students to collect data directly from them.

Although our health promotion research focused on CHWs, we also involved participants who are key stakeholders in the CHW programme including health professionals, the district health team, policymakers, non-governmental organizations and community members, who are the recipients of healthcare services. Involving these wider participants was crucial to ensure that our research with CHWs remained aligned with the existing PHC system at the district and national levels.

14.3 Key Research Findings

14.3.1 Roles of CHWs in Primary Healthcare Delivery

Findings from our research with CHWs showed that they were predominantly involved in communicable diseases (Ilaboya et al., 2018; Musoke et al., 2021) through health education and health promotion, with less pronounced roles in

NCDs. About half of the CHWs in our research were involved in integrated community case management of childhood illnesses (Musoke et al., 2019a, 2021). We also found that CHWs play key roles in addressing antimicrobial resistance and supporting antimicrobial stewardship in human health and animal husbandry through educating community members on good sanitation practices, prescribing antimicrobials in the right dosage and encouraging visits to the appropriate health practitioner for accurate clinical diagnosis and prescription (Musoke et al., 2020a).

Our research showed that the roles of CHWs in breast cancer (Ilaboya et al., 2018) and broader NCD management (Musoke et al., 2021) were constrained by complex health system challenges including lack of training. Although CHWs were aware of different NCDs, our research showed that they had less knowledge of how these diseases could be detected or managed. For instance, in our research that assessed the involvement of CHWs in NCDs, we found that the majority (75.3%) knew about the common NCDs such as cancer, diabetes and high blood pressure, but they had minimal roles in the management of these diseases (Musoke et al., 2021).

It was further evident from our research findings that the roles of CHWs reflect the disease trend and health priorities of the country (Ilaboya et al., 2018). Due to the increasing rate of NCDs in Uganda, CHWs recognized that they were strategically positioned to offer screening, early diagnosis and referral services if adequately trained and supported to do so (Musoke et al., 2021).

14.3.2 Drivers of CHW Performance

From our research, we highlighted three key drivers that facilitate CHW performance in their roles: training, supervision and motivation. Our research, which assessed the performance of 201 CHWs, showed a statistically significant relationship between continuous training and increased CHW performance [COR = 12.54 (95% CI: 2.92–53.8), $p = 0.001$] (Musoke et al., 2019b). In our research on the involvement of CHWs in NCDs, we found a relationship between training CHWs and the ability of the community members to trust their competence (Musoke et al., 2021). The findings from Musoke et al. (2021) showed that community members were more confident to approach CHWs on specific health issues when they knew that the CHWs had received appropriate training regarding the health issue.

In relation to motivation, it was evident from our various research that the provision of financial and non-financial incentives and adequacy of medical supplies motivated CHWs to perform better (Marufu et al., 2017; Musoke et al., 2019a, b). For instance, our research, which assessed the impacts of motivation packages on CHWs, showed that the provision of non-financial incentives such as gum boots, umbrellas and solar equipment enabled CHWs to carry out more home visits for health education and treatment purposes (Musoke et al., 2019a). In addition, our research showed that branded T-shirts reinforced the CHWs' identity as community health practitioners and distinguished them from other members of the community (Musoke et al., 2019a). Whilst valuing non-financial incentives, the CHWs in our research indicated that they would also appreciate financial incentives to be provided (Musoke et al., 2019b).

From our research findings, we also found a relationship between the supervision and performance of CHWs (Musoke et al., 2019a, b). We observed that CHWs performed better when their coordinators were competent in performing their coordination and supervisory roles (Musoke et al., 2019b). Our research further demonstrated that training and provision of motorcycles enhanced the abilities of CHW coordinators to perform their supervisory roles (Musoke et al., 2019b). As a result, the CHWs involved in our research reported that they had better access to the current health information and essential medical supplies to enable them to perform better in their roles.

14.3.3 Impact of Mobile Phones on Community Healthcare Delivery

In our research on the use of mobile phones by CHWs and women (Nchafack, 2016), we found that their use facilitated the delivery of primary care relating to maternal and child health services through provision of consultations and follow-up services. However, there was poor utilization of mobile phones due to cultural and socio-economic issues. We found out that female CHWs were sometimes prevented from owning personal mobile phones by their husbands, which reflects the prevailing patriarchal culture in Uganda. Socio-economic status such as low literacy among the majority of CHWs also impeded their ability to harness mobile phones for healthcare delivery. Despite these challenges, our findings indicated that if adequately maximized, the use of mobile phones has the potential to enhance maternal and child health education and promotion and reduce delays in accessing emergency care.

14.4 How Our Research Enhanced the Capacity Building of CHWs

Through the impact of our research activities, we enhanced the capacity of CHWs to effectively carry out their health promotion roles by focusing on the three key drivers of their performance. As a result, we developed a capacity-building programme for more than 600 CHWs in Wakiso District to strengthen their training, supervision and motivation (Musoke et al., 2019a). Through training, we were able to improve their knowledge and skills to carry out health promotion, education and prevention as well as other roles in their respective communities. We had two major categories of training for the CHWs. The first category of training was related to the overall roles and responsibilities of the CHWs based on the Ministry of Health's guidelines. This training included sessions such as home visits, communication skills, management of childhood illnesses and record keeping. The training was not only useful to the existing CHWs but also to the new ones who were selected by local leaders to replace those who had dropped out of the programme. The second category was refresher training on specific topics of interest to the work of CHWs. For example, due to the changing trends in the disease burden in the country and the gap in CHWs' knowledge, we have recently trained them on NCDs. Our partnership has also recently trained CHWs on antimicrobial stewardship to facilitate proper access and use of antimicrobials in the community as an intervention to reduce antimicrobial resistance. This training was particularly important as some CHWs are involved in managing childhood illnesses in the community. In addition, all CHWs have a key responsibility in health, educating the community about key public health issues including antimicrobial resistance. The design and implementation of all these training initiatives were informed by a prior research carried out by the partnership.

Our partnership trained CHW supervisors in leadership and communication to build their confidence and competence in their role as part of a capacity-building intervention. By training CHW supervisors, our activities fostered a more coherent PHC system and increased the productivity of CHWs. In addition to training, our partnership addressed other related challenges such as the transportation of CHW supervisors through the provision of motorcycles. These motorcycles were instrumental in the supervisors reaching out to CHWs including during reporting as well as the delivery of local supplies including medicines. In addition, these motorcycles supported other activities by the health facilities in the area such as during community outreach initiatives including immunization of children (Musoke et al., 2019a). Most recently, these motorcycles have been used during community response to the COVID-19 pandemic including for community sensitization and contact tracing. These supervision-related activities have all emerged from our research activities.

To enhance motivation of CHWs, our partnership provided them with branded T-shirts, gum boots, solar equipment and umbrellas. In addition, we ensured that all CHWs receive certificates of attendance following the various training sessions conducted. These non-financial incentives were established as key motivators for the enhanced performance of CHWs in the research we conducted earlier. Our partnership work targeted improving the skills, motivation and well-being of CHWs, which has made them preferred partners by different agencies with interest in supporting community health. In addition, our activities also supported the livelihood of many CHWs to better appreciate their role. For instance, a recent evaluation of one of our projects has shown that the solar equipment we provided had served as a means of income for the CHWs through charging mobile phones for community members at a fee. Enhanced motivation of CHWs realized through our partnership work is a major outcome of the research activities we conducted.

14.5 Challenges of Conducting Health Promotion Research Among CHWs

Health promotion research among CHWs, particularly in LMICs, is affected by a myriad of challenges as evidenced for several years (Scott et al., 2018). Some of the notable challenges include lack of funding, language barriers, fragmented research initiatives and minimal translation of research into practice. These challenges were faced by our partnership during the course of our research among CHWs in Uganda as described below.

14.5.1 Funding

As a partnership, we received funding for research on health promotion among CHWs from several agencies including the Tropical Health and Education Trust/the UK Department for International Development/Fleming Fund and Global Challenges Research Fund as part of the Nottingham Trent University Quality Research allocation. These streams of funding enabled us to conduct research on several health promotion components on the work of CHWs as discussed earlier. However, in the broader research funding landscape, low funding priority was given to CHWs as health professionals, with more attention given to higher-level health professionals including doctors and nurses. Indeed, our partnership had previously tapped into funding schemes that had predominantly targeted other health cadres, with community health not being a priority field. It is also worth noting that funding for research (including health promotion) in many LMICs including Uganda heavily relies on international donors, with minimal contribution from respective governments (Grépin et al., 2017). The issue of poor funding for health promotion research is partly a result of meagre health budgets for health ministries in many of these countries. In addition, Uganda's health system, as an example, is faced with several challenges including a high burden of communicable diseases and NCDs. Therefore, research is often not a local priority for the Ministry of Health, with most resources allocated to what seems to be more pressing needs such as curative services. For this reason, the research carried out in Uganda is primarily driven by the interest of donors, which often limits the amount of research conducted on health promotion among CHWs. The high proportion of donor funding in Uganda is also a strong factor in who is determining priorities for interventions including research, which has increasingly become disease-orientated (Ssali, 2018). In addition, tension exists between the provision of curative services (hospital-based and increasingly funded by private financing) and more preventative health services often funded by the external international non-governmental organization sector, which is also reflected in the allocation of resources for research. The problem of marginalization of health promotion research funding is not new as it has also impacted developed countries and has been attributed to the macroeconomic impacts of both globalization and neoliberalism (Baru & Mohan, 2018). Many governments are preoccupied with providing treatment services while viewing health promotion including research as less important (McGinnis et al., 2002). Partnerships such as ours, with a focus and commitment to PHC values and principles, are critical for advocating for research among cadres, such as CHWs, which are heavily involved in health promotion, particularly in LMICs.

14.5.2 Language

One of the requirements to become a CHW in Uganda is the ability to read and write preferably in the local language. In addition, many of the CHWs have completed primary-level education, with a few having reached secondary or tertiary/university level. Most CHWs across the country are particularly fluent in their local language but not always in English. In Wakiso District, where most of our partnership initiatives were conducted, *Luganda* is the local language most commonly used. Therefore, many of the research activities with CHWs were spearheaded by the Uganda team conversant in this language. This ensured direct communication between the CHWs and research teams as part of our work. However, challenges arose when the UK researchers needed to interface directly with the CHWs during partnership activities. For example, some Nottingham Trent University students carried out their master's research in Uganda among CHWs, necessitating them to carry out field work individually. This was challenging and required purposive selection of CHWs fluent in English to participate in such research. In some instances, an interpreter was required in case the CHWs involved were not able to communicate to the researchers in English. Whilst these measures were put in place to address language barriers, there was a possibility of introducing bias in the research process (Squires, 2009). This concern of language during community-based research has also been observed elsewhere (Lee et al., 2014), and, hence, it is important to consider in health promotion (and other health systems) research activities.

14.5.3 Fragmented Research Initiatives

There are many actors, both national and international, carrying out research among CHWs in Uganda on health promotion and beyond including universities (faculty and students), research institutions and government ministries and departments. It is acknowledged that the nature of this research, at various levels, is important to increase the evidence on the work of this cadre in Uganda's health system. However, there is lack of a coordinating mechanism to ensure that all research activities are harmonized to support sharing of experiences and learning as well as to avoid duplication of efforts. It is therefore not surprising to find closely related research being carried out among the same group of CHWs often in the same locality. Such an occurrence could be seen as a burden among the CHWs and can negatively affect their future involvement in research.

The Uganda National Council for Science and Technology is a government body mandated to regulate all research conducted in the country. Therefore, an additional role they could play is to ensure that all research activities across the country are well coordinated as well as keeping track of who is doing what and where. Besides national-level research, coordination of research activities (including health promotion) is supposed to be performed at the district level through the district health office. This office is mandated to oversee all health activities carried out in the district including research. Well-established coordination mechanisms at the district level have been found to be instrumental in supporting the work of CHWs (Nanyonjo et al., 2019). However, the district health office is often minimally involved in research activities implemented by partners. It is also common for some research to be conducted without involving this office, which further jeopardizes their coordination function. It is also worth noting that opportunities for different agencies involved in health promotion research to meet and share findings and experiences as well as to learn from each other are minimal in Uganda (and in other LMICs). Institutions conducting research working more closely together, with adequate support from the relevant authorities at national and sub-national levels, are therefore important to promote health promotion research among CHWs (and beyond).

14.5.4 Research Translation

Research has been conducted among CHWs around the world for several years, particularly in LMICs where they are predominantly situated (Scott et al., 2018). This research has supported the documentation of challenges affecting the work of CHWs in the communities in which they serve. These challenges include those related to training, supportive supervision, remuneration, motivation and availability of equipment and supplies (Kok et al., 2015). The World Health Organization has also recently published guidelines to optimize the performance of CHWs globally, which were partly guided by research evidence gathered for several years (World Health Organization, 2018). Therefore, what is needed to enhance the functioning of CHW programmes is well known locally and globally. For example, the CHW programme in Uganda has been shown for many years to be affected by several challenges including minimal training, insufficient supportive supervision, low motivation and lack of necessities such as medicines (Brunie et al., 2014; Ministry of Health, 2015). However, this knowledge of the issues that need to be addressed to enhance the performance of CHWs has not necessarily led to improvement in the CHW programme. Indeed, such evidence has at times been ignored at the expense of initiating other parallel programmes to enhance PHC. For example, the Ministry of Health has proposed a new Community Health Extension Worker programme in

Uganda to support the community health system as opposed to deliberately enhancing the existing cadre (Ministry of Health, 2016).

Whereas introducing a new cadre in the health system is welcome, doing so without considering the existing structures is likely not to lead to significant improvements (Musoke et al., 2020b). It is for this reason that CHWs are increasingly wondering about the need for continued research among them whilst the translation of findings into practice is hardly being seen. Research fatigue has also been observed elsewhere due to continuous engagement of participants (Clark, 2008); hence, it is critical to be considered for CHWs. The motivation of CHWs to participate in health promotion research is likely to reduce if no tangible benefits are observed over time. If more findings from research are put into practice to support CHW programmes, the attitudes of this health cadre towards health promotion research are likely to improve.

14.6 Key Contributions to Health Promotion Research and Practice

Our research in Uganda contributed to improvement in health promotion work among CHWs. The capacity-building programme for CHWs as part of our partnership highlights the value of improving the competence and performance of CHWs through enhancing training, supervision, motivation and use of mobile phones for health promotion as well as engaging CHWs as key partners in health promotion research. CHWs are important in discharging health promotion and other activities in the community (Meissner & Lyles, 2019). Consequently, it is important that they are adequately supported with the right resources as explained below.

Equal treatment of partners in community-based health promotion promotes efficiency and satisfaction for the parties involved (Zhang et al., 2019). This notion emanated from the 1978 Alma-Ata Declaration, which singled out CHWs as central to PHC in attaining its key target of addressing health inequalities (Lawn et al., 2008). This was to be realized, among others, through involvement of the community and a robust healthcare workforce, which included CHWs (Chan, 2008). Englert et al. (2019) define a "community health worker" as covering a broad range of community-based health service providers "selected, trained and working in their communities". Although the scope of the work they perform may differ from one country to another, they are generally involved in disease prevention and early detection of ill-health, community advocacy, outreach services and home visits among others (Schaaf et al., 2020). In general, the role of CHWs is to act as agents of health promotion, and their comprehensive knowledge of their communities makes them effective health promotion agents (Seutloali et al., 2018). Our research in Uganda spanning a period of 10 years shows that CHWs are central to the continuity of health promotion in the communities they served. Being local people, the CHWs understood the communities they were serving, and they were also respected by the communities. This enabled them to navigate and fully engage with communities during health promotion activities.

Training involves informing or giving instructions to employees on tasks in order to help them improve their knowledge and performance (Kahn et al., 2010). For practitioners to perform their duties to the highest possible standard, they must be effectively and efficiently trained (Morrison et al., 2007). Effective training enables achievement of specific outcomes required. Workers need to gain and maintain the skills and knowledge they need to perform their work as well as instruct and support others. Similarly, lack of training can be attributed to one of the reasons for low quality in performance of tasks and responsibilities. Our research in Uganda proved that effective training should be cost-efficient while also ensuring that time and money is a good investment. As part of maintaining a good quality of health promotion work, CHWs were equipped with key skills to discharge their roles. In addition, the CHWs were supported with continuous refresher training to enhance efficient operation in their health promotion activities.

Motivation for CHWs is important in sustaining health promotion and other activities aimed at supporting the health and well-being of communities (Agarwal et al., 2019). Locke and Schattke (2019) defined motivation as an individual's degree of willingness to exert and maintain an effort towards attaining organizational goals. One of the key constraints in the attainment of the Millennium Development Goals was the absence of a properly motivated workforce (Oxman & Fretheim, 2009). Currently, with the sustainable development goals in place, the presence of motivated workers is critical towards achieving the key outlined targets (Akintoye & Opeyemi, 2014). Poor motivation leads to absenteeism, high turnover, poor work performance and shirking of responsibilities (Fomenky, 2015). Motivation through the provision of financial and non-financial incentives is crucial to increase the recognition and indeed performance of CHWs, especially those who serve voluntarily such as in Uganda (Ormel et al., 2019). Provision of these incentives has seen increased motivation from CHWs to continue participating in discharging the health and well-being of their communities (Haile et al., 2014; Hansen et al., 2002).

During our work in Uganda, motivation of CHWs through different but simple and affordable ways greatly enhanced their performance. In addition, provision of certificates following training also motivated CHWs as they felt confident while undertaking their responsibilities. These motivational strategies were key to mitigate negative factors such as low recognition of CHWs by various stakeholders including non-payment for the services they rendered.

CHWs are an increasingly vital component of many health systems, servicing various communities and participating in a range of health intervention deliveries (Musoke et al., 2019a, b). They also act as first-line managers for sick children and adults through initiatives such as integrated community case management of childhood illnesses. In light of these responsibilities, there is need for adequate supervision of CHWs to ensure high performance, confidence and motivation. Supervision is important, in that communities can hold providers accountable if they have relevant information about the delivery of services (Mallari et al., 2020). In addition, supervision helps create an environment where CHWs are better supported (Tulenko,

2016) and better integrated within the formal healthcare system (Brown et al., 2020). Our work in Uganda showed that supervision for CHWs is often lacking in quality if present at all. In response to this challenge, improved supervision of CHWs during our work in Uganda enhanced their performance including during health promotion.

14.7 Conclusion

This chapter describes carrying out health promotion research among CHWs in Uganda as part of a UK–Uganda interdisciplinary partnership. Our research is an example of the use of both quantitative and qualitative methods to research CHWs as well as the involvement of various stakeholders at national, sub-national and community levels. The methods used in health promotion research come from a range of disciplinary fields, in this case social sciences and public and environmental health. Although the methods used are not unique to health promotion, what makes our research approach distinctive is the interdisciplinary nature of the methods that are appropriate to what we explore and that are inclusive to the communities and stakeholders with whom we work. Methodological pluralism allows the research to be more tailored to the real-world context of the research, and this has enabled us to overcome some of the challenges of working in these settings. A major contribution of this chapter is to demonstrate how our research informed the capacity-building initiatives of CHWs, particularly regarding training, supervision and motivation, which have influenced their health promotion practice. The partners operated from a common value base derived from the Ottawa Charters' principles of empowerment and community action. This aspect of our partnership work has necessitated continuous community engagement and stakeholder involvement over long periods of time both with and in-between funding to support health promotion practice among CHWs in Uganda. Health promotion principles of listening to and working with and in communities informed the research design and the methods used. Our research approach using these principles directly contributed to improving and strengthening the capacity of CHWs; hence, we argue that health promotion research should contribute to bringing about some form of change.

The challenges in carrying out health promotion research identified in this chapter can inform other researchers, particularly those intending to work with CHWs in LMICs. Understanding these challenges is key to using an approach to conducting research that recognizes and reveals those tensions. Some of the tensions we identified are external (donor-driven funding and agendas, paradigmatic biases of funders), local (language, health system/health workforce factors) or are about the practices of the research itself (how research is translated into practice to bring about change). Building deep and trusted partnerships between ourselves as a community of researchers, the grassroots CHWs and our local, national and international stakeholders have helped us negotiate those challenges and tensions and provide an ethic of research practice that we believe is what makes health promotion research distinct.

Acknowledgements We thank all stakeholders who supported our partnership work in the UK and Uganda, including research funders, collaborators, policymakers, practitioners, students, community health workers, local leaders and the community.

References

Agarwal, S., Sripad, P., Johnson, C., Kirk, K., Bellows, B., Ana, J., Blaser, V., Kumar, M. B., Buchholz, K., & Casseus, A. (2019). A conceptual framework for measuring community health workforce performance within primary health care systems. *Human Resources for Health, 17*(1), 1–20. https://doi.org/10.1186/s12960-019-0422-0

Akintoye, V. A., & Opeyemi, O. A. (2014). Prospects for achieving sustainable development through the millennium development goals in Nigeria. *European Journal of Sustainable Development, 3*(1), 33. https://doi.org/10.14207/ejsd.2014.v3n1p33

Baru, R. V., & Mohan, M. (2018). Globalisation and neoliberalism as structural drivers of health inequities. *Health Research Policy and Systems, 16*(1), 91. https://doi.org/10.1186/s12961-018-0365-2

Brown, O., Kangovi, S., Wiggins, N., & Alvarado, C. S. (2020). *Supervision strategies and community health worker effectiveness in health care settings*. NAM perspectives. Paper, National Academy of Medicine. https://doi.org/10.31478/202003c.

Brunie, A., Wamala-Mucheri, P., Otterness, C., Akol, A., Chen, M., Bufumbo, L., & Weaver, M. (2014). Keeping community health workers in Uganda motivated: Key challenges, facilitators, and preferred program inputs. *Global Health: Science and Practice, 2*(1), 103–116. https://doi.org/10.9745/GHSP-D-13-00140

Chan, M. (2008). Return to Alma-ata. *Lancet, 372*(9642), 865–866. https://doi.org/10.1016/S0140-6736(08)61372-0

Clark, T. (2008). 'We're over-researched here!' exploring accounts of research fatigue within qualitative research engagements. *Sociology, 42*(5), 953–970. https://doi.org/10.1177/0038038508094573

Englert, E. G., Kiwanuka, R., & Neubauer, L. C. (2019). 'When I die, let me be the last.' Community health worker perspectives on past Ebola and Marburg outbreaks in Uganda. *Global Public Health, 14*(8), 1182–1192. https://doi.org/10.1080/17441692.2018.1552306

Fomenky, N. F. (2015). The impact of motivation on employee performance. *Global Conference on Business & Finance Proceedings, 10*(1), 332.

Grépin, K. A., Pinkstaff, C. B., Shroff, Z. C., & Ghaffar, A. (2017). Donor funding health policy and systems research in low-and middle-income countries: How much, from where and to whom. *Health Research Policy and Systems, 15*(1), 1–8. https://doi.org/10.1186/s12961-017-0224-6

Haile, F., Yemane, D., & Gebreslassie, A. (2014). Assessment of non-financial incentives for volunteer community health workers – The case of Wukro district, Tigray, Ethiopia. *Human Resources for Health, 12*(1), 54. https://doi.org/10.1186/1478-4491-12-54

Hansen, F., Smith, M., & Hansen, R. B. (2002). Rewards and recognition in employee motivation. *Compensation & Benefits Review, 34*(5), 64–72. https://doi.org/10.1177/0886368702034005010

Ilaboya, D., Gibson, L., & Musoke, D. (2018). Perceived barriers to early detection of breast cancer in Wakiso district, Uganda using a socioecological approach. *Globalization and Health, 14*(9), 1–10. https://doi.org/10.1186/s12992-018-0326-0

Kahn, J. G., Yang, J. S., & Kahn, J. S. (2010). 'Mobile' health needs and opportunities in developing countries. *Health Affairs, 29*(2), 252–258. https://doi.org/10.1377/hlthaff.2009.0965.

Kok, M. C., Dieleman, M., Taegtmeyer, M., Broerse, J. E., Kane, S. S., Ormel, H., Tijm, M. M., & De Koning, K. A. (2015). Which intervention design factors influence performance of community health workers in low-and middle-income countries? A systematic review. *Health Policy and Planning, 30*(9), 1207–1227. https://doi.org/10.1093/heapol/czu126

Lawn, J. E., Rohde, J., Rifkin, S., Were, M., Paul, V. K., & Chopra, M. (2008). Alma-ata 30 years on: Revolutionary, relevant, and time to revitalise. *The Lancet, 372*(9642), 917–927. https://doi.org/10.1016/S0140-6736(08)61402-6

Lee, S. K., Sulaiman-Hill, C. R., & Thompson, S. C. (2014). Overcoming language barriers in community-based research with refugee and migrant populations: Options for using bilingual workers. *BMC International Health and Human Rights, 14*(1), 1–13. https://doi.org/10.1186/1472-698X-14-11

Locke, E. A., & Schattke, K. (2019). Intrinsic and extrinsic motivation: Time for expansion and clarification. *Motivation Science, 5*(4), 277. https://doi.org/10.1037/mot0000116

Mallari, E., Lasco, G., Sayman, D. J., Amit, A. M. L., Balabanova, D., McKee, M., Mendoza, J., Palileo-Villanueva, L., Renedo, A., & Seguin, M. (2020). Connecting communities to primary care: A qualitative study on the roles, motivations and lived experiences of community health workers in the Philippines. *BMC Health Services Research, 20*(1), 1–10. https://doi.org/10.1186/s12913-020-05699-0

Marufu, L., Gibson, L., Ssemugabo, C., Ndejjo, R., & Musoke, D. (2017). Barriers and facilitators of female community health workers when performing their roles: A study in Ssisa sub county, Wakiso district, Uganda. In D. Musoke, R. Ndejjo, T. Mukama, S. T. Wafula, C. Ssemugabo, & L. Gibson (Eds.), *Abstracts from the 1st international symposium on community health workers* (pp. 24–25). *BMC Proceedings, 11*(6), 10. https://doi.org/10.1186/s12919-017-0074-9

McGinnis, J. M., Williams-Russo, P., & Knickman, J. R. (2002). The case for more active policy attention to health promotion. *Health Affairs, 21*(2), 78–93. https://doi.org/10.1377/hlthaff.21.2.78

Meissner, C. A., & Lyles, A. M. (2019). IX investigations: The importance of training investigators in evidence-based approaches to interviewing. *Journal of Applied Research in Memory and Cognition, 8*(4), 387–397. https://doi.org/10.1016/j.jarmac.2019.07.001

Ministry of Health. (1999). National Health Policy (1999). Kampala: Ministry of Health. http://library.health.go.ug/publications/policy-documents/national-health-policy1999. Accessed 11 January 2020.

Ministry of Health. (2015). National Village Health Teams (VHT) Assessment in Uganda. http://library.health.go.ug/publications/health-education/national-village-health-teamsvht-assessment-uganda. Accessed 8 March 2020.

Ministry of Health. (2016). *Community health extension workers strategy in Uganda (2015/16-2019/20)*. Ministry of Health. http://library.health.go.ug/publications/health-education/community-health-extension-workers-strategy-uganda-201516-201920. Accessed 11 Jan 2020

Morrison, G. R., Ross, S. M., Kemp, J. E., & Kalman, H. (2007). *Designing effective instruction*. Wiley.

Musoke, D., Atusingwize, E., Ikhile, D., Nalinya, S., Ssemugabo, C., Lubega, G. B., Omodara, D., Ndejjo, R., & Gibson, L. (2021). Community health workers' involvement in the prevention and control of non-communicable diseases in Wakiso district, Uganda. *Globalization and Health, 17*(1), 1–11. https://doi.org/10.1186/s12992-020-00653-5

Musoke, D., Gibson, L., Mukama, T., Khalil, Y., & Ssempebwa, J. C. (2016). Nottingham Trent University and Makerere University School of Public Health Partnership: Experiences of co-learning and supporting the healthcare system in Uganda. *Globalization and Health, 12*(1), 11. https://doi.org/10.1186/s12992-016-0148-x

Musoke, D., Kitutu, F. E., Mugisha, L., Amir, S., Brandish, C., Ikhile, D., Kajumbula, H., Kizito, I. M., Lubega, G. B., Niyongabo, F., Ng, B. Y., O'Driscoll, J., Russell-Hobbs, K., Winter, J.,

& Gibson, L. (2020a). A one health approach to strengthening antimicrobial stewardship in Wakiso District, Uganda. *Antibiotics, 9*, 764. https://doi.org/10.3390/antibiotics9110764

Musoke, D., Ndejjo, R., Atusingwize, E., Mukama, T., Ssemugabo, C., & Gibson, L. (2019b). Performance of community health workers and associated factors in a rural community in Wakiso district, Uganda. *African Health Sciences, 19*(3), 2784–2797. https://doi.org/10.4314/ahs.v19i3.55

Musoke, D., Ndejjo, R., Atusingwize, E., Ssemugabo, C., Ottosson, A., Gibson, L., & Waiswa, P. (2020b). Panacea or pitfall? The introduction of community health extension workers in Uganda. *BMJ Global Health, 5*(8), e002445. https://doi.org/10.1136/bmjgh-2020-002445

Musoke, D., Ssemugabo, C., Ndejjo, R., Atusingwize, E., Mukama, T., & Gibson, L. (2019a). Strengthening the community health worker programme for health improvement through enhancing training, supervision and motivation in Wakiso district, Uganda. *BMC Research Notes, 12*(1), 812. https://doi.org/10.1186/s13104-019-4851-6

Nanyonjo, A., Counihan, H., Siduda, S. G., Belay, K., Sebikaari, G., & Tibenderana, J. (2019). Institutionalization of integrated community case management into national health systems in low-and middle-income countries: A scoping review of the literature. *Global Health Action, 12*(1), 1678283. https://doi.org/10.1080/16549716.2019.1678283

Nchafack, A. N. (2016). *Exploring the potential of mobile health (mhealth) in improving access to information on maternal and infant HealthCare in a low resource setting. Case study: Ssisa sub county in Wakiso district, Uganda* (Unpublished master's dissertation). Nottingham Trent University.

Ormel, H., Kok, M., Kane, S., Ahmed, R., Chikaphupha, K., Rashid, S. F., Gemechu, D., Otiso, L., Sidat, M., & Theobald, S. (2019). Salaried and voluntary community health workers: Exploring how incentives and expectation gaps influence motivation. *Human Resources for Health, 17*(1), 59. https://doi.org/10.1186/s12960-019-0387-z

Oxman, A. D., & Fretheim, A. (2009). Can paying for results help to achieve the millennium development goals? Overview of the effectiveness of results-based financing. *Journal of Evidence-Based Medicine, 2*(2), 70–83. https://doi.org/10.1111/j.1756-5391.2009.01020.x

Schaaf, M., Warthin, C., Freedman, L., & Topp, S. M. (2020). The community health worker as service extender, cultural broker and social change agent: A critical interpretive synthesis of roles, intent and accountability. *BMJ Global Health, 5*(6), e002296. https://doi.org/10.1136/bmjgh-2020-002296

Scott, K., Beckham, S. W., Gross, M., Pariyo, G., Rao, K. D., Cometto, G., & Perry, H. B. (2018). What do we know about community-based health worker programs? A systematic review of existing reviews on community health workers. *Human Resources for Health, 16*(1), 1–17. https://doi.org/10.1186/s12960-018-0304-x

Seutloali, T., Napoles, L., & Bam, N. (2018). Community health workers in Lesotho: Experiences of health promotion activities. *African Journal of Primary Health Care & Family Medicine, 10*(1), 1–8. https://doi.org/10.4102/phcfm.v10i1.1558

Squires, A. (2009). Methodological challenges in cross-language qualitative research: A research review. *International Journal of Nursing Studies, 46*(2), 277–287. https://doi.org/10.1016/j.ijnurstu.2008.08.006

Ssali, S. N. (2018). Neoliberal health reforms and citizenship in Uganda. In J. Wiegratz, G. Martiniello, & E. Greco (Eds.), *Uganda: The dynamics of neoliberal transformation* (pp. 178–200). Zed Books Ltd.

Tulenko, K. (2016) Supervision of Community Health Workers. CHWCentral. https://chwcentral.org/supervision-of-community-health-workers/. Accessed 7 October 2020.

Uganda Bureau of Statistics. (2016). *The National Population and Housing Census 2014 – Main report*. Uganda Bureau of Statistics.

World Health Organization. (2018). *WHO guideline on health policy and system support to optimize community health worker programmes*. World Health Organization.

Zhang, X., Hailu, B., Tabor, D. C., Gold, R., Sayre, M. H., Sim, I., Jean-Francois, B., Casnoff, C. A., Cullen, T., & Thomas, V. A., Jr. (2019). Role of health information technology in addressing health disparities: Patient, clinician, and system perspectives. *Medical Care, 57*, S115–S120. https://doi.org/10.1097/MLR.0000000000001092

Chapter 15
Intersectoriality and Health Promotion Research: The Perspective of Practitioners from a Brazilian Experience

Maria Cristina Trousdell Franceschini, Marcia Faria Westphal, and Marco Akerman

15.1 Introduction

Intersectoriality is highlighted in agendas, policies and models as a central axis for the development of public policies and as a strategy for social transformations. It is also a key health promotion strategy, based on the recognition of opportunities for the social production of health that reside outside the health sector.

Despite the existence of models built around the importance of intersectoriality, conceiving it as tangible and achievable remains a challenge, particularly for health promotion research. Studies provide few details about the processes, contexts and achievements of intersectoriality and highlight the difficulties in identifying its results (Akerman et al., 2014; Chiari et al., 2018; Kranzler et al., 2013; Shankardass et al., 2011; Tess & Aith, 2014). There exist differing and conflicting conceptual and analytical frameworks aimed at explaining what intersectoriality is and how it is incorporated into public policy processes. Sectoral models do not adequately reflect the problems that are the focus of intersectoral action and the social dynamics that affect them (Franceschini, 2019).

M. C. T. Franceschini (✉)
Maria Cristina Franceschini, Center for Studies, Research and Documentation on Healthy Cities (CEPEDOC-Healthy Cities), Sao Paulo, SP, Brazil
e-mail: cris_franceschini@yahoo.com

M. F. Westphal
Marcia Faria Westphal, School of Public Health, University of São Paulo, São Paulo, SP, Brazil

M. Akerman
Marco Akerman, School of Public Health, University of São Paulo, São Paulo, SP, Brazil

Center for Studies, Research and Documentation on Healthy Cities (CEPEDOC-Healthy Cities), São Paulo, SP, Brazil

L. Potvin, D. Jourdan (eds.), *Global Handbook of Health Promotion Research, Vol. 1*,
https://doi.org/10.1007/978-3-030-97212-7_15

Additionally, the complexity of social problems – health inequities, social exclusion, poverty, etc. – requires the development of new strategies. Such social realities mean that the current intersectoral models that focus on institutional or policy processes are not viable. Strengthening networks (social, community, personal, professional, services) has emerged as an alternative to guarantee effective intersectoral public policies and an integrated view of social problems. As such, understanding the interdependence of intersectoriality and networks in our contemporary society opens up new dimensions for health promotion research.

Between 2017 and 2019, research was conducted to understand how intersectoriality had been incorporated into the actions of the Intersectoral Network "Guarulhos, the City that Protects" (GCP Network) to prevent violence against children and adolescents in the municipality of Guarulhos, São Paulo, Brazil. With this qualitative research, which was based on a health promotion framework and used as a case study approach, the actors who developed it aimed to understand the meanings of intersectoriality and to identify which factors intervened or conditioned the intersectoral processes and the effects of the initiative. The case study was conducted through in-depth interviews with the Network's actors, participant observation of Network activities over a period of 2 years and analysis of available materials produced by the Network since its launch in 2010 (documents, communications, reports, etc.) (Franceschini, 2019).

Considering that intersectoriality, by nature, involves actors from various sectors, the research focused on the interfaces between the fields of education, health, social and development assistance and public safety. Decentralization of actions that are under the responsibility of various sectors, participatory management, empowerment and actors' predisposition to participate in such actions were the objects of this research, and the data produced were the object of reflection by those involved in these practices. The territory – as geographical spaces of life and co-living for children and adolescents – was our empirical base to consider the actions aimed at protecting these populations, conducted by the actors who formed local violence prevention networks. This chapter reflects upon the experience of conducting this research and the lessons that can strengthen health promotion research.

15.1.1 The "Guarulhos, the City That Protects" Intersectoral Network

The GCP Network was formed in 2010 in the municipality of Guarulhos[1] as a school health project led by technical personnel from the municipal health and education departments who worked at the local level (schools and primary healthcare centres).

[1] Guarulhos is 1 of 39 municipalities that form the Metropolitan Area of São Paulo, the largest in Latin America. It is São Paulo state's second most populous municipality, with 1,365,899 inhabitants (2018 estimate). As happens with many cities that experienced rapid and unorganized urban-

It aimed to share information about the types of violence that affected children and adolescents and promote actions to address them (SECEL, 2016). Between 2012 and 2015, districts in four regions of the city were organized as local networks and integrated into the GCP Network.

In 2015, a municipal decree formally established the GCP Network's Intersectoral Committee made up of the Health, Education, Development and Social Assistance and Public Safety departments as well as Boards of Education, the Municipal Council for the Rights of Children and Adolescents and Child Protection Services. By 2019, the GCP Network encompassed 195 representatives (from services, institutions, organizations) and formed a city-wide initiative for violence prevention, mobilizing multiple sectors and strengthening their capacities for action, particularly at the territorial level.

15.1.1.1 Why Did We Study the GCP Network?

An initial assessment was conducted of the local intersectoral initiatives taking place in the state of São Paulo, Brazil, and the GCP Network was selected due to: (1) its express goal of mobilizing various sectors to seek solutions to a common issue; (2) its duration, at the time, of 7 years, which pointed to a capacity to establish sustainable relations, mechanisms, processes and structures that allowed continuity over time and political transitions and (3) its proposal to work across municipal departments and with a territorial basis, which created interesting dimensions to analyze the interfaces between municipal policies and local demands.

15.2 Defining the Research Object: Why Did We Focus on Intersectoriality?

The complex reality, existential problems and multidimensionality of human and social needs require differential approaches from those who look for solutions for a variety of problems: economic, social, political, educational, health, environmental, etc. These problems are embedded in a globalized world, and their solutions demand a new relation between society and each of these fields. In health promotion, the prevention of social problems and disease requires integration and coordination between practices, policies and the sectors responsible for them. Therefore, research focusing on intersectoriality within a health promotion framework is fundamental.

Intersectoriality is a core health promotion strategy, emphasized as essential to tackle the social determinants of health (Jackson et al., 2006; PAHO/WHO, 2011).

---

ization, Guarulhos is marked by high levels of social, economic and health inequalities (GUARULHOS 2008; IBGE 2020).

It is also an approach to broaden the discussion about how to improve quality of life beyond the health sector and is a requirement in development models.

However, in practice, intersectoriality is often uncoordinated and ambiguous, resulting in technical, political and institutional processes that may be contradictory, ineffective and generate resistance instead of synergies. Researchers point to the limited problematization of its conceptual/analytical framework as an obstacle to conduct studies aimed at understanding the intersectoral process, mechanisms and impacts (Cunnil-Grau, 2005; Santos, 2011).

The literature indicates that data regarding intersectoriality are scarce, superficial, descriptive and are presented from isolated perspectives (Shankardass et al., 2011; Akerman et al., 2014). A review of the literature highlighted the various concepts associated with intersectoriality that can lead to confusion about its scope, reach, mechanisms, processes and expected outcomes (Akerman et al., 2014; Cavalcanti & Nicolau, 2012; Junqueira, 1997; Inojosa, 2001). Health promotion researchers highlight the lack of understanding about effective intersectoral mechanisms as a challenge to consolidating models such as Health in All Policies, promoted by the World Health Organization (Kickbush, 2010; McQueen et al., 2012). The challenges identified include the development of theoretical and analytical frameworks for research and evaluation, the documentation of experiences and the construction of evidence.

This research sought to fill in some of these gaps. The theoretical framework was informed by Manuel Castells' discussion on the impact of networks and information to catalyze social transformation in a contemporary society and by Anthony Giddens' social structuration theory, which considers elements such as agent, agency, power, structure and structuration (Castells, 2002; Giddens, 1986). We also considered analytical models for intersectoral action (Solar, 2013; Cunnil-Grau, 2014), how these aligned with the health promotion framework and what the interconnections were between intersectoriality and health-promoting principles such as participation and network development.

15.2.1 The Need to Work on a Common Understanding of the Object of Study

The research was oriented by the question: How are intersectoral relations and actions being constructed within the experience of the Intersectoral Network Guarulhos, the City that Protects, to address violence against children and adolescents in the municipality of Guarulhos, São Paulo?

The objectives that guided the methodological design included:

- Analyzing the intersectoral strategies within the GCP Network, considering the perspectives of all sectors involved
- Identifying factors that affected the consolidation and sustainability of the GCP Network

- Analyzing conceptions related to intersectoriality and networks among the social actors involved
- Understanding whether (and how) collective practices were being institutionalized by the sectors/actors
- Identifying the results and effects of GCP Network activities in relation to intersectoriality

The following definition was proposed as a starting point: "Intersectoriality refers to institutional, technical and political interfaces between governmental and non-governmental sectors, with the goal of overcoming fragmentations and addressing complex social problems beyond the scope of individual public policies. These interfaces potentialize the creation of knowledge and the development of synergetic solutions to social problems. Intersectoriality goes beyond the mere juxtaposition of sectoral actions and aims to promote social development and transformation."

The approach to the object of study considered the following dimensions:

- Structures: How was the GCP Network organized, considering the institutional arrangements, sectoral mandates, legal frameworks and resources?
- Processes: What mechanisms and actions, such as entry points for joint action and planning processes, among others, fostered intersectoriality?
- Effects and results: What did the GCP Network produce, impact or affect, considering dimensions such as relationships, practices, knowledge, resources, leadership, policies and empowerment?

The research design implemented in this study (presented below in Sect. 15.3) represents the end result of a highly dynamic and interactive process. The definition of the object of study and the conceptual framework and the methodological design of the research evolved greatly over the course of the initial stages, as should be the case in health promotion research tackling complex and interconnected issues in the real world, based on feedback from the participants.

As an example, the initial study design focused on intersectoral models developed in the field of public health and health promotion, which often define the improvement of population health as the end result/objective of intersectoral action. When presented with this design, actors of the GCP Network, particularly those who were not from the health sector, reacted strongly against such models. They expressed discontent about what they understood as a hijacking of the intersectoral efforts by the health sector that dismissed their motivations to engage in such initiatives (for example, improving access to education, improving social safety networks and improving access to housing, among others). One discussion was about what we meant by a broader concept of health, which was not understood by most participants, including those from the health sector itself.

The discussions brought to light the actors' various conceptualizations about intersectoriality, its purposes, means and strategies. These were often based on different models and conceptions put forward by their training and field of work. For those from the education sector, the goal of intersectoriality was to promote access to quality education for all; actors from the social development sector understood that the goal of intersectoriality was strengthening social protection networks and poverty prevention; public safety representatives understood intersectoriality as a means to improve community security and decrease determinants of crime; those from the health field pointed to intersectoriality as a strategy to promote population health. These visions, interests and intentions created a series of impasses and pointed to the importance of seeking a conceptual alignment among actors about their stakes, interests and responsibilities and a definition of common goals for their collaboration.

As a result of these discussions, the research team went back to the drawing board and conducted a new review of the literature to better understand the models, epistemologies and strategies related to intersectoriality that permeated the work of the other sectors involved in the GCP Network. This pointed to new understandings of the challenges related to intersectoral action (when considering the inconsistencies and conflicts between sectoral and interdisciplinary models) and led to significant changes in the conceptual framework and methodological design of the study, in order to incorporate a multitude of perspectives beyond what is usually the focus of health promotion research. The final study design is the result of this process; it aims to look at intersectoriality as a multi-stakeholder policy and social process. It does not focus on "health" in itself but considers that it is at the intersection of various dimensions, actors and social dynamics that the social production of health takes place.

Taking time and going through this process of reviewing the conceptual and methodological design of the research, which often meant taking steps back, reflecting upon our own biases and adjusting expectations were all crucial in order to gain the trust of research the participants and to establish a fruitful collaboration with them, thus making them our partners rather than objects of study.

15.2.2 Why Did We Focus on the Actors of the GCP Network?

Over the course of its existence, the GCP Network has been led by technical personnel from municipal departments and local actors. This became a central point in the definition of the research framework: the network did not emerge from policymakers but from those who were caught up in the challenges of implementing policies while being pressured by local demands. The initiative to launch the Network was based on their dissatisfaction with the mechanisms offered by the municipal administration to address violence against children and adolescents, in-depth knowledge of the problems that afflicted each territory and their frustration with a history of attempted collaborative efforts (formal and informal) that they believed were isolated and ineffective.

The proposal to establish the Network was also based on the recognition of intersectoriality as a fundamental strategy to address their common problems and that of the actors' roles, responsibilities, competencies and strengths to be part of the solutions. Each actor that is a part of the GCP Network has their own trajectory, goals and interests. In that sense, understanding their motivations, perceptions and experiences became central to understanding the modes of organization, relationships and strategies to overcome challenges and potentials for the development of more effective intersectoral policies.

15.3 Methodological Design: Approaching the Research Object from Multiple Angles

A qualitative research approach was considered the most appropriate based on the recognition of the subjectivity of human knowledge and experiences. While these are individual and specific, they are also whole, in and of themselves. Knowledge production in social sciences should seek to understand social processes from the perspectives of those immersed in those contexts (DaMatta, 1993). Such understanding depends on the meaning of the world for those who live in it and a "reality" that is made up of multiple, dynamic and simultaneous individual and collective experiences (Victora et al., 2000). Such approach fits in with our research, as intersectoriality is influenced by contextual, social, historical and political factors, and our focus was on understanding this phenomenon through the lenses of those who experienced it and the relationships they developed across social, institutional and political spaces.

The complexity of the research object pointed to the need for multiple methods, namely, social network analysis, content analysis, document analysis and participant observations.

15.3.1 What Was the Contribution of Each Methodological Component?

- Social network analysis (SNA): SNA supports the identification of relational and structural links embedded in social processes through visual representations (Higgins & Ribeiro, 2018). It helped understand how the actors of the GCP Network connected among themselves and with the Network structure as a whole and how relationships were formed, considering institutional affiliations and sectors.
- Qualitative analysis: Analyzing experiences, conceptions and perspectives of the Network participants was a key dimension. This required an in-depth exploration, through semi-structured interviews, of people's ideas, feelings, interests and interpretations related to intersectoriality and the GCP Network. The contents of the interviews were categorized, interpreted and analyzed using Bardin's content analysis methodology (Bardin, 2009).

- Document analysis: Numerous actors and institutions have been involved in the GCP Network. Given that the Network has existed since 2010 and has a high turnover of personnel among the participating institutions, developing a timeline to understand the Network required conducting a thorough assessment of documents, reports, meeting logs, publications and other materials to help reconstruct its history (Cellard, 2012).
- Participant observation: The observation of phenomena allows for direct contact and a better understanding of the research object (Minayo, 2010; Jaccoud & Mayer, 2012). This requires immersion of the researcher in the group or activities being observed. As such, the researcher becomes an actor in the research and interferes with its object and context. The implication of this is the recognition that qualitative research is not a neutral endeavour and must make explicit the relationship between the researcher, the social reality of being investigated and the research subjects. This methodology helped understand the dynamics of the Network and its interactions, contradictions, dilemmas and strategies. This contributed to identifying the processes, structures and strategies related to knowledge production, practices, challenges, barriers and facilitating factors.

15.3.2 What Was the Sampling Methodology?

The research sample was constructed through the snowball technique: an interviewee identified his or her main partners in the GCP Network over a period of 2 years prior to the interview and they were invited to participate in the research. The process started with the identification of an initial group of key informants, and, through their connections, other people were identified and invited to participate in the research. This went on until the process reached a saturation point, at which either no new contacts emerged or these no longer offered relevant information (Vinuto, 2014).

A total of 56 persons were interviewed. They mentioned a total of 90 partners. All sectors and regions of the GCP Network were covered by the interviews.

15.3.3 How Were the GCP Network Actors Involved in the Research Design and Implementation?

Social participation refers to the engagement of state and civil society actors in the development and social control of health promotion actions. It can strengthen community organization and improve resource distribution, access to information and capacity building for those marginalized during decision-making processes, thus creating spaces for social control by citizens (WHO, 1986; Westphal, 2012).

The GCP Network's actors were involved in all phases of the research. In 2016, the project was presented to the Coordinating Committee to assess its interest and to gather inputs. This included representatives from all sectors involved, which was particularly interesting since the group's different perspectives on intersectoriality quickly came into view, sparking reflections about the intentions and motivations that the group had not contemplated until then. The project was also presented to the local networks. Suggestions were incorporated into the project design and helped redirect the research question and methodological framework.

This pattern of interaction accompanied the life cycle of the project. Data collection tools were discussed and field-tested with Network members, the selection of participants included inputs from all sectors and local networks, and document compilation was conducted in conjunction with focal points from municipal departments. Once the results started to come in, they were presented to the group for collective interpretation.

Analyzing the results with the actors was rich and insightful. Their interpretations filled in gaps not previously seen in the research process, redirected the initial analysis and helped shape the research conclusions. These discussions provided insights for the group to rethink through their own actions and led to a reorientation of the strategies related to the GCP Network's development. Therefore, the synergies created by the participatory approach benefitted all sides involved, being in and of itself a generator of knowledge and innovation and a support to the reorientation of practices.

However, this process was not seamless or free of conflict. Often, participants did not agree with the opinions of others, or with decisions made by the group, which led to discussions that were not always productive. Some opinions were quite controversial (such as how to treat patients who did not "comply" with the health personnel or how to deal with parents considered "neglectful"). On many occasions, discussions descended into circular arguments about the root cause of the problems in question, with no consensus among the group. These were in part a consequence of the research object, which was influenced by external and interrelated factors embedded in a complex reality, the scope of which was difficult to grasp. Overall, when situations like these arose, members of the GCP Network who acted as mediators were able to circumvent arguments and negotiate acceptable solutions with the group. In relation to the research, it was often necessary to clarify its purpose, limitations and scope and to guide the discussion towards what the research could answer for, which was not to "solve" all of the Network's problems.

15.4 A Picture Starts to Emerge: Results and Aftermath of the Research

This research aimed to study how a complex, conceptual object was given concreteness and put into practice through a real-life experience. The fact that our empirical base was an intersectoral initiative organized in the form of multi-level, interconnected networks, created an extra but interesting challenge. This confluence – the intersectoral and the network – required an analytical and methodological exercise to delineate the research object in order to capture the dynamics of these two phenomena that were intrinsically connected in their daily practices and effects.

The research unveiled a scenario that was filled with nuances, contradictions, strengths and potentialities. During its course, other themes emerged that had to be considered. As such, the research itself was not only an evolving endeavour that required flexibility, openness and sensitivity but also an attention seeker to maintain the focus of a process that was on the move. Examples of these issues included ethical dilemmas faced by professionals; the mental health of professionals; safety concerns as actions to tackle violence can have unpredictable consequences; and relations with the community, among others.

The results were organized in the following structure:

1. Research participants' profiles (characteristics relevant to the analysis);
2. GCP Network's characteristics (modes of organization, goals, mechanisms, institutional arrangements);
3. GCP Network's structural characteristics (social network analysis);
4. Supporting structures for intersectoriality (institutional arrangements, territorially based planning, information tools, funding mechanisms, partnerships);
5. Perceptions about intersectoriality and networks.

The research uncovered many of the Network's innovative mechanisms to foster an intersectoral process that considered the key health promotion strategies/values as well as the challenges that limited its capacity to advance towards more integrated and sustainable intersectoriality. The analysis of these issues makes up the main body of the research, and, here, we point out the general findings. Limitations included difficulties in mobilizing the interest of policymakers and management, hierarchical and bureaucratic structures that did not support intersectoral actions, little control over decisions and resources, low capacities and competencies for intersectoral work, structural violence that was beyond the Network's capacity to tackle and frustration with the lack of long-term solutions.

Having a health promotion framework as the basis for this research was fundamental in order to focus the methodology and analysis on understanding the context and processes and not merely the end results of policies or institutional actions. This research option also helped highlight the benefits and challenges of investing in health promotion strategies, such as having a focus on territories; on integrating a variety of actors and strengthening their capacities and the potential (or barriers) of promoting system changes.

The inclusion of a statistical methodological tool, social network analysis, emerged as an innovation and highlighted how incorporating methodologies can provide new and out-of-the-box insights into data that emerge from health promotion research.

Through SNA, we concluded that the GCP Network was able to mobilize actors from all of the sectors considered essential, namely, education, health, social assistance and public safety. However, the results pointed to an overwhelming representation of actors from public institutions, compared to civil society. As a result, many of the Network's actions revolved around implementing institutional programmes and mandates with limited inputs from those who lived and worked in the territories in question. Many factors explained this situation, as will be discussed later.

Social network analyses showed a great distribution of intersectoral partnerships within all the territorial networks. However, they also indicated that the connections among local networks were fragile. This means that while the GCP Network was successful in its efforts to spur local intersectoral partnerships and strengthen local networks, it still struggled to constitute an integrated city-wide network that could more effectively tackle broader structural determinants of violence. From a health promotion perspective, such results point to interesting reflections about the challenges of scaling up innovative local initiatives to spur sustained, broader system changes.

The analysis identified 90 partners (actors or institutions) and 170 active partnerships (joint actions). This points to a success of the Network's actions as these partnerships were a direct effect of efforts to promote intersectoral collaboration. An in-depth look at the characteristics and dynamics of these partnerships pointed to their achievements and limitations. Achievements included the establishment of new practices aligned with local needs, development of new strategies for communication and information exchange, design of joint projects and implementation of more appropriate strategies to identify and prioritize local needs. As for limitations, many of these partnerships were short-lived or were focused on solving urgent demands, and there were difficulties in getting managerial buy-in for their development. The results pointed out the potentials that intersectoral partnerships can unlock to redirect efforts and seek joint solutions. However, they also indicated that intersectoriality was perceived and demanded as a strategy to solve specific and/or urgent demands and not necessarily as a strategy to support the development of a common vision to tackle the roots of the problems. For health promotion research, results such as these can point to some of the ingrained, day-to-day factors that affect the feasibility of models that take intersectoriality (and other health promotion strategies) as a central strategy to promote policy and system changes. They lead to a reflection on how to develop models and strategies aimed at tackling such issues at their roots and becoming more fine-tuned, appropriate and applicable in real social and institutional contexts. These results emphasize the importance of fostering intersectoriality not as a utilitarian strategy to achieve sectoral goals but as a logic for the development of public policies with a view to common social goals.

Finally, the research generated insights into the conceptualizations of intersectoriality, networks and their relations. It pointed out how the two phenomena had different dynamics and relevance on each level of the network. While intersectoriality was more emphasized at technical, institutional spheres, with "network formation" being a strategy to achieve it, at the local level, network formation was more valued, with intersectoriality being the secondary outcome. This showed how the two phenomena are different yet intrinsically interconnected, which has important implications in health promotion research. Conceptual frameworks and methodological designs, which look into intersectoral actions that are organized as networks, should seek to delimit clearly and analytically each of these phenomena while also considering their connections and reinforcing attributes.

Initially, our study's conceptual framework focused on intersectoriality alone. Over the course of the study, it became clear that we had to consider its interconnections, conceptually and methodologically, with networks. One consequence of this development was the incorporation of theoretical frameworks such as that of Manuel Castell's and an effort to approach these phenomena separately yet analyze them together with our methodological tools. Social network analysis was a key methodology since it helped understand the network as a structure and how intersectoriality fits into it. The qualitative interviews also considered questions regarding each one of these phenomena, which led to the production of data that helped us understand not only participants' experiences with these concepts separately but also how they interacted.

15.4.1 The Challenges and Benefits of Multiple Methods in Health Promotion Research

Triangulation of data, a process in which researchers draw conclusions by connecting data from various sources related to the same phenomenon, was key to understanding how intersectoriality was taking place within the GCP Network and to relating that to a health promotion framework.

The process meant that the results obtained with one method were complemented, analyzed, validated or questioned by the results obtained via other sources of data. Afterwards, conclusions were drawn. For example, the data from the SNA indicated that there were limited partnerships with civil society organizations (CSOs) and that most collaborations took place between governmental institutions. This presented a research enigma as data from the interviews pointed to participants placing high value on social participation. How could we make sense of this result using the data we had? We looked into the participation levels of the partners in GCP meetings, which we were able to determine by document analysis. We found that CSO representatives rarely attended meetings, and, when they did, it was short-lived. So, one conclusion could be that they were not interested, but, another question was: were they invited/mobilized to participate? The answer again came from document analysis (invitations, memos, electronic communications, reports) as well as from notations from participant observation (field diary), in which some of the internal discussions over the benefits and challenges of engaging in partnerships with CSOs had been reported. This showed that the group was divided and conflicted about the issue, and efforts to mobilize these organizations were sporadic and depended on individual efforts. By reviewing data from the interviews with members of CSOs, we also found mentions of limitations imposed by the GCP Network's legal structure. This led us back to document analysis, where we found that the municipal decree that established the Network specifically defined who could participate in decision-making spaces, that is, who would have a voice in decision-making. This structure emphasized the role of public institutions and placed limits on the participation of CSOs. By being able to connect data from these different sources, we were able to view a fuller picture of the situation and to better analyze the factors that affected intersectoriality for this group. This also allowed us to reflect upon the relationship between health promotion values that are often considered to be reinforcing or complementary but that might not align with real-life experiences – in this case, the value of social participation and of advancing intersectoral efforts.

15.4.2 How Were the Results Used and Disseminated?

Efforts were made to produce results that might make a contribution beyond academic discussions and translate into new practices, policies and knowledge. This required thinking about the various target groups for the data produced, the strategies and opportunities for sharing results and the types of analysis and recommendations that could be developed by the research. Adopting a participatory methodology was crucial to foster strategic thinking and knowledge translation to attain such goals. Throughout 2019, the results of the research were presented to policymakers, Network actors, public sector managers and civil society at various occasions, through seminars or roundtable discussions in order to allow for an active exchange of ideas and reflections. Messages were tailored to suit the audiences, with attention paid to using language that made the information easy to understand. Recommendations for action were also developed, considering what would be feasible and appropriate for each context. In early 2020, efforts were undertaken to hold workshops to develop a logic model of the GCP Network and to think collectively about how to tackle problems and tap potentials identified by the research. This effort was suspended due to the coronavirus pandemic that paralyzed the GCP Network in early March. Contacts were renewed in late 2020, and so, we expect to resume activities in the near future.

15.5 How Does This Research Contribute to Advancing and Structuring the Field of Health Promotion Research?

This research sought to address gaps identified by previous health promotion research and contribute to the discussion about how intersectoriality is brought about, how it connects with other health-promoting concepts and what its contributions are to policies and programmes that ultimately affect people and communities.

The GCP Network offered an excellent case study. The characteristics of the Network, its history, structure and the strong engagement of the actors all offered a unique scenario to understand the implementation of health-promoting practices. The context was also propitious to the generation of knowledge that can contribute to the development of frameworks more attuned to political and social realities. This, in turn, can strengthen health promotion's contribution to the academic, political, social and development arenas.

The research provided elements to reflect upon hybrid/mixed approaches that allow the field of health promotion to advance. This included, for example, the recognition of the changing nature of an object of study during the data production process. This approach allowed for a better understanding of the connections between intersectoral efforts and network formation at various levels and dimensions (social, community, policies, services, etc.). The analytical and methodological design had to be adapted in order to accommodate new data and results. Adopting mixed methods made this process easier and more malleable, though more complex. This experience highlights that health promotion research should allow for flexibility and openness to respond to an evolving situation as well as for sensitivity to maintain focus over the course of the research process.

We demonstrated that participatory methods in the planning, collection and analysis of data can favour the restitution/appropriation of research, where it ceases to be "about" something and becomes something "to be with". This participatory view of a research object helps advance the structuring of health promotion in times of political, institutional, cultural and administrative turbulence. On the other hand, research that aims to work "with" actors requires researchers to be attentive, open to dialogue and willing to listen, negotiate and commit to consider the perspectives of all participants, even when these do not align with their own. This implies being able to look at oneself and the research endeavour and reflect upon one's own biases (personal, epistemological, methodological), looking for ways to transcend them towards inclusive and horizontal relationships.

This leads to reflecting on the role of researchers in participatory research. As we become embedded and involved in the process, some boundaries turn fuzzy. It is important to maintain clarity about the limitations of the research project and to be mindful of one's role in the research itself as well as of the relationships developed in the process. Participatory research carries the idea that the separation of subjects and the researcher, advocated by traditional research methods, is not implemented, given that the distance between the two is considered prejudicial to the research and to the generation of knowledge resulting from this approximation.

The recognition of the role of the researcher as a participant that can affect the research and its object has to be emphasized as part of health promotion research. On the one hand, it allows for immersion with, and a deeper understanding of, the study, which will contribute to better analyses and more relevant results and conclusions. On the other hand, it can create conflicts and methodological confusion as it requires constant attention to issues such as research ethics, delimitation of the study object and proper documentation of processes in order to allow for the identification of potential interferences of the researcher in the results.

Another lesson was the challenge of consolidating intersectoriality models based on health promotion values as a new praxis to guide public policies. The GCP Network was able to achieve important results. However, it could not overcome the barriers imposed by the underlying and overreaching structural, institutional and political contexts of the municipality. This points to the limitations of the strategies that rely on long-term structural and societal transformations and to the need to be aware of transitional periods, such as elections and political changes, which can not only bring about new opportunities but also compromise advances and impose new challenges to intersectoral initiatives.

Finally, this research points to interesting reflections about the relation between health promotion values that are often considered to be mutually reinforcing or complementary but that might not align with real-life experiences. For example, theoretically, increased social participation can lead to more effective intersectoral efforts in the long run. However, while values such as social participation, community empowerment and intersectoral action were called for by the Network's participants, their translation into practice led to dilemmas and actions that underscored social participation and community empowerment in favour of advancing intersectoral efforts while not creating tension within institutional and sectoral structures. Health promotion researchers must be attentive to understand the trade-offs that affect decision-making processes in real-life situations. Yet, as a field that aims to position itself with relevant political and ethical models for social transformation, it is important to continue to advocate for all health promotion core values and to seek to address the underlying factors that can weaken or shift the focus away from the potential and strengths of an integrated health promotion framework to improve society's well-being and development.

Acknowledgements The research described in this chapter was funded by the São Paulo Research Foundation (FAPESP), Grant Number 2016/25409-7.

References

Akerman, M., de Sá, R. F., Moyses, S., Rezende, R., & Rocha, D. (2014). Intersetorialidade? IntersetorialidadeS! *Ciência e Saúde Coletiva, 19*(11), 4291–4300. Available in https://www.scielo.br/pdf/csc/v19n11/1413-8123-csc-19-11-4291.pdf. Access 20 Sep 2020

Bardin, L. (2009). *Análise de conteúdo*. Edições 70 LDA.

Castells, M. (2002). *A sociedade em rede*. Fundação Calouste Gulbenkian.

Cavalcanti P. & Nicolau R. (2012). Estado da arte sobre o conceito de intersetorialidade. Material instrucional. Programa de Pós-Graduação em Serviço Social, Universidade Federal da Paraíba, João Pessoa. APUD: Cavalcanti P. B, Carvalho R. N., Miranda A. P. R. S., Medeiros K. T. & Dantas A. C. S. (2013). *A intersetorialidade enquanto estrategia profissional do servico social na saude. Barbarói, Santa Cruz do Sul,* 39, p. 192–215. Available at https://online.unisc.br/seer/index.php/barbaroi/article/view/3153. Access in 21 Sep 2020.

Cellard, A. (2012). A análise documental. In J. Poupart et al. (Eds.), *A pesquisa qualitativa: enfoques epistemológicos e metodológicos* (pp. 295–316). Vozes.

Chiari, A. P. G., Ferreira, R. C., Akerman, M., Amaral, J. H. L., Machado, K. M., & Senna, M. I. B. (2018). Rede intersetorial do Programa Saúde na Escola: sujeitos, percepções e práticas. *Cad. Saúde Pública, 34*(5), 1–15. Available in: https://www.scielo.br/pdf/csp/v34n5/1678-4464-csp-34-05-e00104217.pdf. Access 2 Oct 2020

Cunill-Grau, N. (2005). La intersectorialidad en el gobierno y gestión de la política social. X Congresso Internacional del CLAD sobre la Reforma del Estado y de la Administración Pública. 2005. Available in: http://cdim.esap.edu.co/bancomedios/Documentos PDF/la intersectorialidad en el gobierno y gestión de la política social.pdf. Access 1 Oct 2020.

Cunnil-Grau, N. (2014). The intersectorality in new social policies: An analytical-conceptual approach. *Gestion y Politica Publica, 23*(1), 5–46. Available at: https://www.researchgate.net/publication/291340068_The_Intersectorality_in_New_Social_Policies_An_Analytical-Conceptual_Approach. Access 1 Oct 2020

DaMatta. (1993). *R. Relativizando: uma introdução à antropologia social*. Rocco.

de Minayo, M. C. S. (Org.). (2010). *Pesquisa social: teoria, método e criatividade. 29. ed.* (Coleção temas sociais). Vozes.

Franceschini M.C.T. (2019). *A construção da intersetorialidade: o caso da Rede Intersetorial Guarulhos Cidade que Protege*. Doctoral Thesis, School of Public Health, University of São Paulo, USP: São Paulo. Available at: https://teses.usp.br/teses/disponiveis/6/6140/tde-09092019-093125/pt-br.php. Access 2 Oct 2020.

Giddens, A. (1986). *The constitution of society: Outline of the theory of structuration*. University of California Press.

GUARULHOS – Prefeitura Municipal de Guarulhos; CEPEDOC – Cidades Saudáveis. Diagnóstico técnico: rosto, vozes e lugares – Guarulhos, São Paulo, Brasil. September 2008. Unpublished report.

Higgins, S., & Ribeiro, A. C. A. (2018). *Análise de redes em ciências sociais*. ENAP.

IBGE – Instituto Brasileiro de Geografia e Estatísticas [webpage]. (2020). Cidades e Estados. Available in: https://www.ibge.gov.br/cidades-e-estados/sp/guarulhos.html. Access Oct 2, 2020.

Inojosa, R. M. (2001). Sinergia em políticas públicas e serviços públicos: desenvolvimento social com a intersetorialidade. *Caderno Fundap, 22*, 102–110. Available at: https://www.pucsp.br/prosaude/downloads/bibliografia/sinergia_politicas_servicos_publicos.pdf. Access 1 Oct 2020

Jaccoud, M., & Mayer, R. (2012). A observação direta e a pesquisa qualitativa. In J. Poupart et al. (Eds.), *A pesquisa qualitativa: enfoques epistemológicos e metodológicos* (pp. 254–294). Vozes.

Jackson, S. F., Perkins, F., Khandor, E., Cordwell, L., Harnann, S., & Buasai, S. (2006). Integrated health promotion strategies: A contribution to tackling current and future health challenges. *Health Promotion International, 21*(Suppl 1), 75–83. Available in: https://academic.oup.com/heapro/article/21/suppl_1/75/770062. Access 1 Oct 2020

Junqueira, L. A. P. (1997). Novas formas de gestão na saúde: descentralização e intersetorialidade. *Saúde e Sociedade, São Paulo, 6*(2), 31–46. Available at: http://www.scielo.br/scielo.php?script=sci_arttext&pid=S0104-12901997000200005. Access 1 Oct 2020

Kickbush, I. (2010). Health in all policies: The evolution of the concept of horizontal health governance. In I. Kickbush & D. K. Buckett (Eds.), *Implementing health in all policies* (pp. 11–25). Government of South Australia.

Kranzler, Y., Davidovich, N., Fleischman, Y., Grotto, I., Moran, D., & Weinstein, R. (2013). A health in all policies approach to promote active, healthy lifestyle in Israel. *Israel Journal of Health Policy Research, 2*(1), 16. Available in: https://pubmed.ncbi.nlm.nih.gov/23607681/. Access 20 Sep 2020

McQueen, D., Wismar, M., Lin, V., & Jones, C. (2012). Introduction: Health in all policies, the social determinants of health and governance. In D. McQueen, M. Wismar, V. Lin, & C. Jones (Eds.), *Intersectoral governance for health in all policies: Structures, actions and experience* (pp. 3–21). World Health Organization.

PAHO/WHO – Pan American Health Organization/World Health Organization. (2011). *Trends and achievements in promoting health and equity in the Americas: developments from*

2003–2011. Washington DC: PAHO/WHO. Available in: http://iris.paho.org/xmlui/handle/123456789/33830. Access 21 Sep 2020.

Santos N. N. (2011) *A intersetorialidade como modelo de gestão das políticas de combate à pobreza no Brasil: o caso do Programa Bolsa Família no Município de Guarulhos*. Master's Thesis. Fundação Getúlio Vargas: São Paulo.

SECEL – Secretaria Municipal de Educação, Cultura, Esporte e Lazer de Guarulhos. (2016). *Ponto a ponto: a trajetória de articulação da Rede Intersetorial "Guarulhos: Cidade que Protege" no enfrentamento às violências contra crianças e adolescentes*. Prefeitura de Guarulhos: Guarulhos. Available at: https://www.guarulhos.sp.gov.br/sites/default/files/ppp_inclusiva_rede_intersetorial_guarulhos_cidade_protege.pdf. Access 2 Oct 2020.

Shankardass, K., Solar, O., Murphy, K., Freiler, A., Bobbili, S., & Bayoumi, A. (2011). Health in all policies: A snapshot for Ontario – Results of a realist-informed scoping review of the literature. In *Report to the Ministry of Health and Long-Term Care (Ontario). Getting started with health in all policies: A resource pack*. Centre for Research on Inner City Health, Keenan Research Centre, Li KaShing Knowledge Institute, St. Michael's Hospital.

Solar, O. (2013). *La construcción de la intersectorialidad: salud en todas las políticas desde la perspectiva de equidad y determinantes sociales de la salud*. Available in: https://www.minsal.cl/sites/default/files/La_construccion_intersectorialidad_salud.pdf. Access 1 Oct 2020.

Tess, B. H., & Aith, F. M. A. A. (2014). Intersectorial health-related policies: The use of a legal and theoretical framework to propose a typology to a case study in a Brazilian municipality. *Ciência & Saúde Coletiva, 19*(11), 4449–4456. Available in: https://www.scielo.br/pdf/csc/v19n11/1413-8123-csc-19-11-4449.pdf. Access 20 Sep 2020

Victora, C. G., Knauth, D. R., & de Hassen, M. N. A. (2000). Metodologias qualitativa e quantitativa. In *Pesquisa qualitativa em saúde* (pp. 33–44). Tomo Editorial.

Vinuto, J. (2014). A amostragem em Bola de Neve na pesquisa qualitativa: um debate em aberto. *Temáticas, Campinas, 22*(44), 203–220. ago./dez. 2014. Available in: https://www.ifch.unicamp.br/ojs/index.php/tematicas/article/view/2144/1637. Access 1 Oct 2020

Westphal, M. F. (2012). *Promoção da Saúde e Prevenção de doenças in Campos, GWS Tratado de Saúde Coletiva*. Hucitec.

WHO - World Health Organization. (1986). *The Ottawa charter for health promotion*. First International Conference on Health Promotion, Ottawa, 21 November 1986. Available at: https://www.who.int/healthpromotion/conferences/previous/ottawa/en/. Access 02 Oct 202.

Chapter 16
Capabilities and Transdisciplinary Co-production of Knowledge: Linking the Social Practices of Researchers, Policymakers, Professionals and Populations to Promote Active Lifestyles

Peter Gelius and Klaus Pfeifer

16.1 Introduction

Participation and knowledge co-production have been suggested as promising approaches to increase the fitness and sustainability of health promotion interventions in real-world settings. This chapter reports on the experience of Capital4Health, a German research consortium that used a participatory approach to promote and research active lifestyles in various settings across the life course. The consortium's concept of knowledge production and sharing was built on transdisciplinary research (Bergmann et al., 2013), which provides a framework for the interaction of research, policy, practice and population groups. A specific approach to knowledge co-production – the cooperative planning approach (Rütten, 1997; Rütten & Gelius, 2013) – was used to implement transdisciplinary exchange at the setting level. In addition, the consortium employed Sen's capability approach as a unifying theory to conceptualize opportunities for active lifestyles across different contexts.

This chapter outlines the structural set-up, theoretical underpinnings and the intervention and evaluation methods of Capital4Health to illustrate its epistemological framework as well as the main implications of this research ecosystem for future health promotion research.

The authors write on behalf of the Capital4Health Consortium.

P. Gelius (✉) · K. Pfeifer
Department of Sport Science and Sport, Friedrich-Alexander-Universität Erlangen-Nürnberg, Erlangen, Germany
e-mail: peter.gelius@fau.de

L. Potvin, D. Jourdan (eds.), *Global Handbook of Health Promotion Research, Vol. 1*,
https://doi.org/10.1007/978-3-030-97212-7_16

16.2 The Problem: Matching Research to the Needs of the Population in the Promotion of Physical Activity

Sustainably promoting health in real-world settings and conditions is one of the central challenges of health promotion. Numerous interventions designed, implemented and evaluated in a research context fail to be "institutionalized" (Finegood et al., 2014; Steckler & Goodman, 1989) or widely implemented, thereby leading to no tangible public health impact (Glasgow et al., 1999).

Consequently, researchers have advocated in favour of more effective solutions to match scientific evidence with the actual prerequisites and demands for health promotion in different settings (Leask et al., 2019). There is growing evidence that health promotion interventions are particularly effective and sustainable when population group members, multipliers and key actors are actively involved in programme planning and implementation (Cornwall, 2008; WHO, 2009; Max-Rubner-Institut, 2013).

Participatory research has been identified as a tool to achieve change by involving end users in creating public health interventions, thereby better adapting them to people's needs and increasing programme adherence, functionality and effectiveness, on the one hand (Green et al., 2016), and reducing health inequalities, on the other (Arcaya et al., 2015; Marmot, 2005; O'Mara-Eves et al., 2015). One important approach in this context is knowledge co-creation, which has its roots in the research aimed at strengthening the evidence base of public health (Ham et al., 1995; WHO, 1998) and in the utilization of scientific knowledge by policymakers (Weiss, 1979). There is agreement among researchers that approaches that attempt to directly "transfer" scientific evidence into policy or to "translate" findings into the language of policymaking are insufficient (Black, 2001; Davies et al., 2008; Nutbeam, 2003) and that more interactions between research, policy and practice are required to ensure that knowledge leads to sustainable action (Brownson et al., 2009; Nutley et al., 2007). Notable theoretical approaches, such as interactive knowledge transfer (Canadian Institutes of Health Research, 2010; Rütten & Gelius, 2013), knowledge co-production (Aeberhard & Rist, 2009) and transdisciplinary research (Bergmann et al., 2013), focus on intervention formats that connect experts and setting representatives to jointly develop strategies for health promotion (Minkler, 2005; Wallerstein & Duran, 2006; Israel et al., 2008).

A thematic area for which these approaches have become increasingly important in recent years is insufficient physical activity, which has been identified as a core public health problem of the twenty-first century (Blair, 2009). Multiple positive health outcomes of physical activity are well documented (WHO, 2009; Lee et al., 2012), and physical activity is considered a key component of a healthy lifestyle (CSDH, 2008). However, despite increasing efforts to promote physical activity and reduce sedentary lifestyles in recent years, physical activity prevalence rates across the world are alarmingly low (Guthold et al., 2018). Further, changing physical activity behaviour is difficult, as it is determined by a variety of factors on multiple levels, including individual (e.g. motivation and competence), social (e.g. support from friends and family), infrastructural (e.g. availability of bike lanes) and political (e.g. existence of national recommendations) variables (Dahlgren & Whitehead, 1991; Sallis et al., 2006). Consequently, researchers and practitioners who aim to promote physical activity are facing the challenge of harnessing knowledge co-production to better tailor interventions to settings and population groups, thereby increasing the impact and sustainability of their efforts (Rütten et al., 2009; Rütten & Gelius, 2013; Zwass, 2010).

16.3 The Capital4Health Consortium

The Capital4Health consortium aims to address the above-mentioned issues by employing knowledge co-production in multiple settings to sustainably promote capabilities for establishing active lifestyles among population groups and other stakeholders. The German Federal Ministry of Education and Research provided funding for a 7-year period (2015–2022), specifically requiring projects to be built on the exchange between different research disciplines and non-academic actors (Bundesministerium für Bildung und Forschung, 2013).

The consortium was developed in 2013 following a call from the Ministry to establish research consortia in the field of primary prevention and health promotion. The call specifically requested the use of interdisciplinary approaches and the inclusion of relevant practitioners from respective fields (Bundesministerium für Bildung und Forschung, 2013). However, the logic of research funding continues to emphasize defining project goals, theories, interventions and measurement tools upfront. Consequently, most major project objectives and tenets of Capital4Health had to be formulated before non-academic actors could be involved. Consortium researchers attempted to offset this problem by building on their previous experience with similar projects and used their own funds to maximize collaboration during project development.

The resulting design process had a primarily interdisciplinary (i.e. academia-oriented) focus. Four preparatory workshops were conducted with potential research partners from a variety of disciplinary backgrounds (including sport science, public health and social science). A representative of the state agency responsible for health promotion also participated in one of these workshops. In addition, external academic experts were invited for several meetings to discuss the theoretical foundations of the consortium. Then, researchers selected key population groups and settings for the promotion of physical activity across the life course and developed initial outlines for the six projects of the consortium. Following this, they approached partners from policy and practice who provided expressions of interest to join Capital4Health in the case of a successful grant application. Once the proposal was accepted, a final kick-off meeting was conducted with partners from academia, policy and practice.

The final set-up of the Capital4Health consortium consisted of four intervention projects dedicated to promoting active lifestyles using co-production in four

Table 16.1 The Capital4Health consortium

Project	Setting	Population group addressed	Main goal
QueB	Fourteen childcare centres	Pre-school children	Creating more physical activity-friendly environments in childcare centres
Health. Edu	Six schools, two universities	Schoolchildren	Enhancing physical literacy among schoolchildren by improving the teaching process of physical education (PE) teaching and providing PE teacher education
PArC-AVE	One car manufacturing company, one public nursing school	Apprentices in vocational training	Improving health competence related to physical activity among young adults in vocational training
Action for men	Two rural communities	Community-dwelling men over the age of 50 years	Improving physical activity offers and infrastructures for men aged over 50 years
CAPCOM	Consortium level	–	Improving theory input, project support and consortium-level knowledge co-production
EVA	Consortium level	–	Supporting consortium-wide evaluation of project results

Adapted from Gelius, P., Brandl-Bredenbeck, H.P., Hassel, H., et al. (2021). Kooperative Planung von Maßnahmen zur Bewegungsförderung. *Bundesgesundheitsbl,* 64, 187–198, Table 1. 10.1007/s00103-020-03263-z, licensed under the terms of the Creative Commons Attribution License (https://creativecommons.org/licenses/by/4.0/)

settings: childcare centres, schools, vocational training and communities (see Table 16.1). In addition, there are two cross-cutting projects that support interaction and co-production among researchers at the consortium level. The CAPCOM project provides theoretical input and practical support and leads an intervention to foster consortium-wide interaction among projects as well as among the areas of research, policy and practice. The EVA (evaluation) project supports consortium-wide evaluation. Thus, Capital4Health provides unique and valuable insights for both students and practitioners of health promotion on how knowledge co-creation and sharing may be used effectively to implement physical interventions in multiple real-world settings across the life course.

Capital4Health is based on the idea that active lifestyles – and, by extension, knowledge related to active lifestyles – are not achieved by individuals alone but are co-produced by a variety of actors and their specific social practices (Rütten et al., 2019). Social practice is a concept that is widely used across disciplinary boundaries and is defined in our context as "everyday actions and interactions in specific settings that shape an individual's agency and choice" (Rütten et al., 2019, p. 48). Capital4Health particularly focuses on the interplay of social practices of four groups of actors:

(1) Academics: The consortium comprises seven core research institutions from Southern Germany that are directly funded by the German government. Seven additional institutions (two German and five international) provide research support to the consortium. Researchers from eight institutions (two German and six international) act as members of the Scientific Advisory Board.

(2) Stakeholders, professionals and (3) policymakers: A total of 49 partners from the fields of health promotion policy and practice are involved in the consortium. These include Bavarian regional ministries and state agencies; city, county or district administrations; national or regional NGOs; chambers of commerce, unions or industry think tanks; private companies and educational institutions (including kindergartens and schools). All policy and practice partners are assigned to one of the four intervention projects of Capital4Health.

(4) Population group representatives: The size of the population groups potentially reached by the Capital4Health projects in different settings amounted to $N = 9247$ (1020 in QueB, 3011 in Health.edu, 2216 in PArC-AVE and an estimated 3000 in Action for Men (A4M)) (Gelius et al., 2021). Members of population groups were not only the addressees of interventions in Capital4Health, but their representatives were involved in the actual measure development. This specifically included secondary school students (in Health.edu), apprentices of automotive mechatronics and nursing (PArC-AVE) and community-dwelling men over the age of 50 years (A4M). In A4M, it was difficult to distinguish professional stakeholders from population group members: several practitioners, policymakers and NGO representatives were members of the involved population group, thereby fulfilling a dual role. Further, PE students participated in measure development in the university setting of health.edu but were not counted as population group members (secondary school students). In QueB, population group members (pre-school children) were considered too young to partake in the planning process.

16.4 The Capital4Health Research Framework

In terms of the interaction and potential co-production processes among population groups, professionals, policymakers and researchers, the Capiatl4Health consortium is built on an interactive exchange between academic and non-academic actors, dubbed in the broader literature as "transdisciplinarity" (e.g. Bergmann et al., 2013; Jahn et al., 2012, 2019; Krohn et al., 2017, 2019; Mittelstraß, 2018). Recently, these ideas have also been picked up by discourses in the public health community, such as knowledge-to-action and interactive knowledge transfer (Holmes et al. 2016; Rütten & Gelius, 2013; Canadian Institutes of Health Research, 2010; Jansen et al., 2012; Stokols et al., 2013).

For Capital4Health, we developed and adapted the concept of transdisciplinary research to initiate knowledge co-production (Rütten et al., 2019) based on different models of aligning the social practices of population groups, practitioners, policymakers and researchers to co-produce knowledge for healthy lifestyles. The scenarios range from traditional push/pull models (Weiss, 1979) – via a pragmatic "development model" that remains research-driven and is mostly focused on co-production among academics, professionals and policymakers – to an "ideal" approach that leads to the creation of an equal partnership among population groups, practitioners, policymakers and researchers. While the consortium aimed at achieving this ideal interaction model, the actual design of the Capital4Health projects most closely matches the development model, with a clear focus on researchers, policymakers and practitioners. As shown below, population group members have been successfully involved in most settings, albeit not as intensely as expected in the design stage.

The other central approach, employed to conceptualize the determinants of physical activity behaviour across domains, was the concept of "capabilities". This approach originated in economics (Sen, 1993) but is increasingly recognized in health promotion as well (Abel & Frohlich, 2012; Ruger, 2010; Van Ootegem & Verhofstadt, 2012). It shifts the focus from people's behaviour ("functioning and being") to the range of options ("capabilities") that they can choose from to live life in the manner they desire. Merely having a greater variety of options is considered to increase well-being, even if an individual eventually does not choose a "healthy" behaviour (Abel & Frohlich, 2012). Sen (1993) considers capabilities to be shaped by both social/structural factors (e.g. material resources, societal norms, laws and regulations and infrastructures) and individual competences (e.g. knowledge, skills and motivation), thereby allowing for linking the capability approach to concepts such as Giddens's structure and agency theory (Giddens, 1984), Weber's concept of lifestyles and Bourdieu's idea of different types of capital (Abel & Frohlich, 2012). An adapted version of the capability approach has been developed in the CAPCOM project for use in Capital4Health, conceptualizing both individuals' capabilities for creating active lifestyles and the potential ("agency") of population groups, health promoters and policymakers to influence the promotion of physical activity in their environments (Frahsa et al., 2020).

16.5 Specific Interventions at the Project/Setting and Consortium Levels

In order to link the social practices of the relevant groups of actors in Capital4Health, the consortium pursued a two-pronged approach with separate interventions at the consortium and the project/setting levels. At the project level, Capital4Health employed the cooperative planning approach (Rütten, 1997; Rütten & Gelius, 2013), which comprises a planning group of representatives from all the four above-mentioned groups of social actors that interact to develop and oversee the implementation of measures tailored to the specific setting and needs of the involved population groups. It employs a predefined sequence of three phases: preparation, development and implementation. The core development phase consists of four to six meetings to brainstorm and prioritize ideas, develop specific measures and agree on an action plan and monitor its implementation. Project researchers typically act in a dual capacity as organizers/moderators of the process and as physical activity experts. Typical outputs may be media campaigns, group-specific programmes, infrastructure development or changes in access rules for physical activity facilities. The concept has been successfully used in a variety of both sport-related contexts – for example, talent identification or the development of a sports facility (Rütten et al., 2005) – and physical activity promotion projects – for example, for women in difficult life situations (Frahsa et al., 2012; Rütten & Pfeifer, 2016) or sedentary older people (Rütten & Gelius, 2013).

Overall, a total of 144 planning sessions were conducted in 22 separate intervention sites across the four participatory intervention projects. A few projects addressed more than one sub-setting (e.g. physical education classes and teacher education, vocational training in automotive mechatronics and nursing) or different geographical regions (childcare centres and communities in different Bavarian counties). Research teams prepared the processes by contacting the key actors well in advance (and occasionally repeatedly), by conducting informational meetings to get to know the partners and raise their awareness of physical activity and by creating systematic context analyses according to the setting.

The four projects' planning groups showed a broad spectrum of group set-ups and processes, ranging from smaller groups in childcare and school settings (with a minimum of four participants) to very large groups of up to 20 individuals in vocational education and community settings. All projects attempted to involve the full spectrum of relevant stakeholders, including both the leadership and "working level" of organizations and representatives of the involved population groups. However, the latter groups were not accessible in all settings, notably the childcare setting, where children were considered too young to participate in a structured planning process. In addition, given the need to limit group sizes, the average number of population group representatives participating in the planning groups remained limited, ranging from one to six representatives. The number of sessions also varied substantially. While a few processes (e.g. in the vocational training setting) required the conduct of the minimum number of sessions prescribed by the cooperative planning approach ($n = 4$), others exceeded this number by far (e.g. the community setting with up to 10 sessions). Most processes took between 6 and 18 months to complete. Projects also adapted the planning process to the needs of the setting – for example, achieving a common understanding of central concepts at the beginning of the project (Health.edu) or the use of certain self-evaluation tools (e.g. a web-based self-check application in QueB).

One central element in cooperative planning is that its impact is not primarily generated by the planning process as such but by the specific measures developed by the planning group, which vary depending on the setting, participants and the course of the process. Across different sites, Capital4Health generated a broad spectrum of measures to promote capabilities for physical activity, ranging from general organizational guidelines (e.g. vision statements or the adoption of a physical activity-friendly language) via one-off events (workshops, info events) to specific physical activity programmes, curriculum changes and monetary subsidies for participation in sports programmes.

At the consortium level, the CAPCOM project developed and implemented a dedicated intervention to foster collaboration among projects, research groups and certain policy/practice partners, which included the following components:

- Ongoing support to the intervention projects, including: (a) regular debriefing interviews with all research teams on the status of their projects, accomplishments and challenges as well as interaction with the project partners; (b) a central digital infrastructure for the consortium with a web-based data repository, an internal Wiki with a glossary of central terminology and a consortium website (www.capital4health.de) and (c) several workshops that were open to all consortium researchers on capabilities, transdisciplinarity, cooperative planning and health economic evaluation.
- A scientific advisory board with eight internationally renowned researchers from the fields of physical activity, health promotion and health economics met annually with the entire Capital4Health research team to discuss project progress, theories, interventions, methods and publications.
- A council of speakers with all principal investigators met every 6 months to discuss consortium strategies, handle project administration and resolve conflicts where necessary.
- A young researchers network was formed to support exchange among graduate students and postdoctoral fellows who were part of the projects. Activities included semi-annual meetings, a summer school and a joint special issue in an international scientific journal.
- A transdisciplinary steering committee, including the principal investigators and select partners from policy and practice recruited from the projects to foster knowledge co-production at the consortium level, was set up. The topics addressed by this committee included problems shared across projects, the practice-oriented dissemination of project results and the creation of permanent structures for the promotion of physical activity beyond the lifetime of the consortium.

16.6 Evaluating Intervention Effects

To evaluate the participatory build-up of new capabilities for physical activity, the consortium collected data from both within each individual project and at the consortium level, using a variety of quantitative and qualitative methods.

To evaluate the effects of their planning processes as well as the resulting measures developed and implemented, all projects conducted their own research. The research foci varied depending on the setting and the researchers' disciplinary backgrounds. The questions researched ranged from the build-up of physical literacy/competences to the build-up of infrastructure and organizational capacities, sport participation and general physical activity behaviour. Projects also used a variety of qualitative and quantitative outcome measures, including self-assessments, qualitative interviews, knowledge tests, surveys, observations and pedometers. The two cross-cutting projects conducted additional evaluations. The EVA project developed and pilot-tested a tool to evaluate the development of organizational capacities during the cooperative planning processes (Sauter et al., 2020). The CAPCOM project conducted a Delphi process to draw joint conclusions on researchers' experiences with the approach (Till et al., under review).

Overall, the results indicate that interventions contributed to improvements in various dimensions of organizational capacity in the PArC-AVE project (Popp et al., 2020) and A4M (Loss et al., 2020). They also helped improve the skills of nursing school teachers in the QueB project (Müller et al., 2019) and significantly improved the physical literacy of high school students in Health.edu (Sygusch et al., 2020; Ptack, 2019). Finally, the measures implemented on the basis of the planning processes in the QueB childcare centres led to a significant increase in the average number of steps per hour among both children and staff (Müller et al., 2019).

At the consortium level, we analyzed project-related documents and took minutes of consortium meetings to document interactions and knowledge co-production over time. In addition, we investigated cooperation and co-production of scientific outputs in the consortium based on Hall et al.'s (2008) model of collaborative readiness, collaborative capacity and collaborative outcomes (Ferschl et al., 2021). For this, we conducted semi-structured interviews with project researchers and analyzed the collaborative products of Capital4Health, such as joint publications and co-supervised MA or PhD theses.

The results indicate that collaborative readiness was fostered by researchers' previous experience with interdisciplinary projects, the geographical proximity of the research groups and a general inclination towards scientific collaboration (Ferschl et al., 2021). On the other hand, scarce resources, a lack of structured planning and limited trust challenged team cooperation in the early project phases. However, by the end of the project, teams reported an increased sense of unity. Scientific publications were mostly produced by individual project teams at the beginning of Capital4Health, but the co-production of outputs increased in the subsequent stages (e.g. Gelius et al., 2020). In addition, project groups perceived the evaluation support received from the EVA project as well as the intervention of the CAPCOM project as important facilitators for the success of the consortium. These findings emphasize the importance of a coordinating entity that provides structured support for exchange and collaboration for complex research initiatives.

The analysis of project documentation revealed that (a) knowledge co-production in the design/proposal-writing phase of the consortium was mostly limited to researchers, while policy and practice partners could be recruited but were not actively involved due to lack of funding; (b) the common theory base was modified by all intervention projects to fit their setting, planning group participants and own disciplinary backgrounds; (c) a common language and understanding was slowly developed with consortium meetings acting as "catalytic events" that stimulated exchange and awareness and (d) involving professionals and policymakers in co-production processes was much more difficult at the consortium level than in individual projects.

16.7 Conclusions

The analysis of Capital4Health provides important insights and lessons for health promotion research and practice. The results from individual projects shed light on the effectiveness and sustainability of specific interventions to promote physical activity in different settings. These results may also help clarify how specific capabilities contribute to healthier lifestyles in different population groups and what professionals and policymakers require to support these groups. At a more general level, the consortium provides important evidence on the utility, feasibility and effects of cooperative planning and other forms of transdisciplinary interaction in health promotion activities. Finally, the results of the consortium may foster the development of health promotion theory (capabilities and transdisciplinarity) and methods (measurement of capabilities, physical literacy, organizational readiness, academic collaboration and health economic aspects).

With regard to the implementation of an approach that fosters co-production, the consortium arrived at the following conclusions (Gelius et al., 2020):

1. Cooperative planning can be effectively utilized to promote health across different settings, but it must be (and can be) adapted to match the respective context.
2. Physical activity (like other health behaviours) does not necessarily take a front seat in many settings, and it is important to raise awareness and build capacities for addressing this aspect.
3. Setting readiness for change is a decisive factor for success, and researchers must ascertain actors' readiness at an early stage (Edwards et al., 2000; Gansefort et al., 2018) and adapt their interventions accordingly.
4. Involving population groups in output-oriented knowledge co-production is challenging, and adapted approaches may be necessary to maximize the number of individuals involved.

Individual actors or "champions" (O'Loughlin et al., 1998; Greenhalgh et al., 2016) may be key to project success. Attempts to identify champions must be made early in the process. With regard to the interaction at the consortium level, a consortium design like the one used in Capital4Health can substantially foster interdisciplinary cooperation among researchers from different disciplines. A common theory and shared methods can be valuable assets for working across different settings and population groups, provided that there is sufficient flexibility that enables adaptations to different contexts and disciplines. However, sufficient resources are required for this. There must be no overly optimistic assumptions regarding the speed of the integration process. In addition, integrating representatives of population groups and other stakeholders into research coordination at the consortium level remains a challenge that must be addressed in future projects.

Acknowledgements The Capital4Health research consortium and its projects CAPCOM, EVA, QueB, Health.eduPlus, PArC-AVE and Action4Men were funded by the German Federal Ministry of Education and Research (BMBF), grant no. 01EL1821 A-H.

References

Abel, T., & Frohlich, K. (2012). Capitals and capabilities: Linking structure and agency to reduce health inequalities. *Social Science and Medicine, 74*(2), 236–244.

Aeberhard, A., & Rist, S. (2009). Transdisciplinary co-production of knowledge in the development of organic agriculture in Switzerland. *Ecological Economics, 68*(4), 1171–1181.

Arcaya, M. C., Arcaya, A. L., & Subramanian, S. V. (2015). Inequalities in health: Definitions, concepts, and theories. *Global Health Action, 8*, 27106. https://doi.org/10.3402/gha.v8.27106

Bergmann, M., Jahn, T., Knobloch, T., Krohn, W., Pohl, C., & Schramm, E. (2013). *Methods for transdisciplinary research: A primer for practice*. Campus Verlag.

Black, N. (2001). Evidence based policy: Proceed with care. *British Medical Journal, 323*(7307), 275. https://doi.org/10.1136/bmj.323.7307.275

Blair, S. N. (2009). Physical inactivity: The biggest public health problem of the 21st century. *British Journal of Sports Medicine, 43*(1), 1–2.

Brownson, R. C., Chriqui, J. F., & Stamatakis, K. A. (2009). Understanding evidence-based public health policy. *American Journal of Public Health, 99*(9), 1576–1583. https://doi.org/10.2105/AJPH.2008.156224

Bundesministerium für Bildung und Forschung (2013). *Bekanntmachung des Bundesministeriums für Bildung und Forschung: Richtlinien zur Förderung von Forschungsverbünden zur Primärprävention und Gesundheitsförderung* [Call by the federal ministry of research and education: Guidelines on funding of research consortia for primary prevention and health promotion]. https://www.bmbf.de/foerderungen/bekanntmachung-859.html. Accessed 14 Apr 2019.

Canadian Institutes of Health Research. (2010). *Knowledge to action: An end-of-grant knowledge translation casebook*. CIHR.

Cornwall, A. (2008). Unpacking "participation": Models, meanings and practices. *Community Development Journal, 43*(3), 269–283. https://doi.org/10.1093/cdj/bsn010

CSDH. (2008). *Closing the gap in a generation: Health equity through action on the social determinants of health. Final report of the commission on social determinants of health*. WHO.

Dahlgren, G., & Whitehead, M. (1991). *Policies and strategies to promote social equity in health*. WHO Regional Office for Europe, (document EUR/icp/rpd 414(2)9866n).

Davies, H., Nutley, S., & Walter, I. (2008). Why "knowledge transfer" is misconceived for applied social research. *Journal of Health Services Research & Policy, 13*(3), 188–190. https://doi.org/10.1258/jhsrp.2008.008055

Edwards, R. W., Jumper-Thurman, P., Plestred, B. A., Oetting, E. R., & Swanson, L. (2000). Community readiness: Research to practice. *Journal of Community Psychology, 28*(3), 291–307.

Ferschl, S., Allmeta, A., Fleuren, T., Weege, M., Abu-Omar, K., & Gelius, P. (2020). Scaling-up auch in der Bewegungsförderung? Konzepte, Handlungsleitfäden und praktische Tipps zur Verbreitung erfolgreicher Interventionen [The role of scaling up in the promotion of physical activity: Concepts, guidelines and practical tips for disseminating successful interventions]. *Bewegungstherapie und Gesundheitssport, 36*. https://doi.org/10.1055/a-1153-5882

Ferschl, S., Till, M., Abu-Omar, K., Pfeifer, K., & Gelius, P. (2021). Scientific cooperation and co-production of scientific outputs for physical activity promotion: Results from a transdisciplinary research consortium. *Frontiers of Public Health*. https://doi.org/10.3389/fpubh.2021.604855

Finegood, D., Johnston, L., Steinberg, M., Matteson, C., & Deck, P. (2014). Complexity, systems thinking, and health behavior change. In S. Kahan, A. Gielen, P. Fagan, & L. Green (Eds.), *Health behavior change in populations* (pp. 435–458). Johns Hopkins University Press.

Frahsa, A., Rütten, A., Röger, U., Abu-Omar, K., & Schow, D. (2012). Enabling the powerful? Participatory action research with local policymakers and professionals for physical activity promotion with women in difficult life situations. *Health Promot International, 29*(1), 171–184. https://doi.org/10.1093/heapro/das050

Frahsa, A., Abel, T., Gelius, P., & Rütten, A. (2020). Locating capabilities and agency for active lifestyle promotion: An analytical framework to guide research on physical activity interventions. *Health Promotion International.* https://doi.org/10.1093/heapro/daaa076

Gansefort, D., Brand, T., Princk, C., & Zeeb, H. (2018). Community readiness for the promotion of physical activity in older adults-a cross-sectional comparison of rural and urban communities. *International Journal of Environmental Research and Public Health, 15*(3). https://doi.org/10.3390/ijerph15030453

Gelius, P., Hassel, H., Loss, J., Sygusch, R., Tittlbach, S., Töpfer, C., Ungerer-Röhrich, U., & Pfeifer, K. (2020). Kooperative Planung zur Erweiterung von Handlungsmöglichkeiten für Bewegung: Ergebnisse aus dem Forschungsverbund Capital4Health [Cooperative planning of measures to promote physical activity: New paths for expanding capabilities – Results from the Capital4Health research consortium]. *Bundesgesundheitsblatt.* https://doi.org/10.1007/s00103-020-03263-z

Gelius, P., Sommer, R., Abu-Omar, K., Schätzlein, V., & Suhrcke, M. (2021). Toward the economic evaluation of participatory approaches in health promotion: Lessons from four German physical activity promotion projects. *Health Promotion International, 36*(S2):ii79–92. https://doi.org/10.1093/heapro/daab158

Giddens, A. (1984). *The constitution of society: Outline of the theory of structuration.* University of California Press.

Glasgow, R. E., Vogt, T. M., & Boles, S. M. (1999). Evaluating the public health impact of health promotion interventions: The RE-AIM framework. *American Journal of Public Health, 89*(9), 1322–1327. https://doi.org/10.2105/ajph.89.9.1322

Green, L. W., O'Neill, M., Westphal, M., & Morisky, D. (2016). The challenges of participatory action research for health promotion. *Promotion & Education, 3*(4), 3. https://doi.org/10.1177/102538239600300401

Greenhalgh, T., Jackson, C., Shaw, S., & Janamian, T. (2016). Achieving research impact through co-creation in community-based health services: Literature review and case study. *The Milbank Quarterly, 94*, 392–429.

Guthold, R., Stevens, G. A., Riley, L. M., & Bull, F. C. (2018). Worldwide trends in insufficient physical activity from 2001 to 2016: A pooled analysis of 358 population-based surveys with 1·9 million participants. *The Lancet Global Health, 6*(10), e1077–e1086. https://doi.org/10.1016/s2214-109x(18)30357-7

Hall, K. L., Stokols, D., Moser, R. P., Taylor, B. K., Thornquist, M. D., Nebeling, L. C., et al. (2008). The collaboration readiness of transdisciplinary research teams and centers: Findings from the National Cancer Institute's TREC year-one evaluation study. *American Journal of Preventive Medicine, 35*(2), S161–SS72.

Ham, C., Hunter, D. J., & Robinson, R. (1995). Evidence based policymaking. *British Medical Journal, 310*(6972), 71–72. https://doi.org/10.1136/bmj.310.6972.71

Holmes, B., Best, A., Davies, H., Hunter, D. J., Kelly, M., Marshall, M., & Rycroft-Malone, J. (2016). Mobilising knowledge in complex health systems: A call to action. *Evidence and Policy, 13*, 539–560.

Israel, B. A., Schultz, A. J., Parker, E. A., & Becker, A. B. (2008). Critical issue in developing and following community based participatory research principles. In M. Minkler & N. Wallerstein (Eds.), *Community-based participatory research for health* (pp. 47–62). Jossey-Bass.

Jahn, T., Bergmann, M., & Keil, F. (2012). Transdisciplinarity: Between mainstreaming and marginalization. *Ecological Economics, 79*, 1–10.

Jahn, T., Keil, F., & Marg, O. (2019). Transdisziplinarität: zwischen Praxis und Theorie [Transdisciplinarity: Between practice and theory]. *GAIA, 28*, 16–20.

Jansen, M., de Leeuw, E., Hoeijmakers, M., & de Vries, N. K. (2012). Working at the nexus between public health policy, practice and research. Dynamics of knowledge sharing in the Netherlands. *Health Research Policy and Systems, 10*(1), 1–12.

King, A., Winter, S. J., Sheats, J. L., Rosas, L. G., Buman, M. P., Salvo, D., Rodriguez, N. M., … Dommarco, J. R. (2016). Leveraging citizen science and information technology for population physical activity promotion. *Translational Journal of the American College of Sports Medicine, 1*(4), 30–44.

Krohn, W., Grunwald, A., & Ukowitz, M. (2017). Transdisziplinäre Forschung revisited: Erkenntnisinteresse, Forschungsgegenstände, Wissensform und Methodologie [Transdisciplinary research revisited: Epistemological interest, objects of research, form of knowledge and methodology]. *GAIA, 26*(4), 341–347.

Krohn, W., Grunwald, A., & Ukowitz, M. (2019). Transdisziplinäre Forschung kontrovers – Antworten und Ausblicke [Controversial transdisciplinary research – Answers and outlook]. *Gaia, 28*(1), 21–25.

Leask, C. F., Sandlund, M., Skelton, D. A., Altenburg, T. M., Cardon, G., Chinapaw, M. J. M., ... Teenage Girls on the Move Research. (2019). Framework, principles and recommendations for utilising participatory methodologies in the co-creation and evaluation of public health interventions. *Research Involvement and Engagement, 5*, 2. https://doi.org/10.1186/s40900-018-0136-9

Lee, I. M., Shiroma, E. J., Lobelo, F., Puska, P., Blair, S. N., Katzmarzyk, P. T., & Lancet Physical Activity Series Working Group. (2012). Effect of physical inactivity on major non-communicable diseases worldwide: An analysis of burden of disease and life expectancy. *Lancet (London, England), 380*(9838), 219–229. https://doi.org/10.1016/S0140-6736(12)61031-9

Loss, J., Brew-Sam, N., Metz, B., Strobl, H., Sauter, A., & Tittlbach, S. (2020). Capacity building in community stakeholder groups for increasing physical activity: Results of a qualitative study in two German communities. *International Journal of Environmental Research and Public Health, 17*(7), 2306. https://doi.org/10.3390/ijerph17072306

Marmot, M. (2005). Social determinants of health inequalities. *Lancet, 365*(9464), 1099–1104. https://doi.org/10.1016/s0140-6736(05)71146-6

Max-Rubner-Institut (2013) *Evaluation des Modellvorhabens „Besser essen. Mehr bewegen. KINDERLEICHT-Regionen". Zentrale Ergebnisse und Empfehlungen für Entscheider, Projektförderer und Projektnehmer* [Evaluation of the pilot program „Better eating. More physical activity. KINDERLEICHT Regions". Central results and recommendations for policymakers, funding agencies and applicants]. Max-Rubner-Institut.

Minkler, M. (2005). Community-based research partnerships: Challenges and opportunities. *Journal of Urban Health : Bulletin of the New York Academy of Medicine, 82*(2 Suppl 2), 3–12.

Mittelstraß, J. (2018). Forschung und Gesellschaft. Von theoretischer und praktischer Transdisziplinarität [Research and society: On theoretical and practical transdisciplinarity]. *GAIA, 27*(2), 201–204.

Müller, C., Foitzik, E., & Hassel, H. (2019). Bewegte Kitas durch Organisationsentwicklung [active childcare centers through organizational development]. *Prävention und Gesundheitsförderung, 15*, 50–55. https://doi.org/10.1007/s11553-019-00737-0

Nutbeam, D. (2003). How does evidence influence public health policy? Tackling health inequalities in England. *Health Promotion Journal of Australia, 14*(3), 154–158. https://doi.org/10.1071/HE03154

Nutley, S. M., Walter, I., & Davies, H. T. O. (2007). *Using evidence: How research can inform public services* (Vol. 16). Policy Press.

O'Loughlin, J., Renaud, L., Richard, L., Gomez, L. S., & Paradis, G. (1998). Correlates of the sustainability of community-based heart health promotion interventions. *Preventive Medicine, 27*, 702–712.

O'Mara-Eves, A., Brunton, G., Oliver, S., Kavanagh, J., Jamal, F., & Thomas, J. (2015). The effectiveness of community engagement in public health interventions for disadvantaged groups: A meta-analysis. *BMC Public Health, 15*, 129. https://doi.org/10.1186/s12889-015-1352-y

Popp, J., Carl, J., Grüne, E., Semrau, J., Gelius, P., & Pfeifer, K. (2020). Physical activity promotion in vocational education: Does capacity building work? *Health Promotion International, daaa014*. https://doi.org/10.1093/heapro/daaa014

Prochaska, J. M., Prochaska, J. O., & Levesque, D. A. (2001). A Transtheoretical approach to changing organizations. *Ad Policy Men Health, 28*(4), 247–261.

Ptack K. (2019). Eine Interventionsstudie zum Thema Gesundheit im Sportunterricht: Evaluation eines kooperativen Planungsprozesses in der Health.edu-Studie [An intervention study on the topic of health in physical education: Evaluation of a cooperative planning process in the health.edu study]. Feldhaus.

Ruger, J. P. (2010). Health capability: Conceptualization and operationalization. *American Journal of Public Health, 100*(1), 41–49.

Rütten, A. (1997). Kooperative Planung und Gesundheitsförderung. Ein Implementationsansatz [Cooperative planning and health promotion: An implementation approach]. *Zeitschrift für Gesundheitswissenschaft*, 257–272.

Rütten, A., & Gelius, P. (2013). Building policy capacities: An interactive approach for linking knowledge to action in health promotion. *Health Promotion International, 29*(3), 569–582.

Rütten, A., & Pfeifer, K. (Eds.). (2016). *National recommendations for physical activity and physical activity promotion*. FAU University Press.

Rütten, A., Ziemainz, H., & Röger, U. (2005). *Qualitätsgesichertes system der Talentsuche, –auswahl und -förderung* [Quality-assured system of talent selection, identification and development]. Sport und Buch Strauß.

Rütten, A., Abu-Omar, K., Frahsa, A., & Morgan, A. (2009). Assets for policy-making in health promotion: Overcoming political barriers inhibiting women in difficult life situations to access sport facilities. *Social Science and Medicine, 69*, 1667–1673.

Rütten, A., Frahsa, A., Abel, T., Bergmann, M., de Leeuw, E., Hunter, D., Jansen, M., King, A., & Potvin, L. (2019). Co-producing active lifestyles as whole-system-approach: Theory, intervention and knowledge-to-action implications. *Health Promotion International, 34*(1), 47–59.

Sallis, J. F., Cervero, R. B., Ascher, W., Henderson, K. A., Kraft, M. K., & Kerr, J. (2006). An ecological approach to creating active living communities. *Annual Review of Public Health, 27*, 297–322.

Sauter, A., Lindacher, V., Rueter, J., Curbach, J., & Loss, J. (2020). How health promoters can assess capacity building processes in setting-based approaches – Development and testing of a monitoring instrument. *International Journal of Environmental Research and Public Health, 17*(2), 407. https://doi.org/10.3390/ijerph17020407

Sen, A. (1993). Capability and Well-being. In M. Nussbaum & A. Sen (Eds.), *The quality of life*. Clarendon Press.

Steckler, A., & Goodman, R. M. (1989). How to institutionalize health promotion programs. *American Journal of Health Promotion, 3*(4), 34–43. https://doi.org/10.4278/0890-1171-3.4.34

Stokols, D., Hall, K. L., & Vogel, A. L. (2013). Trasdisciplinary public health: Core characteristics, definitions, and strategies for success. In D. Haire-Joshu & T. D. McBride (Eds.), *Transdisciplinary public health: Research, methods, and practice* (pp. 3–30). Jossey-Bass Publishers.

Strobl, H., Brew-Sam, N., Curbach, J., Metz, B., Tittlbach, S., & Loss, J. (2020). ACTION for men: Study protocol of a community capacity building intervention to develop and im-plement gender-sensitive physical activity programs for men 50 plus. *Frontiers in Public Health, 8*, 4.

Sygusch, R., Brandl-Bredenbeck, H.P., Tittlbach, S., Ptack, K., Töpfer, C. (2020). *Gesundheit in Sportunterricht und Sportlehrerbildung. Bestandsaufnahme, Interventionen und Evaluation im Projekt "Health.edu"* [Health in physical education and physical education teacher education: Stock-taking, interventions and evaluation in the "Health.edu" project]. Springer VS.

Till, M., Abu-Omar, K., Ferschl, S., Abel, T., & Gelius, P., on behalf of the Capital4Health consortium (under review). Using the capability approach in health promotion projects: A framework for implementation.

Van Ootegem, L., & Verhofstadt, E. (2012). Using capabilities as an alternative indicator for Well-being. *Social Indicators Research, 106*(1), 133–152.

Wallerstein, N. B., & Duran, B. (2006). Using community-based participatory research to address health disparities. *Health Promotion Practice, 7*(3), 312–323.

Weiss, C. H. (1979). The many meanings of research utilization. *Public Administration Review, 39*(5), 426–431. https://doi.org/10.2307/3109916

WHO. (1998). *Health promotion glossary*. World Health Organization. Retrieved from: https://www.who.int/healthpromotion/about/HPR%20Glossary%201998.pdf?ua=1

WHO. (2009). *Interventions on diet and physical activity: What works: Summary report*. World Health Organization. Retrieved from: https://apps.who.int/iris/bitstream/handle/10665/44140/9789241598248_eng.pdf;jsessionid=C539D2462C7161E245BE11E825A9AD4F?sequence=1

Zwass, V. (2010). Co-creation: Toward a taxonomy and an integrated research perspective. *International Journal of Electronic Commerce, 15*(1), 11–48. https://doi.org/10.2753/JEC1086-4415150101

Chapter 17
Conducting *Embedded* Health Promotion Research: Lessons Learned from the Health On the Go Study in Ecuador

Irene Torres, Daniel López-Cevallos, and Fernando Sacoto

17.1 Introduction

Embedded research has gained traction in recent years, as a form of acknowledging implementation actors as important stakeholders in knowledge creation, in the health programmes in which they work and for which they are ultimately responsible. In addition, it is considered that having "insider" perspectives makes information more relevant and also more attuned to the needs of decision-makers (Varallyay et al., 2020). However, similar to other fields, while embedded research holds promise to award the necessary importance to local knowledge and capacities, it seems to be dominated by reflections and work from high-income country researchers, as signalled by their affiliations in publications (Reidpath & Allotey, 2019; Collyer, 2018). Concurrently, embedded research has largely focused on health care systems and health care delivery and less on health promotion. The aim of this chapter is to identify the values, opportunities, challenges and limitations of conducting embedded research with allied health professionals (Slade et al., 2018; Harris et al., 2020) from our experience in a study of the Health On the Go (*Salud Al Paso*) Program in Quito, Ecuador.

I. Torres (✉)
Fundación Octaedro, Quito, Ecuador
e-mail: irene.torres@octaedro.edu.ec

D. López-Cevallos
School of Language, Culture and Society, Oregon State University, Corvallis, OR, USA

F. Sacoto
Ecuadorian Society of Public Health, Quito, Ecuador

L. Potvin, D. Jourdan (eds.), *Global Handbook of Health Promotion Research, Vol. 1*,
https://doi.org/10.1007/978-3-030-97212-7_17

17.2 Context

In Ecuador, a country of 17 million, about 65% of the population (19 years of age and older) is overweight or obese (both considered risk factors for non-communicable diseases, NCDs, such as heart disease, diabetes and stroke) with direct and indirect costs estimated at about 4.3% of the annual Gross Domestic Product (GDP) (Fernandez & Martínez, 2017, p. 9). The situation is exacerbated by a powerful and well-connected processed food and alcohol industry, leading to a saturation of highly processed foods, tobacco and electronic cigarettes, with limited controls due to lax regulations that are incompatible with their health effects. The health actors' landscape depicts parallel private and public health systems, where the private sector is available to those with private health insurance and/or the ability to pay out of pocket. In turn, the public sector operates in a fragmented and, at the same time, centralized manner through two systems: (a) different social security regimes (Social Security Institute, Peasant Social Security) and (b) the Ministry of Health network of community health centres and hospitals (Torres & López-Cevallos, 2018). A curative care model prevails in Ecuador, limiting health promotion and disease prevention approaches that have been shown to have the largest benefits to tackle NCDs (Beaglehole et al., 2011; Mikkelsen et al., 2019).

In this context, health policies are often implemented following political rather than evidence-based arguments and are therefore hostage to political calculus, inertia or are formulated at the discretion of elected officials preoccupied more on the next election cycle rather than operating along scientific, institutional goals (Mejia Acosta, 2019; Pribble, 2013; Campos Herrera & de Reguero, 2019).

The Metropolitan District of Quito (DMQ), the seat of Ecuador's central government, with 2.5 million inhabitants, constitutes the largest and one of the most unequal urban areas in the country. The municipal government has had relatively limited health competencies (given by the law to the national health authority, the Ministry of Health), such as managing three Metropolitan Health Units, one of which focused on maternal and neonatal care (discontinued in 2019), and, most recently, a temporary hospital to identify and treat COVID-19 patients ("Pop-up hospital in Quito is taking COVID-19 patients", 2020).

The DMQ has also implemented a few health promotion interventions aimed at filling the void left by limited capacity in primary care services in Quito. For example, Ordinance 494 enabled the local government to undertake actions of "promotion, prevention and provision of health and surveillance services… for the development of a healthy territory in the DMQ, as a guarantee for the exercise of the right to health of its inhabitants" (Municipality of the Metropolitan District of Quito, 2014). In spite of this ordinance, health promotion initiatives have been limited in scope, geared primarily towards a "captive" population, under municipal responsibility, which represents less than 5% of the population of Quito. This subset of the DMQ population included populations served by their network of social and educational services (children attending their network of childcare centres; older adults participating in their network of elderly care services; K-12 students attending municipal schools; merchants operating in municipal markets; DMQ employees and patients served by municipal health units who have been diagnosed with cardiometabolic risk) (Municipality of the Metropolitan District of Quito, 2019).

17.3 Conducting Embedded Research

Ideally, "embedded" research aims to improve an existing policy, programme or service and therefore informs programme improvement or reform (Cheetham et al., 2018; Newbury-Birch & Allan, 2019). This study aimed to analyze whether preliminary results could justify continuation of the programme and, if that were the case, how sustainability could be achieved. One underlying assumption was that these types of interventions (with included screening and nutritional counselling) are necessary to prevent non-communicable diseases and promote healthy lifestyles (Bock et al., 2012; Afshin et al., 2014). Another underlying assumption was that research that is embedded in the institution, i.e. having an "internal" view, may be able to find how the programme can remain sustainable or decision-makers who have a vested interest in the continuation of the programme can learn how it may continue, by undertaking changes that can positively influence its continuity and accomplishments.

Conceptually, an embedded research approach has the potential to facilitate more interactive and horizontal engagement and knowledge co-production, enable collaborative/two-way relationships between researchers and allied health professionals and decision-makers and encourage end users' involvement in research (facilitating their timely access to current evidence and best practices while allowing researchers to experience the worldviews of the end users and their organization). At the same time, these studies demand negotiating interests or concerns involved in the different relationships that are established with institutions and individuals (Harding, 2019).

Conducting research on policy, programmes and services with the support of decision-makers in an "embedded" study may help ensure that the topic of study is well-identified and relevant in terms of its applied benefit. An embedded study centred on knowledge exchange can hold greater relevance for policy and practice and their reforms (Cheetham et al., 2018; van der Graaf et al., 2017). However, it is likely that decision-makers would not have a clear "on-the-ground" programming knowledge, and, therefore, partial understanding of the research needed to inform change. In addition, community participation, i.e., co-creation of knowledge, is an important tenet of health promotion research (Woodall et al., 2018). As such, from our point of view, at least two conditions are necessary to carry out an embedded health promotion research study: (1) the health personnel are supported to become partners in the research process, and (2) as the health personnel become co-creators of knowledge, researchers have less vertical control over the study.

An embedded research approach would have the potential benefit that recommendations arising from such research would be in a better position to be considered, and perhaps effectively implemented by local authorities. However, it is necessary to take into account some aspects of this premise: (a) the selection of the topic under study is crucial, and it is advisable for embedded research teams to make decisions based on local data that point to more prevalent public health issues, which may affect large segments of the population that are potentially beneficiaries of the study results; (b) the active involvement of decision-makers is critical, but it may also be necessary to take precautions both due to frequent limitations in the exercise of authorities in our countries, related to instability in management positions, and limitations of preparation for such efforts, possibly more accentuated for conducting research, which in turn could conspire for a proper conduct of studies and subsequent use of results, and (c) it would also be necessary to consider the feasibility of decision-makers effectively implementing changes suggested by the findings, whether because it is within their reach or because influence at other levels is required (Koon et al., 2013).

In this context, the participation of health workers in the study of a programme or policy in which they work also generates some reflections. In principle, this could be motivated by the interest to include a research and evaluation component to their work. As is the case in much of the Global South, there are limitations to conducting research in general and research on health policies, systems and services in particular (Franzen et al., 2019). One important element of embedded research is that stakeholders' opinions are considered from the very beginning of the studies, analyzing topics or contents that in their perspective would be relevant to examine. Concurrently, taking their contributions into account can be stimulating for them, as they believe that they contribute to improving the policy or programme analyzed and that their suggestions are included in the conclusions and recommendations. Their active involvement can also help to look more objectively and critically at the programme's performance, to contrast their perceptions and opinions with those of their colleagues, with other stakeholders and service users.

In contrast, it could also be true that, depending on the commitment required to participate in such studies, there may be resistance due to the additional time and effort that it would represent beyond their usual tasks. The type of institutional culture that exists should also be considered, since in hierarchical environments, participation of allied health professionals could represent a threat to their job security, even more so if work relationships are not stable, a common issue across health institutions in countries such as Ecuador. Hence, their assessment or opinions about the programme or policy could be biased towards what may be desirable by supervisors, elected officials or other powerful/influential stakeholders.

17.4 The Health On the Go Study

17.4.1 Original Focus of the Research

Our study focused on the Health On the Go (*Salud Al Paso*) Program, which aimed to promote healthier lifestyles through decentralized and mobile attention units on demand in key sites across the DMQ. In compliance with Ordinance 494, the Quito Ten-Year Health Plan (2015–2025) included the goal of "promoting the adoption of healthy lifestyles that contribute to preventing or controlling NCDs" (Municipality of the Metropolitan District of Quito, 2015). In this context, during the 2014–2019 municipal administration, the Health On the Go (*Salud Al Paso*, SAP) Program was created in May 2015 intending to prevent cardiovascular diseases and type 2 diabetes mellitus. Its strategies included screening for the detection of risk factors and intervention in low-risk people to improve their diet, especially by encouraging the consumption of fruits and vegetables and promoting physical activity. Those with higher identified risk were referred to the metabolic units of municipal health services. Nutrition consultants saw participants across service points located in high traffic areas (10 fixed service points and 4 semi-fixed points) and 11 mobile units that served peripheral or rural areas or functioned during outdoor events. Despite promising preliminary results, the Program's scope was significantly reduced when a new municipal administration took office in 2019 (Municipality of the Metropolitan District of Quito, 2019).

In this context, our study analyzed the conditions and possibilities of permanence of the SAP Program following the mayoral change in 2019. For this purpose, we consulted 69 of its 72 contracted nutritionists and 90 local leaders (decision-makers and opinion leaders) that would have a stake and potentially influence/inform its continuity ("as is" or with reforms), and the new authorities, including the recently appointed Secretary of Health of Quito.

17.4.2 Research Conditions

The study was funded by a small competitive grant ("Improving Program Implementation through Embedded Research") from the Pan American Health Organization (PAHO), intended to support embedded research on health policies and programmes in the region, with the participation of institutional decision-makers. This is why they required that the study be designed and conducted together with officers with decision-making capacity, which for this research was the Secretary of Health of the DMQ. The purpose of the study was to analyze the potential for continuity and improvement of the Program because there was the possibility that the new administration would dismantle it, without specifically considering its potential benefits or impact. This aim was defined between the external researchers and the public officials and advisors involved. Ultimately, if Health On the Go continued, then the decision-makers would have information and recommendations for improvement.

17.4.3 Research Approach

We used a pragmatic research paradigm, with the assumption that this study would require a mixed methods approach to answer the question of what would be required for the continuity of a health prevention programme with elements of health promotion strategies. Allied health workers participated as active stakeholders, while community leaders (opinion and political leaders) and new authorities acted as the key informants. Quantitative analysis centred on screening results and intervention outcomes, to adoption, cost per person and coverage (Fig. 17.1). Through a memorandum of understanding, the study team had access to the SAP database (from April 2015 to May 2019), which included 525,252 people (accounting for 1,058,880 visits); most were adults aged 19 years and older (n = 444,990; 934,525 visits). Additional information was obtained through a meeting with the new authorities, including the Secretary of Health of the DMQ, and from the documentation provided by them. Due to our small research budget, the quantitative component was limited to a descriptive analysis, whereas the qualitative analysis did not include the opinions of SAP users. In either case, both gaps point to opportunities for future research.

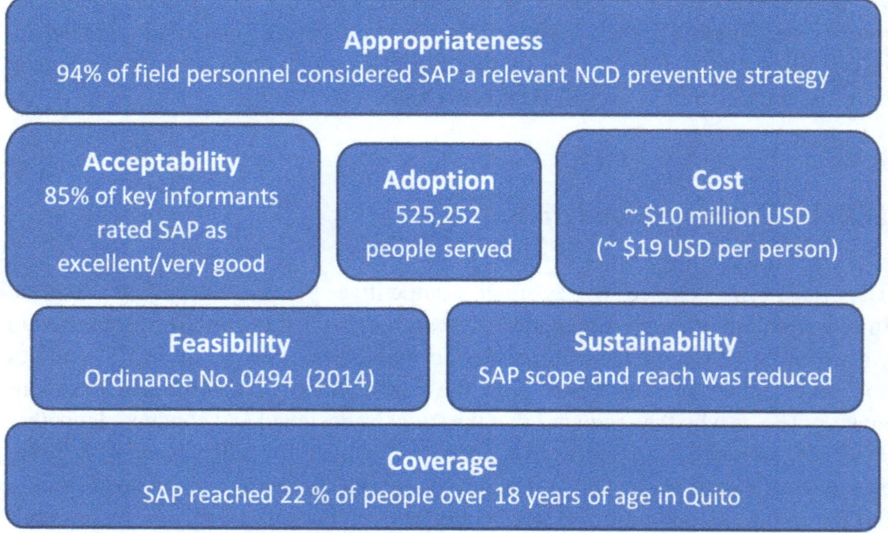

Fig. 17.1 Implementation outcome variables studied in the *Salud Al Paso* (SAP) Program (Appropriateness, acceptability, adoption, feasibility cost, sustainability, and coverage. The outcome variables are further described in Peters et al. (2013, p. 30)

A link to a structured self-administered survey was sent to SAP field personnel via email so that they could send their individual answers confidentially. A list of instructions and informed consent statements preceded the questions. The survey included open- and close-ended questions, with a focus on the working conditions, perceptions and perspectives of the SAP Program and their own performance. A brief survey with local leaders was applied by a member of the research team; of 90 participants, 17 were presidents of local rural councils, which are at a lower level of government than the municipality. The majority of participants answered on their own through a virtual form, and the rest did so by telephone. Informed consent was secured prior to starting the survey. The research team decided to conduct a survey to try to reach as many participants as possible, since, based on initial outreach, it seemed that the participants were more open to a survey (virtual or by phone) than to an interview. The leaders' survey included open- and close-ended questions and was aimed at identifying their general knowledge about the SAP Program, non-communicable diseases, their perspectives on the performance of the SAP Program and their opinions about its continuation.

After the tabulation of the surveys, a day-long feedback workshop was held with 69 health workers, of which 62 were nutritionists who served as SAP field personnel, 5 were supervisors and 2 were logistics workers. The group discussions and presentations focused on analyzing and deepening our understanding of both positive and negative perspectives, mainly on organizational aspects, their perceptions of user opinions and the future of the SAP Program. The participants first worked in two groups divided at random, and, then, we hosted a plenary session. With their permission, their de-identified oral opinions and written statements were collected and transcribed for further analysis. During the workshop, discussion workers were able to learn about the results of our survey and share feedback that they believed was necessary to improve the Program. This was extremely helpful because we strived to create a "safe space", free of judgement, or fear of prejudice or jeopardizing their jobs, for them to provide their opinions and perspectives, individually and collectively, and the evaluation that was produced provided valuable recommendations for other health promotion strategies in the future. Nevertheless, it is worth noting that workers mentioned that their untenured status affected their sense of belonging to or how they identified with the Program and felt influenced by their answers.

All participants were informed of their rights, before giving their consent to participate. The study protocol was approved by the Ethics Committee of the Pan American Health Organization (PAHO-2019-01-0003) and by the Bioethics Committee of the Universidad Internacional del Ecuador (CEU-082-19).

17.4.4 Data Analyses

Opinion leaders' telephone surveys were transcribed verbatim and combined with the responses sent through the virtual form. Quantitative responses of the two surveys were disaggregated and tabulated by questions, whereas qualitative responses were compiled by questions and coded in an open and inductive way in a matrix. To ensure the rigor and validity of the analysis, data from the different sources were compared and contrasted and the researchers discussed possible discordant interpretations. Answers to open-ended questions were coded and compiled by similarity according to thematic categories, and their frequency was tabulated to identify the common opinions among participants.

Applicable data were analyzed according to the outcome variables of Peters et al.'s (2013) guide, which the PAHO requested participating research teams to use. Following these recommendations, which considered SAP as a "novel intervention", our analysis focused primarily on issues of acceptability, adoption, appropriateness and feasibility, although we also considered coverage and costs (Fig. 17.1). Both quantitative and qualitative data provided further context to contrast the new administration's decision to discontinue the SAP Program as originally designed and rather reduce the scope and reach of the Program.

By applying Peters et al.'s (2013) framework, we assessed the effectiveness of the SAP Program and potentially informed its sustainability and continuity during the transition from one mayoral administration to the next. We found that a majority (94%) of field personnel saw the SAP Program as an *appropriate* strategy for prevention of non-communicable diseases in the DMQ. Similarly, most key informants' (85%) *acceptability* of the SAP Program was excellent/very good. From its inception until the time of this study, SAP was widely *adopted*, with over half a million people served, at a *cost* of $10 million US dollars (~$19 per person), *covering* over one in five adults (22%) in the DMQ. Although its *feasibility* was supported by a 2014 city ordinance (No. 0494), its *sustainability* scope of action was undoubtedly in question following elections and the transition to a new mayoral administration.

Following the structure outlined by Cheetham et al. (2018), Table 17.1 shows the three main steps the research team took and considerations for each one during the Health On the Go study. First, we started out/negotiated the research process by developing a trusting relationship between the researchers and the Secretariat of Health. Buy-in in the study was strengthened by including the Secretary of Health advisor in the team and jointly applying for funding from the PAHO. Additional senior personnel, such as the SAP Program coordinator, also provided support. However, throughout the study, the research team did struggle with limited organizational culture valuing research and evaluation.

Second, we moved forward with the study, starting with the signing of a formal MOU (memorandum of understanding) outlining the research collaboration, including granting access to the SAP database. Following this formal step, we met with the key city government team members to explain the ethical approval process and what it means to adhere to its principles. We then jointly engaged in the development of the SAP survey and group discussion questions, incorporating feedback from those with responsibility in the redesign of the SAP scope and services. Following a change in leadership (post-mayoral election), we engaged in constant communication with city officials during the transition period. During this uncertain time, we did find that there was a mixed welcoming/apprehensive environment by

Table 17.1 Embedded research with allied health professionals involved in the continuity study of the Health On the Go (*Salud Al Paso*) Program in Quito, Ecuador: steps and considerations (for the analysis, we apply Cheetham et al.'s framework (2018))

Steps	Considerations
1. Starting out/ negotiating the research process	Trusting relationship between the researchers and the Secretary of Health, who served as study co-Principal Investigators (PIs) Funding by the PAHO through a competitive process, along with support from the senior personnel at Quito's Secretary of Health office, including the Secretary of Health advisor and the SAP Program coordinator, which increased buy-in Shared agreement between the city officials, research consultants and PAHO representatives to identify gaps in the current evidence Limited organizational culture valuing research and evaluation
2. Moving forward with the research process	Signed an MOU to access the SAP database for descriptive purposes Explained the ethical approval process and what it means to adhere to its principles Joint development of the SAP survey and group discussion questions Engaged in ongoing communication with the city officials during the transition period following a change in leadership A mix of welcoming/apprehensive environment by the new city officials Incorporating feedback from those with responsibility in the redesign of the SAP scope and services
3. Working in co-production, making sense of findings, generating recommendations	Jointly identified the key stakeholders to be invited for this study Negotiated access to the key informants (staff and opinion leaders) Recognized that participants may have preconceived reservations about participating in this study Jointly discussed the implications of survey findings in a follow-up gathering with the SAP staff and new officials Cautious of being drawn into taking sides, particularly given the change in city officials following election results and the decision to discontinue the SAP Program as originally planned

the new city officials, which we had to get acquainted with to renew trust in the research.

Finally, we worked in knowledge co-production, making sense of findings and generating recommendations for outgoing and incoming city officials. Together with the Secretary of Health staff, we jointly identified the key stakeholders to be invited for this study and negotiated access to the key informants (staff and opinion leaders), recognizing that participants may have preconceived reservations about participating in this study (e.g. potential consequences for the current staff; community standing/political repercussions for opinion leaders). We also discussed the implications of survey findings in a follow-up meeting with the SAP staff and new officials. All of this was done while being cautious about staff perception of taking sides (outgoing vs. incoming administration), particularly given the change in city officials following election results, and the ultimate mayoral decision to discontinue the SAP Program as originally envisioned.

17.5 Lessons Learned

It is expected that health promotion research be adaptive to the needs of a study or a particular setting (Woodall et al., 2018) and therefore have the potential to overcome barriers as it is being carried out. However, there are a number of challenges to conducting embedded research, e.g. concerning institutional barriers to knowledge exchange and the potential for subjectivity, including conflicts of interest (Vineis & Saracci, 2015). Our research derived from the vested interest of the (eventually outgoing) Secretary of Health of the DMQ in the continuation of the SAP Program, especially since the intervention was based on the perspective that it was relevant within the competencies, priorities and budget of the municipal government. As researchers, the potential for a conflict of interest and the possibility that we could be advocating for a particular stance was clear (i.e., sustainability of the SAP Program), which in turn could influence the integrity and credibility of the study (Vineis & Saracci, 2015). In our case, a team member (and a co-author of this chapter) was the advisor to the outgoing Secretary of Health. Although he did not have a direct influence on the future of the SAP Program, we continuously raised the need to be aware and reflect on our personal viewpoints. It is therefore relevant to highlight that the focus of the SAP study was shaped to some extent by the overarching goals of the funding agency (in this case, the PAHO), including the integration of public officials and the use of the analytical framework.

In an embedded research study, researchers need to consider not only the differing expectations of participants but also those of the authorities involved. The municipal authorities could not guarantee the extent to which the opinions of the study participants could or would be taken into consideration in possible adjustments to the Program following our research. This depended not only on the immediate decision-making capacity of the Secretary of Health but also on bureaucratic and budget limitations. Finally, public institutions in Ecuador (as may be the case in other countries) have high personnel rotation at the decision-making and operational levels. Such instability may erode efforts to integrate evidence into health promotion practices. In the current study, the continuity, sustainability and improvement possibilities of a community-wide intervention, such as the SAP Program, was indeed challenged in the transition to a new slate of local elected officials, ultimately leading to a major change in SAP Program priorities.

Differences in priorities, concerns and incentives to participate, or the appreciation of the researchers' purposes, may influence how a study is conducted in collaboration with health professionals at their place of work (van der Graaf et al., 2017). In our study, participants admitted being afraid of giving their opinions in the survey and were relieved to be able to not hold back as much during the group discussions. At the same time, some of the comments steered towards labour demands that we had to carefully redirect towards the focus of the conversation: the SAP Program.

Government planning in Ecuador and, in particular, at the office of the Secretary of Health of the DMQ, does not include research activities for departments that are not strictly dedicated to data analysis, and, even then, staff members are not supported to collect additional information. In other words, research is not included in staff position descriptions, except for pre-programmed monitoring activities of a specific intervention, which may thwart novel research initiatives or, worse, sideline concerns that arise during interventions. Furthermore, funding is also not assigned to expenses involved in collecting additional data that may be needed, much less for analysis, which also means that institutions rely on offers of external research support or none at all. In this study, the embedded research approach allowed us to work with the Secretary of Health, also creating a "safe space" for the Program personnel to interact with each other and the research team. We were thus able to gather useful information with relatively minimal research and project resources.

It is important to instil in allied health personnel and illustrate to them the mechanisms and relevance of research for policy and practice so that they become more appreciative and proficient in research. In fact, training health personnel in research can facilitate their involvement as partners in a study. This would also make researchers value their contributions to a study and not see them as solely informants. However, this is dependent upon job stability and work contracts, ensuring that the staff view themselves as key stakeholders.

Concurrently, working with personnel to have them make suggestions may also be stimulating for them since it shows that all health staff opinions are valued, without distinction on their contract status, and may even help them reflect on their own work. Emphasizing the academic or formative nature of a study on a particular health intervention may enable health workers to see a programme differently and not "settle" only into following orders or instructions. Focus groups can be useful for participants to contrast their own perceptions and opinions with those of their colleagues and also see the importance of jointly assessing processes and practices within the program.

Although asking workers for their perspectives may open the door to labour demands, their participation in group discussions where findings are explained, and further analyzed in a collaborative effort, can constitute valuable space for allied health professionals to learn about this part of the research process and gain further insights into the applicability on their own work.

17.6 Conclusions

This chapter presents embedded research as a relevant alternative to health promotion studies. To do so, we reflect on our experience conducting an embedded research study regarding the Health On the Go (Salud al Paso, SAP) Program in Quito, Ecuador. Building on the embedded research framework proposed by Cheetham et al. (2018), our approach included three steps: 1) starting out/negotiating the research process; 2) moving forward with the research process and 3) working in co-production, making sense of findings and generating recommendations (see Table 17.1).

In the first step, researchers developed a trusting relationship between the researchers and city government officials, building on existing connections (so that we wouldn't have to start building a relationship of trust from scratch) and building new ones. This relationship was further solidified by jointly applying for external funding to conduct the study and by following (at times extremely lengthy) bureaucratic processes to formalize the partnership and data sharing.

In the second step, following the signing of a formal MOU (memorandum of understanding) outlining the research collaboration, the research team and city government representatives engaged in the development of data collection instruments (surveys/interviews/group discussion questions) and maintained constant communication with the city officials during the transition period from the outgoing and incoming administration.

In the third step, the research team worked in knowledge co-production, making sense of findings and generating recommendations for outgoing and incoming city officials. We jointly discussed the implications of survey findings in a follow-up gathering with the SAP staff and new officials while taking extra precautions to avoid perceptions of taking sides.

In conclusion, our study contributes to the field of health promotion research by describing the process and lessons learned from conducting an embedded research project in Quito, Ecuador. Such an approach has the potential to inform future approaches that strive to more systematically integrate evidence into health promotion practices. While our study was conducted in a particular setting, our embedded research process has the potential to guide future studies elsewhere, particularly when the motivation of the research endeavour is to more meaningfully engage governmental and community agencies and stakeholders in knowledge co-production and real-world application of such findings (Büyüm et al., 2020; Erondu et al., 2020). Ultimately, an embedded approach to health promotion research has the potential to increase localized understanding of organizational/systems culture and awareness of social, political and economic realities in which research findings would be actualized.

References

Afshin, A., Micha, R., Khatibzadeh, S., Schmidt, L.A., Mozaffarian, D. (2014). Dietary policies to reduce non-communicable diseases. In G.W. Brown, G. Yamey & S. Wamala *The handbook of global health policy*. https://doi.org/10.1002/9781118509623.ch9.

Beaglehole, R., Bonita, R., Horton, R., Adams, C., Alleyne, G., Asaria, P., et al. (2011). Priority actions for the non-communicable disease crisis. *The Lancet, 377*(9775), 1438–1447. https://doi.org/10.1016/S0140-6736(11)60393-0

Bock, C., Diehl, K., Schneider, S., Diehm, C., & Litaker, D. (2012). Behavioral counseling for cardiovascular disease prevention in primary care settings: A systematic review of practice and associated factors. *Medical Care Research and Review, 69*(5), 495–518. https://doi.org/10.1177/1077558712441084

Büyüm, A. M., Kenney, C., Koris, A., Mkumba, L., & Raveendran, Y. (2020). Decolonising global health: if not now, when? *BMJ Global Health, 5*(8), e003394. https://doi.org/10.1136/bmjgh-2020-003394

Campos-Herrera, G., & de Reguero, S. U. (2019). Populism in Latin America: Past, present, and future. *Latin American Politics and Society, 61*(1), 148–159. https://doi.org/10.1017/lap.2018.63

Cheetham, M., Wiseman, A., Khazaeli, B., Gibson, E., Gray, P., Van der Graaf, P., & Rushmer, R. (2018). Embedded research: A promising way to create evidence-informed impact in public health? *Journal of Public Health, 40*(suppl 1), i64–i70. https://doi.org/10.1093/pubmed/fdx125

Collyer, F. M. (2018). Global patterns in the publishing of academic knowledge: Global North, global South. *Current Sociology, 66*(1), 56–73. https://doi.org/10.1177/0011392116680020

Erondu, N. A., Peprah, D., & Khan, M. S. (2020). Can schools of global public health dismantle colonial legacies? *Nature Medicine, 1–2*. https://doi.org/10.1038/s41591-020-1062-6

Fernández, A., & Martínez, R. (2017). *The cost of the double burden of malnutrition: Social and economic impact. Summary of the pilot study in Chile, Ecuador and Mexico*. UN Economic Commission for Latin America and the Caribbean (ECLAC). Available at: https://reliefweb.int/sites/reliefweb.int/files/resources/wfp291993.pdf

Franzen, S. R. P., Chandler, C., & Lang, T. (2019). Health research capacity development in low and middle income countries: reality or rhetoric? A systematic meta-narrative review of the qualitative literature. *BMJ Open, 2017*(7), e012332. https://doi.org/10.1136/bmjopen-2016-012332

Harding, S. (2019). After Mr. Nowhere: New proper scientific selves. In *Objectivity and Diversity*. University of Chicago.

Harris, J., Grafton, K., & Cooke, J. (2020). Developing a consolidated research framework for clinical allied health professionals practising in the UK. *BMC Health Services Research, 20*(1), 1–15. https://doi.org/10.1186/s12913-020-05650-3

Hospital temporal en Quito ya recibe a pacientes COVID-19 [Pop-up hospital in Quito is taking COVID-19 patients] (2020, May 23). *El Universo*. https://www.eluniverso.com/noticias/2020/05/23/nota/7850127/hospital-temporal-quito-ya-recibe-pacientes-covid-19

Koon, A. D., Rao, K. D., Tran, N. T., & Ghaffar, A. (2013). Embedding health policy and systems research into decision-making processes in low- and middle-income countries. *Health Research Policy and Systems, 11*, 30. https://doi.org/10.1186/1478-4505-11-30

Mejia Acosta, A., & Meneses, K. (2019). Who benefits? Intergovernmental transfers, subnational politics and local spending in Ecuador. *Regional & Federal Studies, 29*(2), 219–247. https://doi.org/10.1080/13597566.2018.1556644

Mikkelsen, B., Williams, J., Rakovac, I., Wickramasinghe, K., Hennis, A., Shin, H. R., et al. (2019). Life course approach to prevention and control of non-communicable diseases. *British Medical Journal, 364*, l257. https://doi.org/10.1136/bmj.l257

Municipality of the Metropolitan District of Quito. (2014). *Ordenanza 494*. Concejo Metropolitano de Quito. http://www7.quito.gob.ec/mdmq_ordenanzas/Ordenanzas/ORDENANZAS%20MUNICIPALES%202014%20ADMINISTRACI%C3%93N%20BARRERA/ORDM%200494%20-%20ACCIONES%20DE%20SALUD-SUSTITUTIVA%20ORD.%20205.pdf

Municipality of the Metropolitan District of Quito. (2015). *Plan Decenal de Salud 2015-2025*. Secretaría Metropolitana de Salud, Alcaldía del Distrito Metropolitano de Quito.

Municipality of the Metropolitan District of Quito. (2019). *Propuesta de Reestructuración del Proyecto Salud Al Paso*. Secretaría de Salud - Dirección Metropolitana de Promoción, Prevención y Vigilancia de la Salud.

Newbury-Birch, D., & Allan, K. (Eds.). (2019). *Co-creating and co-producing research evidence: A guide for practitioners and academics in health, social care and education settings*. Routledge.

Peters, D. H., Tran, N. T., & Adam, T. (2013). *Implementation research in health: A practical guide*. Alliance for Health Policy and Systems Research, World Health Organization.

Pribble, J. (2013). *Welfare and party politics in Latin America*. Cambridge University Press.
Reidpath, D. D., & Allotey, P. (2019). The problem of 'trickle-down science' from the Global North to the Global South. *BMJ Global Health, 4*, e001719. https://doi.org/10.1136/bmjgh-2019-001719
Slade, S. C., Philip, K., & Morris, M. E. (2018). Frameworks for embedding a research culture in allied health practice: A rapid review. *Health Research Policy and Systems, 16*(1), 29. https://doi.org/10.1186/s12961-018-0304-2
Torres, I., & López-Cevallos, D. F. (2018). Institutional challenges to achieving health equity in Ecuador. *The Lancet Global Health, 6*(8), e832–e833. https://doi.org/10.1016/S2214-109X(18)30245-6
van der Graaf, P., Forrest, L. F., Adams, J., Shucksmith, J., & White, M. (2017). How do public health professionals view and engage with research? A qualitative interview study and stakeholder workshop engaging public health professionals and researchers. *BMC Public Health, 17*, 892. https://doi.org/10.1186/s12889-017-4896-1
Varallyay, N. I., Bennett, S. B., Kennedy, C., Ghaffar, A., & Peters, D. H. (2020). How does embedded implementation research work? Examining core features through qualitative case studies in Latin America and the Caribbean. *Health Policy and Planning, 35*(2 suppl), ii98–ii111. https://doi.org/10.1093/heapol/czaa126
Vineis, P., & Saracci, R. (2015). Conflicts of interest matter and awareness is needed. *Journal of Epidemiology and Community Health, 69*, 1018–1020. https://doi.org/10.1136/jech-2014-205012
Woodall, J., Warwick-Booth, L., South, J., & Cross, R. (2018). What makes health promotion research distinct? *Scandinavian Journal of Public Health, 46*(20 suppl), 118–122. https://doi.org/10.1177/1403494817744130

Chapter 18
Doing Collaborative Health Promotion Research in a Complex Setting: Lessons Learned from the COMPLETE Project in Norway

Torill Larsen, Ingrid Holsen, Helga Bjørnøy Urke, Cecilie Høj Anvik, and Ragnhild Holmen Waldahl

18.1 Introduction

Education and health are intertwined: young peoples' educational success may depend on the health-promoting conditions in school, but, educational success also has an impact on health, living conditions, social mobility and societal participation throughout the life course (Pillas and Suhrcke, 2009; Poulton et al., 2002). This duality of the school setting underscores its role as a crucial but complex health promotion arena (Larsen, 2016), both in terms of research and practice.

The COMPLETE project – a health promotion research intervention in Norway aimed at increasing participation, equity and educational success among upper secondary school students – is distinctive of health promotion research. The project was implemented and evaluated in Norway from 2016 to 2019, and this chapter will present the results – and our experiences – of conducting health promotion research in such a complex setting.

During the last few decades, the field (and social science research, in general) has experienced two parallel, yet different, trends within evaluation. The first is the recognition that research should be more societally relevant through collaboration with, and for, society. For example, the collaborative initiatives taken to reduce school dropouts and to enable robust youth generation by promoting mental

T. Larsen (✉) · I. Holsen · H. B. Urke
Department of Health Promotion and Development, Faculty of Psychology, University of Bergen, Bergen, Norway
e-mail: torill.larsen@uib.no

C. H. Anvik
Faculty of Social Sciences, Nord University, Bodø, Norway

R. H. Waldahl
Nordland Research Institute, Bodø, Norway

L. Potvin, D. Jourdan (eds.), *Global Handbook of Health Promotion Research, Vol. 1*,
https://doi.org/10.1007/978-3-030-97212-7_18

well-being and positive youth development. Within collaborative innovations, the methods used are often qualitative and formative in nature. The second trend is to determine the effects of specific interventions (e.g. to reduce dropouts) by utilizing randomized controlled trials (RCTs), a trend that is also evident in the European Union (EU) and the United Kingdom (Pearce & Raman, 2014). The rationale for the use of RCTs is that when aiming for a change in a social environment (to be more health promoting), cost effectiveness and causal effects should also be identified (Henry, 2009). With its roots in evidence-based medicine, an RCT is the preferred method for research findings to be as conclusive as possible and to rule out alternative explanations (Henry, 2009). One could argue that these two trends have their origins in different research traditions and different paradigms. RCTs have long been the gold standard for determining causality in medical research, and it is increasingly used in the social sciences as well (Cartwright, 2010, p. 59). RCT studies are characterized by controlling and keeping track of both known and unknown variables between treatment and control groups to measure the effects of interventions (Grossman & Mackenzie, 2005). To ensure that the effect is attributable to the intervention, it is important to secure "purity" that the participants are not affected by each other or exposed to other conditions that may influence the effect (Grossman & Mackenzie, 2005).

Collaborative innovation (and research), however, is characterized by the intention to find better solutions to societal challenges, in a joint effort between a field of practice and research communities (Sørensen & Torfing, 2011). The idea is that extended interaction between different actors or stakeholders will increase the quality of scientific knowledge production. One important element of collaborative innovation is a close dialogue and interface between research and practice. The common ground is the aim for both initiating and capturing the change in practice.

Although the COMPLETE project from the beginning was not explicitly designed as a collaborative innovation, this feature became more and more evident through the co-creation and collaboration during the project period. Thus, the COMPLETE project (Larsen et al., 2018) can be seen as an example of how both trends are evident in health promotion research.

In this chapter, we aim to discuss the synergies and tensions/challenges involved in the process of implementing COMPLETE – a collaborative innovation project involving an RCT and a process evaluation.

18.2 The COMPLETE Project

18.2.1 Background

In Norway, there is an increasing acknowledgement that the educational goals in schools should not only focus on literacy and numeracy but also have a broader approach aiming at educating the "whole child". It is statutory that all children have the right to a safe and sound school environment that promotes health, well-being and academic competence (Larsen, 2016). The Norwegian school system is further set up with the aim of being an important contributor to the efforts to reduce social inequalities (Ministry of Education, 2006). For schools to function as a health-promoting support system for young people's positive development, there is a need to shift the focus more in the direction of how to emphasize and strengthen young people's resources as an integrated part of a school day (Larsen, 2016). Many upper secondary schools and counties in Norway already do a lot of good work, for example, related to psychosocial learning environments and dropout prevention. Nevertheless, a more systematic approach to the existing work could contribute to improved quality of this work (Larsen, 2016). This position is supported by Lillejord et al. (2015), who confirm that schools need to employ more systematic and planned efforts in order to succeed in reducing the number of youths dropping out of school.

The context outlined above was the background for the development and design of the COMPLETE project. The main purpose was to investigate whether systematic work in the class and school psychosocial environment affected students' experience of the psychosocial environment, mental health, school performance, absenteeism, dropout and completion of upper secondary education. The project came about as a result of a dialogue tender announced by the Norwegian Ministry of Education, where researchers and counties (school owners) together were to develop projects to be eligible for applying for funding. COMPLETE can therefore be seen as a collaborative innovation project involving four counties, one university and two research institutes, in addition to the organization Adults for Children and the Mental Health Support Team (MHST) at an upper secondary school. An important prerequisite was that research should be developed and carried out together *with* practice and not just *in* or *on* practice.

Specifically, the research design within the COMPLETE project was an RCT combined with a process evaluation addressing the intervention. The schools implemented two measures, the Dream School Program and the Mental Health Support Team, to help address and improve the psychosocial learning environment in a more systematic manner (Larsen et al., 2018). A total of 16 schools (11 intervention and 5 control schools) participated in the project over a 3-year period.

18.2.2 The Health Promotion Intervention

The Dream School Program (measure 1) is a universal programme aimed at improving the learning environment, increasing student participation and building an inclusive culture in the whole school (Adults for Children, 2017). In addition, the measure is intended to function as a quality assurance of the transition from lower secondary school to upper secondary school, to ensure that all students are included in the psychosocial learning environment from the start. Peer leaders are a core component of the programme and function as facilitators of the activities. Student participation paired with teacher support and guidance are found to have a range of positive outcomes, including increased motivation, better peer relations and a more inclusive school climate (Griebler et al., 2014).

The Mental Health Support Team (measure 2) is a selective/indicated measure that provides an opportunity to highlight and strengthen the roles, routines and interaction of various health and social pedagogical professions in prevention and follow-up at the school. Close follow-up is highlighted in the literature as an effective measure for better completion and in this way prevent young people from being left out of school and work life (Lillejord et al., 2015). At the same time, the need is pointed out for better collaboration and coordination of services around the young people and for a better learning environment for the school as a whole (Lillejord et al., 2015).

The purpose of combining the two described measures was to gain more knowledge about whether a multi-tier prevention model consisting of universal, selective and indicated measures would be (more) effective in reaching the entire student population in schools. This is in line with the concept of proportionate universalism presented by Sir Michael Marmot in "Fair Society: Healthy Lives" 2010. According to Marmot et al. (2010), in order "to reduce the steepness of the social gradient in health, actions must be universal, but with a scale and intensity that is proportionate to the level of disadvantage" (Marmot et al., 2010, p. 16).

18.2.3 The Collaborative Innovation Processes

As COMPLETE was developed and operated as a dialogue project, research and practice were to work closely together and contribute to synergies. It is clear that the project could not have been implemented to this extent without the expert knowledge of each of the collaborating partners. More concretely, within the COMPLETE project, the partnership was facilitated over the research project period by regular meetings with the Project Council. These meetings were key to continuous development and collaboration. The Project Council consisted of one representative from each of the nine partners and four county project coordinators (see Fig. 18.1).

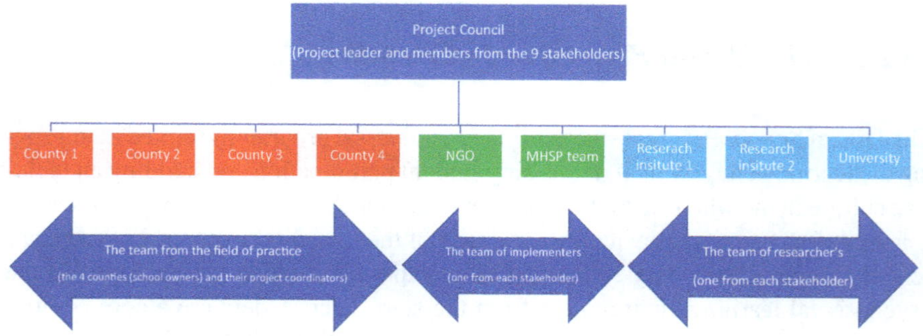

Fig. 18.1 Organization of the COMPLETE project

The Project Council was the arena in which the complexity of the project was discussed and where different interests emerged most clearly. It was also a forum where challenges associated with the project were addressed and discussed. The Project Council was important in the continuous anchoring of the various parties' engagement and ownership. It was also the forum where the tension between the considerations of the RCT design, the process evaluation and the dynamics of the practice was most clearly expressed. Thus, within the Project Council, an important aim was to negotiate and produce knowledge to tie together research and practice. All reports from the project findings were developed within the setting of the Project Council to enable stakeholder involvement and ownership of the communication of the results.

18.2.4 The Objectives and Results from the RCT and Process Evaluation of COMPLETE

In Table 18.1, we summarize the overall objectives and results from the RCT and process evaluation of the COMPLETE project.

In the following section, we discuss the synergies, tensions and knowledge gained related to the process of leading what became a collaborative innovation project involving an RCT and a process evaluation.

18.3 Collaborative Innovation in School Health Promotion Research: Tensions, Synergies and Lessons Learned

The experience from COMPLETE as a collaborative innovation project is that at times it was demanding to reconcile a) the different expectations of the school stakeholders in the practice field and the boundaries inherent in the research design and b) the two methodological approaches of the project (RCT and process evaluation). First, while school development depends on close dialogue and continuous change/adjustment of the interventions implemented based on return of knowledge throughout the intervention process, research more often takes a comparably more distant approach. Second, tensions between different research approaches, in this case qualitative process evaluation and quantitative RCT, can arise, e.g. regarding how different types of data are interpreted and weighted. One could argue that both approaches to research have a common goal of capturing change that helps improve the quality of practice through an intervention. Nevertheless, combining the approaches in a practical setting will challenge both methodological and ethical aspects. We will here highlight some of the tensions we experienced between the desire to return knowledge and ensure learning along the way and the expectation that the intervention would take place in controlled forms and with the least possible noise (to ensure purity). We also highlight the ethical challenges related to this.

Table 18.1 Summary of the project objectives and results of COMPLETE

Objectives	Results	
	RCT	Process evaluation
Assess statistical (RCT) and experienced (process evaluation) effects of measures (Dream School and Mental Health Support Teams)	No statistically signifciant effect on mental health (mental health complains, life satisfaction and loneliness) across the project period.	In all groups of informants (students, teachers, school management and resource teams), positivity and appreciation of working more systematically with the psychosocial learning environment was expressed. Schools experienced that they had been given a tool for such systematic work through the Dream School Programme and the Mental Health Support Teams, and that such work no longer was dependent on the individual teacher. The aspect of student participation and involvement was experienced as a great value.
Assess relationship between implementation and effects	Schools with interprofessional Mental Health Support Team that had high fidelity and high integration had a significantly higher proportion of students who after three years had either completed and passed upper secondary education or where in practice compared to schools with low fidelity and integration (but not for other outcome measures).	

(continued)

Table 18.1 (continued)

Objectives	Results	
	RCT	Process evaluation
Assess extent of implementation in classrooms and schools, and identify facilitators and barriers to implementation		The degree of implementation varied between schools, but overall, both the Dream School Programme and the Mental Health Support Teams were relatively well integrated in the schools' mangement and structures. However, the implementation and integration as a "whole school effort" was challenging for most of the schools, and required considerable efforts. Schools did to a very limited extent manage to link the two interventions together. Identified barriers: time, resources, the degree of anchoring at top and bottom level, the organization's stability, visibility and communication about the measures. Organisational changes related to change of leadership, staff, merging with other schools etc. On part of the project organisation and communication, more focus on the measures as part of a longterm school development process could have benfitted implementation. For example, it was found that the Dream School Programme was not sufficiently anchored among all teachers/staff at some schools. Further, the theoretical basis and the focus on a resource perspective was perhaps not communicated sufficiently.
Assess whether there was a difference between the different measures (Dream School only vs. Dream School + Mental Health Support Teams) in the proportion of pupils who had quit, and whether pupils who had quit school were in any form of formal activity as a replacement for school	Only 112 (5.1%) of the total sample of 2203 (both control and intervention schools) dropped out of upper secondary education. Of these, only 1.2 per cent were registered not to be in any form of activity or follow-up at project closure. In our sample, there were a total of only 26 students who are not at school or in activity at project end. At the closure of the project, we could not conclude that there was a statistically significant difference in the proportion of students who had quit depending on measure combination.	

18.3.1 The Negotiation on the Research Process

The co-creation that occurred during the early stages of the project contributed to a strong sense of ownership of the project among all the stakeholders. This was expressed through the presence and loyalty of all the stakeholders throughout the 4-year-long project.

However, among the stakeholders, there also existed several different worldviews, which we had to integrate. When it comes to research, the two different methodological approaches in this project have their scientific and theoretical roots in different paradigms or worldviews on knowledge. The RCT is rooted within the positivist paradigm with a focus on the objective and the measurable and embedded in this are explicit understandings of validity and reliability. On the other hand, the process evaluation approach we chose in this project has its origin in the interpretive and interactionist paradigm, which premises that data are experiences and that the interpretations of these are produced in the interaction between the researcher and informant. In recent times, however, combining these methodological approaches has often been rooted in a pragmatic paradigm. According to Creswell (2016), the pragmatic paradigm is concerned with the research problem and which methods are best available to study and understand the problem. In a mixed methods approach, one can choose whether one method should have more weight or if the two should have equal weight (Creswell, 2016). In the COMPLETE study, both methods were equated – a so-called convergent parallel design (Creswell, 2016), where the aim was to merge the qualitative (process evaluation) and quantitative (RCT) findings in order to obtain a richer interpretative basis.

One challenge we experienced was that the research part within COMPLETE was designed as a mixed methods design without having explicitly entered discussions about the scientific–theoretical basis of the study. This led to tensions and discussions of a scientific and theoretical nature as the project progressed, including balancing the various understandings of validity and reliability in the interconnection of the findings from the process evaluation (qualitative) and the RCT (quantitative). Initially, as mentioned before, the project was not designed as a collaborative innovation but was organized as two sub-studies, where one team was responsible for the quantitative part and another team the qualitative part of the study. Data were then linked through dialogue meetings between the researchers focusing on how to enable a joint presentation of the findings. To merge the different approaches, one had to negotiate a common understanding of the validity and reliability of the different methods to gain a common understanding of what is valid knowledge and how it helped illuminate the same or different sides of the problem area. Where the RCT measured the effect of the intervention, the process evaluation focused on the experience of the implementation of the intervention from the view of the informants. The tension between the different scientific and theoretical approaches was expressed in concrete terms, in that the effect analyses based on the RCT design did not find significant changes in the predefined outcome measures, whereas the intervention from the informants' point of view was perceived as changes in practice.

There was thus a tension between the "objective" and the "experienced" change, which became necessary to negotiate an agreement in the project.

To complicate the picture even more, the knowledge from the practice field contributed to challenging the researchers' stand as the practice field had their own perceptions of what kind of change had happened within the different schools. To some degree, these reflections supported and represented the more subjective perception of change, but they also challenged both the quantitative and the qualitative findings. Practical knowledge was important and valuable for interpreting the findings as it originated from those who knew the context in depth, and, although it created discussions about the findings, we consider it as contributing substantially to synergy in the project. Already from the design phase of the project, the methodological knowledge that the researchers possessed was paired with the practical knowledge from the counties to enable access to the field for data collection at the right time to ensure data quality. However, we would recommend that future projects make their different worldviews explicit and negotiate right from the beginning to enable an even stronger integration of the different types of knowledge.

Another aspect that became evident in our project is that the distinction between proximity and distance to the research field is challenged by combining the methods. Where in a process evaluation, researchers are in closer contact with the study setting and informants, researchers in an RCT can and will have a more distant role without direct interaction with the informants in the field of practice. Meetings in the Project Council with all the nine partners and stakeholders made an arena for challenging and negotiating proximity and distance. This could be illustrated by the stakeholders from the county and non-governmental organization (NGO) being more hands on and closer to the schools during the project period, while the researchers were more in and out collecting data. The experience from the COMPLETE project is that these negotiating processes had a positive effect on the whole team and made us understand each other's viewpoints in a better way. This is also supported by scholars, such as Krogh and Nielsen (2017), who argue that having a closer relationship between research and practice can strengthen the entire research process. Similarly, Van de Ven (2007) claims that collaborative processes can contribute to more focused problem identification, easier access to the field of study and strengthen the interpretation of data through the inclusion of diverse forms of knowledge and expertise. This is also our experience throughout the project and again a contributor to synergy in process and outcome.

However, close collaboration over time can challenge the role of the actors, and the research team also focused particularly on the researchers' relationship with and the ownership of the interventions. Both measures that were tested in COMPLETE were developed over time and through previous projects. Some of the researchers in COMPLETE were involved in this prior development process, and this has led to reflections on whether individual researchers can gain too much ownership of the interventions as well as an awareness of the value of keeping some distance from the interventions. The same goes for the implementers in the project, namely, the NGO and the Mental Health Support Team (MHST), which also had a close ownership of the measures implemented.

18.3.2 The Negotiation on the Ethical Issues

Ethical considerations are of vital importance in health promotion research. The main ethical standards that should guide any project are to do no harm, ensure informed consent and confidentiality and secure anonymity (Helsinki declaration). The COMPLETE project fulfilled these standards, but, some were at times challenged, mainly due to the collaborative and co-creative nature of the project that involved different stakeholders representing practice and research.

One important ethical issue related to the negotiation of knowledge was the amount of details from the research results that was possible to be fed back into practice without jeopardizing the ethical standards of informed consent, confidentiality and anonymity and, at the same time, enabling a good implementation process within practice. From the stakeholders' point of view (the county and the implementation teams), there was a desire to obtain detailed and concrete information on the consecutive findings from the researchers to make necessary adjustments to improve the practice, interventions and implementation. For example, the counties wanted information about how individual schools had implemented the measures and whether there were special conditions at each school that the counties should be aware of. For the counties, representing school owners as stakeholders, it is quite understandable that they wanted concrete feedback on their specific schools to enable more tuned implementation processes.

However, there are particularly two reasons of an ethical nature as to why it was difficult to accommodate this on the part of the researchers. First, the whole data collection was based on confidentiality and freely informed consent. All informants who either responded to a questionnaire or were interviewed were provided with information on how the information obtained should be used and how the presentation of the data should be done in a way that it was not possible to trace the information back to the individual informant. At the same time, it is in the "contract" between the researcher and informant that the information that is disclosed must also be given back to society but that this should not happen so that it threatens confidentiality or causes harm. According to Hartley et al. (2013), implementation of new and bold solutions can be improved when different resources are mobilized, exchanged and coordinated and joint ownership is created through participation and dialogue. The assessment made by the researchers in the project was that it was not possible to provide information about the individual school to the counties without breaking the preconditions for confidentiality. Such ethical considerations are important to negotiate at the beginning of a project to avoid tensions and misunderstandings.

The second reason is the prerequisite for purity, which is a key element of an RCT. The county's desire to obtain information about the individual school was based on the desire to be able to guide the schools more precisely and thus influence the interventions. However, this challenged the logic of the experiment, which lies as a backdrop for the RCT. The implementation teams also wanted information obtained from the data collection to implement the interventions more accurately. It was challenging to balance these desires for information with the structure of the RCT.

Another ethical aspect related to ownership relates to the financial interests that the NGO had as the programme owner and the interest that the school owners had in their schools "doing well" in the project. Both the NGO and the school owners had a clear self-interest in the project, which was a positive driving force in the project as both actors were highly committed throughout the project and insisted that the implementation ought to be as good as possible for the schools to succeed. However, both these driving forces might have influenced the purity of the RCT through introducing changes or modifications to the interventions.

The negotiations on the ethical issues were often about finding a balance between feeding back information, keeping confidentiality and the need for keeping "purity" in the RCT. Although the Project Council could have been a natural channel to feed knowledge back to the counties and the implementation teams, the ethical elements mentioned above put limitations on its ability to do so. The restrictions that an RCT imposes on the use of formative elements (e.g. feeding back knowledge) have consequences on the opportunities for learning during the project. A lack of learning during the process could make the interventions less targeted and thus reduce the quality of outcomes. For example, in COMPLETE, questions could have been asked about whether the degree of implementation, which is one of the performance goals, would have been better if the project had placed greater emphasis on the formative elements. This could in turn influence the RCT's need for control and fidelity. At the same time, we have learned that the dissemination of the results during the project influenced the interventions and their implementation and thus had an impact on the purity of the RCT.

In summary, we agree with Hartley et al. (2013, p. 826) who claim that collaboration is a strength in all the stages of an innovation cycle, especially when new and creative solutions are developed, combined, challenged and built on. However, the degree of details in the feedback, findings and dissemination of results can be challenged by the ethical research standards, a challenge also evident in the COMPLETE project. As with the negotiation of knowledge, the ethical negotiation took place within the Project Council. Thus, having a sound project organization with a stakeholder council for negotiating knowledge and ethics was vital for succeeding with this project. However, it is recommended that these challenges be addressed in the planning phase of the project to avoid tensions later on.

18.4 Lessons Learned from the COMPLETE Project as a Health Promotion Research

The COMPLETE project was an ambitious health promotion research project, which illustrates how true partnerships between researchers, NGOs and educational practice fields can be constructed and maintained throughout an intensive research process.

In line with the understanding of schools as "living" organizations, the project was designed as a mixed methods approach including an RCT and a process evaluation. This combination was determined for understanding the outcomes. As such, the COMPLETE project makes valuable contributions to further similar research endeavours in the educational setting. Specifically, we want to highlight the aspects related to the use of an RCT in this setting. RCTs with a "whole school approach" aimed at psychosocial factors are challenging for a variety of reasons. The complexity of the upper secondary school as a "living" organization means that many factors will not be considered, and this challenges the strict RCT design. Our recommendation through the COMPLETE project's thorough process evaluation is that research on interventions in (upper secondary) schools must include parallel process evaluations to capture the challenges in implementation, which in turn provides valuable explanatory information on effect results. For example, our findings indicate that schools with Mental Health Support Teams, which scored high on implementation, benefitted more from the measure than did those schools with Mental Health Support Teams that scored low on implementation, which shows both the importance of good implementation and having knowledge of the implementation itself to better assess the overall value of the measure.

Schools, local environments and regions are different, and the value of understanding how different conditions are reflected in different ways of running a school is important in further research. We recommend that future research also apply research designs other than RCTs, such as quasi-experimental studies and/or other types of qualitative studies, which could be important contributions to knowledge about adolescents' school life related to the psychosocial environment and completion of upper secondary education in various contexts in Norway. It is also to engage young people themselves as researchers in their own environment through the use of more creative research methods (e.g. photovoice), which is something that we believe should be used more in the future. This is to lend a clearer voice to the target group itself.

Another recommendation is to design a more explicit project as a collaborative innovation from the beginning to enable a more systematic approach to leading and running such complex projects. One of the core elements of collaborative innovations taking place between stakeholders and researchers is that the research is not only supposed to be relevant to society (such as the counties and upper secondary schools) but also to be produced *in collaboration with* the society and stakeholders. Collaborative innovation research must be made relevant and able to respond to the challenges existing in the field of practice (e.g. concerns around young people dropping out of school, greater focus on psychosocial learning environments). This can take place through engagement and commitment from the stakeholders experiencing these challenges and through their involvement in the design and implementation of the project. Thus, combining a process evaluation with an RCT within the frame of collaboration innovation is possible as we have shown here, but it requires a well-designed project organization, inclusive to all stakeholders and with defined roles, as well as the willingness to negotiate knowledge and ethics between the different stakeholders to enable transforming practice.

Finally, based on the findings from the COMPLETE project, we also recommend that school owners and schools conduct systematic work in the psychosocial environment. Although the COMPLETE project has not been able to demonstrate statistically significant effects of the Dream School Program or the combination of the Dream School Program and the Mental Health Support Team, this does not mean that these programmes cannot have or have had some positive effect. Based on the findings from the process evaluation, we believe that there is a basis for recommending systematic work in the psychosocial environment, especially systematic work with the group of students who are vulnerable. We recommend that work in the psychosocial environment must have a long-term perspective and must be framed as a school development project with a clear anchoring early in the process at all levels, from county to teachers and students.

18.5 Concluding Remarks

To sum up, research on outcomes of health promotion interventions in a complex setting such as a school is possible, but it should be done collaboratively with stakeholders who are actively involved to ensure that relevant and valid knowledge is created. For a comprehensive research design including, for example, both an RCT and a process evaluation, there is a need from early on to establish an openness for discussion among partners. From our experience, aspects like opinions and negotiation of findings and explicitly addressing different worldviews and epistemological positions that could have implications in the interpretation of findings etc. are particularly important to raise. This can enable an even stronger integration of different types of knowledge and ethical considerations faced.

Practically, we recommend a firm planning process up front together with designing planned regular meetings in a project council, which has a broad representation of project members, to discuss each other's role in the project, expectations of the findings, the theoretical frame and worldviews as well as ethical issues related to conducting research within a complex health-promoting setting like a school. To enable this, we also recommend building a programme theory and a logical project model to guide these discussions.

References

Cartwright, N. (2010). What are randomised controlled trials good for? *Philosophical Studies, 147*(1), 59.

Creswell, J. (2016). *Research design* (4th ed.). Sage.

Griebler, U., Rojatz, D., Simovska, V., & Forster, R. (2014). Effects of student participation in school health promotion: A systematic review. *Health Promotion International*, first published online January 6, 2014. https://doi.org/10.1093/heapro/dat090

Grossman, J., & Mackenzie, F. J. (2005). The randomized controlled trial: Gold standard, or merely standard? *Perspectives in Biology and Medicine, 48*(4), 516–534.

Hartley, J., Sørensen, E., & Torfing, J. (2013). Collaborative innovation: A viable alternative to market competition and organizational entrepreneurship. *Public Administration Review, 73*(6), 821–830.

Henry, T. (2009). When getting it right matters: The case for high-quality policy and program impact evaluations. In S. I. Donaldson, C. Christie, & M. M. Mark (Eds.), *What counts as credible evidence in applied research and evaluation practice?* (pp. 32–50). Sage.

Krogh, A. H., & Nielsen, M. V. (2017). Succeeding with interactive research: How to manage research with and about society. *Research for All, 1*(2), 351–364.

Larsen, T. (2016). Shifting towards positive youth development in schools in Norway – Challenges and opportunities. *International Journal of Mental Health Promotion, 18*(1), 8–20.

Larsen, T., Urke, H. B., Holsen, I., Anvik, C. H., Olsen, T., Waldahl, R. H., … Hansen, T. B. (2018). COMPLETE – A school-based intervention project to increase completion of upper secondary school in Norway: Study protocol for a cluster randomized controlled trial. *BMC Public Health, 18*(340).

Lillejord, S., Halvorsrud, K., Ruud, E., Morgan, K., Freyr, T., Fischer-Griffiths, P., et al. (2015). *Frafall i videregående opplæring: En systematisk kunnskapsoversikt* [Student dropout in upper secondary education–A systematic review]. Kunnskapssenter for utdanning.

Marmot, M., Atkinson, T., Bell, J., Black, C., Broadfoot, P., Cumberlege, J., et al. (2010). *Fair society, healthy lives. The Marmot review*. Institute of Health Equity. https://www.instituteofhealthequity.org/resources-reports/fair-society-healthy-lives-the-marmot-review

Pearce, W., & Raman, S. (2014). The new randomised controlled trials (RCT) movement in public policy: Challenges of epistemic governance. *Policy Sciences, 47*(4), 387–402. https://doi.org/10.1007/s11077-014-9208-3

Pillas, D., & Suhrcke, M. (2009). *Assessing the potential or actual impact on health and health inequalities of policies aiming to improve Early Child Development (ECD) in England* (Background report to marmot review). Monograph. https://ueaeprints.uea.ac.uk/id/eprint/15293/. Accessed 3 Oct 2020.

Poulton, R., Caspi, A., Milne, B. J., Thomson, W. M., Taylor, A., Sears, M. R., & Moffitt, T. E. (2002). Association between children's experience of socioeconomic disadvantage and adult health: A life-course study. *The Lancet, 360*(9346), 1640–1645. https://doi.org/10.1016/S0140-6736(02)11602-3

Sørensen, E., & Torfing, J. (2011). Enhancing collaborative innovation in the public sector. *Administration & Society, 43*(8), 842–868.

Van de Ven, A. H. (2007). *Engaged scholarship: A guide for organizational and social research*. Oxford University Press.

Voksne for Barn [Adults for Children]. (2017). Drømmeskolen. Retrieved Sept 7, 2017, from http://www.vfb.no/no/vart_arbeid/psykisk_helse_i_skolen/drommeskolen/Dr%C3%B8mmeskolen.b7C_wtLM4L.ips

Ministry of Education. (2006). *White paper 16. (2006-2007) Tidlig innsats for livslang læring* [Early intervention for lifelong learning]. Accessed 3 Oct 2020 from https://www.regjeringen.no/no/dokumenter/stmeld-nr-16-2006-2007-/id441395/.

Chapter 19
Researching the Process of Implementing Mental Health Promotion: Case Studies on Interventions with Disadvantaged Young People

Margaret M. Barry, Tuuli Kuosmanen, and Katherine Dowling

19.1 Introduction

Mental health promotion is an interdisciplinary area of research and practice within health promotion, underpinned by the same fundamental concepts and principles (Barry, 2009). Mental health promotion is concerned with strengthening protective factors for good mental health, enhancing supportive environments and enabling access to skills, resources and life opportunities that promote the mental health and well-being of individuals and populations (Barry et al., 2019). Mental health promotion is integral to promoting population health and well-being and contributes to the functioning of individuals, communities and society and the global health development agenda (UN, 2015; WHO, 2013). A health promotion approach reframes the challenge of improving mental health from a deficit model of illness to a broader understanding of mental health as a positive concept and as a resource for living with relevance for the whole population. Mental health promotion interventions intervene at the level of strengthening individuals and communities, reorienting health services and promoting intersectoral actions to remove the structural barriers to mental health at a societal level (Herrman et al., 2005; Friedli, 2009) Current policy frameworks endorse a whole-of-government and a whole-of-society approach (WHO, 2013) and call for universal actions across the life course to ensure that the conditions that create good mental health and reduce inequities are accessible to all (WHO Calouste and Gulbenkian Foundation, 2014).

Mental health promotion research has focused primarily on establishing a sound evidence base to inform practice and policy. Evidence syntheses show that

M. M. Barry (✉) · T. Kuosmanen · K. Dowling
WHO Collaborating Centre for Health Promotion Research, National University of Ireland Galway, Galway, Ireland
e-mail: margaret.barry@nuigalway.ie

L. Potvin, D. Jourdan (eds.), *Global Handbook of Health Promotion Research, Vol. 1*,
https://doi.org/10.1007/978-3-030-97212-7_19

comprehensive interventions for promoting mental health, when implemented effectively, can enhance protective factors for good mental health, reduce risk factors for mental disorders and lead to lasting positive effects on a range of health, social and economic outcomes (Barry et al., 2019; Petersen et al., 2016; WHO, 2013). Despite the large number of mental health promotion interventions that have been developed and tested in efficacy and effectiveness trials in recent decades, there is a science-to-practice gap in implementing evidence-based approaches, especially in low-resource settings. The majority of evidence-based interventions have been developed in high-income countries, and these interventions have not been subjected to rigorous implementation and evaluation in more diverse socio-cultural and health systems (Barry et al., 2017a). Research on systematically assessing the process and quality of implementation, reach, sustainability and scaling up is underdeveloped in most countries.

Bridging this science-to-practice gap requires critical consideration of how best to generate and apply evidence that is congruent with the principles of mental health promotion practice and is inclusive of the realities of intervention implementation across diverse cultural and socio-economic settings (Barry & McQueen, 2005). As mental health promotion is an interdisciplinary area of practice, evaluation methods are needed that will cross the disciplinary and methodological boundaries, embracing multi-method evaluation approaches to develop an "evidence-into-practice-into-evidence" cycle that will generate an understanding not only of what works but also of how, why, when and with whom.

Case studies of the effective implementation of mental health promotion interventions in diverse socio-economic and cultural contexts demonstrate the practical realities and challenges of implementing complex multifaceted interventions in real-world practice (Barry et al., 2019). Implementation within complex systems requires a clear understanding of the multiple interacting factors that can influence the quality of implementation within the local context and ultimately their impact on outcomes. The complexity of implementation in different settings calls for a focus on systematically examining the factors influencing the "how" of effective implementation in order to maximize the quality and impact of evidence-based approaches in practice.

This chapter examines the importance of implementation research in the field of mental health promotion. Based on a review of current implementation concepts, frameworks and empirical studies, this chapter sets out to consider the critical role of implementation research in deepening our understanding of the relationship between the process of implementing mental health promotion interventions, contextual factors in the local setting and intended intervention outcomes. The distinctive features of implementation research are examined and findings from mental health promotion intervention studies are presented, which illustrate the use of different research methods for systematically assessing the quality of implementation and determining its impact on intervention outcomes.

19.2 Researching the Process of Implementation

Implementation is concerned with the central question of how interventions are put into practice (Durlak, 2016). Implementation research systematically assesses the process of implementing interventions in complex naturalistic settings and identifies the factors and conditions that can facilitate high-quality implementation. Research approaches are employed that permit a better understanding of the actualities of intervention activities and lead to a better-informed assessment of implementation processes and outcomes. A science of implementation has been developed to examine the adoption and implementation of evidence-based interventions, including those that are scaled up (Fixsen et al., 2005). Implementation science has been defined as the scientific study of methods to promote the uptake of research findings and evidence-based strategies into routine practice (Eccles & Mittman, 2006). This growing body of research is concerned with developing an evidence base to guide implementation practice, identifying the how-to of implementation as distinct from effectiveness outcomes. The overall goal of implementation research is, therefore, to improve the quality, reach and impact of evidence-based interventions that will promote population health and well-being.

To assess implementation adequately, information is needed on specific intervention activities or components, how they are delivered and the characteristics of the context or settings in which the intervention is conducted (Durlak, 2016). Implementation studies from across multiple areas have confirmed that one of the most important factors affecting intervention outcomes is the quality of implementation (Durlak, 2016; Fixsen et al., 2005). Among the key components of implementation quality that have been identified are fidelity, dosage, quality of delivery, adaptation, participant responsiveness, programme differentiation, monitoring of control conditions and programme reach (Dane & Schneider, 1998; Durlak & DuPre, 2008). These components have been assessed using both quantitative and qualitative methods, with fidelity and dosage receiving the most research attention to date. However, a relatively small number of evaluation studies systematically assess the quality of implementation and even fewer studies have related implementation quality to intervention outcomes (Durlak & DuPre, 2008; Rojas-Andrade & Bahamondes, 2019). Research examining the relationship between implementation quality and outcomes is essential for the accurate interpretation of intervention outcomes.

19.2.1 Characteristics of Implementation Research

From a health promotion perspective, implementation research brings a focus on the core aspects of practice, including attention to process, local contexts, resources and systems, and the importance of stakeholder engagement in co-producing knowledge on how and why change processes work. The distinctive features of implementation research with particular relevance to mental health promotion are now outlined.

Concern with Process Implementation research documents how interventions are actually delivered in practice, assessing the variability across settings and change agents and interpreting how the quality of implementation influences outcomes (Dane & Schneider, 1998; Greenberg et al., 2005). A focus on process is also critical to implementing mental health promotion, as the principles of collaborative practice, including participation and empowerment, are integral to the practice of community mental health promotion (Barry et al., 2019). Mental health promotion implementation research, therefore, has a clear focus on assessing the process of delivering interventions and how they engage end users in the process of bringing about change.

Context Matters The importance of context-specific factors is highlighted in the implementation literature, including organizational structures and policies, capacity and readiness to implement the interventions, mobilization of support and the ecological fit of the intervention in the local context (Chen, 1998; Durlak, 2016). Similarly, context is critically important in implementing mental health promotion interventions. For example, adopting a whole-school approach entails addressing the context of the school's environment and ethos, organization, management structures, relationships with parents and the wider community and the taught curriculum and pedagogic practice (Samdal & Rowling, 2013). Understanding the complex interaction of influencing factors within the wider context plays an important role in determining the quality of implementation and hence intervention effectiveness, especially in disadvantaged and low-resource settings.

Pluralistic and Pragmatic Approach to Research Implementation research employs a range of empirical methods to test the feasibility, adoption and acceptance of interventions and their reach, quality, equity, efficiency, scale and sustainability (Theobald et al., 2018). A pragmatic approach to research selects the methods that are best suited to answer the research question. Although randomized controlled trials (RCTs) are regarded as the gold standard for research questions concerning what works, these study designs typically provide limited information about how to implement interventions within the existing systems and settings. More practice-oriented studies and qualitative approaches are employed to elucidate the factors influencing which interventions and implementation strategies work best in particular settings.

Participatory Research Approach Implementation research draws on different types of knowledge from the perspectives of knowledge producers, including researchers from different disciplinary traditions, and knowledge users, such as programme participants, practitioners, policymakers and funders. This entails adopting more participatory research approaches and user-engaged methods and processes for knowledge production. Through the adoption of participatory research methods, the knowledge base of programme implementers and participants can be integrated into the research process, thereby incorporating tacit knowledge into the evidence base. Participatory research methods facilitate collaboration between researchers, practitioners and intervention participants and are, therefore, congruent with the principles of mental health promotion practice.

Implementation in Complex Contexts and Real-World systems Implementation research is concerned with the adoption and integration of evidence-based interventions into complex real-world systems that are constantly adapting to change (Lobb & Colditz, 2013). While many evidence-based interventions have been developed under relatively controlled conditions, there is a need to determine whether they can be feasibly implemented across more diverse populations and settings, especially those that are most disadvantaged. Embedding mental health promotion interventions within complex settings, such as communities, schools and workplaces, is not a simple linear process as it involves an ongoing process of synergistic change producing effects at different levels in different spheres. Such settings-based approaches bring a focus on systems, how they operate and the dynamics of change, including the influence of wider system factors at an organizational, policy and community level. Assessing the implementation of interventions in complex organizational settings calls for research approaches that can capture the extent of systems change and transformation and not just individual-level outcomes as in more traditional research designs. A systems approach to research involves the use of a broad spectrum of methods that can assess change at a whole systems level, capturing multiple interacting factors within the system that can shape a desirable set of outcomes (Rutter et al., 2017).

19.3 Models and Frameworks for Understanding Implementation Systems and Strategies

Conceptual models and theoretical frameworks have been developed to advance an understanding of the dynamic nature of implementation and the systems and processes involved. These frameworks describe the main influences on implementation processes and outcomes, drawing on syntheses of the literature and direct experience from practice. The overall conceptualization that emerges from the literature is that implementation is a systematic, multistage and multilevel process that requires a coordinated series of planned actions, requiring different activities and skills at different stages of the process, together with collaboration among multiple stakeholders for positive outcomes to be achieved (Aarons et al., 2011; Fixsen et al., 2005; Greenhalgh et al., 2005; Meyers et al., 2012; Tabak et al., 2012). Although there are a large number of frameworks, there is considerable overlap in the concepts and theoretical constructs that are identified, which mainly relate to enabling contexts, implementation drivers and implementation stages, alongside the characteristics of implementation teams, improvement cycles and effective innovations (Fixsen & Fixsen, 2016).

The importance of multilevel ecological frameworks for understanding implementation has also emerged from systematic reviews (e.g. Greenhalgh et al., 2005; Stith et al., 2006; Wandersman et al., 2008). These frameworks adopt a systems approach, whereby the influencing factors are recognized as operating at multiple interacting levels. For example, a socio-ecological model developed by Durlak and DuPre (2008) underscores the importance of variables related to the characteristics of the intervention (activities, core components, quality of materials, adaptability and contextual fit with the local organization and setting); the characteristics of the implementer (knowledge, skills and motivation); the implementing organization (e.g. structure, ethos, history, resources, leadership); participants (identifying, recruiting, engaging and retaining the target population) and the specific context (environment, policies, politics, agencies and collaborations) as well as those associated with the intervention delivery and support system. The complex interaction between individual- and organizational-level factors and how these in turn interact with the characteristics of the interventions to be implemented has been emphasized and supported in a number of studies (Greenhalgh et al., 2005; Fixsen et al., 2005; Durlak & DuPre, 2008).

It is clear from the existing frameworks that effective implementation is dependent on the favourable interaction of multiple factors operating within the implementation system, including the delivery and support systems specific to the local context (Flaspohler et al., 2008; Wandersman et al., 2008). Socio-ecological frameworks have particular relevance for implementing mental health promotion interventions, which tend to take place in complex interactive settings such as communities, schools, workplaces and health settings. For such settings-based interventions, the focus is not solely on the implementation of a single discrete intervention activity but also on the broader context of the school or community within which the implementation is taking place. The capacity of the setting for change is an important determinant including organizational and structural changes so that the implementation process addresses change in the settings itself as well as change for the individuals within the setting (Dooris & Barry, 2013; Dooris, 2005).

Frameworks, such as the Consolidated Framework for Implementation Research (CFIR) developed by Damschroder et al. (2009), are used to guide the systematic assessment of multilevel implementation contexts, bringing a focus on factors in both the inner setting (e.g. organizational structure, communication, culture, readiness) and the outer setting (e.g. external policy and incentives, resources), which interact with the characteristics of the intervention, the individuals involved and the stages of the implementation process. While the CFIR is widely used, a review by Kirk et al. (2016) found that it has been primarily used to guide analysis and few studies have investigated any outcomes. Kirk et al. (2016) recommended integrating the CFIR throughout the research process and linking the determinants of the implementation process to outcomes. The use of effectiveness–implementation hybrid study designs have also been proposed for analyzing the relationship between implementation processes and intervention outcomes (Curran et al., 2012). These designs have a dual focus on assessing both implementation and effectiveness outcomes, integrating traditional experimental designs with more qualitative approaches for process evaluation. However, such hybrid designs are quite rare in the literature.

19.3.1 Researching Implementation Outcomes

While there is consensus in the literature concerning the key factors in the implementation process, there is a lack of evidence concerning the relative importance of each factor and how they may interact to influence implementation for any given intervention in a given context. Few of the conceptual models have been subjected to empirical testing in a comprehensive manner, where aspects of implementation at different levels within multiple systems are assessed. Proctor et al. (2011) advanced the concept of implementation outcomes (such as acceptability, appropriateness, feasibility, fidelity) as distinct from intervention outcomes, which serve three key purposes: as indicators of implementation success, proximal indicators of implementation processes and intermediate outcomes in effectiveness research. Proctor et al. (2011) suggested that advancing research on implementation outcomes will help specify the causal mechanisms and relationships within implementation processes and thereby advance the evidence base on successful implementation.

Evaluating the complexity of multifaceted and multicomponent interventions presents a particular methodological challenge. Mental health promotion interventions are typically composed of multiple components that are designed to be delivered across different ecological levels, e.g. individual, interpersonal, organizational, community and macro-policy levels. These types of multicomponent interventions require an implementation and evaluation model that is capable of capturing the sequence of events needed for effective outcomes at each level. The complexity of the evidence debate in health promotion is well documented, and researchers have called for rules of evidence that take into account the diverse, multidisciplinary and contextualized nature of health promotion practice (McQueen, 2001; Rootman et al., 2001; Potvin & McQueen, 2008; McQueen & Jones, 2007). In response to these developments, there is a need to expand the current range of evaluation methodologies and analytical frameworks applied in mental health promotion and to widen the evidence base to be more inclusive of the realities of practical applications, especially in low-resource settings.

19.4 Researching Implementation Processes in Mental Health Promotion

There is a limited body of research on implementation within the field of mental health promotion. The existing studies show that the effective implementation of evidence-based mental health promotion interventions across diverse settings is possible but requires supportive implementation structures, including wider policy support, leadership, ongoing training and technical support, integrated delivery, capacity development and organizational supports (Barry et al., 2019).

Research on the implementation of school-based mental health promotion interventions has received particular attention (Barry et al., 2017b; Durlak & DuPre, 2008; Durlak, 2016; Greenberg et al., 2005). Evaluations of school-based programmes clearly show that the level of programme implementation is variable across sites, is significantly associated with student outcomes and that positive academic and social and emotional well-being outcomes are not achieved when the quality of implementation is low (Battistich et al., 2000; Clarke et al., 2014; Dix et al., 2012; Kam et al., 2003; Rimm-Kaufman et al., 2014; Slee et al., 2009). Meta-analyses and reviews of social and emotional learning programmes (Durlak et al., 2011), bullying prevention programmes (Smith et al., 2004) and youth mentoring programmes (DuBois et al., 2011) have reported effect sizes two to three times greater for youth participating in interventions implemented with high quality, characterized by high levels of intensity, clarity, consistency and fidelity. Understanding the importance of implementation quality and the wide range of influencing factors is, therefore, critical to effective evidence-based practice.

19.5 Case Studies

Two case studies are presented to illustrate how different research approaches can be used to elucidate the factors influencing implementation quality and to determine the relationship between context, process and intervention outcomes.

19.5.1 Case Study 1: The Implementation of the SPARX-r Computerized Program with Disadvantaged Young People

Digital interventions show potential in improving young people's mental health and well-being (Clarke et al., 2015). However, low engagement and high dropout rates remain a challenge when implementing these interventions in real-life settings (Fleming et al., 2016). This study explored the implementation of a computerized intervention, SPARX-r, to improve the mental health and well-being of young people (15–20 years of age) attending an alternative education programme in Ireland. SPARX-r is a revised version of the evidence-based SPARX cognitive behavioural therapy intervention for treating anxiety and depression (Fleming et al., 2011; Merry et al., 2012). SPARX-r is designed for universal use and uses strategies from computer games and storytelling to facilitate young people in learning skills for improving their mental health. The Youthreach[1] alternative education centres cater for young people who have fallen out of mainstream education, many of whom experience social, economic and educational disadvantages and higher levels of poor mental health and well-being. This study examined the feasibility and effectiveness of delivering SPARX-r in Youthreach settings.

Methods The study design consisted of a qualitative requirements analysis (Kuosmanen et al., 2018a) and a randomized controlled trial with integrated implementation research (Kuosmanen et al., 2017, 2018b).

Requirements Analysis Prior to the RCT study, user needs and preferences in relation to digital mental health promotion intervention delivery were examined by applying the requirements development approach (Van Velsen et al., 2013). This approach highlights the importance of the fit between the technology, the requirements of the key stakeholders and the context of delivery in determining programme uptake and impact. The requirements analysis explored what digital mental health promotion programmes should look like, what they should do and how they should be implemented in the context of an alternative education setting. There were two main elements to the requirements analysis: (1) mapping the context of delivery using an online staff survey and (2) exploring the needs and preferences of Youthreach students and staff in student and staff group discussions. The data from the requirements analysis were used to inform the implementation and process evaluation of SPARX-r within the overall RCT study, including programme selection, the selection of outcome measures and the development of process evaluation questionnaires and implementation manuals. Implementation questionnaires were tailored to measure how well the programme met the specific requirements expressed by the students and staff. Further details on the study can be found in a previously published paper (Kuosmanen et al., 2018a).

RCT and Implementation Research Students from 21 Youthreach centres were randomized to two groups: a SPARX-r intervention group and no-intervention control. SPARX-r was delivered during class time by the Youthreach staff in all but two centres, where the programme was delivered by the researcher. Implementation research was integrated into the study to examine the factors, whether student-, programme- or context-related, which may have influenced programme implementation and student engagement. Student views on SPARX-r were explored via a post-intervention implementation questionnaire and open-ended verbal or written feedback. Furthermore, process evaluation questionnaires completed after each level of SPARX-r examined the views of students throughout the study, including those who dropped out before completing the intervention. Staff views were explored through a post-intervention questionnaire and interviews. For further information on the measures employed, please refer to Kuosmanen et al. (2017) and (2018b).

[1] For further information, please see https://www.education.ie/en/Schools-Colleges/Services/Further-Education-and-Training/Youthreach/Youthreach.html

Findings The findings from the requirements analysis indicated that alternative education students and staff have quite specific requirements that need to be met in order for digital interventions to be delivered successfully (Kuosmanen et al., 2018a). These requirements reflect the specific needs of young people, including low literacy levels, issues with concentration and the unstructured nature of the alternative education setting. The student participants valued programmes that are student-centred with an attractive design and limited amount of text-based content. They also reported a preference for positively framed content that teaches practical skills on improving mental health and well-being. Students also valued user control and autonomy, expressing the need for optional attendance and privacy, and a tailored programme look and content. In order to deliver digital interventions successfully, staff considered both flexibility and careful planning and timetabling essential to support student engagement. The staff wanted to be able to integrate the programme into the curriculum while also allowing students to progress at their own pace. Staff training in intervention delivery was also considered critical.

In terms of intervention outcomes, the findings from the RCT indicated that SPARX-r had a positive impact on emotion regulation strategies, with expressive suppression decreasing significantly in the intervention group in comparison to the controls (Kuosmanen et al., 2017). However, low engagement and high dropout rates were reported, with 55% dropping out before completing the post-intervention assessment and only 30% completing the entire programme. Technical limitations, lengthiness and lack of positive focus were the main reasons for disengagement reported by the students (Kuosmanen et al., 2018b).

Although most participants considered SPARX-r easy to use, the findings indicate that increased personalization of the programme look and content may be necessary to improve the engagement rates and the relevance of the programme for all students (Kuosmanen et al., 2018b). Although the majority of the participants agreed that the activities in SPARX-r made sense to them, less than half agreed that they related well to their lives or considered the programme useful/worth doing. The staff and the majority of young people preferred universal rather than targeted delivery of SPARX-r, which highlights the importance of providing intervention content that can be tailored to meet the different levels of mental health needs among young people.

The staff referred to the need for improved flexibility and complementing digital interventions with face-to-face activities and discussions for digital interventions to better fit into the context of the alternative education setting, accommodating student absenteeism, literacy issues, irregularities in the curriculum and the need to provide individual support to students (Kuosmanen et al. 2018b). The feedback from the staff and students illustrates the influence of the programme characteristics on engagement and highlights the need for staff training in supporting effective implementation in the local context, even in the case of implementing fully automated digital interventions.

Implications The study findings draw attention to several factors that may influence the successful integration of evidence-based programmes into youth settings and that need to be taken into account in programme development and implementation to improve engagement and uptake. Within the alternative education setting, increased tailoring of the programme look and content, together with a focus on positive mental health and building social and emotional skills, could improve the relevance of such programmes when delivered universally to all students. Furthermore, the findings highlight the importance of contextual factors in determining programme engagement and uptake and call for further guidelines on optimizing the implementation of such programmes in youth settings. Providing a more structured and supported environment for programme delivery by integrating such programmes into a dedicated mental health curriculum, along with developing training and programme manuals that would provide guidelines for programme delivery and a format for discussion, could increase sustainable delivery. The findings have helped inform the development of subsequent versions of SPARX-r, with improved technical performance, which has been shown to be effective as a universal intervention for the prevention of depression in secondary school students (Perry et al., 2017).

19.5.2 Case Study 2: Implementing the MindOut Programme in Schools

MindOut is a social and emotional well-being programme for adolescents aged 15–18 years, designed to be delivered as a universal programme in school or youth settings. MindOut aims to strengthen young people's social and emotional skills and competencies for healthy development (Dowling et al., 2016). A cluster randomized controlled trial (c-RCT) outcome evaluation was conducted on the MindOut programme with 675 post-primary students in 32 schools designated as being of disadvantaged status in Ireland (Dowling et al., 2019). This study revealed significant intervention effects on students' emotional skills (e.g. improved coping skills and emotional regulation) and mental health (e.g. reduced stress and depression scores). However, there was considerable variability in implementation quality between schools. A process evaluation was integrated into the c-RCT study, which allowed for a closer examination of the implementation processes and the relationship between implementation quality and outcomes. This case study reports on the evaluation of implementing the MindOut programme and the relationship between the level of implementation quality and programme outcomes.

This study had three main objectives:

1. To investigate the variability in implementation quality across multiple dimensions
2. To identify contextual factors that were likely to contribute to this variability in implementation quality
3. To examine how the level of implementation quality impacted participants' outcomes

Further details of the study can be found in two previously published papers (Dowling & Barry, 2020a, b).

Methods Employing a mixed methods approach, quantitative and qualitative implementation data were collected from teachers and students who participated in the MindOut programme. Implementation was measured quantitatively through teacher and student measures using indicators, which were selected based on their ability to assess one of the four dimensions of implementation quality: Dosage, Fidelity/Adherence, Quality of Delivery and Participant Responsiveness (Dane & Schneider, 1998). These indicators formed an implementation quality index. Each indicator was scored separately, and these scores were then averaged within each dimension to produce four total dimension scores. A reliability analysis was carried out on the four dimension scores and high internal consistency was found. The four total dimension scores were combined to produce an overall Total Implementation Quality score. Following this, a visual binning procedure, as used in a previous study (Dix et al., 2012), was performed on each of the total scores in order to determine schools' implementation-level grouping (e.g. high-implementing or low-implementing).

The qualitative data were used to identify the key factors that may have affected implementation quality as reported by teachers and students. These data were obtained through interviews, participatory workshops with students and open-ended questions in the teacher and student implementation questionnaires. All of the qualitative data were coded and subjected to thematic analysis. The reported implementation factors (qualitative) were examined according to schools' group allocation (quantitative), which allowed for the exploration of the similarities and differences between high- and low-implementing schools in relation to the reported implementation factors.

Finally, the relationship between the level of implementation quality and outcomes was examined. The outcome data from the initial c-RCT study (Dowling et al., 2019) were linked to the implementation data and comparisons were made. Due to the clustered nature of the data, linear mixed model (LMM) techniques were employed, examining intervention outcomes across all three implementation groups (high-implementation, low-implementation, controls) at post-intervention and 12-month follow-up. To assess the relationships between the total dimension scores and outcomes, additional LMMs were completed.

Findings Variability in total implementation quality was evident between schools even when the training and resources that the schools received were identical. A total of eight schools were assigned as high implementers and another eight as low implementers, based on their implementation scores. There was also evidence of variability within schools across different dimensions of implementation quality. Of the 16 intervention schools in this study, 7 consistently scored either high or low across all four implementation dimensions, while all other schools varied, scoring high in certain dimensions and low in others.

Influencing factors identified by the teachers and students were categorized into five themes: (i) programme factors (e.g. relevance, materials and resources, user-friendliness, etc.); (ii) participant factors (e.g. group dynamics, engagement, responsiveness, etc.); (iii) teacher factors (attitudes towards the programme, comfort with the content, facilitation skills, etc.); (iv) school contextual factors (timing of the sessions, year group the programme was delivered to, access to resources and technology) and (v) organizational capacity factors (e.g. external supports, support from the school management and staff support). Several differences between high and low implementers were found in relation to these influencing factors, which are reported in further detail in a previously published research (Dowling & Barry, 2020a).

The findings related to implementation quality and outcomes (Dowling & Barry, 2020b) revealed that the positive effects of the programme found during the initial c-RCT study (i.e. reduced suppression of emotions, reduced avoidance coping, increased social support coping, reduced levels of stress and depressive symptoms) were only significant with the high-implementation but not with the low-implementation group at post-intervention. At 12-month follow-up, reduced avoidance coping was the only sustained outcome. With regard to implementation dimensions, "Quality of Delivery" was the only dimension to have a significant effect on all of the tested outcomes.

Implications Overall, these findings demonstrate that although the MindOut programme can be effective in producing positive outcomes for students of disadvantaged status, this is only true when the programme is delivered with high quality. This finding highlights the importance of implementation quality in the overall success of a programme. Considerable variability in implementation quality was evident both between schools and within schools across different dimensions. Certain dimensions (e.g. Quality of Delivery) were found to have contributed more to outcomes than other dimensions, such as dosage, which are more commonly reported in the literature (Domitrovich & Greenberg, 2000; Durlak & Dupre, 2008; Rojas-Andrade and Bahamondes 2019). These findings demonstrate the need to consistently monitor implementation quality alongside programme outcomes, particularly through the assessment of multiple dimensions. The study also identified several factors that were likely to have contributed to the schools' quality of programme implementation. In order to increase the likelihood of best outcomes for participants, strategies need to address these contextual factors in order to support higher quality implementation and, in turn, better outcomes. The findings have clear implications for policy, practice and future research, highlighting the importance of implementation and the need to ensure its quality for positive outcomes to be achieved.

19.6 Conclusions

Implementation research generates knowledge of the process, context and factors that influence the quality, reach and equity of evidence-based interventions in diverse settings. The distinctive features of implementation research have been outlined in this chapter, with a particular focus on how they relate to the principles and practice of mental health promotion. These include a concern with process and the contextualized nature of practice, necessitating the use of participatory research approaches and a pluralistic range of methods to assess the process of implementing change in complex systems. Current conceptual frameworks and empirical findings underscore the importance of systematically researching the process of implementation, including variables related to the characteristics of the intervention, the needs and views of the participants and implementers and the specific contextual factors operating in the local setting. The findings from the case studies clearly illustrate the importance of process-oriented research and its critical function in documenting the factors that influence the quality of implementation and its impact on intervention outcomes in specific settings. A comprehensive evaluation of the implementation process is critical to determining whether the intervention is meeting the needs of end users and leading to the intended outcomes. Ensuring that interventions have positively framed content and empowering processes is particularly important for mental health promotion, as the focus is on enabling positive mental health through a strengths-based, competency enhancement approach. Ensuring high levels of participant engagement and participation is key to effective practice.

The case studies also illustrate how participatory research methods can be used in the context of larger evaluation frameworks to incorporate the perspectives of the key stakeholders in the research process. This is a fundamental aspect of implementation research, as ignoring the knowledge base of the programme implementers and participants is detrimental to effective intervention delivery and undermines the ability of evaluation studies to lead to accurate interpretation of intervention outcomes. The importance of contextual factors in the local setting is also clearly highlighted, as the case study findings show how the quality of implementation is heavily influenced by organizational and system factors in different school and youth sector settings. Evaluation studies need to include an assessment of these wider implementation system factors in order to understand how they influence the quality of intervention delivery and outcomes.

The systematic study of implementation research in mental health promotion can strengthen not only the body of research knowledge but ultimately contribute to more effective and sustainable practice and policy. The literature reviewed in this chapter points to a number of key characteristics of implementation research including employing participatory research methods that engage the key stakeholders from the outset, systematically assessing the process of implementation and its quality across multiple dimensions, employing pluralistic methods to gain a deeper understanding of the contextualized nature of mental health promotion practice and implementing interventions in complex naturalistic settings. Fundamentally, implementation research enhances knowledge of the relationship between the process and outcomes and increases an understanding of the critical connections between the local context, intervention activities and the intended intermediate and long-term outcomes. Implementation research calls for research methods and analytical frameworks that can integrate the process and outcome data in meaningful ways so that clear statements can be made about how and why intervention changes have come about.

Understanding the implementation process is, therefore, critical to the effective adoption, replication and scaling up of evidence-based interventions. Innovative research approaches are needed to examine how processes and outcomes operating within complex systems may drive synergistic change. Increased attention to implementation research will strengthen the health promotion evidence base and lead to the development of more effective interventions for promoting population mental health and well-being and there by contribute to advancing global health and sustainable development.

Acknowledgements We gratefully acknowledge funding from the Hardiman Research Scholarships, National University of Ireland Galway, provided for the SPARX-r research study and the Irish Research Council (IRC) and the Health Service Executive (HSE) Health Promotion and Improvement in Ireland for funding the research on the MindOut evaluation study. The views expressed in this chapter are those of the authors only.

References

Aarons, G. A., Hurlburt, M., & Horwitz, S. M. (2011). Advancing a conceptual model of evidence-based practice implementation in public service sectors. *Administration and Policy in Mental Health, 38*, 4–23.

Barry, M. M. (2009). Addressing the determinants of positive mental health: Concepts, evidence and practice. *International Journal of Mental Health Promotion, 11*(3), 4–17.

Barry, M. M., & McQueen, D. V. (2005). The nature of evidence and its use in mental health promotion. In H. Herrman, S. Saxena and R. Moodie (Eds.), *Promoting mental health: Concepts, emerging evidence, practice,* (pp. 108–119). A report of the World Health Organization, Department of Mental Health and Substance Abuse in collaboration with the Victorian Health Promotion Foundation and University of Melbourne. World Health Organization.

Barry, M.M., Kuosmanen, T., & Clarke A.M. (2017a). *Implementing effective interventions for promoting adolescents' mental health and wellbeing and preventing mental health and behavioural problems: A review of the evidence in the WHO European Region.* A report produced for the WHO European Regional Office by the World Health Organization Collaborating Centre for Health Promotion Research, National University of Ireland Galway.

Barry, M. M., Clarke, A. M., & Dowling, K. (2017b). Promoting social and emotional well-being in schools. *Health Education, 117*(5), 434–451. https://doi.org/10.1108/HE-11-2016-0057

Barry, M. M., Clarke, A. M., Petersen, I., & Jenkins, R. (2019). *Implementing mental health promotion* (2nd ed.). Springer. https://www.springer.com/in/book/9783030234546

Battistich, V., Schaps, E., Watson, M., Solomon, D., & Lewis, C. (2000). Effects of the child development project on students' drug use and other problem behaviors. *The Journal of Primary Prevention, 21*(1), 75–99.

Chen, H. T. (1998). Theory-driven evaluations. *Advances in Educational Productivity, 7*, 15–34.

Clarke, A. M., Bunting, B., & Barry, M. M. (2014). Evaluating the implementation of a school-based emotional well-being programme: A cluster randomized controlled trial of Zippy's friends for children in disadvantaged primary schools. *Health Education Research, 29*(5), 786–798.

Clarke, A. M., Kuosmanen, T., & Barry, M. M. (2015). A systematic review of online youth mental health promotion and prevention interventions. *Journal of Youth and Adolescence, 44*(1), 90–113.

Curran, G. M., Bauer, M., Mittman, B., Pyne, J. M., & Stetler, C. (2012). Effectiveness-implementation hybrid designs: Combining elements of clinical effectiveness and implementation research to enhance public health impact. *Med Care, 50*(3), 217–226. https://doi.org/10.1097/MLR.0b013e3182408812

Damschroder, L. J., Aron, D. C., Keith, R. E., Kirsh, S. R., Alexander, J. A., & Lowery, J. C. (2009). Fostering implementation of health services research findings into practice: A consolidated framework for advancing implementation science. *Implementation Science, 4*(1), 50. https://doi.org/10.1186/1748-5908-4-50

Dane, A. V., & Schneider, B. H. (1998). Program integrity in primary and early secondary prevention: Are implementation effects out of control*? Clinical Psychology Review, 18*(1), 23–45.

Dix, K. L., Slee, P. T., Lawson, M. J., & Keeves, J. P. (2012). Implementation quality of whole-school mental health promotion and students' academic performance. *Child and Adolescent Mental Health, 17*, 45–51.

Domitrovich, C. E., & Greenberg, M. T. (2000). The study of implementation: Current findings from effective programs that prevent mental disorders in school-aged children. *Journal of Educational and Psychological Consultation, 11*(2), 193–221. https://doi.org/10.1207/S1532768XJEPC1102_04

Dooris, M. (2005). Healthy settings: Challenges to generating evidence of effectiveness. *Health Promotion International, 21*(1), 55–65.

Dooris, M., & Barry, M. M. (2013). Overview of implementation in health promoting settings. In O. Samdal & L. Rowling (Eds.), *The implementation of health promoting schools* (pp. 14–23). Routledge.

Dowling, K., & Barry, M. M. (2020a). Evaluating the implementation quality of a social and emotional learning program: A mixed methods approach. *International Journal of Environmental Research and Public Health, 17*(9), 3249. https://doi.org/10.3390/ijerph17093249

Dowling, K., & Barry, M. M. (2020b). The effects of implementation quality of a school-based social and emotional well-being program on students' outcomes. *European Journal of Investigation Health, Psychology and Education, 10*(2). https://doi.org/10.3390/ejihpe10020044

Dowling, K., Clarke, A. M., & Barry, M. M. (2016). *The re-development of the MindOut programme: Promoting social and emotional wellbeing in post-primary schools*. WHO Collaborating Centre for Health Promotion Research, National University of Ireland Galway.

Dowling, K., Simpkin, A. J., & Barry, M. M. (2019). A cluster randomized-controlled trial of the MindOut social and emotional learning program for disadvantaged post-primary school students. *Journal of Youth and Adolescence, 48*(7), 1245–1263. https://doi.org/10.1007/s10964-019-00987-3

DuBois, D. L., Portillo, N., Rhodes, J. E., Silverthorn, N., & Valentine, J. C. (2011). How effective are mentoring programs for youth? A systematic assessment of the evidence. *Psychological Science in the Public Interest, 12*(2), 57–59. https://doi.org/10.1177/1529100611414806

Durlak, J. A. (2016). Program implementation in social and emotional learning: Basic issues and research findings. *Cambridge Journal of Education, 46*(3), 333–345. https://doi.org/10.1080/0305764X.2016.1142504

Durlak, J. A., & DuPre, E. P. (2008). Implementation matters: A review of research on the influence of implementation on program outcomes and the factors affecting implementation.

American Journal of Community Psychology, 41(3-4), 327–350. https://doi.org/10.1007/s10464-008-9165-0

Durlak, J. A., Weissberg, R. P., Dymnicki, A. B., Taylor, R. D., & Schellinger, K. B. (2011). The impact of enhancing students' social and emotional learning: A meta-analysis of school-based universal interventions. *Child Development, 82(1)*, 405–432. https://doi.org/10.1111/j.1467-8624.2010.01564.x

Eccles, M. P., & Mittman, B. S. (2006). Welcome to implementation science. *Implementation Science, 1*, 1. https://doi.org/10.1186/1748-5908-1-1

Fixsen, D. L., & Fixsen, A. A. M. (2016). *An integration and synthesis of implementation frameworks.* Accessible at: https://www.activeimplementation.org/wp-content/uploads/2018/11/Fixsen-and-Fixsen-IntegrationAndSynthesisImplementationFrameworks-2016.pdf

Fixsen, D. L., Naoom, S. F., Blasé, K. A., Friedman, R. M., & Wallace, F. (2005). *Implementation research: A synthesis of the literature*. University of South Florida, Louis de la Parte Florida Mental Health Institute, The National Implementation Research Network.

Flaspohler, P., Stillman, L., Duffy, J. L., Wandersman, A., & Maras, M. (2008). Unpacking prevention capacity: An intersection of research-to-practice models and community-centered models. *American Journal of Community Psychology, 41*, 182–196.

Fleming, T., Dixon, R., Frampton, C., & Merry, S. (2011). A pragmatic randomized controlled trial of computerized CBT (SPARX) for symptoms of depression among adolescents excluded from mainstream education. *Behavioural and Cognitive Psychotherapy, 40*(5), 529–541.

Fleming, T. M., De Beurs, D., Khazaal, Y., Gaggioli, A., Riva, G., Botella, C., … Riper, H. (2016). Maximizing the impact of e-therapy and serious gaming: Time for a paradigm shift. *Frontiers in Psychiatry, 7*, 65.

Friedli, L. (2009). *Mental health resilience and inequalities*. WHO Regional Office for Europe.

Greenberg, M. T., Domitrovich, C. E., Graczyk, P. A., & Zins, J. E. (2005). The study of implementation in school-based preventive interventions: Theory, research, and practice. In *Promotion of mental health and prevention of mental and behavior disorders* (Vol. 3). U.S. Department of Health and Human Services.

Greenhalgh, T., Robert, G., Bate, P., Kyrakidou, O., MacFarlane, F., & Peacock, R. (2005). *Diffusion of innovations in health service organisations: A systematic literature review.* Blackwell Publishing.

Herrman, H., Saxena, S., & Moodie, R. (eds.) (2005). *Promoting mental health: Concepts, emerging evidence, practice.* A report of the World Health Organization, Department of Mental Health and Substance Abuse in collaboration with the Victorian Health Promotion Foundation and University of Melbourne. World Health Organization.

Kam, C. M., Greenberg, M. T., & Walls, C. T. (2003). Examining the role of implementation quality in school-based prevention using the PATHS curriculum. *Prevention Science, 4*, 55–63.

Kirk, M. A., Kelley, C., Yankey, N., Birken, S. A., Abadie, B., & Damschroder, L. (2016). A systematic review of the use of the consolidated framework for implementation research. *Implementation Science, 11*, 72. https://doi.org/10.1186/s13012-016-0437-z

Kuosmanen, T., Fleming, T. M., Newell, J., & Barry, M. M. (2017). A pilot evaluation of the SPARX-R gaming intervention for preventing depression and improving wellbeing among adolescents in alternative education. *Internet Interventions, 8*, 40–47. https://doi.org/10.1016/j.invent.2017.03.004

Kuosmanen, T., Fleming, T. M., & Barry, M. M. (2018a). Using computerized mental health programs in alternative education: Understanding the requirements of students and staff. *Health Communication, 33*(6), 753–761. https://doi.org/10.1080/10410236.2017.1309620

Kuosmanen, T., Fleming, T. M., & Barry, M. M. (2018b). The implementation of SPARX-R computerized mental health program in alternative education: Exploring the factors contributing to engagement and dropout. *Children and Youth Services Review, 84*, 176–184. https://doi.org/10.1016/j.childyouth.2017.11.032

Lobb, R., & Codlitz, G. A. (2013). Implementation science and its application to population health. *Annual Review of Public Health, 34*, 235–251.

McQueen, D. V. (2001). Strengthening the evidence base for health promotion. *Health Promotion International, 16*(3), 261–268.

McQueen, D. V., & Jones, C. M. (Eds.). (2007). *Global perspectives on health promotion effectiveness*. Springer.

Merry, S. N., Stasiak, K., Shepherd, M., Frampton, C., Fleming, T., & Lucassen, M. (2012). The effectiveness of SPARX, a computerised self help intervention for adolescents seeking help for depression: Randomized controlled non-inferiority trial. *BMJ, 344*(e2598), 1–16.

Meyers, D. C., Durlak, J. A., & Wandersman, A. (2012). The quality implementation framework: A synthesis of critical steps in the implementation process. *American Journal of Community Psychology, 50*, 462–480.

Perry, Y., Werner-Seidler, A., Calear, A., Mackinnon, A., King, C., Scott, J., … Batterham, P. J. (2017). Preventing depression in final year secondary students: School-based randomized controlled trial. *Journal of Medical Internet Research, 19*(11), e369. https://doi.org/10.2196/jmir.8241

Petersen, I., Evans-Lacko, S., Semrau, M., Barry, M. M., Chisholm, D., Gronholm, P., Egbe, C. O., & Thornicroft, G. (2016). Promotion, prevention and protection: interventions at the population- and community-levels for mental, neurological and substance use disorders in low- and middle-income countries. *International Journal of Mental Health Systems, 10*(30). https://doi.org/10.1186/s13033-016-0060-z

Potvin, L., & McQueen, D. V. (Eds.). (2008). *Health promotion evaluation practices in the Americas: Values and research*. Springer.

Proctor, E., Silmere, H., Raghavan, R., Hovmand, P., Aarons, G., Bunger, A., Griffey, R., & Hensley, M. (2011). Outcomes for implementation research: conceptual distinctions, measurement challenges, and research agenda. *Administration and Policy in Mental Health, 38*, 65–76.

Rimm-Kaufman, S. E., Larsen, R. A. A., Baroody, A. E., Curby, T. W., & Ko., M., Thomas, J. B. & DeCoster, J. (2014). Efficacy of the responsive classroom approach: Results from a 3-year, longitudinal randomized controlled trial. *American Educational Research Journal, 51*, 567–603.

Rojas-Andrade, R., & Bahamondes, L. L. (2019). Is implementation fidelity important? A systematic review on school-based mental health programs. *Contemporary School Psychology, 23*(4), 339–350. https://doi.org/10.1007/s40688-018-0175-0

Rootman, I., Goodstadt, M., Hyndman, B., McQueen, D.V., Potvin, L., Springett, J., Ziglio, E. (Eds.) (2001). *Evaluation in health promotion: principles and perspectives*. European series, no.92. World Health Organization Regional Publications/WHO Regional Office for Europe.

Rutter, H., Savona, N., Glonti, K., Bibby, J., Cummins, S., Finegood, D. T., … White, M. (2017). The need for a complex systems model of evidence for public health. *Lancet*. https://doi.org/10.1016/SO140-6736(17)31267-9

Samdal, O., & Rowling, L. (2013). *The implementation of health promoting schools: Exploring the theories of what, why and how*. Routledge.

Slee, P. T., Lawson, M. J., Russell, A., Askell-Williams, H., Dix, K. L., Owens, L., Skrzypiec, G., & Spears, B. (2009). *KidsMatter primary evaluation final report* (pp. 1–120). Centre for Analysis of Educational Futures, Flinders University of South Australia.

Smith, J. D., Schneider, B. H., Smith, P. K., & Ananiadou, K. (2004). The effectiveness of whole-school antibullying programs: A synthesis of evaluation research. *School Psychology Review, 33*(4), 547–560.

Stith, S., Pruitt, I., Dees, J., Fronce, M., Green, N., Som, A., & Linkh, D. (2006). Implementing community-based prevention programming: A review of the literature. *The Journal of Primary Prevention, 27*(6), 599–617. https://doi.org/10.1007/s10935-006-0062-8

Tabak, R. G., Khoong, E. C., Chambers, D. A., & Brownson, R. C. (2012). Bridging research and practice: Models for dissemination and implementation research. *American Journal of Preventive Medicine, 43*, 337–350.

Theobald, S., Brandes, N., Gyapong, M., El-Saharty, S., Proctor, E., Diaz, T., … Peters, D. H. (2018). Implementation research: New imperatives and opportunities in global health. *The Lancet, 392*, 2214–2228. https://doi.org/10.1016/S0140-6736(18)32205-0

United Nations (2015). *Transforming our world: The 2030 Agenda for Sustainable Development.* Sustainable Development knowledge platform. United Nations. https://sustainabledevelopment.un.org/post2015/transformingourworld Accessed 13 Aug 2020.

Van Velsen, L., Wentzels, J., & Van Gemert-Pijnen, J. (2013). Designing eHealth that matters via a multidisciplinary requirements development approach. *JMIR Research Protocols, 2*(1), e21.

Wandersman, A., Duffy, J., Flaspohler, P., Noonan, R., Lubell, K., Stillman, L., Blachman, M., Dunville, R., & Saul, J. (2008). Bridging the gap between prevention research and practice: The interactive systems framework from dissemination and implementation. *American Journal of Community Psychology, 41*, 171–181.

World Health Organization. (2013). *Mental health action plan 2013-2020.* World Health Organization.

World Health Organization and Calouste Gulbenkian Foundation. (2014). *Social determinants of mental health.* World Health Organization.

Chapter 20
Skills-Based Health Education for Health Promotion Among School Adolescents Through Participatory Action Research: A Case from Nepal

Sudha Ghimire and Bhimsen Devkota

20.1 Introduction

The hegemony of the positivist research paradigm has ruled Nepali higher education for a long time. It is taken for granted in most educational practices (Guatam, 2019). To break that commanding domination, we adopted participatory action research (PAR) while researching in the public schools of Nepal. PAR is a collaborative approach to research in which researchers aim to carry out research "with" practitioners (as research partners) rather than "on" practitioners (as research objects) (Wright, 2021). This method empowers both the researcher and the research participants, which conventional research has failed to do. PAR is a non-coercive participatory type of action research; knowledge is created through collaborative activities between the researcher and research participants and is known as co-researcher (Zuber-skerritt, 2018). In PAR, both researcher and research participants' (so-called in the positivist paradigm) involvement is considered to be "mainstream" to the study. Epistemologically, PAR assumes that knowledge is based on experience and people's real life. This understanding is made with cooperation among researchers and co-researchers (Jacobs, 2016). We considered early adolescents and school teachers as co-researchers and worked explicitly with them.

Skills-based education has shown a significant positive impact on contributing to the healthy development of children and adolescents in addressing their health risk behaviours (Clarke et al., 2006); however, there is still a gap between the skills provided to the adolescents and the skills they need. Adolescents have very little voice in communities, families and even in schools; either their ideas are ignored or are not

S. Ghimire (✉) · B. Devkota
Tribhuvan University, Kirtipur, Nepal
e-mail: sudha.ghimire@gc.tu.edu.np

L. Potvin, D. Jourdan (eds.), *Global Handbook of Health Promotion Research, Vol. 1*,
https://doi.org/10.1007/978-3-030-97212-7_20

prioritized (Samuels & Ghimire, 2013). In the context of a classroom, the vast majority of teaching related to health includes didactic teacher-centred lectures that encourage rote learning and reproduction by students rather than increasing their knowledge and creating appropriate skills. Such irrelevant and disempowering teaching and learning fails to directly link the children's everyday lives and acts as an obstacle for transformation (Acharya et al., 2018). However, a health needs assessment report highlights that parents, students and teachers prefer collaborative health education activities in schools and in the community (Baidya et al., 2001). We tried to understand the actual health-related needs of early adolescents and the ways of managing those needs by imparting skills-based health education through PAR, using situations in which they were listened to and could participate. In this chapter, we describe the process, challenges and lessons learned while conducting PAR in a public school setting in Nepal. The aim of the project was twofold: developing meditation skills to relieve adolescents' stress and making improvised homemade reusable pads for better management of menstruation hygiene among adolescent girls.

We explain how we identified the needs for health education skills among early adolescents (10–14 years of age) and how they learned the skills in a participatory way. Additionally, this study provides evidence on students' needs and how teachers could acquire pedagogical skills in identifying the students' needs in order to provide evidence-based education. The educational manual and the teaching and learning materials developed using a participatory action research approach could be used and scaled by different educational agencies.

20.2 The Nature of Intervention and the School Context

This chapter is based on one of the school-level interventions conducted by the Rupantaran Project, a project jointly implemented by the consortium of Tribhuvan University, Kathmandu University and the Norwegian University of Life Sciences, funded by the Norwegian Agency for Development Cooperation (NORAD) (2016–2021). The project aims to strengthen the motivation and capacity of a range of stakeholders at the local and higher education levels. The project consists of several interrelated phases: Phase I – Stakeholder engagement to establish the action research cycle; Phase II – Assessment of school needs, including physical infrastructure and curricular needs; Phase III – Piloting innovative approaches to improve education, health and livelihood outcomes and Phase IV – Evaluation of the project schools relating to the intervention provided.

During the first phase, eligible PhD students from Tribhuvan University were selected. The project developed the PhD scholars' capacity to undertake participatory action research (PAR) by involving them in different workshops, conferences and theoretical and practical sessions on PAR. In the second phase, to ensure a relevant approach and community ownership for the project, a robust, multilevel stakeholder engagement strategy was developed. The project created a working environment with a PhD student, teachers from the project school, parents and local community members jointly identifying the needs of the school's adolescents. They also addressed the planning and implementing of the skills-based health education programme as well as the intensive teacher and leadership training for teachers and head teachers to further their professional development. Students' needs were then identified, in this phase, with the help of various qualitative and quantitative data collection tools. Based on the needs identified in the third phase, a range of interventions were implemented with the school personnel, PhD scholars, teachers, parents and the community. In the fourth phase, attempts were made to replicate the project's success in other schools near the project school. The project has referred to these schools as reference schools. Finally, the project is planning to disseminate the intervention package and the PAR process in the public schools of Nepal. The project is collaborating with the Curriculum Development Center (CDC) under the Ministry of Education. The outcome and lessons learned from this PAR are being used to revise school-level curricula in the future. The project partners envision that the teaching manuals and policy briefs developed in the course of the PAR process will act as reference materials for curriculum planners to make the school-level health education curriculum responsive, demand-driven and needs-based.

The project has chosen four reference schools in the Chitwan District and one action or project school. Chitwan district is located in the south-western part of Nepal, 98 kilometres from the capital city of Kathmandu. The district consists of seven municipalities. One is a metropolitan city, five are urban municipalities and one is a rural municipality – the project selected the project school based on predefined criteria. The school should be government-funded and have low academic performance, with students from marginalized and disadvantaged communities and ultra-poor families.

20.3 Participatory Action Research (PAR): For Health Promotion

Participatory action research (PAR) is an approach to research that emphasizes participation and action to build research participants' capacity to solve self-identified problems and promote health and social justice through collaboration with researchers (Marincowitz, 2003). In PAR, researchers become facilitators or catalysts and participants become co-learners. Nobody is considered an expert and the work is collaborative.

PAR is a dynamic, multidisciplinary, multiform, life-enhancing qualitative inquiry (Jacobs, 2016; Macdonald, 2012; Reason & Hilary, 2008) that proceeds in a spiral of steps composed of planning and evaluation of the results of the action. In the context of health promotion, PAR has an extremely short history. In earlier decades, very little research using PAR was found in health journals (Baum et al., 2006); however, these days, it is widely applied, as evidenced by people's participation in improving health, highlighted in Alma Ata (in 1978) through to Ottawa (in 1986) and Jakarta (in 1996) (Wallerstein & Duran, 2008). People's participation in emancipation and transformation is the primary goal of PAR. Furthermore, PAR differs from most other conventional positivist approaches in public health research because it is based on reflection, data collection and action that aims to improve health and reduce health inequities by involving the people who, in turn, take action to improve their own health. Additionally, PAR helps reduce the gap between knowledge and practice by embedding problem solving and action for better health outcomes (Choudhry et al., 2002).

In this research, we embodied PAR with a democratic approach, where all stakeholders (teachers, parents, students) worked collaboratively to empower each other in the process of co-generating context and responsive performative knowledge related to skills-based health education. In this research, participants acted as co-creators of knowledge rather than passively providing information to the researcher. Therefore, in the PAR process, the research participants participate as co-researchers.

20.4 Methodology

In this section, we detail how we conducted the PAR process, beginning with how we developed the collaborative, balanced power dynamics. This is the first cycle of PAR, containing multiple microcycles. During this cycle, we introduced ourselves to the school stakeholders. In cycle II, we involved the multiple and diverse stakeholders of the school in open discussions regarding the research objectives and process. Throughout this cycle, we regarded the "power dynamic" as an opportunity and also as a challenge. During this cycle, we (researcher and co-researchers) agreed on a common understanding to further process design needs. We started working together from this point. Cycle III was about discovering the key skills required by early adolescents, and to do this, we conducted focus group discussions and workshops. In cycle IV, we designed and implemented the curriculum developed through the participatory method, focusing on stress management through classroom meditation and on menstruation hygiene management via awareness and improvised reusable homemade cotton pads. In the current cycle V of the project, we are planning to evaluate the effectiveness of the skills acquired by early adolescents (refer to Fig. 20.1).

Cycle I	Cycle II	Cycle III	Cycle IV	Cycle V
Collaboration and trust building, PAR committee formation, continue filed engagement	Involving multi and diverse stakeholder in school-based program	Finding key skills needed by early adolescents	Designing and implementing Participatory curriculum on skill-based health education	Effectiveness of skilled based health education

Fig. 20.1 PAR cycle of study

The data presented in this chapter are part of the PhD project and one of five PhD student projects. It focuses on the first author's research on transformative skills-based health education among early adolescents. The entire process of identifying the skill needs of early adolescents in the local context of Chitwan is presented here.

20.4.1 Collaboration and Trust Building

PAR focuses on conducting research "with" people, not "for" people (Jacobs, 2016; Liamputtong, 2019). Considering this, we involved teachers, students and parents beginning with the early stage of the PAR, from identifying the issues to be studied to planning and implementing the intervention. From the beginning, we collaborated and co-worked with them to develop trust and a feeling of ownership. We helped them understand the objectives and nature of the study and that it was targeted for their skills development.

In order to make everyone comfortable and establish connections, PhD scholars from the university and teachers from their formal setting, we started sharing a table in the canteen during lunch break, held informal conversations in our free time and visited the school's catchment area communities with the teachers to gain contextual knowledge. We discussed with the teachers what would be the best way to identify the skills the adolescents required. Apart from these, we also built rapport with the students who were research participants using play-based child-focused activities. It took more than 6 months for us to develop this rapport and create a working environment.

20.4.2 Involving Multiple and Diverse Stakeholders in School-Based Programmes

Initially, we developed 1 PAR committee with 21 members from different fields. This included representatives from the parents, the community, health workers from health centre school management committees (SMCs), school teachers, local farmers, local leaders and social leaders. This committee was the learning community to co-work together on the school project. This group performed a series of activities, prioritizing needs-based problems through skills-based health education. During the meeting, a representative of the school management committee (SMC) made the following statement:

> In our community, many people come and ask us questions about health, hygiene, food habits, and our socio-cultural practices, but we never know what they do after asking us; they never come back to us. But this is the first time we know that you are working with our children and us to make them better in their health and education. We will help you to learn different skills that are required for our better health. (45-year-old female, SMC)

Adding to this, a head teacher shared:

> Most of the time scholars, policymakers, journalists, and advocates come and indicate our weakness, most of the time they talk about the negative things. They give big suggestions but never work with us … giving suggestions is an easy job; anyone can suggest. Working with us to solve the existing problem for our children is most important. We know learning can't take place overnight. It takes time. So, we need to have patience. We need to teach the skills required by our children, not based on textbook or expert advice alone... How can outsiders know our problem unless they work with us? (Head teacher, JJ School)

These comments from the different stakeholders made us realize that they were in favour of the PAR. They suggested that the expertise they have, through the health post-in-charge, can involve teaching the skills of menstruation hygiene and the ward chair can support the logistics and awareness sessions. Though they agreed to work voluntarily, the power differential and reluctance to take on responsibilities were the main challenges in this stage.

20.4.3 Power Dynamics

Knowledge symbolizes power, and there is never a perfect equilibrium of power within society. It is important to understand power relations before initiating the PAR process (Dworski-Riggs & Langhout, 2010). Power relationships are also central to understanding the dynamic relationships between researchers and communities. The school where we were working had its own hierarchical system. First, permanent school teachers who were in the job as government employees considered themselves more powerful than a part-time teacher or contract teacher.

> We are the senior government teachers; we can be transferred to any place and can work. Our job is not insecure like part time or contract teachers, so no one can force us to do any work we don't want to do. We should have priority in all work or in all facilities, otherwise what's the meaning of permanent teacher? (Permanent teacher)

We included a representative of both the permanent government teachers and the temporary teachers in PAR meetings to mitigate this gap during the planning and implementing phase. Both types of teachers were treated equally, irrespective of the nature of their jobs. Similarly, a teacher who teaches math and science is generally considered more important when compared to the other teachers. Teachers believe that math and science are technical subjects and only experts can teach them but anyone can teach subjects like languages and health. In our observations, the value given to health teachers is comparatively less than that given to math and science teachers. The main objectives of this study were to develop health-related skills among early adolescents. Thus, health teachers were more engaged and empowered throughout the PAR process.

The majority of the Nepalese societies live under a patriarchal system, where men are the head of the family and women are generally considered subordinate to them. This is reflected in family and professional life (Shrestha & Gartoulla, 2017).

During our field engagement, women teachers shared that sometimes they feel dominated by their male counterparts. They further added that most of the time the administration takes suggestions from only the male teachers while ignoring the female teachers. The female teachers were only expected to follow the instructions they were provided rather than giving suggestions or making any decisions.

> We got involved in the activities just to fulfill the quota of females; otherwise, they (males) would never involve us in any program, though they give space to us, they rarely listen to us. At last, males make one team or tie-up with some political parties, and we females are left behind. (Female, primary teacher)

In our project, we involved women teachers equally in the PAR meeting, and a woman teacher led each meeting. Though in the early days, women teachers were very active and attended all the meetings, by the middle of the PAR process, some teachers were no longer participating because of family responsibilities. So, to remedy this, we conducted meetings at times that were best suited to the women teachers.

> Sometimes it's hard to include a female teacher in training and other activities. They can't give their full attention because most of the time they have their own problems, small children, family, so sometimes they request not to be involved in some activities. (Head teacher)

Furthermore, there was a different power dynamic between the school personnel and the school management committee (SMC). SMC members consider themselves more powerful because they belong to that particular community and continually work voluntarily for school progress. At the same time, teachers think being part of the SMC is a political position and shouldn't interfere with the school schedule and school teachers.

> SMC overburdens us; we are getting a salary from the government, not from SMC, they are volunteers and volunteers do not have full responsibilities. They are here for a short time, and they want to impress society so that their future political relationships will be good. But we are different because we have been in this profession for a long time. (School teacher)

Whereas the SMC representatives shared that "we belong to this community and teachers should work under us. The main purpose of the SMC committee is to observe the activities of the teacher and take necessary action." We observed this in the field. We conducted an open discussion and came to a consensus on the importance of skills-based education for adolescents. As we worked with the adolescents, we realized that they had the least power and were compelled to do whatever they were assigned. Most of the time, the programmes were designed for them without their involvement. So, we involved them actively throughout the study by addressing their ideas and suggestions. Similarly, we felt that another power dynamic existed within our group of researchers. The school personnel and teachers said that there was a gap between school teachers and university scholars. One of the school teachers replied to us, "You people are from a university with high qualification and positionality, but we are just school teachers. We are yet to learn how to have academic discourse with you." (A female basic school teacher). Such strong feelings were difficult to overcome in order to collaborate on the work to be done. We decided to switch our role in this process from "being there" to "becoming with them" in order to change the power dynamics. We began to visit the school during regular hours, we had food with the teachers in the canteen, we began to have different contextual conversation and spent a lot of time with them. Slowly, they accepted us as part of their school and community.

20.4.4 Finding the Key Skills Needed by Early Adolescents

We conducted a workshop and had focus group discussions with the representatives of the students, parents and teachers to understand their perception of health-related skills (refer to Fig. 20.2).

> For me, skill means the ability to perform in a good way. If people can do work effectively, using the proper steps then that is a skill and learning is the key to acquiring skill (Member, SMC, 48-year-old female).

The parents shared that being knowledgeable about health means their children would avoid bad habits like smoking, drinking alcohol and drug addiction; they should be able to share what they learned in school with their parents at home; they should respect and listen to their parents as well as help others in need in an empathetic manner and they should be able to communicate effectively. The head teacher from the school shared:

> In school, everyone (different agencies) comes and teaches our students and us what to do and why … but they never teach us how to do it…. (Head teacher, school)

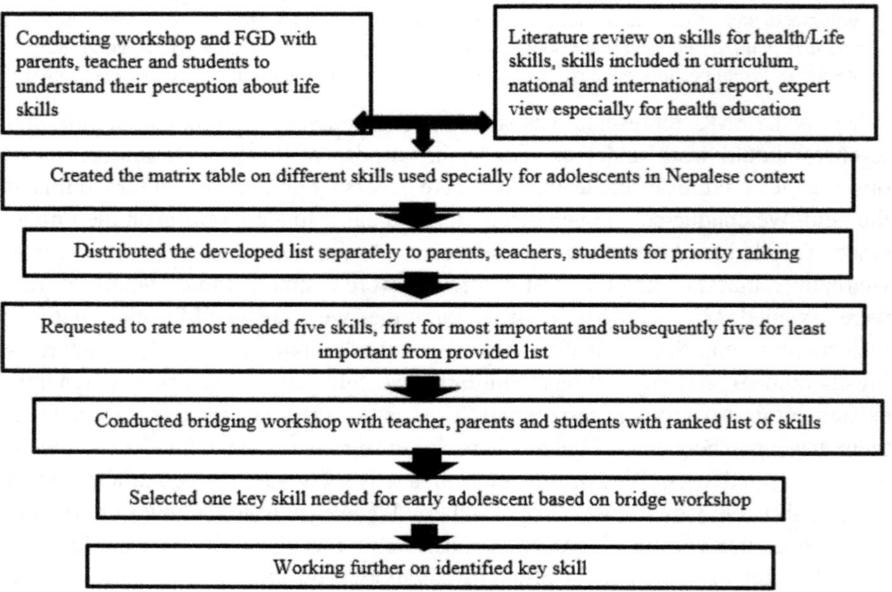

Fig. 20.2 Process adopted to discover the most needed skills by early adolescents

Based on the focus group discussion and a literature review, we developed a list of skills that were identified in different studies targeting adolescents. We allowed the parents, teachers and students to choose and then rank any five skills from the given list that they considered important to learn. After collecting the separate lists from the students, parents and teachers, the researchers conducted a bridging workshop with the parents, student representatives and teachers and shared their recommended list. In a participatory discussion, they jointly selected the key skills important to the adolescents; however, the process is still evolving and is interactive.

The bridging workshop attended by the teachers, students and parents led to a common understanding that students should learn problem-solving skills and stress management skills.

20.4.5 Designing Curriculum Development Through the Participatory Method

Researchers and health teachers discussed the relevant literature related to health skills during the first stage of curriculum development. Subsequently, provisional teaching concepts, methods for delivering the new skills, integrating the contents into the existing curriculum and the credit hours needed for teaching were all discussed. All subjects of basic education were explored. The skills were planned to be introduced in an integrated way, such as blending the menstruation hygiene management (MHM) content (refer to Fig. 20.3) with the health subject. Making

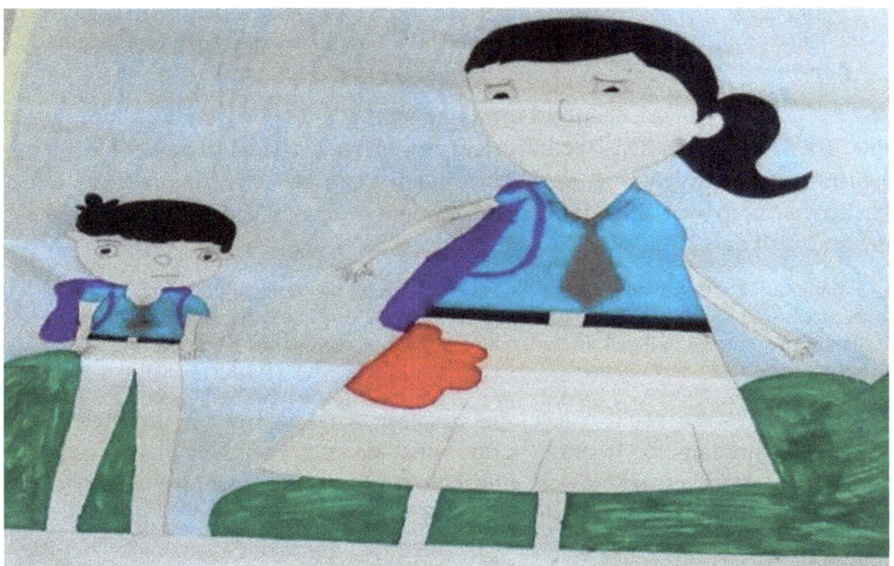

Fig. 20.3 Art by students depicting the sensitivity of teaching the content of menstruation

sanitary pads was incorporated into the knitting and sewing chapter titled Occupation Business and Trade (OBT).

Similarly, the psychological changes in early adolescents were blended with the health subject, whereas doing meditation for the purpose of relieving stress was incorporated into the physical education subject. Parents and members of the PAR were also included as experts to deliver related contents. Representative students were also involved with their suggestions and were empowered to develop peer teaching. After adapting the content, the students were involved in developing teaching materials based on their interests, like drawing pictures, writing poems and writing theatrical scripts, which were later used in teaching.

20.4.6 Implementing Skills-Based Health Education Sessions

First, we assessed the awareness and sensitivity around the reasons for adolescents' stress and their potential health impacts. This was done at the personal, family and community levels through the school fair, school drama, a puppet show and Parents' Day programmes. An awareness rally with the students, teachers and parents on International Yoga and Meditation Day was carried out in the school's catchment area to highlight the importance of meditation for stress management.

> Involving students in such awareness sessions via the rally is effective. Parents give more attention to their children when they see their children walking with the placard in their hands. This is how learning at school can be disseminated to the community. Such activities directly link the school with the community. We have been trying to educate people on the importance of meditation for stress relief. Involving people is difficult because they are busy with their own lives. But if we involve their children as 'change agents' I think that people will give more attention to them. (Ward President, KHR Municipality, Chitwan)

Second, activities were conducted involving teachers, focusing on the concept of a child-friendly school. This included learning about the legal aspects of corporal punishment, active learning, apperceive inquiry and the art of living to help the teachers develop their skills for better classroom pedagogy and also to reduce their stress as well as the students' stress.

> From group discussion and in my personal experience, I can say that first teachers should be stress-free to create a positive learning environment. We know that we need to create a happy environment in the classroom, but … uummn … because of many reasons, we are unable to do so. Hope this training will be effective in doing so… (Health teacher, JJ School)

Third, students were taught to develop meditation as a skill. This was done in school, early in the morning, for 10 min to reduce their stress and improve their concentration. The meditation sessions were guided by adults using public loudspeakers connected to each classroom. They provided guiding instructions for meditation. The students were further asked to follow the meditation practices at home when they felt exhausted or stressed. Furthermore, the causes of stress, the effectiveness of meditation and the methods used to resolve tension were provided and then integrated into the regular health education classes.

> .. allowing students to have meditation within their regular class is a wonderful idea. We don't need a sophisticated yoga hall. Students can do meditation sitting on their regular desk bench. I think this is the best skill that anyone requires to be healthy. (President, School Management Committee)

Fourth, female students participated in making reusable cotton sanitary pads for hygienic management of menstruation. After learning to make reusable pads, they also developed one procedural video about the process of pad making, which was later used as a resource material for teaching other students.

Initially, a group of students (8 girls and 4 boys) were taught to make reusable cotton pads. Later, they taught the remaining students. A separate teaching manual was developed in collaboration with the regular teachers. The entire process of problem identification through skills delivery to adolescents was included.

20.4.7 Effectiveness of Skills-Based Health Education

The intervention has been recently completed while writing this chapter. Evaluation of the educational sessions on skills will be made immediately after 3 months of intervention and then 6 months after the first evaluation in order to document the changes and transformation over time among the school adolescents. Both qualitative and quantitative methods and tools will be used for assessing the effectiveness of the skills-based health education sessions. However, some initial evaluations after the intervention show that the students are happy. They have started working with their peers. Teachers have become conscious of reducing and/or preventing stress in collaboration with the students, other teachers and parents.

20.5 Discussion

We have considered the research participants as co-researchers who can engage and balance research and action in a participatory way (Liamputtong, 2019; Madrigal et al., 2016). The case study by Simovska (2012), in participatory health promotion in school children, shows that, if given sufficient guidance, children can act as agents of health-promoting changes; their experience with active participation seems to have empowered them, giving them a feeling of ownership, efficacy and success in working with "real-life" problems. Reflected in our study as well, adolescents and their parents and teachers were actively involved in identifying the issues to be studied and the skills to be learned. A study by Tomokawa et al. (2020), on the Kenyan Comprehensive School Health Program (KCSHP) project, identified that activities such as a school health checklist, organizing teacher training on health education, the presence of an active child health club and school-based health check-ups improve the health-related knowledge, attitudes and practices among students and teachers. Considering this, we also created one child health club, which acted as a "change agent" for behaviour modification and skills teaching.

Similarly, Fidan and Balcı (2017) described schools as "complex adaptive systems" that comprise a population of diverse rules-based agents and multilevelled and interconnected systems. In our study, we have considered "school personnel as unique in themselves" whose problems and ideas to solve those problems are distinct in themselves. Furthermore, the school culture, environment, school size, teacher and student profiles and school administrators' leadership skills make each school a different and individual unit of the community (Fidan & Balci, 2017). In our study, we have considered the school personnel as unique in themselves. As such, they were given an equal chance to provide their views and suggestions, which we included from the beginning, for the implementation of the intervention. People from different levels and an expert from the community identified the adolescents' basic health-related skills.

Similarly, this study is equally helpful in understanding how the multilayers of society can participate in the participatory action research (Sokhanvar & Salehi, 2018). A study by Rentala et al. (2019) argued that academic stress is among the significant stresses in adolescents. They addressed this in a holistic group health promotion programme as an intervention for better health, whereas, in our school context, we used meditation and skills for making reusable menstrual pads to address the real problems of the school adolescents.

20.6 Conclusions

In the participatory action research process, the participants were the co-researchers who worked together throughout the study. We found the school personnel unique in themselves, and, if given a chance, they can equally collaborate for knowledge generation and action planning. Furthermore, the participatory action research process provided a venue for the adolescents to co-create knowledge based on their expressed needs rather than becoming passive receivers of information. It provided a platform for engaging multilayers of the society for knowledge creation and to deal with their day-to-day health problems. It created a context-specific evidence base for identifying and addressing the health problems of school adolescents. However, we observed that power dynamics played a significant role and had to be managed throughout the research process. Furthermore, if we ask the community to identify their problems, they indicate a specific problem that is sometimes not considered to be a problem at the macro level; for example, in our case, the stakeholders, including early adolescents, identified academic stress as a major problem they were facing. However, if we consider national data and programmes, only reproductive health-related issues are stressful among adolescents. So, PAR helps find the context-specific ground-level problem of the community.

We conclude that the PAR approach is essential for health promotion research. It helps uncover the hidden health-related problem, which is sometimes overlooked by other conventional researches where the researcher assumes full power. Furthermore, this study provided insights into how we can make the research process with school adolescents more participatory. The research findings will inform ways of sustaining the learned skills, revisiting curricula and defining the teacher's role in bringing about desirable changes among school-going adolescents.

Acknowledgements We thank the teachers, students and SMC members for their participation as part of the collaborative learning. This chapter was prepared with support from the NORHED/ Rupantaran project implemented by Tribhuvan University, Nepal. Ms. Jenn Weidman deserves special thanks for copyediting the manuscript.

References

Acharya, D., Thomas, M., & Cann, R. (2018). Nepalese school students' views about sexual health knowledge and understanding. *Educational Research, 60*(4), 445–458. https://doi.org/10.1080/00131881.2018.1525304

Baidya, P., Chhetri, H., & Devkota, B. (2001). *A study on health needs assessment and school health program in Nepal* (trans. N. H. R. Council). (pp. 1–46).

Baum, F., Macdougall, C., & Smith, D. (2006). Participatory action research. *Journal of Epidemiol Community Health, 60*, 854–857. https://doi.org/10.1136/jech.2004.028662

Choudhry, U. K., Jandu, S., Mahal, J., Singh, R., & Mutta, B. (2002). Health policy and systems research with South Asian women. *Journal of Nursing Scholarship, 34*(1), 75–81.

Clarke, D., Maier, C., Birdthistle, I., & Buckland, P. (2006). *Skills for health: Infromation series on school health, docunmnet 9* (pp. 90–90). WHO.

Dworski-Riggs, D., & Langhout, R. D. (2010). Elucidating the power in empowerment and the participation in participatory action research: A story about research team and elementary school change. *American Journal of Community Psychology, 45*(3–4), 215–230. https://doi.org/10.1007/s10464-010-9306-0

Fidan, T., & Balcı, A. (2017). Managing schools as complex adaptive systems: A strategic perspective. *International Electronic Journal of Elementary Education, 10*(1), 11–26. https://doi.org/10.26822/iejee.2017131883

Guatam, S. (2019). *Letter to professor Auguste Comte* (pp. 61–73). Brill|Sense.

Jacobs, S. (2016). The use of participatory action research within education-benefits to stakeholders. *World Journal of Education, 6*(3), 48–55. https://doi.org/10.5430/wje.v6n3p48

Liamputtong, P. (2019). *Handbook of research methods in health social sciences* (1st ed.). Springer.

Macdonald, C. (2012). Understanding participatory action research : A qualitative research methodology option. *Canadian Journal of Action Research, 13*(2), 34–50.

Madrigal, D. S., Minkler, M., Parra, K. L., Mundo, C., Enrique, J., Gonzalez, C., et al. (2016). Improving Latino youths ' environmental health literacy and leadership skills through participatory research on chemical exposures in cosmetics : The HERMOSA study. *International Quarterly of Community Health Education, 36*(4), 231–240. https://doi.org/10.1177/0272684X16657734

Marincowitz, G. J. O. (2003). How to use participatory action research in primary care. *Family Practice, 20*(5), 595–600. https://doi.org/10.1093/fampra/cmg518

Reason, P., & Hilary, B. (2008). *The SAGE handbook of action research participative inquery and practice* (2nd ed.). SAGE.

Rentala, S., Hi, B., Lau, P., Aladakatti, R., & Thimmajja, S. G. (2019). Effectiveness of holistic group health promotion program on educational stress, anxiety, and depression among adolescent girls – A pilot study. *Journal of Family Medicine and Primary Care, 8*, 1082–1089. https://doi.org/10.4103/jfmpc.jfmpc

Samuels, F., & Ghimire, A. (2013). *Understanding key capability domains of adolescent girls and gender justice. Findings from Nepal.*

Shrestha, A., & Gartoulla, R. P. (2017). Socio-cultural causes of gender disparity in Nepalese Society. *Journal of Advanced Academic Research, 2*(1), 100–111. https://doi.org/10.3126/jaar.v2i1.16601

Simovska, V. (2012). Case study of a participatory health – Promotion intervention in school. *Democracy and Eduactaion, 20*(1), 1–10.

Sokhanvar, Z., & Salehi, K. (2018). Participatory action research to promote educational quality: A literature review. *Research & Reviews: Journal of Educational Studies, 4*(2), 23–34.

Tomokawa, S., Asakura, T., Njenga, S. M., Njomo, D. W., Takeuch, R., Akiyama, T., et al. (2020). Examining the appropriateness and reliability of the strategy of the Kenyan Comprehensive School Health Program. *Global Health Promotion*, 1–10. https://doi.org/10.1177/1757975920917976

Wallerstein, N., & Duran, B. (2008). The theoretical, historical, and practical roots of CBPR. In M. Minkler & N. Wallerstein (Eds.), *Community-based participatory research for health: From process to outcomes*. Wiley.

Wright, P. (2021). Transforming mathematics classroom practice through participatory action research. *Journal of Mathematics Teacher Education, 24*(2), 155–177. https://doi.org/10.1007/s10857-019-09452-1

Zuber-skerritt, O. (2018). An educational framework for participatory action learning and action research (PALAR). *Educational Action Research, 0792*(May), 1–20. https://doi.org/10.1080/09650792.2018.1464939

Part III
Researching the Practices of Policy Makers and Institutions

Chapter 21
Evaluating Health Promotion in Schools: A Contextual Action-Oriented Research Approach

Nina Bartelink, Patricia van Assema, Hans Savelberg, Maria Jansen, and Stef Kremers

21.1 Introduction

Improving health promotion in the school setting is challenging. To create a meaningful impact, it requires introducing, managing and sustaining health-promoting changes in all aspects of the school including individual health behaviour, school environment, policies and curriculum and even in families and the local community (Deschesnes et al., 2003; Lee, 2009; Langford et al., 2014; Mohammadi, 2010). This system-wide change is a complex task to fulfil (Mohammadi, 2010; Deschesnes et al., 2003). It implies a need for more context-specific evaluation to understand the implementation and impact of health promotion in such a complex system (Darlington, 2016; Moore et al., 2015; Patton, 2011). To align the research of school health promotion with this complexity, we translated the principles of action

N. Bartelink (✉) · P. van Assema · S. Kremers
Department of Health Promotion, Care and Public Health Research Institute (CAPHRI), Maastricht University, Maastricht, The Netherlands

Department of Health Promotion, School of Nutrition and Translational Research in Metabolism (NUTRIM), Maastricht University, Maastricht, The Netherlands

Academic Collaborative Centre for Public Health Limburg, Public Health Services, Heerlen, The Netherlands
e-mail: n.bartelink@maastrichtuniversity.nl

H. Savelberg
Department of Nutrition and Movement Sciences, Nutrition and Translational Research Institute Maastricht (NUTRIM), Maastricht University, Maastricht, The Netherlands

M. Jansen
Academic Collaborative Centre for Public Health Limburg, Public Health Services, Heerlen, The Netherlands

Department of Health Services Research, Care and Public Health Research Institute (CAPHRI), Maastricht University, Maastricht, The Netherlands

L. Potvin, D. Jourdan (eds.), *Global Handbook of Health Promotion Research, Vol. 1*,
https://doi.org/10.1007/978-3-030-97212-7_21

research into a contextual action-oriented research approach (CARA). This research approach builds on previous experiences in school health promotion and on the international literature regarding new insights into complex systems thinking. In this chapter, we explain how CARA is applied as a research approach in a Health Promoting School initiative. The methods used as well as the insights obtained from the CARA-based evaluations are discussed. At the end of this chapter, we elaborate on the consequences for researchers when applying CARA as well as on the consequences for the study design and data collection and analysis of the research.

21.2 Health Promotion in Schools

Schools can play an important role in promoting healthy behaviours in children, since a significant proportion of a child's day is spent there and schools reach all children from a variety of socio-economic and ethnic backgrounds (Bonell et al., 2013). Health promotion in schools has therefore the potential to reduce the gap in health disparities among children (Oosterhoff et al., 2019). Moreover, a school is also one of the diversities of microsystems, which interact to shape child development and well-being: the impact of changes in the school may also interact with the child's behaviour in other microsystems, e.g., the home setting and neighbourhood, which could enhance the effects of health promotion in the school (Gubbels et al., 2014; Lohrmann, 2008). Moreover, since healthy behaviours also improve academic achievements, school health promotion can contribute to achieving a school's primary educational goals (Hollar et al., 2010). However, education and health are often not combined in school systems. Worldwide, school health promotion has long been characterized by relatively low priority, fragmentation and a lack of coordination, partly due to the absence of a legal obligation (WHO, 1997). This created a situation in which all kinds of external organizations developed health-promoting interventions to improve a specific aspect of a child's health and well-being (Mohammadi, 2010). It was hereby assumed that an intervention only impacts a small part of the school and will produce predicted effects in each school context. The primary focus of these interventions was often on increasing knowledge through classroom-based health education, and this resulted in limited integration of the interventions as implementation stopped after the last lesson. As a result of this situation, schools were overloaded with externally developed health-promoting interventions. Teachers perceived themselves as a "dumping ground" for all these interventions and complained about the high workload as all these well-intended interventions were added to their regular work (Mohammadi, 2010). Studies that investigated the implementation and effects of these interventions recommended to use a whole-school approach and to involve the people in the school when developing health-promoting interventions (Deschesnes et al., 2003). This should create more ownership for the changes, and, in this way, the changes can be better adapted to the school's context.

The Health Promoting School (HPS) approach aims for such a whole-school approach. The World Health Organization (WHO) defines the HPS approach as "a school that is continuously strengthening its capacity as a healthy setting for living, learning and working" (WHO, 2009). Even though different definitions of the HPS approach exist worldwide, they all have similar underpinning principles (Deschesnes et al., 2003; Turunen et al., 2017) and a focus on six essential components: 1) healthy school policies, 2) the school's physical environment, 3) the school's social environment, 4) individual health skills and action competencies, 5) community links, and 6) health services (WHO, 2009; Turunen et al., 2017). Several reviews have been published on the effectiveness of the HPS approach in improving the health and well-being of schoolchildren. Overall, school initiatives that were inspired by the HPS approach showed some promising effects, such as improved health behaviours of children, a decline of children's body mass index (BMI) and improved aspects of mental and social well-being (Langford et al., 2014; Stewart-Brown, 2006). However, these findings were not uniform across the included studies: achieving successful implementation and sustaining the positive health benefits has proven to be challenging (Mohammadi, 2010). Translating the HPS approach successfully into practice has been considered a complex task to fulfil since it requires change in both the people in the school and the school system itself. Very little is known yet about this system-wide change (Mohammadi, 2010), which has resulted in a considerable gap between the vision of the HPS and its implementation (Deschesnes et al., 2003; Mohammadi, 2010).

21.3 Schools as Complex Adaptive Systems

New insights have led to the suggestion to consider schools as complex adaptive systems (CASs) (Mohammadi, 2010). A CAS consists of many interacting components and has the capability to self-organize and adapt. The system has typically non-linear relations between components: it may respond in different ways to the same input, depending on the context. The behaviour of the system is also not easily controlled or predicted, and it tends to self-organize to a state of stability (Turunen et al., 2017; Mohammadi, 2010). Embracing this perspective of considering schools as CASs means that a school acts in a unique way and can react differently to changes, since each school has its own context. The school context can be defined as *the specific circumstances and characteristics of each school, which relate to the social, political, economic, and physical environment; the characteristics, behaviours, wishes, and needs of the people in the school; the wider community in which the school is located; as well as the history and organization of the school* (Damschroder et al., 2009; Bartelink et al., 2019b). This definition shows that a school context consists of many different aspects. Previous studies have shown that some specific aspects might be of importance for school health promotion efforts. They include the characteristics of the school population (demographics, current health behaviours, health and well-being) (Poland et al., 2009); health-promoting practices of the teachers (Darlington et al., 2018); perceived barriers to the implementation of health-promoting initiatives, which can be categorized into barriers related to the users, innovation, support, organization and socio-political environment (Fleuren et al., 2014); current health-promoting elements in the school (school routine, policy, education and environment) (WHO, 2009) and dominating organizational issues (e.g., merger process) (Poland et al., 2009).

21.4 A Contextual Action-Oriented Research Approach (CARA)

Embracing the perspective of schools as complex adaptive systems implies a need for more context-specific evaluation of health-promoting initiatives in schools (Darlington, 2016; Moore et al., 2015; Patton, 2011). Therefore, to align the research of school health promotion with the complex and adaptive nature of school systems, we translated the principles of action research into a contextual action-oriented research approach (CARA). This research approach builds on our previous experiences in school health promotion and on the international literature regarding new insights into complex systems thinking. The purpose of CARA for researchers is not only to evaluate a Health Promoting School initiative but also to support the process of change in the participating schools, with a specific focus on the contextual differences. This means that researchers are able to contribute to the initiative and at the same time conduct a thorough evaluation of the process and effect. CARA is an adaptation of the action research principles, whereby the traditional linear steps of needs assessment, development, implementation, monitoring and evaluation of change are let go as they suggest a logical, causal process. In contrast, CARA aims to identify where changes interact with the contextual aspects of the school. The basic properties of CARA are its specific focus on the contextual differences and the use of monitoring and feedback to both support and evaluate the process of change. The approach centres around four key questions: 1) What is the pre-existing context of each school? 2) How does the process of change in each school evolve, and which factors affect this process? 3) How can research contribute to the process of change? 4) Do children's health and health behaviours improve as a result of the health-promoting changes? Table 21.1 illustrates the development of CARA and its main features. It shows how the traditional steps of action research (column 1) are combined with new insights into complexity thinking (column 2) to form CARA (column 3).

Table 21.1 The development and main features of a contextual action-oriented research approach (CARA)

Traditional steps of action research	New insights into complexity thinking	Contextual action-oriented research approach
Assessment of needs, interests and opportunities ↓ **Development of change** ↓ **Implementation of change** ↓ **Monitoring (change in) each context** ↓ **Evaluation**	- The school system itself is a complex system as it is characterized by a large number of interacting institutional elements (Patton 2011). - Besides the contextual differences between schools, each implemented change will also work differently at each school; there is always an interaction between intervention and context (Darlington et al., 2017; Moore et al., 2015). - The willingness to participate in a process of change depends on motivation, capacity and opportunity (Michie et al., 2011). - A process of change in a complex system does not have a linear cause–effect relationship: e.g. small changes can produce large effects at the so-called "tipping points" (non-linearity) (Patton, 2011; Van Kann et al., 2015). - How suitable a change is depends on the school context (Darlington et al., 2018; Moore et al., 2015). - A variety of factors can influence the implementation of a change in the school setting, such as factors relating to the implementers, innovation, organization and socio-political context (Fleuren et al., 2014). - An intervention that is conceived as an add-in rather than an add-on to the existing school system is more likely to be implemented and sustained successfully (Bentsen et al., 2018). - Implementation of a change will be more successful and will lead to greater ownership and commitment if it involves a process of mutual adaptation, where a change is modified to suit the needs, interests and opportunities of the school and where the people in the school are open to (major) adjustments and will adapt to meet the requirements of the change (Reiser et al., 2000). - A bottom-up approach is needed as teachers, children and their parents know best which changes are most appropriate for their school, and this approach will create greater ownership of the changes (Laverack & Labonte, 2000; Van Kann et al., 2015). - A top-down approach is needed as the external experts involved have specific health promotion knowledge, skills and experiences, which may lead to more effective changes (Laverack & Labonte, 2000; Van Kann et al., 2015). - Monitoring and evaluation is no longer merely an external observation of strategies to implement changes but becomes one of the strategies itself (Patton, 2011). - The attitude of the researchers is no longer neutral and fully objective but involves joining in the discussions and providing support to the innovators whenever possible using their specific knowledge, skills and experiences (Patton, 2011). - Regular feedback provides valuable guidance to the process of change in the schools (Waterman et al., 2000).	**Aim:** To identify where and how changes interact with the contextual aspects in the school system **Main features:** - Evaluate and support the process of change. - Specific focus on the contextual differences. - Monitoring and feedback loops. **Four key questions:** 1. What is the pre-existing context of each school? 2. How does the process of change in each school evolve, and which factors affect this process? 3. How can research contribute to the process of change? 4. Do children's health and health behaviours improve as a result of the health-promoting changes?.

Adapted from Bartelink et al., (2018).

21.5 Example of a Health Promoting School Initiative: The Healthy Primary School of the Future

The Healthy Primary School of the Future (HPSF) is a Dutch Health Promoting School initiative and was developed by three collaborating organizations: the regional educational board "Movare", the regional Public Health Services and Maastricht University. The aim of HPSF was to sustainably integrate health and well-being into the school system. The initiative builds upon the principles of the HPS approach and considers schools as complex adaptive systems (Bartelink, 2019). HPSF intends to go beyond the traditional, temporary and superficial top-down solutions and aims to systematically incorporate health and well-being, which ideally leads to sustained changes that become embedded in the DNA of the school. Moreover, HPSF intends to establish a co-creation movement in schools by including top-down and bottom-up processes to develop and implement health-promoting changes in all aspects of the school system. On top of the HPS approach, the aim of HPSF is to create some form of positive disruption in the schools by initiating two health-promoting top-down changes: 1) a free healthy lunch each day and 2) daily structured physical activity and cultural sessions after lunch. Realizing that these changes were only possible by extending the school day, the schools now finish at 15.30/15.45 p.m. instead of 15.00 p.m. Moreover, to avoid increasing the workload of teachers, both changes were implemented by external pedagogical employees (PEs) provided by childcare organizations. This integration of the childcare organizations during school hours is intended to change the school's organization in a sustainable way. The aim for the future is to bring school and childcare closer together and thereby create an integrated day for children, whereby children are supervised by the same people prior, during and after school hours. While in other national school systems the two changes may represent usual practice, they were hypothesized as positively disruptive to the Dutch school system because the provision of school lunches and structured physical activity sessions are not the usual practice in Dutch schools. The two changes were contextualized bottom-up and hypothesized to lead to momentum for more bottom-up processes to implement additional health-promoting changes in the schools.

Participant involvement was a key feature of HPSF. Teachers and parents were involved from the start in the adoption decision and the process of adapting the several changes into the school context. The participating four pilot schools decided to only start implementation of HPSF if they had full teacher support and at least 80% parental support. All four schools used a children's voice group, with representatives from each class in the school, to get insights into the opinion of children regarding HPSF. Each school selected a teacher as a school coordinator, who managed HPSF in their school. Overarching the four schools, the HPSF initiative was led by a project leader from Movare and an executive board with representatives of Movare, the regional Public Health Services and Maastricht University, including the project leader. These organizations, together with several other external partners, cooperated with HPSF to support the schools in the development and implementation of the health-promoting changes. A PE coordinator per school acted as the contact person for all external PEs in that school. Lunch products were provided by a catering service (Sodexo). Instructions for the physical activity sessions were provided by a sports and leisure organization (the Move Factory). The Move Factory also supported the external PEs during implementation when needed, and, after a year, they provided a training course (8 sessions of 2 hours each) to supply them with additional tools on how to motivate children to participate actively during the physical activity sessions. A health promoter from the regional Public Health Services was assigned to each school to provide support when needed. Researchers from Maastricht University monitored and fed back results to the schools to support the process of change. The provincial authorities supported the initiative financially. Regular meetings were held at the school level and overarching the four schools to keep each other updated, provide feedback and discuss the process of change. Each school initiated regular meetings between the school coordinator and PE coordinator, working groups with teachers and parents and children's voice groups. The health promoters of the four schools met regularly to keep each other updated on the ongoing processes in each school. A project team was created with representatives of all partners involved: the four schools, Movare, regional Public Health Services, Maastricht University, the Limburg provincial authorities, childcare organizations, the caterer, and the sports and leisure organization.

21.6 Applying CARA in the Example of HPSF

To study the process and effects of HPSF in the four schools, we applied CARA as our research approach. This enabled us to deal with the differences between the school contexts and helped us not only evaluate HPSF but also support the implementation process. As part of applying CARA, the evaluation methods had to be sensitive to the dynamics of the local context (Hawe, 2015; Darlington et al., 2017; Rutter et al., 2017). Therefore, we used different methods to combine the accuracy of quantitative methods and the in-depth insights of qualitative methods. To be able to deal with the unpredictability of the system, we had to make decisions regarding the appropriate methods along the way instead of only preparing a research proposal beforehand to be able to react to unexpected changes or effects. In general, the following methods were used to assess the four (pre-existing) school contexts and to facilitate the ongoing process of change in each school.

Semi-structured interviews were conducted annually with the school coordinator and the health promoter in each school. The aim of the interviews was to draw up an overview of the health-promoting elements in the school, to get a broad understanding of any dominating organizational issues in the school and to discuss the health-promoting changes in the school, their development and implementation and the influencing factors associated with them.

Observations were conducted in the four schools with the aim of learning about the school's dynamics and to see and hear the influencing factors of HPSF (rather than as a form of fidelity assessment). The same researcher also participated, observed and took notes in all meetings related to HPSF.

Minutes were collected of the meetings of the project team, health promoters, working groups with parents and teachers and children's voice groups. Data derived from these minutes provided qualitative, in-depth information about the development and implementation of HPSF in each school and any experienced influencing factors.

A *barrier questionnaire* was used to examine which factors in the context were perceived to be (potential) barriers to the process of change. All teachers and external pedagogical employees were asked to complete the barrier questionnaire twice a year. The questionnaire contained statements related to innovation-, implementers-, organization-, and socio-political context-related barriers for HPSF affecting innovation adoption, implementation and integration.

A *practices questionnaire* was used to examine annually the health-promoting practices of teachers at school and parents at home, e.g., modelling behaviour, encouragement and availability.

Anthropometry, accelerometry and several health behavioural questionnaires were used to examine children's health and health behaviours. The measurements were carried out by researchers during 1 week at the beginning of the school year at all the four HPSF schools and four control schools.

The collected data were used to provide feedback and recommendations to the schools to guide their actions and help them adapt to the health-promoting changes. Examples of feedback were written summaries of the most important results of the interviews; overviews of the perceived barriers to the teachers and external pedagogical employees and short, easily understandable animated videos of the most important results of the health and behavioural measures. Other contributions on top of the feedback were suggestions for possible behavioural goals and the offer of a selection of relevant, previously developed and evidence-based additional changes for the schools. To be able to offer this as a range of possibilities, a so-called "fruit basket model" is introduced. This "basket" consists of a continuously expanding overview of the available evidence-based additional health-promoting changes ("fruits") that schools can introduce. Examples of such changes are gardening activities, energizers in the lessons and creating a physical activity-friendly schoolyard. According to the school's needs, interests and opportunities, the school coordinator can decide together with the working groups what the school's focus will be and which specific "piece of fruit" – additional change – fits their school. The change can then be adapted to the specific school context, with the help of external experts, before implementation starts.

The collected data were also used to conduct an extensive process and effect evaluation. The process evaluation was conducted to better understand implementation processes (Schaap et al., 2018). In line with the recent debates in this research area (Hawe, 2015; Moore et al., 2015; Patton, 2011; Rutter et al., 2017), the focus of the process evaluation was not on the fidelity of the intervention components in purely compositional terms but on the adaptation of the intervention and system to one another and the factors crucial to sustained change (Bartelink et al., 2019b). The evaluation explored the processes through which HPSF and the school context adapted to one another in the four schools. The aim was to generate knowledge and experiences on how to implement health-promoting changes in the complex adaptive school system. An effect evaluation was carried out to examine whether HPSF led to changes in children's health and health behaviours. A quasi-experimental design with the four control schools was used for this evaluation (Willeboordse et al., 2016; Bartelink et al., 2019d, e). However, since changes may have different effects in different contexts, we also investigated where, for whom and under which circumstances HPSF had the greatest effect (Bartelink et al., 2019a, c). This was done by combining the results of the effect evaluation with relevant implementation and contextual factors of the schools. This integration of process and effect data was done by the use of moderator analyses and qualitative comparisons. Not only to remain objective towards these scientific evaluations but also to be involved in and give support to the process of change, we had to be close enough to the practice to know and understand what was happening but distant enough to evaluate the bigger picture. By conducting the process evaluation prior to the effect evaluation, we were involved in the process of change without knowing the effects. Using the principle of data triangulation for the process evaluation and a quasi-experimental design for the effect evaluation helped us study the process and effects as objectively as possible.

21.7 CARA-Based Evaluation of HPSF: Insights

The CARA-based evaluation of HPSF has provided us with an insight into the interaction between the effects of HPSF and the school context (Bartelink et al., 2019a). Findings have shown that even when schools implemented similar health-promoting changes, this did not lead to similar effects due to the moderating role of the school context. These findings demonstrate that studying the effects of a Health Promoting School initiative cannot be done in isolation from its context, which is in line with the complex adaptive systems' perspective and the recommendations of other researchers (Darlington et al., 2018; Hawe et al., 2009; Moore et al., 2019). Moreover, since the contextual aspects on different levels of the school system (i.e. level of the children, level of the teacher and level of the school organization) seem to moderate the effects of HPSF, a broad understanding of the school context is crucial. The moderating role of the contextual aspects of the school system suggests that when analyzing the effects of changes in a complex adaptive system, they need to be examined separately for each context to prevent over- or underestimation. The findings also suggest that effect sizes of outcomes do not provide a full answer regarding the effectiveness of health-promoting changes (Burton, 2012; Kremers et al., 2018). Larger effects can also be achieved due to the interaction with specific contextual aspects. Therefore, the

CARA-based evaluation of HPSF has provided us with the insight that when evaluating the effectiveness of health-promoting changes, the focus should not only be on the effect sizes and outcomes but also on the aspects in the context that interacted with the health-promoting changes. This context-oriented evaluation may contribute to explaining the variation in effects across schools when implementing a comparable health-promoting school initiative. This also means that due to the moderating role of the context, it does not automatically lead to similar effects when transferring specific health-promoting changes to another school. Therefore, in the HPSF initiative, a flexible concept was created to enable schools to fully adapt it to their situation. In this way, the initiative can provide guidance on how to adapt health promotion into the whole school system but leaving room for adaptation to the specific school context.

The CARA-based evaluation of HPSF has also provided us with a better insight into how to successfully integrate health promotion into a specific school (Bartelink et al., 2019b). One of the main insights we obtained was that a co-creation process was crucial to adapt the health-promoting changes in a way that fits best to the specific school context (Bartelink et al., 2019b). This co-creation should consist of a continuous process of trial and error, feedback loops and communication between all internal and external people involved. This means continuous interactions between bottom-up involvement, top-down advice and external practical support. This co-creation process was perceived as crucial to the integration of HPSF into the schools, as together they include all the required knowledge, experiences and resources. Bottom-up involvement was needed as teachers, children and their parents knew best which health-promoting changes fit best in their school, and this helped to create ownership and school-wide support. Top-down advice from external experts was needed since they possess the scientific knowledge from previous research about evidence-based health-promoting changes or conditions and how to integrate health promotion into the schools. External partners were able to provide support in terms of personnel, money and materials but also had specific practical knowledge and experience to share. This combination of bottom-up involvement, top-down advice and external practical support shows how top-down and bottom-up forces meet, with the local context being respected whilst making use of the knowledge and support of the broader system. This co-creation process also demonstrates that integrating health promotion into a school system is rather a non-linear, complex and dynamic process instead of a linear trajectory with a beginning and an end. This means that a one-size-fits-all does not exist and that a standardized programme package with a form that looks the same in each school will not work (Hawe et al., 2004; Moore et al., 2019). Although the importance of implementation fidelity is recognized (Elliott & Mihalic, 2004; Schaap et al., 2018), enough flexibility could create a better fit of health-promoting changes within a specific school context, as the needs, wishes and opportunities of the context in which the changes are implemented could be addressed (Darlington et al., 2017).

21.8 Applying CARA: Consequences for Research

CARA is a novel way to evaluate a health-promoting school initiative. This means that applying CARA also has some consequences for conducting research. Applying CARA implied that we, as researchers, were actively participating partners in the HPSF initiative. We joined in the discussions and provided support to the schools whenever possible on the basis of our professional knowledge, skills and experiences as well as the results of the monitoring data. This is comparable to the role of researchers in developmental evaluation (Fagen et al., 2011; Patton, 2011). As a consequence of this more involved role, the research on HPSF was more time-consuming, as, for example, a thorough insight into the school context was necessary, which required a relationship of trust with the schools and all other partners involved. This took time to build. Moreover, a more flexible time planning was needed. We had to react quickly to what happened in each school. To be able to give relevant support, analysis of the data had to be done quickly to translate it into real-time feedback for the schools. At the same time, the feedback process needed to take place in a careful manner, as both the initiative and the research benefitted from an open discussion of the real situation of those involved without losing the trust of the informants. On top of these consequences, for the role of researchers, applying CARA also has several consequences for the study design and data collection and analysis of the research.

21.8.1 Study Design

It was not perceived as desirable or feasible to randomize a population-level intervention, such as HPSF, as it attempts to factor out the system's context (Pommier et al., 2010; Rutter et al., 2017). Therefore, a quasi-experimental study design was used to evaluate the effects of HPSF on children's health and health behaviours. The design enabled us to examine the effects over time and to enrol schools on the basis of their motivation. We did not include any randomization, which has resulted in significant baseline differences between the intervention and control group. However, to deal with the limitation of no randomization, all analyses were controlled for relevant covariates, e.g., gender, age and BMI at baseline. In addition, the inclusion of only four intervention schools was a result of the research approach. Due to limitations in resources (money, time, manpower), it was perceived as undesirable to include more schools in the implementation of HPSF. Including only four intervention schools created the possibility to really get to know the people in the schools and to obtain a detailed understanding of each school context. It also created the time to assess the effects of HPSF on all children in these schools without overburdening the researchers. This had the advantage that more effort could be put into the recruitment of children and their parents for participation in the measurements in each school, which has resulted in a high number of children who enrolled in the study and a low dropout rate over the years.

21.8.2 Data Collection

Applying CARA required a thorough insight into the school context. Fully assessing and understanding all aspects of each school context was deemed impossible. Therefore, we followed research suggestions and focused on the contextual aspects that were indicated as relevant to school health promotion. Even though more insights, e.g., leadership of the school coordinators, could have contributed to an even better understanding of the school context, the contextual aspects that were assessed provided a deep insight into the four school contexts. We combined appropriate quantitative and qualitative methods and were able to employ the principle of data triangulation, which is a strategy that facilitates the validation of data through cross-verification from different sources (Boonen et al., 2009). In addition, to evaluate the effects of HPSF, many different outcomes were assessed rather than just one. This provided us with a thorough understanding of the effects of HPSF on different aspects. Again, a combination of data sources was used to obtain information about children's health and health behaviours. For example, accelerometers were used, which objectively measured children's physical activity (PA) behaviours, along with parent and child questionnaires. These different sources helped to gain a better insight into the actual dietary and PA behaviours of children throughout the day. To deal with possibly overburdening the participating children, parents and teachers, we scheduled all annual effect measurements in a school in a single week. Since we used the same weeks each year to conduct the measurements, seasonal effects were reduced. The disadvantage of this measurement schedule was that the researchers were present in the school for the whole week. This could have influenced the children's health behaviours during that measurement week and might have biased the effects, for example, on their PA behaviours. However, the researchers' influence was reduced by the quasi-experimental study design since their presence in school was comparable in the intervention and control schools.

21.8.3 Data Analysis

Applying CARA is time-consuming, which means that choices have to be made. Since we focused on a thorough understanding of the contexts and changes in the four intervention schools, we had only a limited focus on the specific school context in the control schools. To evaluate the effects of HPSF, the control schools were combined into one "control group" in the analyses. This means that their unique contexts were not taken into account, which can be seen as a limitation, since each school can be considered as a complex adaptive system and therefore the control schools should ideally also be considered as such. Moreover, linear mixed model analyses were conducted to study the longitudinal intervention effects of HPSF. This analysis technique deals with the dependency in the data that is created by the repeated measurements of participants. But it suggests a linear cause–effect relationship, which is in contrast to the non-linearity of intervention effects in a school system. Thus, it is actually suboptimal for evaluating complex adaptive systems, but a better option was not yet embedded in our way of working. Recently, system dynamics modelling has been increasingly suggested as a promising innovative method (Owen et al., 2018). This method has already been applied successfully to other sectors, such as engineering, economics, defence, ecology and business, and is underpinned by a mathematical theory of non-linear dynamics (Atkinson et al., 2015). System dynamics modelling makes use of causal loop diagrams, which aim to represent the feedback structure of a system by identifying the key variables and indicating the causal relationships between them. Systems modelling in public health research is still in its early stages and includes several limitations linked to, amongst others, model validity (Xue et al., 2018). Future studies should deal with these limitations and investigate whether this method can properly analyze the health-promoting initiatives in schools.

21.9 Conclusions

Creating system-wide change in the school setting is a challenging task, since schools can be considered as complex adaptive systems. To understand the implementation and impact of health promotion initiatives in such systems, there is a need for more context-specific evaluation. Therefore, to align the research of school health promotion with this complex and adaptive nature of schools, we translated the principles of action research into a contextual action-oriented research approach (CARA).

In this chapter, we explained how CARA has been applied as a research approach in the Healthy Primary School of the Future, a Dutch Health Promoting School initiative. By applying the research approach, we were able to support the participating schools in their process of change and to conduct a thorough evaluation of the process and its final outcomes while addressing the importance of the implementation context. Furthermore, we discussed the important insights obtained from the CARA-based evaluations and elaborated on the consequences for researchers when applying CARA as well as on the consequences for the study design and data collection and analysis of the research. Overall, this chapter illustrates the use of the CARA research framework, which is typical of health promotion research as CARA provides a solution to align the health promotion research with new insights into complex systems thinking.

References

Atkinson, J.-A., Wells, R., Page, A., Dominello, A., Haines, M., & Wilson, A. (2015). Applications of system dynamics modelling to support health policy. *Public Health Research and Practice, 25*(3), e2531531.

Bartelink, N. (2019). *Evaluating health promotion in complex adaptive school systems: The healthy primary School of the Future*. Maastricht University.

Bartelink, N., van Assema, P., Jansen, M., Savelberg, H., Willeboordse, M., & Kremers, S. (2018). The healthy primary School of the Future: A contextual action-oriented research approach. *International Journal of Environmental Research and Public Health, 15*(10), 2243.

Bartelink, N., van Assema, P., Jansen, M., Savelberg, H., & Kremers, S. (2019a). The moderating role of the school context on the effects of the healthy primary School of the Future. *International Journal of Environmental Research and Public Health, 16*(13), 2432.

Bartelink, N., van Assema, P., Jansen, M., Savelberg, H., Moore, G., Hawkings, J., et al. (2019b). Process evaluation of the healthy primary School of the Future: The key learning points. *BMC Public Health, 19*(1), 698.

Bartelink, N., van Assema, P., Kremers, S., Savelberg, H., Gevers, D., & Jansen, M. (2019c). Unravelling the effects of the healthy primary School of the Future: For whom and where is it effective? *Nutrients, 11*(9), 2119.

Bartelink, N., van Assema, P., Kremers, S. P., Savelberg, H. H., Oosterhoff, M., Willeboordse, M., et al. (2019d). Can the healthy primary School of the Future offer perspective in the ongoing obesity epidemic in young children? A Dutch quasi-experimental study. *BMJ Open, 9*(10).

Bartelink, N., van Assema, P., Kremers, S. P., Savelberg, H. H., Oosterhoff, M., Willeboordse, M., et al. (2019e). One-and two-year effects of the healthy primary School of the Future on Children's dietary and physical activity Behaviours: A quasi-experimental study. *Nutrients, 11*(3), 689.

Bentsen, P., Bonde, A. H., Schneller, M. B., Danielsen, D., Bruselius-Jensen, M., & Aagaard-Hansen, J. (2018). Danish 'add-in'school-based health promotion: Integrating health in curriculum time. *Health Promotion International.*

Bonell, C., Parry, W., Wells, H., Jamal, F., Fletcher, A., Harden, A., et al. (2013). The effects of the school environment on student health: A systematic review of multi-level studies. *Health & Place, 21*, 180–191.

Boonen, A., de Vries, N., de Ruiter, S., Bowker, S., & Buijs, G. (2009). *HEPS guidelines. Guidelines on promoting healthy eating and physical activity in schools*. NIGZ.

Burton, C. (2012). Heavy tailed distributions of effect sizes in systematic reviews of complex interventions. *PLoS One, 7*(3), e34222.

Damschroder, L. J., Aron, D. C., Keith, R. E., Kirsh, S. R., Alexander, J. A., & Lowery, J. C. (2009). Fostering implementation of health services research findings into practice: A consolidated framework for advancing implementation science. *Implementation Science, 4*(1), 1.

Darlington, E. (2016). *Understanding implementation of health promotion programmes: Conceptualization of the process, analysis of the role of determining factors involved in programme impact in school settings*. Clermont-Ferrand 2,

Darlington, E., Simar, C., & Jourdan, D. (2017). Implementation of a health promotion programme: A ten-year retrospective study. *Health Education Journal, 117*(3), 252–279.

Darlington, E., Violon, N., & Jourdan, D. (2018). Implementation of health promotion programmes in schools: An approach to understand the influence of contextual factors on the process? *BMC Public Health, 18*(1), 163.

Deschesnes, M., Martin, C., & Hill, A. J. (2003). Comprehensive approaches to school health promotion: How to achieve broader implementation? *Health Promotion International, 18*(4), 387–396.

Elliott, D. S., & Mihalic, S. (2004). Issues in disseminating and replicating effective prevention programs. *Prevention Science, 5*(1), 47–53.

Fagen, M. C., Redman, S. D., Stacks, J., Barrett, V., Thullen, B., Altenor, S., et al. (2011). Developmental evaluation: Building innovations in complex environments. *Health Promotion Practice, 12*(5), 645–650.

Fleuren, M. A., Paulussen, T. G., Van Dommelen, P., & Van Buuren, S. (2014). Towards a measurement instrument for determinants of innovations. *International Journal for Quality in Health Care, 26*(5), 501–510.

Gubbels, J. S., Van Kann, D. H., de Vries, N. K., Thijs, C., & Kremers, S. P. (2014). The next step in health behavior research: The need for ecological moderation analyses-an application to diet and physical activity at childcare. *International Journal of Behavioral Nutrition and Physical Activity, 11*(1), 52.

Hawe, P. (2015). Lessons from complex interventions to improve health. *Annual Review of Public Health, 36*, 307–323.

Hawe, P., Shiell, A., & Riley, T. (2004). Complex interventions: How "out of control" can a randomised controlled trial be? *BMJ, 328*(7455), 1561.

Hawe, P., Shiell, A., & Riley, T. (2009). Theorising interventions as events in systems. *American Journal of Community Psychology, 43*(3–4), 267–276.

Hollar, D., Lombardo, M., Lopez-Mitnik, G., Hollar, T. L., Almon, M., Agatston, A. S., et al. (2010). Effective multi-level, multi-sector, school-based obesity prevention programming improves weight, blood pressure, and academic performance, especially among low-income, minority children. *Journal of Health Care for the Poor and Underserved, 21*(2), 93–108.

Kremers, S. P., Visscher, T. L., & Schuit, A. J. (2018). Effect in zijn context [Effect in its context]. *Tijdschr Gezondheidswetenschappen, 96*(3–4), 128–131.

Langford, R., Bonell, C. P., Jones, H. E., Pouliou, T., Murphy, S. M., Waters, E., et al. (2014). The WHO health promoting school framework for improving the health and well-being of students and their academic achievement. *Cochrane Database of Systematic Reviews, 4*(4), CD008958.

Laverack, G., & Labonte, R. (2000). A planning framework for community empowerment goals within health promotion. *Health Policy and Planning, 15*(3), 255–262.

Lee, A. (2009). Health-promoting schools. *Applied Health Economics and Health Policy, 7*(1), 11–17.

Lohrmann, D. K. (2008). A complementary ecological model of the coordinated school health program. *Public Health Reports, 123*(6), 695–703.

Michie, S., van Stralen, M. M., & West, R. (2011). The behaviour change wheel: A new method for characterising and designing behaviour change interventions. *Implementation Science, 6*(1), 42.

Mohammadi, N. K. (2010). *Complexity science, schools and health: Applications for management of change in schools to promote health and education*. Lambert Academic Publishing.

Moore, G. F., Audrey, S., Barker, M., Bond, L., Bonell, C., Hardeman, W., et al. (2015). Process evaluation of complex interventions: Medical Research Council guidance. *BMJ, 350*, h1258.

Moore, G. F., Evans, R. E., Hawkins, J., Littlecott, H., Melendez-Torres, G., Bonell, C., et al. (2019). From complex social interventions to interventions in complex social systems: Future directions and unresolved questions for intervention development and evaluation. *Evaluation, 25*(1), 23–45.

Oosterhoff, M., Joore, M. A., Bartelink, N. H., Winkens, B., Schayck, O. C., & Bosma, H. (2019). Longitudinal analysis of health disparities in childhood. *Archives of Disease in Childhood, 104*(8), 781–788.

Owen, B., Brown, A. D., Kuhlberg, J., Millar, L., Nichols, M., Economos, C., et al. (2018). Understanding a successful obesity prevention initiative in children under 5 from a systems perspective. *PLoS One, 13*(3), e0195141.

Patton, M. Q. (2011). *Developmental evaluation: Applying complexity concepts to enhance innovation and use*. Guilford Press.

Poland, B., Krupa, G., & McCall, D. (2009). Settings for health promotion: An analytic framework to guide intervention design and implementation. *Health Promotion Practice, 10*(4), 505–516.

Pommier, J., Guével, M.-R., & Jourdan, D. (2010). Evaluation of health promotion in schools: A realistic evaluation approach using mixed methods. *BMC Public Health, 10*(1), 43.

Reiser, B. J., Spillane, J. P., Steinmuler, F., Sorsa, D., Carney, K., & Kyza, E. (2000). Investigating the mutual adaptation process in teachers' design of technology-infused curricula. *Fourth International Conference of the Learning Sciences*, 342–349.

Rutter, H., Savona, N., Glonti, K., Bibby, J., Cummins, S., Finegood, D. T., et al. (2017). The need for a complex systems model of evidence for public health. *Lancet*.

Schaap, R., Bessems, K., Otten, R., Kremers, S., & van Nassau, F. (2018). Measuring implementation fidelity of school-based obesity prevention programmes: A systematic review. *International Journal of Behavioral Nutrition and Physical Activity, 15*(1), 75.

Stewart-Brown, S. (2006). *What is the evidence on school health promotion in improving health or preventing disease and, specifically, what is the effectiveness of the health promoting schools approach?* World Health Organization, Regional Office for Europe.

Turunen, H., Sormunen, M., Jourdan, D., Von Seelen, J., & Buijs, G. (2017). Health promoting schools—A complex approach and a major means to health improvement. *Health Promotion International, 32*(2), 177–184.

Van Kann, D. H., Jansen, M., De Vries, S., De Vries, N., & Kremers, S. (2015). Active living: Development and quasi-experimental evaluation of a school-centered physical activity intervention for primary school children. *BMC Public Health, 15*(1), 1315.

Waterman, H., Tillen, D., Dickson, R., & De Koning, K. (2000). Action research: A systematic review and guidance for assessment. *Health Technology Assessment, 5*(23), iii–157.

WHO (1997). Promoting health through schools: Report of a WHO expert committee on comprehensive school health education and promotion.

WHO. (2009). *Health promoting schools: A framework for action*. World Health Organization Western Pacific Region.

Willeboordse, M., Jansen, M., van den Heijkant, S., Simons, A., Winkens, B., de Groot, R., et al. (2016). The healthy primary School of the Future: Study protocol of a quasi-experimental study. *BMC Public Health, 16*(1), 1.

Xue, H., Slivka, L., Igusa, T., Huang, T., & Wang, Y. (2018). Applications of systems modelling in obesity research. *Obesity Reviews, 19*(9), 1293–1308.

Chapter 22
Developing School Health Promotion Through Research: An Example of a Participatory Action Research Project

Marjorita Sormunen

22.1 Introduction

Schools are communities with their own mission and obligations to be fulfilled. They are formal organizations that have objectives for learning and structures for teaching. A national curriculum defines the content for learning, and, depending on the country, local curricula can include learning activities that are specific to an area. Furthermore, schools have a hidden curriculum that can generate values, attitudes and skills within students. Schools also represent a workplace for several professionals who contribute to building a school climate and have roles in school health promotion. Finally, schools are in close interaction with the outside community.

Schools are ideal settings for health promotion but are also found to be challenging social environments from the viewpoint of conducting research (Turunen et al., 2017). As Cohen et al. (2018) point out, there is no one way to conduct research or a single truth to be found. Consequently, there are several ways to approach a school-based health promotion research. The knowledge generated in schools through research is multidisciplinary and is based on different methodological approaches. The ultimate aim of school health research is to produce knowledge that can be applied in ever-changing school environments.

The school community includes pupils/students (children/adolescents), teaching and non-teaching staff (the principal, teachers, school health nurses, psychologists, social workers, cleaners, janitors, canteen workers, etc.) and parents/caregivers. Much research has been conducted where school-aged children and adolescents have been the informants or participants, very often being asked about their

M. Sormunen (✉)
Faculty of Health Sciences, Institute of Public Health and Clinical Nutrition, University of Eastern Finland, Kuopio, Finland
e-mail: marjorita.sormunen@uef.fi

L. Potvin, D. Jourdan (eds.), *Global Handbook of Health Promotion Research, Vol. 1*,
https://doi.org/10.1007/978-3-030-97212-7_22

perceptions related to healthy policies or practices or tracking their health behaviours (e.g. Eskola et al., 2018, Illøkken et al., 2017, Sormunen & Miettinen, 2017). Furthermore, teachers' and principals' perceptions of, for example, their occupational well-being (Laine et al., 2017) or teachers' role in health promotion (Byrne et al., 2018) have been explored as well as parents' perspectives on home–school collaboration in various contexts (e.g. Bordalba & Bochaca, 2019, Bendixsen & Danielsen, 2020). Less research has been conducted where a broader perspective has been taken into account by also including representatives of non-teaching staff, such as in the study by Parikh et al. (2019), where adolescents, parents, teachers, school counsellors and clinical psychologists/psychiatrists were the participants. Moreover, in addition to principals, teachers, school nurses and doctors and counsellors, the study by Jourdan et al. (2010) also included administrative, maintenance, canteen and cleaning staff, which truly provides a welcome and needed perspective in school health promotion research. Health promotion in the school environment is not merely a curriculum-based activity but includes strong informal daily input from all members of the school community. It is equally important to include non-teaching staff in research activities if the research design allows it.

This chapter contributes to the multidimensional research of school health promotion by introducing a research study conducted using a participatory and pragmatic approach that is relevant to school contexts. This chapter also examines the reasons behind the chosen approach and reflects the role of the researcher in an action-oriented intervention study. At all stages, the practical knowledge and experience of the members of the school community are assessed to provide understanding and insight concerning contextual factors.

22.2 Participatory Action Research in Four Comprehensive Schools in Finland

22.2.1 General Description of the Project

Four schools comprising grades 1– took part in a participatory action research project over the course of four semesters (Sormunen, 2012; Sormunen et al., 2012, 2013b). The purposes of the study were to (1) examine the prevailing practices and experiences of collaboration between the home and school and in children's health education, (2) investigate and develop practices related to collaboration in areas of children's health learning and (3) evaluate the effects of a 2-year intervention. In addition, the research and development project was intended to strengthen pupils' knowledge and skills regarding health-related issues in their age groups. One cohort of pupils, starting at the beginning of grade 5 and ending at the end of grade 6, along with their parents and classroom teachers, was chosen from the participating schools as the target group. The school principals, school nurses and health education teachers participated in the planning and development process of the intervention. The development activities were carried out as participatory processes in two

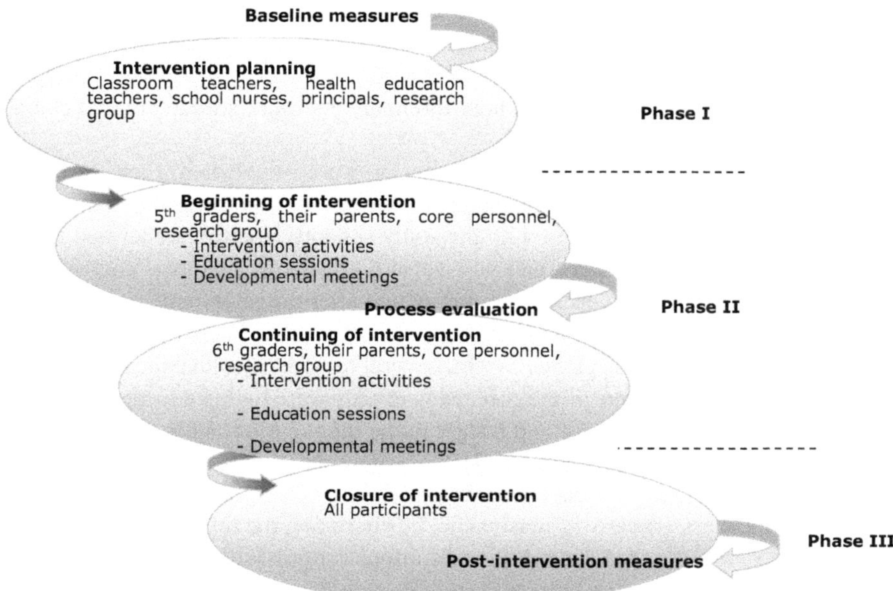

Fig. 22.1 Phases of the study (Adapted from Sormunen, 2012)

intervention schools, whereas two control schools followed the national core curriculum without extracurricular activities, increased parental involvement and strengthened home–school collaboration.

The study consisted of three phases under which four research questions were set (Fig. 22.1). Phase I involved identification of the current stage of the home–school collaboration and homes' and schools' responsibilities in children's health education with the following research questions: "What was the current stage of the home–school collaboration from the viewpoint of parents, pupils, classroom teachers and principals?" and "What was the current stage of homes' and schools' roles in children's health education from the viewpoint of parents?" Phase II included developmental activities through intervention implementation. A related research question was "How was the intervention implemented in schools from the viewpoint of classroom teachers and families in a mid-intervention process evaluation?" The last phase (III) was an outcome evaluation with the research question: "What were the main outcomes of the 2-year intervention study as evaluated by parents?"

22.2.2 *School Selection*

The criteria for school selection were set using five components: 1) school location inside the country, 2) type of school (comprehensive schools, including grades 1–9), 3) obligation to use the national core curriculum, 4) having more than one parallel class in the fourth grade and 5) having no other ongoing home–school initiatives or about to start during the study period. The reasons for setting these criteria were derived from the study design and the assessment of having the highest possible potentiality to conduct the study without too many confounding factors that could affect the intervention negatively.

The following justifications for each criterion were established. First, *location* was restricted to a certain geographical area, since a PAR approach requires ongoing interactions and involvement with the study schools. The researcher had to be able to reach the schools easily, and vice versa. Furthermore, the two intervention schools could connect with each other during and after the intervention, which can add motivation and commitment to the study of both schools. Second, *type of school* was chosen to include class grades 1–9 for several reasons. Health education teachers were invited as members of the core team, as they were highly educated specialists who could bring experience and insight to the intervention. As health education teachers only worked in upper grades (7–9) of comprehensive schools, but the intervention group of pupils and their parents was from grade 5, choosing schools that covered all the class grades was reasonable. Furthermore, the research team wished to include a school nurse as an expert on health promotion with a view and experience of pupils' developmental process, and this would be possible in schools where school nurses have seen pupils from the start of their school path to the end of compulsory education. Including schools with the broadest variety of class grades also made it easier to prepare the pupils and their families to transition to the upper grades of comprehensive schools (after the sixth grade), which is often an exciting phase for families. Third, *obligation to use the national curriculum* excluded schools that may have different curricula because of the pedagogy or special assignment of the school. That alternative curricula could have had effects on the home–school relationship, which was the key variable measured in the study. Fourth, *having more than one parallel class* in the fourth grade was important for ensuring a sufficient number of participants in the study and preparing for loss of pupils and their parents after 2 years of the intervention. Moreover, it gave an opportunity to concentrate on one age cohort and follow the cohort more closely from the fifth to the sixth grade. Extending the study to other age cohorts would have entailed larger developmental differences among study participants and most likely led to challenges in tailoring the intervention. Fifth, the criterion that *no other home–school initiatives were ongoing or about to start* was simply set to minimize the extraneous variables in the study design, which could have threatened the internal validity of the experiment. In addition to the criteria above, both rural and urban schools were selected to find out whether school location would affect the outcomes, which turned out to be the case. After the selection process, the study included four study schools, which were divided into groups of two intervention and two control schools.

22.2.3 Study Design

The study used a quasi-experimental design, which differs from a true experiment by selection of participants in the experimental and control/comparative groups using purposive sampling without randomization (Shek & Wu, 2018). Although there has been debate on using experimental designs in school health research, there is also strong support for such use (e.g. Langford et al., 2015). A quasi-experimental design was selected to be able to answer the fourth research question: "What were the main outcomes of the 2-year intervention study as evaluated by parents?" Specifically, an untreated control group design with a pre-test and a post-test (Cook & Campbell, 1979, p. 103–112) was used. In this design, the study groups (intervention and control) are expected to be as similar as possible before the beginning of the intervention. Finding out the similarity between the groups at the starting point is an important step to be able to assess the effect of the intervention, and it is done using statistical methods in the pre-test/baseline measure (e.g. Sormunen et al., 2013a, b). If the two groups are similar in their pre-test scores but differ in their post-test scores, the indication of the results' effectiveness increases (Shek & Wu, 2018).

As Shek and Wu (2018) summarize, quasi-experimental designs are alternatives when it is impossible to meet the requirements for a true experiment, which is often the case in school environments. They continue to say that, in real life, educational field settings are complex for several reasons, such as difficulties in determining a population or randomizing participants to an experimental or a control group. However, as Langford et al. (2015) present, experimental research, such as cluster randomized control trials, can contribute greatly to the body of evidence and bring valuable insight to understand the components of school health promotion. Moreover, in the broad field of education, conducting experiments has gone from being underrepresented to having considerable prominence (Cohen et al., 2018).

As in this study, experimentation is possible when the essential requirements are met. However, even if clear steps for the conduct of the experiment have been set (e.g. Cohen et al., 2018, p. 411) and optimal conditions for meeting the rigorous standards of experimental study have been met, key persons can drop out from the study, implementation can fail or some other important piece of the process may change. The odds of unexpected situations occurring may even grow alongside intervention length. Moreover, as in this study, one highly unpredictable aspect was the participatory approach, with its fascinating but demanding characteristics.

22.3 Application of PAR in School Health Promotion Research

As schools have become more participatory in nature – i.e. as pupils/students are increasingly involved with processes related to, for example, the school physical or social environment – knowledge production can also be guided in a more participatory manner. In addition to personal effects on students, the review by Griebler et al. (2017) showed that student participation had positive effects on a school as an organization and improved interactions and social relationships in the school. Participation is also a central concept and key value in health-promoting schools (HPSs).

According to Kemmis (2009), action research (AR) aims to change people's practices, their understandings of their practices and the conditions in which they work or act. As Baum et al. (2006) evince, participatory action research (PAR) is collective and empowering, and power is a crucial underpinning concept of PAR. As in health promotion, PAR seeks to achieve empowerment of those involved. Baum (2006, p. 855) continues with an important notion that can be applied to research conducted in schools: "When communities seek control of research agendas, and seek to be active in research, they are establishing themselves as more powerful agents." PAR involves academic researchers and participants working collaboratively: the researcher and appropriate persons in a school community define the problem(s) to be examined, seek relevant knowledge and experience, implement actions in the school and interpret the results of the actions on the basis of what they learn.

In this study, participatory processes were present from the beginning to the end of the study (Fig. 22.2). The cyclical process of PAR enabled joint planning of the study's steps and finding the natural reflection points during it. As Bradbury Huang (2010) points out, an essential feature of action research is combining the context of practice and collaboration of researchers and practitioners with a purpose to generate knowledge, develop competencies and empower stakeholders by planning, acting, observing and reflecting the practice, as illustrated in the figure. The rationale

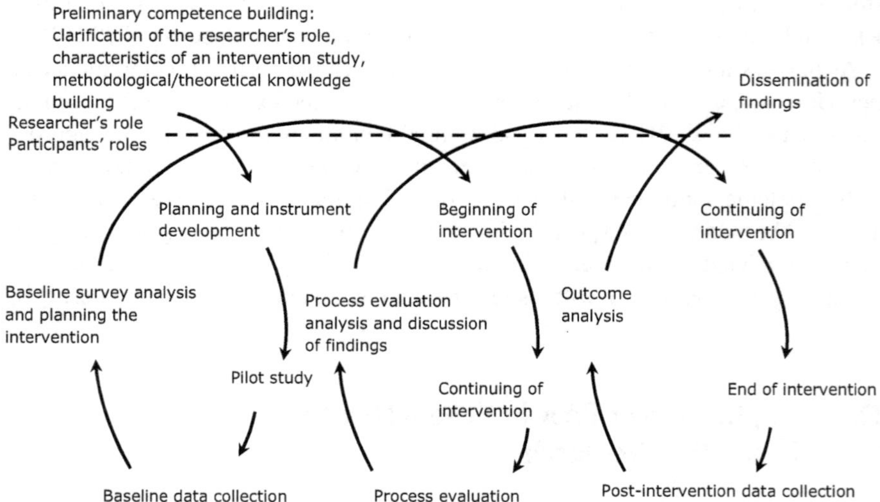

Fig. 22.2 The cyclical process of action research of a school health intervention (Adapted from Sormunen, 2012)

for using PAR in this study was based on collaborative development of health learning in the school setting using the experience and expertise of school staff, researchers and parents and the views of pupils at different stages of the intervention. Applying PAR in the study most likely increased the intervention schools' parents' and teachers' interest in and motivation towards the intervention. PAR is therefore a highly recommended and well-reasoned approach for school health interventions.

As the intervention was concretely intended to inform teachers and other school personnel about supportive communication with parents, to give parents information about the lives of 11 – 13-year-old children and their health issues, to develop new material for interactive health education between the school and home and to build pupils' knowledge and skills regarding multiple health-related issues, it required multiple components. Different activities were planned, scheduled and executed in two intervention schools during 2 school years. The majority of the activities were built on baseline findings, and some developmental activities were started on the basis of the process evaluation findings. The schools themselves prioritized their developmental needs after the researcher analyzed the findings and shared them with the schools.

Although PAR is used widely in health promotion as well as in educational research, the combination of these two areas was a novel approach, especially in this study employing experimental methods. It included an intensive planning phase, followed by several cycles of action, evaluation and reflection that formed a relatively demanding process. The main advantage of a PAR is its characteristic of involving academic researchers and study participants working together, as in the example study: the researcher together with teachers and principals prioritized the problem(s) that emerged from the baseline data, sought relevant knowledge and experience to find solution(s), implemented the tailored actions in the school community and interpreted the results of the actions on the basis of what they learned (see Kindon et al., 2009). Even though some children or their parents did not participate in the surveys, they were able to participate fully in the developmental activities. Families were invited to actively participate in the process, and pupils had their own continuous roles as developers and evaluators.

It was essential to understand that all developmental needs could not be addressed in one participatory cycle. In fact, during one cycle, other, more urgent needs can be discovered, requiring either immediate responses or changing already-scheduled processes. Moreover, the cycles are not identical in their duration, nor are intervention components similarly feasible.

The combination of PAR and experimental design raises several important issues that require attention. One essential characteristic of experimental design is comparison, which means the use of a control/comparison group. In our study, the control group comprised the pupils, their parents and classroom teachers in the two control schools that did not participate in any developmental activities. Their role was simply to follow their normal school routine. This admittedly raises ethical and practical issues that need to be addressed during the study planning phase. Furthermore, in this study, all contacted schools were offered the option to refuse or participate either in the intervention or in the control group, i.e. participation and group selection were voluntary. With a long-lasting intervention in particular, schools may not be keen to participate in the intervention group but are happy to contribute in a less demanding role. Finally, though the intervention was implemented in two schools, materials developed during the intervention were offered to control schools after the intervention.

Naturally, the intervention with a PAR approach had broader benefits for the intervention school participants, since they were involved with the collaborative process. For example, decisions concerning developmental procedures were thoroughly discussed with the core participants, making the decision-making a highly shared process (Sormunen et al. 2012).

22.4 Methodological Choice

As PAR aims to develop practice, the approach that most emphasizes the practical aspect of knowledge, mixed methods research (MMR), was chosen as the most suitable methodological approach for this study (Johnson & Onwuegbuzie, 2004; Johnson et al., 2007; Creswell & Plano Clark, 2011). Although combining qualitative and quantitative methods in the same study can be recommended for school health research on account of capturing the multifaceted nature of school life, there is still ongoing discussion on MMR use, largely based on philosophical differences (e.g. Bryman, 2008; Leech & Onwuegbuzie, 2009; Creswell & Plano Clark, 2011; Ghiara, 2020).

Similar to PAR, MMR also has roots in pragmatism. While PAR is used to improve practice, MMR opens options for answering research questions in the most practical and useful way (Flemming, 2007; Creswell & Plano Clark, 2011); in the study described here, MMR was designed to gather the views of the school personnel as well as those of pupils and their parents on a topic that concerns them all. The chosen qualitative and quantitative methods (questionnaires, interviews, attendance logs) complemented each other, providing breadth and depth in the findings and an increased understanding of the phenomenon. Moreover, mixing methods in the mid-intervention process evaluation phase offered a rich and concrete description of the intervention activities, and the various perspectives analyzed helped find the advantages and deficiencies of the implementation (Sormunen et al., 2012).

In this study, using only a quantitative approach would not have reached the actual root cause(s) of the problems that emerged during the 2-year intervention. Conversely, without a quantitative approach and an experimental design, the extent of the changes in the home–school health partnership would have remained unknown. Exploring and combining quality and quantity is worth considering and also may encourage researchers with different worldviews but a shared research interest to work together (Sormunen et al., 2013a). Different methods have various strengths and weaknesses, and recognizing those can create larger possibilities in research.

In addition to selecting a method from either a quantitative or a qualitative research approach, answering research questions may require combining both approaches, as was the case in our study: pupils and their parents filled out a questionnaire before and after the 2-year intervention, whereas school principals, classroom teachers, school health nurses and health education teachers were interviewed using semi-structured interviews. In addition, during the intervention, families and teachers were interviewed and event attendance logs were reviewed.

22.5 Role of the Researcher

Action research emphasizes the importance of understanding the organizational, cultural and social contexts of the study environment. In a school-based research, prior knowledge and understanding of the dynamics of the ever-changing school environment is essential. Further, the analytical and reflective role of the researcher is meaningful during the process (Greenwood & Levin, 1998). On the basis of experiences from this research study and the earlier literature, several key characteristics can define the role of a researcher conducting participatory health promotion research in a school community.

22.5.1 Discretion

Schools are not laboratories where researchers enter, take the needed measures, analyze and interpret the results and move to another set of measurements. Instead, schools are live settings wherein the researcher *asks* to be included, *negotiates* how to conduct research and what would be the ideal timing for it and *keeps* the key personnel, with whom one is working, *up-to-date*. The way the researcher takes care of these actions undoubtedly influences the motivation of the school personnel for involvement in the study as well as the inclusion of future researchers later. This characteristic also refers to how the relationship between participants and the researcher appears, referring to the epistemological nature of the research. As Cohen et al. (2018) insightfully lay out, planning and conducting research is like art: it is an iterative and often negotiated process between people. The researcher explains what knowledge would be ideal to obtain and – when applied to a school community – the school sets the ultimate boundaries by stating what is possible and in which condition. Making compromises is natural in a school-based research.

22.5.2 Ability to Justify and Confirm – And Be Patient

As always, justifying the research – why it is conducted – is important. The researcher has to be specific and state clearly why a particular school should take part in a study. Furthermore, could it be "our project" instead of "my project"? Even more justifications are needed if the approach is participatory and needs substantially more time than responding to a cross-sectional survey. On the other hand, the outcomes of the research are important to any research study, and, therefore, the steps of the research process have to be executed as planned.

The findings of the process evaluation in our study revealed that although the uncertainty of the intervention development process and its outcomes puzzled the teachers – despite being a normal characteristic in the participatory approach – they appreciated the researcher listening to and speaking with them as well as assuring them that they are not expected to perform miracles. Sigurdardottir and Puroila (2020, p. 85–86) summarize this excellently, stating, "- - *the researcher cannot have complete control over the research process and therefore should remain patient, open, creative, and responsive. The researcher is challenged to allow the research to be process-driven, while also being prepared for unexpected events.*" This description of the reality of action research exemplifies the demands of this approach. A key point of the action-oriented, participatory approach is the necessity of conversing with the study participants before the intervention or activity begins to be able to clarify the process sufficiently for them.

22.5.3 Ability to Listen

Schools work under given policies and working practices and a schedule that structures their annual work. The ability to listen refers to at least three equally important key characteristics.

1. *Listening to schools' wishes* to optimally combine research activities and regular schoolwork, including teaching and non-teaching staff schedules, exam and holiday periods and other major events. If the researcher is unaware of the issues concerning school schedules, it can negatively affect someone's motivation or possibility of participation in the research and can thus damage the validity of the study. For example, it may not be appropriate to invite teachers for an interview a week before a holiday season starts or to send a survey to pupils during their examination week.
2. *Listening to the personnel's experiences and views* regarding ways to "navigate" the school to gain insights into school life. Research in schools is multidisciplinary, meaning that a variety of researchers with different scientific orientations conduct research in schools and naturally cannot have updated knowledge about the continuously changing school life. It is equally important to do "homework" before entering a school or communicating with a contact person: finding out the key characteristics of education as well as schools' features is vital to be able to understand and speak the same "language".
3. *Listening to pupils/students' voices* throughout the study to be able to develop and/or fine-tune the activities that are planned or ongoing in the school. Regarding intervention studies, process evaluation measures are often based on listening to the study participants, which, on that point, is an extremely vital skill to have.

22.5.4 Ability and Motivation to Communicate Findings

Far too often, researchers concentrate on disseminating research within academia through scholarly journals and conference presentations, although the starting point should be how schools could best benefit from the studies in which they participated. Taking part in a research takes time and effort from the school personnel and pupils/students and/or their parents, so opening a discussion about the school's needs at the beginning of the collaboration is recommended. For instance, in addition to academic publications, our study used several techniques to disseminate the findings, such as: (1) sending the key results to the schools in an understandable way using a graphic presentation (PowerPoint) that they could incorporate into their own presentations and embed on their website, (2) presenting the findings at various events at the schools, (3) having a workshop for pupils based on the findings and (4) embedding the findings in educational materials. Moreover, the findings were shared with the municipality policymakers, who were able to justify their actions on the basis of actual data.

22.5.5 Understanding the Principles That Guide (Modern) Health Promotion in Schools

In addition to the generic knowledge and skills that a researcher masters in the context of school research, understanding the unique setting of schools as places where health promotion is embedded both in daily work and in curriculum can be considered an essential starting point. The values underlying health-promoting schools need to be operationalized and shared. Before even starting intervention planning, it is valuable to consider how a researcher and advocate for school health promotion sees the values of equity, sustainability, inclusion, empowerment and democracy (Dadaczynski et al., 2020) being applied to, and further supported in and through, the research project. Furthermore, for schools, health promotion is not necessarily the most important or obvious priority – at least over educational purposes. The language specific to health promotion may also contain concepts that cause insecurity and confusion in participants; therefore, keeping the message understandable to each is vital.

Keeping up with the methodologies, latest advances in research and ongoing discussions in the field as well as reacting to emerging situations are demanding tasks and require active involvement. Moreover, justifying and applying this knowledge in schools in a way that does not impose an additional burden but ultimately offers appropriate tools and creates supportive conditions is important. As written in the Ottawa Charter (WHO, 1986), "At the heart of this process is the empowerment of communities, their ownership and control of their own endeavours and destinies."

22.6 Conclusions and Reflections on Future Research

Based on this experience, school health promotion research benefited from combining methodologies and by applying a participatory approach. Mixed methods research enabled a rich and complementary picture of a school as a community, and participatory action research was intended to bring about social change and develop practices collectively with the participants. Further, measuring the change in an intervention study was numerically possible by tailoring the study design accordingly. Based on our study results, this combination turned out to be successful, leading to positive intervention outcomes and achieving "practical significance" on three intervention components: parental involvement ethos, health education knowledge and health support. Inside these large components were several intervention activities that resulted in greater understanding of the phenomenon and also positive organizational changes that decreased the workload of teachers (Sormunen et al., 2013b).

As Turunen et al. (2017) point out, expected achievements in health promotion and prevention programmes are multilevel and complex, containing many variables that cannot be controlled comprehensively. They see the challenges in school health promotion research related to transferability and the difficulty of replicating interventions and suggest tailoring programmes to better fit each context. These observations were relevant several years ago, and they still are. Moreover, schools have encountered extreme global threats, which, on the one hand, pose challenges to equal schooling and conducting research at schools and, on the other hand, create a need to conduct research in schools to be able to acquire knowledge and transform it into practice.

References

Baum, F., MacDougall, C., & Smith, D. (2006). Participatory action research. *Journal of Epidemiology and Community Health, 60*, 854–857.

Bendixsen, S., & Danielsen, H. (2020). Great expectations: Migrant parents and parent-school cooperation in Norway. *Comparative Education, 56*(3), 349–364. https://doi.org/10.1080/03050068.2020.1724486

Bordalba, M. M., & Bochaca, J. G. (2019). Digital media for family-school communication? Parents and teachers' beliefs. *Computers & Education, 132*, 44–62. https://doi.org/10.1016/j.compedu.2019.01.006

Bradbury Huang, H. (2010). What is good action research? Why the resurgent interest? *Action Research, 8*(1), 93–109.

Bryman, A. (2008). *Social research methods* (3rd ed.). Oxford University Press.

Byrne, J., Rietdijk, W., & Pickett, K. (2018). Teachers as health promoters: Factors that influence early career teachers with health and wellbeing education. *Teaching and Teacher Education, 69*, 289–299. https://doi.org/10.1016/j.tate.2017.10.020

Cook, T. D., & Campbell, D. T. (1979). Quasi-Experimentation. Design and Analysis Issues for Field Settings. Boston, MA. Houghton Mifflin.

Cohen, L., Manion, L., & Morrison, K. (2018). *Research methods in education* (8th ed.). Routledge.

Creswell, J.W., & Plano Clark, V.L. (2011). Designing and conducting mixed methods research (2nd). : Sage Publications, Inc.

Dadaczynski, K., Bruun Jensen, B., Grieg Viig, N., Sormunen, M., von Seelen, J., Kuchma, V., & Vilaça, M. T. (2020). Health, well-being and education. Building a sustainable future. The Moscow statement on health promoting schools. *Health Education, 120*(1), 11–19. https://doi.org/10.1108/HE-12-2019-0058

Eskola, S., Tossavainen, K., Bessems, K., & Sormunen, M. (2018). Children's perceptions of factors related to physical activity in schools. *Educational Research, 60*, 410–426. https://doi.org/10.1080/00131881.2018.1530948

Flemming, K. (2007). The knowledge base for evidence-based nursing. A role for mixed methods research? *Advances in Nursing Science, 30*(1), 41–51.

Ghiara, V. (2020). Disambiguating the role of paradigms in mixed methods research. *Journal of Mixed Methods Research, 4*(1), 11–25. https://doi.org/10.1177/1558689818819928

Greenwood, D. J., & Levin, M. (1998). *Introduction to action research*. Sage Publications.

Griebler, U., Rojatz, D., Simovska, V., & Forster, R. (2017). Effects of student participation in school health promotion: A systematic review. *Health Promotion International, 32*, 195–206. https://doi.org/10.1093/heapro/dat090

Illøkken, K.E., Bere,E., Øverby, N.C., Høiland, R., Petersson, K.O., Vik, F.N. (2017). Intervention study on school meal habits in Norwegian 10−12-year-old children. Scandinavian Journal of Public Health, 45, 485−491.

Johnson, R. B., & Onwuegbuzie, A. J. (2004). Mixed methods research: A research paradigm whose time has come. *Educational Researcher, 33*(7), 14–26.

Johnson, R. B., Onwuegbuzie, A. J., & Turner, L. A. (2007). Toward a definition of mixed methods research. *Journal of Mixed Methods Research, 1*(2), 112–133.

Jourdan, D., Mannix McNamara, P., Simar, C., Geary, T., & Pommier, J. (2010). Factors influencing the contribution of staff to health education in schools. *Health Education Research, 25*(4), 519–530. https://doi.org/10.1093/her/cyq012

Kemmis, S. (2009). Action research as a practice-based practice. *Educational Action Research, 17*(3), 463–474.

Kindon, S., Pain, R., & Kesby, M. (2009). Participatory action research. In R. Kitchin & N. Trift (Eds.), *International encyclopedia of human geography* (pp. 90–95). Elsevier. https://doi.org/10.1016/B978-008044910-4.00490-9

Laine, S., Saaranen, T., Ryhänen, E., & Tossavainen, K. (2017). Occupational well-being and leadership in a school community. *Health Education, 117*(1), 24–38. https://doi.org/10.1108/HE-02-2014-0021

Langford, R., Bonell, C., Jones, H., Pouliou, T., Murphy, S., Waters, E., Komro, K., Gibbs, L., Magnus, D., & Campbell, R. (2015). The World Health Organization's health promoting schools framework: A Cochrane systematic review and meta-analysis. *BMC Public Health, 15*, 130. https://doi.org/10.1186/s12889-015-1360-y

Leech, N. L., & Onwuegbuzie, A. J. (2009). A typology of mixed methods research designs. *Quality & Quantity, 43*, 265–275.

Parikh, R., Michelson, D., Sapru, M., Sahu, R., Singh, A., Cuijpers, P., & Patel, V. (2019). Priorities and preferences for school-based mental health services in India: A multi-stakeholder study with adolescents, parents, school staff, and mental health providers. *Global Mental Health, 6*, e18. https://doi.org/10.1017/gmh.2019.16

Shek, T., & Wu, J. (2018). Quasi-experimental designs. In *The SAGE encyclopedia of educational research, measurement, and evaluation*. SAGE.

Sigurdardottir, I., & Puroila, A.-M. (2020). Encounters in the third space: Constructing the researchers' role in collaborative action research. *Educational Action Research, 28*(1), 83–97. https://doi.org/10.1080/09650792.2018.1507832

Sormunen, M. (2012). *Toward a home-school health partnership. A participatory action research study, 2008-2010*. Doctoral dissertation. Publications of the University of Eastern Finland. Dissertations in Health Sciences 127.

Sormunen, M., & Miettinen, H. (2017). Health behavior tracking via mobile game: A case study among school-aged children. *Cogent Education, 4*, 1311500. https://doi.org/10.1080/2331186X.2017.1311500

Sormunen, M., Saaranen, T., Tossavainen, K., & Turunen, H. (2012). Process evaluation of an elementary school health learning intervention in Finland. *Health Education, 112*(3), 272–291. https://doi.org/10.1108/09654281211217795

Sormunen, M., Saaranen, T., Tossavainen, K., & Turunen, H. (2013a). Monimenetelmätutkimus terveystieteissä (Mixed methods research in health sciences). *Sosiaalilääketieteellinen Aikakauslehti (Journal of Social Medicine), 50*, 312–321. (In Finnish).

Sormunen, M., Tossavainen, K., & Turunen, H. (2013b). Finnish parental involvement ethos, health support, health education knowledge and participation: Results from a 2-year school health intervention. *Health Education Research, 28*(2), 179–191. https://doi.org/10.1093/her/cyt005

Turunen, H., Sormunen, M., Jourdan, D., von Seelen, J., & Buijs, G. (2017). Health promoting schools – A complex approach and a major means to improvement. *Health Promotion International, 32*(2), 177–184. https://doi.org/10.1093/heapro/dax001

WHO (1986). *Ottawa charter for health promotion*. https://www.euro.who.int/__data/assets/pdf_file/0004/129532/Ottawa_Charter.pdf. Accessed 22 Mar 2021.

Chapter 23
Fourth-Generation Realist Evaluation: Research Practice to Empower the NGO – A Reflection on the Case of Sport for Social Change

Alex Richmond, Evelyne de Leeuw, and Anne Bunde-Birouste

23.1 Introduction: Research that Accounts for the Voice of the NGO

Research, evidence and action are integral dimensions of ways to address the social determinants of health and support the achievement of health equity (Baum, 2007). With the launch of the Ottawa Charter in 1986, they have been considered critical to engaging its action areas to promote and sustain health in a community (cf. the Ottawa Charter WHO, 1986; de Leeuw, 2020). It stands thus to reason that the methodologies employed in health promotion research should be aligned with the premises of the Ottawa Charter and take into account the complexity of conditions and associated stakeholders in the health promotion process (de Leeuw & Skovgaard, 2005; Potvin & McQueen, 2008). How this is enacted, however, remains a poignant question in health promotion research practice.

This chapter puts this question into practice in a review of a health promotion study on key stakeholders that are integral to achieving health for all, particularly at the community level. These are specifically, community-based organizations or non-profit non-governmental organizations (NGOs). Referred to in this chapter as

A. Richmond (✉) · A. Bunde-Birouste
School of Population Health, University of New South Wales, Sydney, New South Wales, Australia
e-mail: alex.richmond@unsw.edu.au

E. de Leeuw
Centre for Health Equity Training, Research and Evaluation, University of New South Wales, Sydney, New South Wales, Australia

Local Health District & Ingham Institute, Liverpool, NSW, Australia

Healthy Urban Environments Collaboratory of Maridulu Budyari Gumal SPHERE, Sydney, New South Wales, Australia

L. Potvin, D. Jourdan (eds.), *Global Handbook of Health Promotion Research, Vol. 1*,
https://doi.org/10.1007/978-3-030-97212-7_23

NGO's, these organizations are ideally connected to their community, crafting programme responses correlated with their community needs (Anbazhagan & Surehka, 2016). Yet, these organizations face a key challenge. They often fall subject to the whims of external stakeholders, even researchers, as service providers to institutional interests including governments, corporations, intergovernmental bodies and philanthropies (Anheir et al., 2007).

The Helsinki Statement on Health in All Policies (WHO, 2014) asserts the importance of collaboration, and it is the nature of this collaboration between an NGO and a researcher that is at the core of this chapter. In a review conducted by Corbin, Jones and Barry (2018), the authors assert that collaboration is a negotiation, a promotion of synergy for a common agenda. Health promotion research is not just about collaboration focused on measuring how and if these organizations reach their objectives but how we can better support them to achieve this (Potvin & McQueen, 2008). This requires identifying the right question that the research needs to ask.

Fourth-generation realist evaluation (4GE) is an approach that advocates the negotiation, query and binding of a study's trajectory by working alongside the stakeholders being evaluated, as experts on the socio-ecological intricacies impacting health and well-being in a specific context (Guba & Lincoln, 1989). The research is carefully designed using open-ended interviews structured according to the rules of a Hermeneutic Dialectic Circle (HDC). By following this structure, the study trajectory is defined by the stakeholders under evaluation rather than the researcher. In practice, what we find is that by following this protocol, the NGO is guiding the study to ask the right question. This chapter surmises that health promotion research can draw on the foundations of this methodology to ensure that the research remains credible and relevant to the NGO.

What follows is an explanation on "why" this research methodology is important to the field of health promotion and "how" it can be practised. This chapter draws on a current study exploring a unique case of a community-based organization known as Sport for Social Change (S4SC). Situated against the backdrop of this growing field, this chapter first reviews the concept of methodology against the challenges facing health promotion research. The principles of 4GE are introduced in practice, explaining how the constructivist paradigm structures an appropriate method to create negotiation between the researcher and NGO. This, in turn, illustrates the iterative nature of the research in practice and why it is important. What we can consider in conclusion is that research is not only done to produce evidence on impact but to produce the insight organizations need to support them in delivering sustainable impact within their communities.

23.2 The Methodology Comes First: What Is the Logic Behind Researching the International NGO?

Methodology is the logic behind the methods we use to address pertinent questions (de Leeuw, 2012). The problem influences the question, which, to no surprise, influences the answer. This is why it is pertinent for research to identify the "right" problem, to develop the "right" question and to then facilitate the "right" answer to solve the problem at hand. Yet, what we have to remember is that problems and the socio-ecological environment in which they exist are complex (Rootman & Goodstadt, 2001). Particularly for the NGO, these problems are connected in a dynamic interplay between multiple stakeholders, action, environments for health, community characteristics and potential, individual behaviours and the role of the health system. Therefore, it should be reasonable to expect this complexity across the phases of the research design and in the answers it yields. It is also reasonable to expect that those on the ground with the lived experience of this complexity are best situated to identify the problems. Recognition of this logic in research practice has not always been simple though. We use the case of S4SC to explain this.

23.3 Unpacking the Importance of Methodological Choice: Examining the Logic of Researching NGOs in the Field of Sport for Development and Social Change

Sport for Social Change (S4SC) is the umbrella term encompassing community-based programmes that employ specifically designed sports interventions to yield a "positive influence on [the] public health" of often marginalized and vulnerable communities to increase social inclusion, build capacity, and foster social change (Lyras & Peachey 2011 p. 311; Bunde-Birouste et al., 2010). A significant early contribution towards the practice and visibility of S4SC was made in 2001 by the inauguration of a United Nations task force on Sport for Development and Peace (UNICEF, 2003). Its launch secured early international interest in what was deemed the power of sports to meet development objectives.

By mid-2020, more than 900 community programmes, spanning 120 countries across low-, middle- and high-income contexts, intentionally use sports to deal with the social determinants of health and well-being (Whitley et al., 2019; Bunde-Birouste et al., in press); Schulenkorf, Sherry, and Rowe, 2016). The design and delivery of S4SC programmes hinge on the core practices of health promotion action, specifically embracing and working towards Ottawa Charter parameters: mediation and advocacy (Spaaij & Schulenkorf, 2014), developing supportive environments (Nathan et al., 2010) and building community action for the empowerment of disadvantaged communities (Hancock et al., 2013). These organizations build on the health promotion principles of participatory action, inclusion and empowerment to connect individuals and engage sports' values of fair play, sportsmanship and belongingness (Kauffman & Wolfe, 2010). S4SC programme examples include the use of sports as a health promotion tool to face the HIV/AIDs epidemic in South Africa (Fuller et al., 2010), as a foundation for life skills development in the United Kingdom and Australia (Bunde-Birouste et al., in press), to remove the barriers to equitable gender participation of youth in community sports (Chawansky & Hayhurst, 2015), football for peace building in Myanmar (Shwe &

Bunde-Birouste, 2018) and to promote the employability of the disenfranchised youth in The Netherlands (Spaaij et al., 2016).

The S4SC field has been seen as a fertile ground for evolving research. However, in a review of the field's research practices, early research on S4SC programmes aimed to legitimize growing interest in the power of sports amongst a series of global stakeholders, ranging from community-based organizations to global aid initiatives, corporations and sports governing bodies (Svensson & Hambrick, 2019). The pertinent question seemed to be, what is the impact of these programmes? However, who asked this question? What interest did they have in the answer?

The research parameters for S4SC have been challenged by scholars from its genesis. They claimed that research interests were pursued in a top-down manner by powerful institutions seeking straightforward and easily consumed evidence that would prove S4SC is worthy of their interest and investment into this practice. This placed S4SC programmes as recipients and beneficiaries to the existing agendas (Bruening, 2015; Coalter, 2015). In the past 5 years, we have seen a dynamic shift in S4SC's research methodology. This is a change of focus on "what" is being researched in hopes to better support community organization needs. Even so, we find that studies remain constrained by existing, preconceived frameworks, which may or may not always reflect the contextual nuances of on-the-ground practice (Clutterbuck & Doherty, 2019; Svensson & Hambrick, 2019).

Skills development, community action and empowerment are the core values in health promotion. They connect to the social dynamics that create good health promotive systems (Johansson et al., 2018; Potvin & McQueen, 2008). Yet, what we find in this review of S4SC is that the understanding and appreciation of the dimensions of the research are limited and possibly biased. This is due to the framing of the research by agents higher up in the pecking order rather than by the communities themselves. This disconnect is a moral and ethical challenge. There is a degree of knowledge and expertise that is required for complex research processes, and some of the research is legitimately carried out by credentialed evaluators. However, this possible academic perspective on research must not stand in the way of fully engaging the dynamic communities and their institutions in programme development and assessment.

In health promotion programmes, stakeholders under evaluation should have a vital role in the research, particularly to ensure that the knowledge generated by the programme adequately describes the actual reality lived by the programme's social actors (de Leeuw & Harris-Roxas, 2016). This is where paradigmatic underpinnings of the fourth-generation realist evaluation (4GE) ensure that empowerment and participation support (1) the questions we ask, (2) for whom we ask the question and (3) how we action the answers.

23.4 The Principles of Fourth-Generation Realist Evaluation (4GE): An Overview of the Concepts and an Examination of the Research in Practice

Fourth-generation realist evaluation (4GE) aims to reduce the practice of top-down-driven research by including intensive stakeholder participation in determining the course of evaluation. The methodology embraces the parameters of empowerment and participation through a set of specific approaches applied to better understand and frame a specific reality; but, in contrast to other research traditions, it is a reality massaged and moulded by the stakeholders seeking answers to questions that they deem pertinent (Guba & Lincoln, 1989). In further contrast to other research approaches, the central argument of 4GE is that research should be an act of inclusion, a means to minimize exploitation of NGOs rather than contribute to it (Guba & Lincoln, 1989).

Engagement in 4GE principles results in two constructions of a phenomenon, one based on merit and one based on worth. The merit construction is a convergence of all different means to how the stakeholders make sense of a phenomenon. It describes the intrinsic qualities of the phenomenon, while worth constructions describe the extrinsic qualities, those that describe its usefulness and applicability in each setting (Guba & Lincoln, 1989). Ultimately, the aim is to identify what the issue is, reflective of all stakeholder voices, and to develop an agenda to approach it. In the next section, we address the key characteristics of the 4GE methodology. Each of these will be illustrated by an explanation of a current study on the case of S4SC.

Research Context The emergent practice of social enterprise in S4SC provides a unique case to explore how researchers develop studies that better support community organizations. The following explanation of 4GE draws on the collaborative study between the S4SC research team, i.e. the authors of this chapter, at the School of Population Health at the University of New South Wales (Sydney) and the largest S4SC network, Streetfootballworld (SFW).[1] The network facilitates knowledge exchange and capacity-building processes to support member organizations. Social Enterprise Assist (SEA), (www.social-enterprise-assist.org) is the social enterprise capacity-building arm of the SFW network. This study furthers the efforts of the SEA to educate and support organizations about the application of social enterprise to move towards sustainability. A research question was developed, and a preliminary insight into the problem was gained. While we initially queried "How does social enterprise contribute towards the financial sustainability of S4SC organizations?" we soon found that this was not the right question to ask. How we reached this conclusion is explained in each subsequent section while drawing on the principles of 4GE.

[1] SFW is a global network of 135+ S4SC organizations, together employing 8000+ staff and reaching more than 2 million youths around the globe (www.streetfootballworld.org).

The Research Paradigm Context is unique to each NGO. Yet, often researchers impose a priori assumptions to try to make sense of a concept or a particular phenomenon. This can result in denying the relevance of the context, as the assumption may be incongruent to the lived reality of the organization. Constructivism underpins the 4GE methodology as a means to face this challenge and account for each reality. Therefore, in this study, it underpins the development a study trajectory relevant to the concerns and interests of each NGO in the field. In order to achieve this, we ground our work in the three assumptions informing the constructivist approach (Guba & Lincoln, 1989) (see Table 23.1). Overall, these assumptions refer to how we interpret the qualities of the concept relative to each individual, the relationship of an individual with that concept and the process and rules to follow for inquiry into this.

Together, these assumptions reflect a progressive shift in the methodological repertoire of the researcher (Lincoln, 2003). What is interesting are the findings that this shift uncovers. According to Guba and Lincoln (1989) "the algorithm" for conducting research is a process that starts with "a method for determining what questions are to be raised" (p. 39). By considering the interests and concerns of these stakeholders, research first and foremost unpacks what the issue is and then reflects upon this to better define the research processes.

What we find at the heart of constructivism is accountability to those under evaluation. Rather than being passive participants, answering questions in carefully structured and controlled realities, these stakeholders are in the driver's seat. Each of these participants educates and negotiates with the researcher on the concept as well as shares their own experience with other stakeholders. This facilitates a system of mutually beneficial knowledge exchange, which results in data. The role of the researcher is to listen, digest and interpret the parameters each stakeholder uses to bind the concept under review. While the researcher is encouraged to facilitate these conversations with his or her own knowledge of the concept, these preconceptions should not negate those of the stakeholders (Guba & Lincoln, 1989).

Table 23.1 Core assumptions of the constructivist paradigm

Assumption	Type	Explanation
Relativism	Ontological assumption	The means to identify the relative nature of a concept. Rather than suggesting that "anything goes", the researcher understands that "anything" exists and that it exists according to each individual's process to organize and make sense of that concept.
Transactional subjectivism	Epistemological assumption	This assumption suggests that what we know is according to the information available to us.
Hermeneutic dialecticism	Methodological assumption	This assumption suggests that the concept constructed is based on the perspectives of several individuals and stakeholders because the research has travelled through a process of identifying, interpreting and juxtaposing conflicting and similar ideas to form a holistic representation of those involved.

In the case study presented in this chapter, such accountability was not initially included in the study's core design. The authors initially began the study to better understand "social enterprise" as a key parameter to the research question: "How does social enterprise contribute towards the financial sustainability of S4SC organizations?" Initial assumptions regarding the concept stemmed from the authors' own experience with social enterprise development as well as interaction with other SFW network members.

A pilot survey was an integral building block to this assumption. This survey of 125 SFW network members aimed to map the sustainable funding mechanisms that support these organizations (see Elkington & Bunde-Birouste, 2017). A total of 27 organizations indicated the constant financial stress that hinders organizations' capacity to foster lasting social change, scale their impact and maintain a dedicated workforce (Rottkamp & Bahazhevska, 2016). Thus, at this stage, it was believed that social enterprise was a mechanism to deal with the perennial challenge of financial sustainability (Elkington et al., 2019).

It is possible that our assumption was based on the way we framed the initial question. We were searching for sustainable funding mechanisms, so it should not have surprised us that we aligned our interpretation with theoretical assumptions that social enterprises are non-profit organizations that move "away from reliance on more traditional forms of income" by developing their own businesses to approach revenue generation (Arpinte et al., 2010, p. 154). In-depth exploration using open-ended interviews with participants, asking them to explain the mandate of their enterprise and its role in the programme, challenged our assumption and merited further engagement with the network to unpack this concept (see Table 23.2).

Social enterprise is fraught with the unknown and plagued by an inconsistency of definitions (Defourny & Nyssens, 2017; Litrico & Besharov, 2019). Social enterprise definitions vary to reflect specific research questions, to describe operations in a specific context or for clarity within a policy agenda (Pestoff & Hulgard, 2016). This yields an almost infinite number of understandings and operationalizations falling under the umbrella of social enterprise. It is not a matter of picking and choosing one but putting the question to the stakeholders. Here is where we started to be accountable to their voice and turned towards the paradigmatic underpinnings of 4GE to guide this process.

23.5 Hermeneutic Dialecticism: Unpacking Key Issues to Identify the Right Question

A question now arises: How do we ensure that accountability to the programme stakeholders is embedded in the research methods? We needed to structure this accountability. The answer was to draw on the principles of hermeneutic dialecticism and interpret the juxtaposition of the multiple experiences within the SFW network, including our own as researchers. 4GE uses an interview protocol known

Table 23.2 SFW network member responses to social enterprise operationalization

Organization	Country of operations	Description of the enterprise	Defined role of the enterprise
Organization A	St. Lucia	Social enterprise is the management of farmland. The enterprise was initially started to generate jobs for the youth beneficiaries coming through the programme as the beneficiaries approached the organization asking for this opportunity to be created. The youth initiated and developed the programme as a life skills pathway.	The role of the enterprise is twofold: to generate employability for the programme youth upon graduation from the programme and to generate income for the organizations.
Organization B	Colombia	The organization maintains several social enterprises including a guest house, a print shop and a bakery. These enterprises are to create income for the S4SC programme and to provide unique life skills development training for the youth. Their enterprises also support other needs of the organizations in the network, such as screen printing of jerseys.	The role of the enterprise is twofold: to generate employability for the programme youth upon graduation from the programme and to generate income for the organizations.
Organization C	South Africa	The organization contracted with the federal government to fill the gaps in youth education and treatment of HIV/AIDS. They supply a unique approach to identify vulnerable youth and provide a safe place for engagement in activity, education and treatment.	The role of the enterprise is to fill the gap left by public services by contracting with government departments for the purpose of harnessing engagement with the local youth.
Organization D	United Kingdom	The social enterprise provides resources for events throughout the region of their operations. This is specifically a smoothie bicycle machine hired out by individuals, corporations and private parties. The current management of this business is only handled by staff rather than as an employment opportunity for programme beneficiaries.	The role of the social enterprise is to generate income for the social programme.
Organization E	Portugal	The organization operates several social enterprises to ensure job creation for the vulnerable population in their region. This includes Airbnb cleaning services, mobile car wash and a café.	The role of the social enterprise is to generate employability pathways for programme beneficiaries and to directly support their community.

as the Hermeneutic Dialectic Circle (HDC). This protocol falls within the responsive constructivist paradigm as the research *constructs* the concept from three different types of perceptions, being sure to *respond* and consider each stakeholder voice as relevant to the study (Guba & Lincoln, 1989).

The initial step is to identify the relevant stakeholders. In the case of the study on S4SC, it was the SFW network. However, we wanted to engage those with experience in social enterprise. To ensure that we did not identify organizations solely based on our assumption of the term, we returned to the network and asked members to nominate others across the SFW Network who currently operate social enterprises and who they would like to learn from. There were 40 respondents from the 129 organizations. Respondents nominated a total of 16 organizations, with multiple organizations receiving 2 or more nominations. We triangulated the nominations against the pilot survey responses and found organizations nominated that had clearly stated that they were NOT social enterprises. Following the principles of 4GE, we had to determine what created the inconsistencies. Were we asking the right question?

Engaging the guiding principles of the HDC requires a continuous interplay of discovery and assimilation. Discovery comes first. The researcher uses an open-ended interview structure to identify the unique perceptions held by each stakeholder on the phenomenon under review. Upon completion of the interview, each stakeholder identifies the next stakeholder who they believe will broaden the parameters on the researcher's current understanding of the interrogative field (Guba & Lincoln, 1989; Mathison, 2005). Discovery is the process to identify each unique perception of the study's relevant stakeholders. Throughout this process, assimilation occurs to ensure ongoing analysis of the stakeholder's perceptions. Ideally, interviews become increasingly more structured, with each answer by previous stakeholders serving as a prompt to new stakeholders until discussion on each construct reaches redundancy (Koch, 2000). Assimilation incorporates each new discovery yielded by the stakeholders into the existing knowledge about the evaluand, or as we tend to refer to it, the phenomenon under review. By the end of the circle, the researcher gains a holistic understanding of the topic under review, an understanding of a concept framed by those with the greatest stake in the phenomenon (see Fig. 23.1). The principle that is most notable here is that the interview processes require ongoing development of the phenomenon to further interpret the experiences of the next participants.

We pursued the initial series of semi-structured key informant interviews with six network member organizations to identify the inconsistencies of nominations and assumptions. Informants were asked to describe social enterprise and given their perception of the term, i.e., why they believe they were nominated. Here, we thought we might start addressing what was the core challenge of our initial question. Following this, the authors and interviewees engaged in a discussion about the organizations' social purpose, their practices, the organization and/or enterprise structure and how they achieve their success.

This early analysis was conducted using an inductive thematic approach that permitted us to create early analytical interpretations of what was being said during the interviews to unpack the inconsistencies and identify what about these organizations made them notable to others in their network. These early observations showed that there are key activities across these organizations that enable them to maintain a consistent level of conditions, which not only progress their social mission but

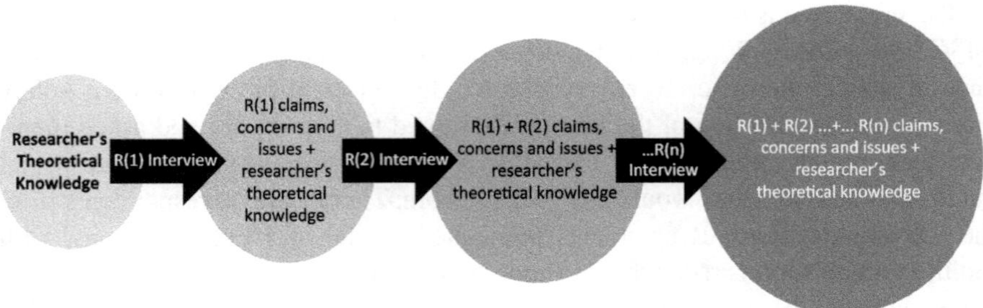

Fig. 23.1 Generalized description of the HDC

also substantiate the longevity of that mission. This notion of "longevity" mirrored a parameter in our study's research question – sustainability.

Sustainability is a fuzzy concept, particularly for the NGO. Swerissen and Crisp (2004) have asserted that it is the gold star outcome of these organizations, while others assert that it is the processes and procedures they must engage with to survive (Phillips & Hebb, 2010). Perhaps, the challenge is more in line with Baldwin's (2020) assertion that research just understands sustainability as many things including an item, an outcome or a strategy; thus, it is a concept that merits further review. For this study, we once again had to face an a priori assumption regarding the nature of a concept. While initially this was social enterprise, the processes and procedures of the nominated organizations were much more than just financial processes, so, perhaps, our assumption that sustainability is solely financial was incongruent to the network's reality as well.

We thus shifted the lens of our analysis to interpret the study stakeholders and what they were saying about sustainability. This involved incorporating the experiences of each nominated organization into a holistic representation of sustainability (see Fig. 23.2).

23.6 A Concept Reflective of the Stakeholder Voice: How Did We Get Here and for What Purpose?

What follows is an explanation of how we interpreted sustainability in a manner reflective of the stakeholders' voices. We do this for the purpose of highlighting the notion of *representative*. While not all stakeholders elicited claims regarding each of the dimensions highlighted in Fig. 23.2, we did not negate any outliers. The concept needed to be reflective of each voice. Following this, we could continue negotiating with the SFW network to develop and refine the concept, constantly recycling this process until we understand any conflicting perceptions and how we can action these findings within a common agenda (Guba & Lincoln, 1989).

According to the study stakeholders, sustainability involves two major components, one internal and inherent to the construct of sustainability in the operations of

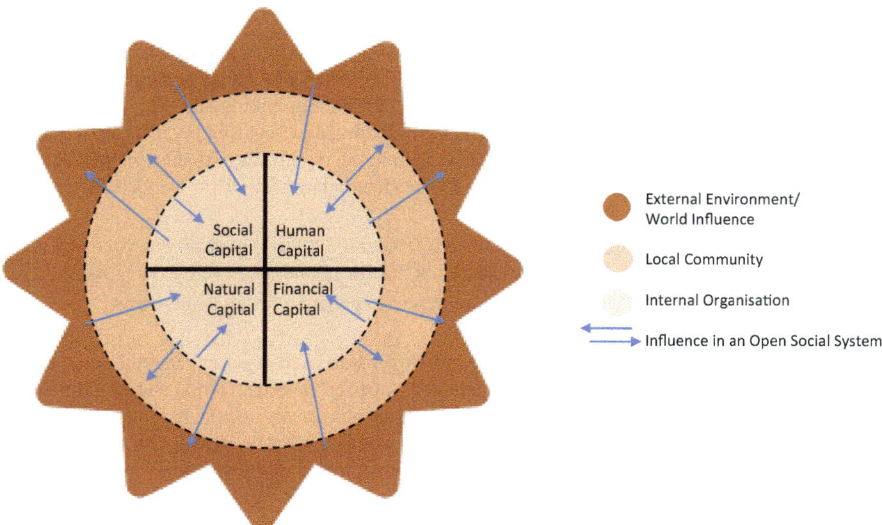

Fig. 23.2 Sustainability framework representative of the dialectic circle

the organization and the other driven by external forces. This is illustrated in the framework as the two inner circles, respectively. The internal dimensions of the framework are financial capital, social capital, natural capital and human capital (see Table 23.3). We have used these terms because "capital" implies a component of the organization, which supports the delivery of their programme and reflects their capacity to meet their goals. Each capital is situated within the same internal circle, indicating that these capitals do not exist within their own unique silo.

Following this example, we believe that we had to "silo-bust" and articulate the internal component of sustainability as a series of interconnected constructs. The challenges, as well as the opportunities faced by these organizations, are complex and multifaceted, such that there is a multiplier effect. This suggests that when one capital is acted upon, changes may result in another (The Secretariat of Catalyst 2030, 2020). Given this, the capitals are all situated within a single circle to account for this interplay.

Moving outwards in the framework, we see that an organization sits within the external dimensions of the framework, the second circle. This dimension is context-based depending on the organization under analysis. The external dimension represents the socio-ecological complexities inherent within a community such as individual behaviour, the overall environment for health and community characteristics (Vermeulen et al., 2016). We have included this dimension because organizations revealed that their primary focus was to meet the community needs and act upon the social determinants as outlined in the organization's objective and mission. Rather than the day-to-day needs and complexities in which organizations exist, additional external influences may impact the programme and community. We have illustrated these as the outer ring in Fig. 23.2. During the interviews, one

Table 23.3 Defining the capitals of internal sustainability

Social capital	This is the co-creation of social networks and relationships amongst an organization's workforce, which generates specific value for an organization and external environment. It reflects elements of bonding, linking and bridging capital, i.e. how the organization bonds similar individuals such as employees, works with the community in reciprocity such as linking the organization to the community and provides bridges to external environments beyond immediate networks (Claridge, 2018; Bhaandari & Yasunobu, 2009).
Natural capital	This is the stock of resources gathered from our natural (physical) surroundings, which are used to generate greater value for the organization (Olewiler, 2006).
Financial capital	This is anything with monetary value used to generate future value for an organization (Coleman, 2007).
Human capital	This is the total accumulation of knowledge, skills and development embodied in an organization's workforce, which creates value for the organization and its external environment/stakeholders. This term focuses on the value of the individual rather than the value of the group. Therefore, this term is often confused with the "hired talent" of an organization. However, organizations do not just appreciate the talent upon which an employee arrives at the organization but also their capacity to innovate, grow and adapt to the organization and its goals (Pasban & Nojedeh, 2016).

organization spoke about the impact of governmental regime changes on their programme delivery, funding, capacity to develop government partnerships and influence policy. This discussion with one stakeholder illustrated that there are external influences, which do not have constant impact on the organization. A timely example at the writing of this chapter would also be the COVID-19 pandemic. These are changes in the external macro environment, which influence organizations.

We have placed arrows within the framework to further account for the interplay of stakeholder interests, resources and external influences, which impact and/or drive the capacity of organizations to facilitate social change. It would be foolish of us to claim that the internal and external elements components exist independently. This would not only be incompatible to the overall integration and construction within the 4GE protocol but also, contrary to our understanding of community-based programmes, as open social systems (Potvin & McQueen, 2008). Community-based organizations need to respond to and interact with their direct community and potentially external stakeholders across the world. Our research indicates that civil society organizations require an ongoing exchange of capitals between the organization and society and communication and engagement with the community to not deplete their capacity to deliver their mission. This, in turn, is a holistic view of sustainability. For a civil society organization to do good in perpetuity, they need to draw on their core capitals while responding with equal emphasis to their community and its needs. If we fail to consider this interplay, we would be reinforcing many of the current challenges to the concept of sustainability (Baldwin, 2020) and, additionally, develop a concept on sustainability, which may be incompatible with some of the stakeholders' values and voices. This is vitally important when we start to think about how this framework may be implemented.

Though this framework is notable to research on the NGO, the framework development is a result of *hermeneutic dialecticism*. If we agree that "the algorithm" for conducting research is a process that starts with "a method for determining what questions are to be raised" (Guba & Lincoln, 1989 p. 39), then it stands to reason that the concept of sustainability is our question and the associated framework is the next step in the process. This framework is the research agenda to address our question. It will guide all further negotiations on interpreting and conceptualizing this complex system of sustainability within the NGO. We therefore pursue this study by asking "what is sustainability?" and "how does social enterprise contribute to it?"

Analysis The reality of the researcher and that of the NGO may not always agree, but what shapes health promotion research is its propensity to understand and answer to communities and, of particular interest to this chapter, the NGOs supporting them. Community-based participatory research is one of the critical research designs in health promotion to identify needs and address health inequities. It invites multiple stakeholder groups, including community leaders, health officials, researchers, funders and governments just to name a few, to the table to identify the disproportionate health outcomes across vulnerable communities and how to address them (Oetzel et al., 2018). This model of engagement reflects the values of the Ottawa Charter and distinguishes health promotion research (Potvin & McQueen, 2008). However, what this chapter discovers is that the initial nature of collaboration and conversation between these relevant stakeholders and the researcher may continue to be imbalanced if we do not structure it properly.

This study's initial failure to engage the principles of 4GE revealed this imbalance. Once this study recognized that notable S4SC organizations were turning to social enterprise to financially support their programme delivery, we thought we had the answer to a significant challenge experienced across the network – we would research social enterprise and how to operationalize it across the field. It also stood to reason that our research remained inclusive. We were designing research that was reflecting both a need (financial inconsistency) and an appropriate action to face this (social enterprise). This, we thought, was listening to the network on the back of the survey findings. What resulted was a study that sought to learn more about the concepts of social enterprise and financial sustainability. However, what we failed to realize was that there was a bigger picture. While organizations struggle financially, their overarching aim is a more holistic approach to sustainability, one in which they aim for perpetuity of their impact.

Participation amongst stakeholder groups requires a strong paradigmatic foundation that structures how we lend our voice and give accountability to those living the experiences. This includes all the relevant stakeholders, as it is not appropriate to discount different groups. However, without the right processes and procedures, the nature of participation may not yield the right research agenda. A *constructivist paradigm* provides rules. It provides a foundation to structure the engagement between the researcher and study stakeholders. And, most importantly, *hermeneutic dialecticism*, the structured protocol behind this engagement, reduces the inclination of researchers to impose assumptions onto the experiences of other stakeholders.

What this yielded in this study was a new research agenda. This is the final purpose of 4GE: to develop a shared agenda appreciative of the experiences of those involved in addition to maintaining a shared commitment for all further negotiations. When we can commit to this, we commit to an iterative nature within health promotion research to untangle and understand the complexity of our communities and what it means to achieve health for all.

23.7 Conclusions

Fourth-generation evaluation can render health promotion research more useful to the NGO. The underpinning constructivist paradigm ensures that the researcher is accountable to each stakeholder, interprets the realities of each stakeholder according to the field at large and employs a continuous interplay of data collection and analysis. This imparts an iterative nature to the research, allowing the researcher to continually negotiate with those about the best practice moving forward in the research. When health promotion research draws on this methodology, it is feasible for the study to embrace the values of health promotion set forth in the Ottawa Charter.

The principles expounded on throughout this chapter are critical to ensuring that the participatory nature of health promotion research is not constrained by the assumptions of a research team. What is witnessed throughout this chapter is that we can be critical of our research practices and that we must be critical to continually make ourselves accountable to those we aim to support. To achieve this, how we define the role of the researcher must continue shifting away from managerialism, whereby the researcher is extraneous to the findings (Guba & Lincoln, 1989). This ultimately starts with the questions we ask. If we structure our entry into the research process through intensive negotiations with those under review, then, moving forward, health promotion research questions will be indicative of the lived experiences of those working with the complexity of health and health equity.

References

Anbazhagan, S., & Surekha, A. (2016). Role of non-governmental organizations in global health. *International Journal of Community Medicine and Public Health, 3*(1), 17.

Anheier, H., Simmons, A., & Winder, D. (2007). *Innovation in strategic philanthropy*. Springer Science+ Business Media, LLC.

Arpinte, D., Cace, S., & Cojocaru, S. (2010). Social Economy in Romania: Preliminary Approach. *Revista de cercetare si interventie sociala, 31*, 64–79.

Baldwin, L. (2020). Sustainability in health promotion. *Health Promotion in the 21st Century: New approaches to achieving health for all*, 12.

Baum, F. (2007). Cracking the nut of health equity: top down and bottom up pressure for action on the social determinants of health. *Promotion & Education, 14*(2), 90–95.

Bhandari, H., & Yasunobu, K. (2009). What is social capital? A comprehensive review of the concept. *Asian Journal of Social Science, 37*(3), 480–510.

Bruening, J., Peachey, J., Evanovich, J., Fuller, R., Murty, C., Percy, V., & Chung, M. (2015). Managing sport for social change: The effects of intentional design and structure in a sport-based service learning initiative. *Sport Management Review, 18*(1), 69–85.

Bunde-Birouste, A. W., Bull, N., & McCarroll, B. (2010). Moving beyond the Lump-Sum: Football United and JP Morgan as a case study of partnership for positive social change. *Cosmopolitan Civil Societies: An Interdisciplinary Journal, 2*(2), 92–114. Retrieved from http://epress.lib.uts.edu.au/ojs/index.php/mcs/article/view/1533

Bunde-Birouste, A., Richmond, A., & Kemp, L. (in press). Social Inclusion as a Mechanism and an Outcome in Sport for Good: Football United, Handbook of Social Inclusion, Research and Practices in Health and Social Care, Pranee Liamputtong, Editor, Springer

Catalyst 2030. (2020). *Getting from crisis to systems change Advice for leaders in the time of COVID*.

Chawansky, M., & Hayhurst, L. (2015). Girls, international development and the politics of sport: Introduction. *Sport in Society, 18*(8), 877–881.

Claridge, T. (2018). Criticisms of social capital theory: And lessons for improving practice. *Social Capital Research*, 1–8.

Clutterbuck, R., & Doherty, A. (2019). Organizational capacity for domestic sport for development. *Journal of Sport for Development, 7*(12), 16–32.

Coalter, F. (2015). Sport-for-change: Some thoughts from a sceptic. *Social Inclusion, 3*(3), 19–23.

Coleman, S. (2007). The role of human and financial capital in the profitability and growth of women-owned small firms. *Journal of Small Business Management, 45*(3), 303–319.

Corbin, J., Jones, J., & Barry, M. (2018). What makes intersectoral partnerships for health promotion work? A review of the international literature. *Health Promotion International, 33*(1), 4–26.

De Leeuw, E. (2012). Do healthy cities work? A logic of method for assessing impact and outcome of healthy cities. *Journal of Urban Health, 89*(2), 217–231.

De Leeuw, E. (2020). Health promotion. In J. Firth, T. Cox, & C. Conlon (Eds.), *Oxford textbook of medicine* (5th ed.).

de Leeuw, E., & Harris-Roxas, B. (2016). Crafting health promotion: from Ottawa to beyond Shanghai. *Environnement, Risques & Santé,15*(6), 461–464

De Leeuw, E., & Skovgaard, T. (2005). Utility-driven evidence for healthy cities: problems with evidence generation and application. *Social Science & Medicine, 61*(6), 1331–1341.

Defourny, J., & Nyssens, M. (2017). Fundamentals for an international typology of social enterprise models. *Voluntas: International Journal of Voluntary and Nonprofit Organizations, 28*(6), 2469–2497.

Elkington, M., & Bunde-Birouste, A. (2017). *Exploring sustainable funding mechanisms of sport for social change organisations*. Streetfootballworld.

Elkington, M., Bunde-Birouste, A., & Apoifis, N. (2019). Sustainable funding mechanisms used by sport for social change organisations. *International Journal of Sport & Society, 10*(4).

Fuller, C. W., Junge, A., DeCelles, J., Donald, J., Jankelowitz, R., & Dvorak, J. (2010). 'Football for Health'—a football-based health-promotion programme for children in South Africa: a parallel cohort study. *British Journal of Sports Medicine, 44*(8), 546–554.

Guba, E., & Lincoln, Y. (1989). *Fourth generation evaluation*. Sage.

Hancock, M., Lyras, A., & Ha, J. (2013). Sport for development programs for girls and women: A global assessment. *Journal of Sport for Development, 1*(1), 15–24.

Johansson, A., Ericsson, I., Boström, M., Björklund, A., & Fristedt, S. (2018). A participatory evaluation of the health promotion programme "more healthy years of life" programme among senior citizens in Sweden. *Cogent Medicine, 5*(1), 1521085.

Kauffman, P., & Wolffe, E. (2010). Playing and protesting: Sport as a vehicle for social change. *Journal of Sport & Social Issues, 34*(2), 154–175.

Koch, T. (2000). 'Having a say': negotiation in fourth-generation evaluation. *Journal of Advanced Nursing, 31*(1), 117–125.

Lincoln, Y. (2003). Fourth generation evaluation in the new millennium. In *Evaluating social programs and problems: Visions for the new millennium* (pp. 77–90).

Litrico, J., & Besharov, M. (2019). Unpacking variation in hybrid organizational forms: Changing models of social enterprise among nonprofits, 2000–2013. *Journal of Business Ethics, 159*(2), 343–360.

Lyras, A., & Peachey, J. (2011). Integrating sport-for-development theory and praxis. *Sport management review, 14*(4), 311–326.

Mathison, S. (2005). *Encyclopedia of evaluation* (Vol. 1-0). Sage Publications, Inc.. https://doi.org/10.4135/9781412950558

Nathan, S., Bunde-Birouste, A., Evers, C., Kemp, L., MacKenzie, J., & Henley, R. (2010). Social cohesion through football: A quasi-experimental mixed methods design to evaluate a complex health promotion program. *BMC Public Health, 10*(1), 587.

Olewiler, N. (2006). Environmental sustainability for urban areas: The role of natural capital indicators. *Cities, 23*(3), 184–195.

Oetzel, J. G., Wallerstein, N., Duran, B., Sanchez-Youngman, S., Nguyen, T., Woo, K., Alegria, M., Wang, J., Schulz, A., Kaholokula, J. K., & Israel, B. (2018). Impact of participatory health research: A test of the community-basedparticipatory research conceptual model. BioMed Research International, 2018, 1–12.

Pasban, M., & Nojedeh, S. (2016). A review of the role of human capital in the organization. *Procedia-Social and Behavioral Sciences, 230*, 249–253.

Pestoff, V., & Hulgård, L. (2016). Participatory governance in social enterprise. *Voluntas: International Journal of Voluntary and Nonprofit Organizations, 27*(4), 1742–1759.

Phillips, S., & Hebb, T. (2010). Financing the third sector: Introduction.

Potvin, L., & McQueen, D. (2008). Practical dilemmas for health promotion evaluation. In *Health promotion evaluation practices in the Americas* (pp. 25–45). Springer.

Rootman, I., & Goodstadt, M. (Eds.). (2001). *Evaluation in health promotion: principles and perspectives*. (No. 92). WHO Regional Office Europe.

Rottkamp, D., & Bahazhevska, N. (2016). Financial sustainability of not-for- profits. *The CPA Journal, 86*(4), 20.

Schulenkorf, N., Sherry, E., & Rowe, K. (2016). Sport for development: An integrated literature review. *Journal of Sport Management, 30*(1), 22–39.

Shwe, T., & Bunde-Birouste, A. (2018). Football United, Myanmar, Football for Peace 2017-18 Project Evaluation, UNSW, ISBN-13 - 978-0-7334-3840-0.

Spaaij, R., & Schulenkorf, N. (2014). Cultivating safe space: Lessons for sport-for-development projects and events. *Journal of Sport Management, 28*(6), 633–645.

Spaaij, R., Oxford, S., & Jeanes, R. (2016). Transforming communities through sport? Critical pedagogy and sport for development. *Sport, Education and Society, 21*(4), 570–587.

Svensson, P., & Hambrick, M. (2019). Exploring how external stakeholders shape social innovation in sport for development and peace. *Sport management review, 22*(4), 540–552.

Swerissen, H., & Crisp, B. (2004). The sustainability of health promotion interventions for different levels of social organization. *Health Promotion International, 19*(1), 123–130.

UNICEF. (2003). *Sport for development and peace: Towards achieving the millenium development goals*. United Nations.

Vermeulen, F., Minkoff, D., & van der Meer, T. (2016). The local embedding of community-based organizations. *Nonprofit and Voluntary Sector Quarterly, 45*(1), 23–44.

Whitley, M., Massey, W., Camiré, M., Blom, L., Chawansky, M., Forde, S., … Darnell, S. (2019). A systematic review of sport for development interventions across six global cities. *Sport Management Review, 22*(2), 181–193.

WHO (1986, November). Ottawa Charter for health promotion. In *First international conference on health promotion* (pp. 17–21).

World Health Organization. (2014). *Health in all policies: Helsinki statement*. Framework for country action.

Chapter 24
A Successful Intervention Research Collaboration Between a Supermarket Chain, the Local Government, a Non-governmental Organization and Academic Researchers: The *Eat Well @ IGA* Healthy Supermarket Partnership

Miranda R. Blake, Gary Sacks, Josephine Marshall, Amy K. Brown, and Adrian J. Cameron

24.1 Introduction

There is increasing interest within health promotion research and practice in co-design approaches that involve multiple stakeholder groups in intervention development. The involvement of retailers and/or consumers as part of the process of developing health promotion interventions in food retail environments can increase the relevance of the intervention to implementors and increase the likelihood of findings being integrated into practice (Greenhalgh et al., 2019). However, there have only been a limited number of food retail initiatives globally that have involved co-design approaches.

Interventions designed to encourage healthy purchases in the food retail setting are based on an underlying socio-ecological understanding (Dahlgren & Whitehead, 1991) of the strong influence that these retail environments have on food choice. It is now well recognized that unhealthy food environments have been the prevailing drivers of unhealthy diets and global weight gain seen in the last three decades (Swinburn et al., 2011). With supermarkets accounting for a large proportion of all food and grocery spending (67% in Australia in 2019, for example (Euromonitor International, 2020)), they represent a key setting for the promotion of healthy diets

M. R. Blake (✉) · G. Sacks · J. Marshall · A. J. Cameron
Global Obesity Centre, Institute for Health Transformation, Deakin University, Geelong, Victoria, Australia
e-mail: miranda.blake@deakin.edu.au

A. K. Brown
Healthy Greater Bendigo, Bendigo, Victoria, Australia

L. Potvin, D. Jourdan (eds.), *Global Handbook of Health Promotion Research, Vol. 1*,
https://doi.org/10.1007/978-3-030-97212-7_24

and for addressing obesity. Supermarket retailers and food manufacturers make extensive use of marketing techniques in store, modifying product, price, promotion and placement to encourage customers to buy and eat more (Dawson, 2013; Hawkes, 2009). Foods high in salt, fat and sugar, which are recommended to constitute only a small proportion of the overall diet, are frequently the focus of these marketing efforts (Cameron et al., 2013; Charlton et al., 2015; Grigsby-Duffy et al., 2020; Thornton et al., 2013). However, the potential to promote a healthy diet using the same in-store marketing techniques has been increasingly recognized (Cameron et al., 2016; Chandon & Wansink, 2012; Hawkes, 2009). A diverse range of marketing strategies have been tested to encourage healthy purchases in supermarkets, including shelf tags (indicating product healthiness), product placement, in-store signage, price discounts and taste testing (Cameron et al., 2016).

This chapter describes the development of the *Eat Well @ IGA* initiative. Established in 2013, it involved a collaborative relationship between academic researchers, the local government, a non-governmental organization and Australian supermarket retail partners with the aim of testing the impact of a range of low-cost and scalable supermarket marketing interventions on the healthiness of consumer food purchases. This chapter describes the development of the partnership, the research approach and methodology and the lessons learnt from the *Eat Well @ IGA* initiative. We aim to enhance the understanding of the process, benefits and challenges of a co-design approach to health promotion research involving supermarkets.

24.1.1 Setting

The research was conducted with supermarkets located in or near the City of Greater Bendigo, a regional centre approximately 150 km to the north of the state capital Melbourne, in the state of Victoria, Australia. In the latest census in 2016, the Greater Bendigo municipality was home to 110,000 residents (Australian Bureau of Statistics, 2017). Bendigo faces a substantial burden from non-communicable diseases: just 6% of adults met the national fruit and vegetable consumption guidelines in 2014 and 27% of the adult population are affected by obesity compared to 19% of the total Victorian population (Department of Health and Human Services, 2018).

The retail partner Independent Grocers of Australia (IGA) is the fourth largest supermarket retailer in Australia (~1400 stores and 8% market share) (Euromonitor International, 2020). IGA is a particularly prominent chain in the Bendigo region with more IGA stores there than any of the other three major Australian supermarket retailers. The initiators of the initiative and the main IGA contact were "Champions IGA", which owns five supermarkets in the Greater Bendigo region and nine stores in total.

24.1.2 Study Origin and Formation of the Partnership

The primary motivator for the creation of the partnership was the desire of the retailer to improve the health of the communities served by their stores. Bendigo was one of 12 sites included in a state-wide obesity prevention trial called *Healthy Together Victoria* from 2011 until 2015 (Strugnell et al., 2016). *Healthy Together Victoria* facilitated increased awareness and readiness to take action to improve population diets for both the retailer (Champions IGA) and local government (City of Greater Bendigo). Of relevance, senior representatives of both the retailer and local government had an existing professional relationship. In 2014, the academic partners became aware (via the *Healthy Together Victoria* network) of the desire of the local government to initiate a supermarket healthy purchasing intervention and became involved based on their history of supermarket-related research. A co-development approach to an initial trial was taken whereby, through several meetings, the academic, local government and retail partners contributed their expertise on previous research evidence and the value of evaluation, study design considerations, likely public health impact, logistical considerations and feasibility from a retailer's perspective.

The three initial partners successfully applied for funding from the Victorian Health Promotion Foundation (VicHealth) to conduct three short-term Phase 1 pilot trials in 2015–2016 to test the effects of a series of single interventions on supermarket purchases of healthier foods. Retailer and local government contributions were both in kind, with the retailer providing no funding to support this study. The key collaborator from the City of Greater Bendigo was the primary local contact who acted as a liaison between the retailer and academic partner. Based on the success of two of the three pilot trials, funding (from an Australian government grant, VicHealth and Deakin University) was obtained for a larger and multicomponent randomized controlled trial (RCT) involving 11 stores (5 intervention and 6 control stores) (2017–2018). The timeline of development of the *Eat Well @ IGA* partnership and studies is shown in Fig. 24.1.

24.1.3 Conflict of Interest Management

In collaborating with a commercial operator that makes a profit on sales of a range of foods (including healthy and unhealthy products), the partnership included an inherent conflict of interest. Specifically, the supermarket retailer could be expected to be reluctant to implement changes that would decrease unhealthy food sales in absolute terms, even though this would likely be beneficial from a public health perspective. However, the collaborators agreed that if the initiative aimed to increase sales of healthy foods, this would likely result in a "win-win", whereby the relative healthiness of customer purchases would increase and any loss in profit associated

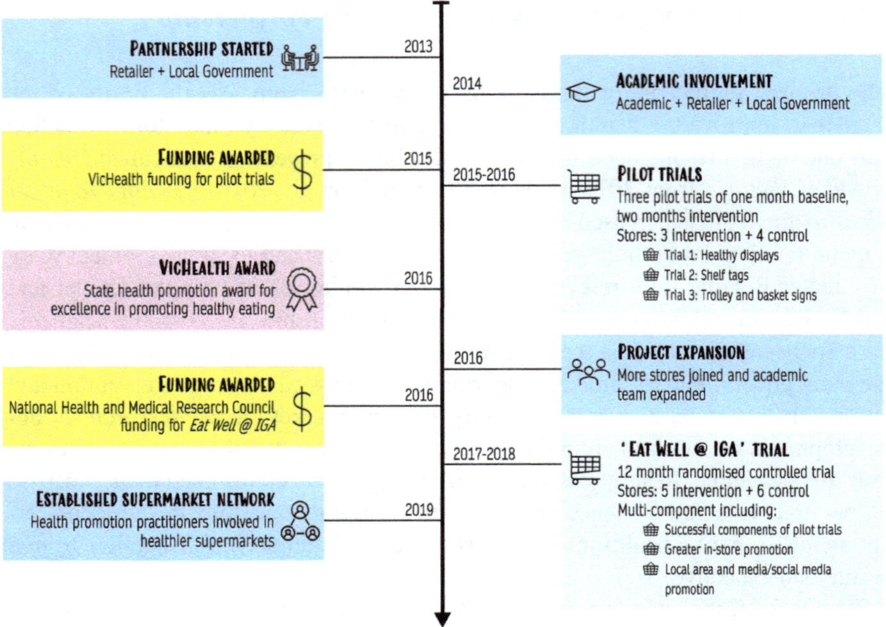

Fig. 24.1 Timeline of the *Eat Well @ IGA* partnership and studies

with decreased sales of unhealthy foods would be offset. The conflict of interest was managed by a clear delineation of partner roles, the provision of external funding to maintain researcher financial independence, the inclusion of the local government in a liaison role, and acknowledging multiple stakeholder priorities and outcomes. Analysis of the results was conducted independently without involvement of the retailers.

24.2 Research Approach

24.2.1 Theoretical Basis

A programme logic model was developed by the research team and used to guide the development and evaluation of the project (Fig. 24.2). The programme logic model summarizes the process of development for Phase 1 (12-week pilot trials) and Phase 2 (a multicomponent 12-month RCT), the underlying assumptions about the mechanism of effect and predicted short-term (less than 6 months), medium-term (6 months) and long-term outcomes (more than 6 months) of the intervention, and the data sources used to capture each outcome. Programme logics are useful tools for demonstrating how an intervention attempts to address an identified

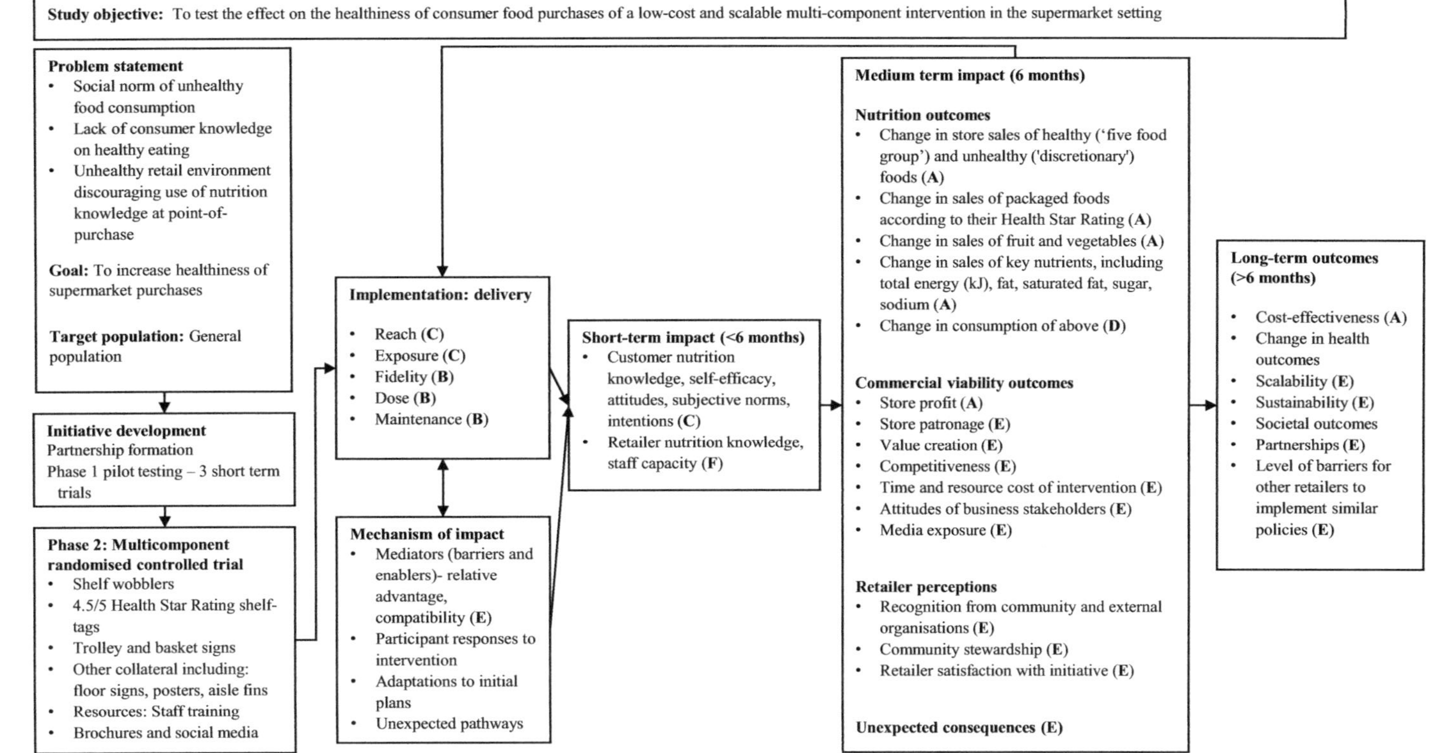

Fig. 24.2 *Eat Well @ IGA* programme logic. Data sources: (**a**) sales data, (**b**) monitoring data, (**c**) customer surveys, (**d**) consumption data, (**e**) qualitative interviews with stakeholders and (**f**) staff surveys

problem and the design of an evaluation to assess if and how the intervention is effective in addressing the problem.

The project used a rigorous controlled trial design and embodied several aspects of the "collective impact" approach including (i) collaboration between multiple actors from different sectors; (ii) solutions developed in real-world conditions of complexity; (iii) continuous learning based on feedback; (iv) multiple organizations looking through the same lens to see change and e) a "backbone" coordinating organization (Kania & Kramer, 2013).

24.3 Phase 1: Pilot Trials

The Phase 1 pilot trials consisted of three 8-week controlled trials in three intervention and four control stores between May 2015 and April 2016. They aimed to test the effects of a series of single interventions on supermarket purchases of healthy and unhealthy foods. The interventions were collectively agreed upon by all partners (retailer, academic, government). The decision to conduct short-term pilot trials rather than a multicomponent intervention was based on the desire to know about the individual effects of specific interventions, to build retailer trust in the interventions, and the feasibility of preparing for a single intervention rather than multiple interventions simultaneously.

24.3.1 Intervention

Designing and selecting intervention components was informed by the previous literature demonstrating their potential to positively impact the purchasing behaviour of healthy products (Cameron et al., 2016; Nakamura et al., 2014; Payne et al., 2015). Where there was insufficient empirical literature, planning was guided by the theory of planned behaviour (Ajzen, 1991) to alter the retail environment through signage, in order to influence social norms and nutrition knowledge. Furthermore, the components were chosen based on their feasibility of implementation and the likelihood that they would be both scalable and sustainable in alignment with the strategic objectives of the retailer (including profitability and customer acceptability). Importantly, increasing the sales of fresh foods (fruits, vegetables, meat, deli products and dairy) was identified as a priority for the retailer because of the relatively higher profit margins on some of these foods, the potential for product spoilage or wastage if these products remain unsold and because their purchase typically encourages "whole store shopping" (i.e. customers who buy these products typically also buy other accompanying products such as other fresh foods, condiments, drinks, pantry items, etc.).

The individual components trialled were: (i) a placement intervention designed to increase the proportion of healthier products at end-of-aisle and island bin displays; (ii) prominent shelf tags (7×10 cm^2) for all packaged products considered

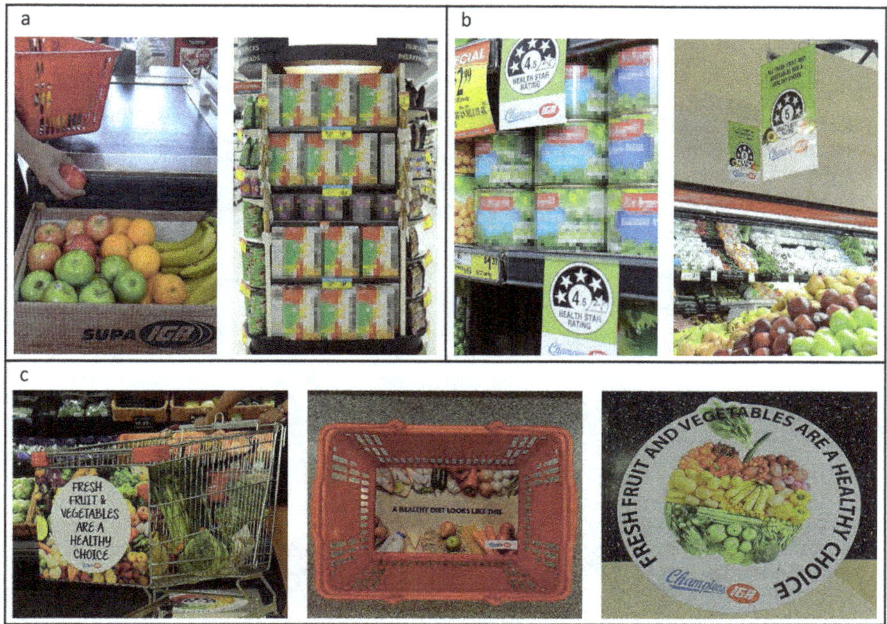

Fig. 24.3 Phase 1 intervention components. (**a**) Trial 1: Healthier end-of-aisle and island bin displays. (**b**) Trial 2: Shelf tags and posters. (**c**) Trial 3: Trolley and basket signs and floor signs

healthy as well as posters promoting fruits and vegetables and (iii) custom-developed signage in all trolleys and baskets promoting healthy purchasing. Healthiness was classified using the Australian government-endorsed Health Star Rating (HSR) system that rates products from 0.5 (least healthy) to 5 (healthiest) (Department of Health, 2019). For the trial, products receiving 4.5 or 5 stars were considered healthy, representing approximately 6–7% of all packaged food items. Examples of interventions are presented in Fig. 24.3.

24.3.2 Evaluation

The Phase 1 evaluation focused on gathering feedback on the potential effectiveness and process of implementing individual intervention components in the context of a complex supermarket environment. The well-established RE-AIM framework (Glasgow et al., 1999) guided the evaluation approach. Specifically, we quantitatively assessed the "Reach" of the interventions (via customer surveys), "Effectiveness" in changing customer purchasing (via sales data) and the way that the interventions were "Adopted", "Implemented" and "Maintained" (via store monitoring and stakeholder interviews with the key local government, academic and retail stakeholders). Lessons learnt from the Phase 1 evaluation were used to inform the development of the Phase 2 randomized controlled trial (Fig. 24.4).

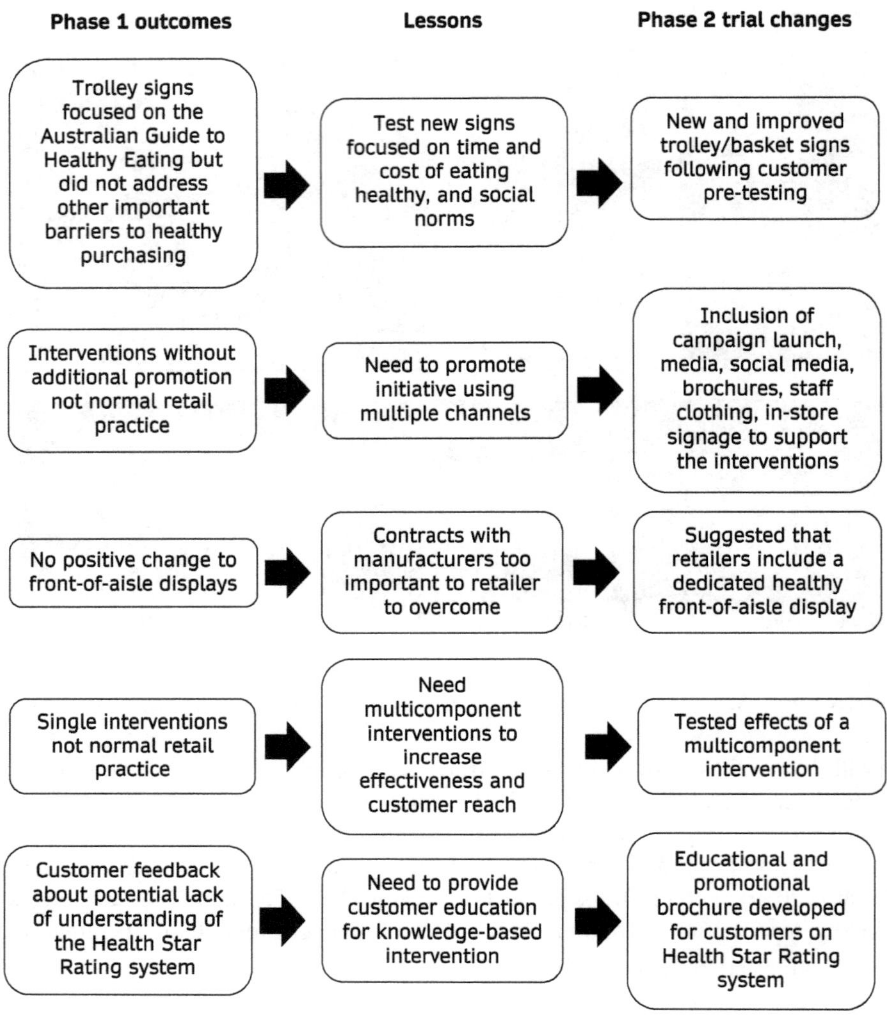

Fig. 24.4 Development of the Phase 2 supermarket trial based on lessons learnt in Phase 1

24.3.3 Lessons from the Phase 1 Trials

Trial 1: Product Placement Intervention

The product placement intervention was unable to be implemented as planned. A nutritionist attended the retailer's regular weekly product placement planning meetings with the aim of assisting the retailer to select healthy items for placement at end-of-aisle and other promotional displays. Although this resulted in a 12.3% decrease in the proportion of unhealthy items at back-of-aisle displays (at the rear of the store), in intervention stores (control stores: +5.9%), there was no reduction in the proportion of unhealthy food products displayed at island bin or front-of-aisle displays. In front-of-aisle displays (near registers), there was actually an increase in unhealthy items displayed in both the intervention (+25.0%) and control stores (+4.9%). Unsurprisingly, given the inability of the intervention to improve the healthiness of front-of-aisle displays, the percentage of healthy foods sold (as classified by the Australian Dietary Guidelines) decreased by 1% more in the intervention stores compared to the control stores between the baseline and intervention periods, with a corresponding 1% increase in unhealthy foods sold (as classified by the Australian Dietary Guidelines (National Health and Medical Research Council, 2013)).

Nevertheless, interviews and customer surveys revealed the positive aspects of the approach. The majority of 754 customers surveyed indicated strong support for healthier end-of-aisle and island bin displays and indicated that this would influence them to purchase more of these products. This intervention was also seen by store managers as a public good. One store manager felt that this was good training for department managers, who themselves noted that they learned a lot about which foods were healthier. Academics and a local council representative felt that, despite the overall problems with implementing the intervention as planned, the implementation of the intervention improved over time with learning from all sides. All interviewed staff noted the tension between this intervention and the necessity to meet the needs of supermarket suppliers, particularly in relation to front-of-aisle displays. Quite apart from the challenges in effecting change in practices, the sustainability and ongoing commitment to this intervention by the retailer were uncertain due to the additional effort required for implementation, including longer weekly meetings.

Trial 2: Shelf Tag Intervention

Overall, the proportion of products sold that were promoted with shelf tags increased by 9.3% in the intervention stores compared to the control stores between the baseline and intervention periods. In all, 35% of the customers surveyed reported that they noticed the shelf labels or posters in the stores, of which 63% believed that it influenced their purchasing behaviours. Interviewed retail staff were extremely positive about this intervention, with good customer feedback and little work involved for the retailer (albeit some missing tags were replaced by the researchers). Food industry representatives had passed on comments that they were happy with this intervention, with the marketing/merchandizing manager commenting that this was his favourite intervention. No significant barriers to ongoing maintenance were identified.

Trial 3: Trolley Signage Intervention

The trolley signage intervention was considered successful from several perspectives. Trolley signage was maintained throughout the intervention period. The retailer reported overwhelmingly positive customer feedback regarding the trolley signage that was consistent with the results of the customer surveys conducted by the researchers. The basket signs were seen by store managers to make the baskets appear cleaner. This intervention required minimal time and resources from the retailer. The signs were noted as being extremely well built with no sign of deterioration 6 months post intervention, with many signs remaining in place in the intervention stores for at least 2 years post intervention. A non-significant increase of 1.1% in the volume (kg) of healthy foods sold (as a proportion of all food purchases) was observed between the baseline and intervention periods, in the intervention compared to the control stores.

24.3.3.1 Summary of the Lessons Learnt and Progression to the Phase 2 Large Randomized Controlled Trial

Lessons learnt from Phase 1 informed the design of Phase 2 (see Fig. 24.4). The Phase 1 trials assisted in overcoming initial supermarket staff scepticism about health-related changes in the supermarket environment. The retailer noted no negative commercial outcomes from either the signage or shelf tag interventions, with both resulting in promising changes in sales of targeted products. An important observation by the retailer was that single interventions without any additional promotion are not a normal supermarket practice, with large changes usually accompanied by substantial promotion in store and in the media. All interventions had the advantage of encouraging purchases of healthy products without using a price discount, which is normally a challenge in retail. The retailer was noted by all partners as being extremely cooperative. All parties felt that the project had strengthened the existing relationships between the retail and government partners.

24.4 Phase 2: A Large Randomized Controlled Trial

24.4.1 Development

The strong and growing relationships, the early success of the pilot trials and the importance of the public health issue led the consortium to submit a grant application to build on the Phase 1 trials. Phase 2 of the project was an RCT funded by a competitive grant from the Australian National Health and Medical Research Council, VicHealth and Deakin University. The study aimed to test a multicomponent supermarket intervention designed to promote healthy purchasing over a longer period in more stores. Stakeholders included an advisory group (eight scientific investigators and representatives from the City of Greater Bendigo), a retailer advisory group of all store owners, the VicHealth representatives are not part of the retailer advisory group.

24.4.2 Intervention

The full multicomponent intervention incorporated the successful pilot interventions (shelf tags, trolley signage) plus additional promotions in store, local area and in media and on social media. Online media promotion included a study website describing and promoting the intervention, and Instagram, Twitter and Facebook posts including recipes and healthy weekly specials. Letterbox drops of 40,000 brochures were made, promoting the intervention in the local area. In-store posters, floor signs, aisle fins and 58,000 additional brochures promoted the *Eat Well @ IGA* brand as well as echoing messages on shelf tags, shelf wobblers and trolley signs. Examples of each component are found in Fig. 24.5.

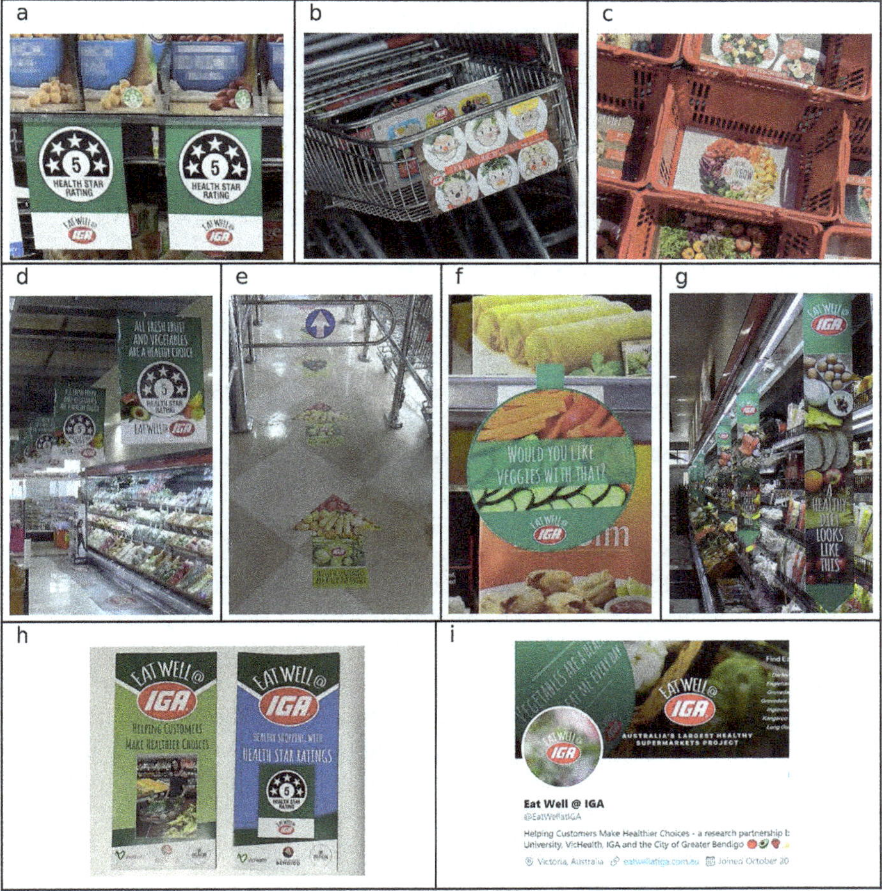

Fig. 24.5 Phase 2 *Eat Well @ IGA* intervention components. (**a**) Shelf tags. (**b**) Trolley signs. (**c**) Basket signs. (**d**) Posters. (**e**) Floor signs. (**f**) Shelf wobblers. (**g**) Aisle fins. (**h**) Brochures. (**i**) Social media

After a 12-month baseline period (May 2016–May 2017), five stores were allocated to a 12-month intervention (May 2017–May 2018). In order to assist with retailer engagement and store recruitment, the six control stores were wait-listed, and they all received the intervention after the trial was completed.

24.4.3 Evaluation Overview

A variety of data sources were used to assess intervention efficacy, sustainability and scalability. The aims, methods and analysis of data sources are summarized in Table 24.1.

The primary outcomes for the trial were the differences between the intervention and control stores in percentage sales of (i) healthy and unhealthy foods; (ii) fruits and vegetables and (iii) key nutrients, including total energy (kJ), fat, saturated fat, sugar and sodium.

Secondary outcomes were assessed in a thorough process evaluation and included (i) fidelity to the original implementation plan and reported adaptations; (ii) project reach to customers; (iii) stakeholder perceptions of *Eat Well @ IGA*, including those of the junior staff, management and customers; (iv) factors that enabled or inhibited initiative implementation and may affect maintenance and scalability and (v) cost-effectiveness of the intervention. At the time of writing, the cost-effectiveness evaluation had not yet been completed.

24.4.4 Results from the Phase 2 Randomized Controlled Trial

24.4.4.1 Purchasing Behaviour Outcomes

At time of writing, full analyses of the primary outcomes were yet to be completed. However, preliminary results based on multilevel modelling show that the *Eat Well @ IGA* RCT resulted in no significant change in healthy food sales overall but in a significant 0.22% increase in the sales for products with a Health Star Rating of 4.5 or higher and a 0.81% increase in the sales of fruits and vegetables (in the intervention stores compared to the control stores in the intervention vs. baseline period). The large volume of data and the associated time for data cleaning, matching nutrition data to purchasing data, and analysis proved to be extremely time-consuming and contributed to an inability to report results back to the stakeholders in a timely manner. Although formal analyses have not yet been completed, the retailer indicated that the profits did not appear to have been negatively impacted.

Table 24.1 Data sources for the key *Eat Well @ IGA* evaluation outcomes of interest

Data source; aim	Brief methods	Outcomes	Participants	Analysis
Sales data To assess the impact of the *Eat Well @ IGA* intervention on sales of key food groups and nutrients	Electronic sales data were collected weekly or monthly from all the intervention and control stores from 12 months pre to 12 months post intervention. Data included products sold, sales price, product weight and the number of items sold. These were mapped by a dietician to an equivalent product in a nutrient database to obtain (i) nutrient data; (ii) Health Star Rating and (iii) healthy and unhealthy food categories.	Differences between the intervention and control stores in store sales of healthy and unhealthy foods, sales of fruits and vegetables and sales of key nutrients, including total energy (kJ), fat, saturated fat, sugar and sodium content and store revenue and profit	N/A	Analysis was conducted comparing the differences in outcomes between the intervention and control stores. Additional analysis based on monthly sales was conducted using linear mixed models.
Monitoring data To monitor fidelity to the original implementation plan and report any adaptations	The intervention stores were monitored weekly for maintenance throughout the 12-month intervention and then again at 3- and 6-months follow-up.	Fidelity of the Health Star Rating tag display (monitored weekly) and shelf wobblers display (monitored monthly); new store initiatives that might promote healthy purchasing and fidelity of other programme components including trolley and basket signage	N/A	Descriptive statistics described the initial extent of implementation and weekly or monthly fidelity to the original implementation plan, per store.

(continued)

Table 24.1 (continued)

Data source; aim	Brief methods	Outcomes	Participants	Analysis
Customer surveys To investigate composition of the customer base and responses to the initiative	Anonymous exit surveys were conducted at 6 months into the intervention. Surveys addressed customer demographics; frequency and use of the target supermarket and competitors, and awareness of, perceived purchasing impact of and attitudes towards *Eat Well @ IGA* (measured on 7-point Likert scales).	(i) Customer demographics; (ii) recall of the intervention; (iii) perceptions of the intervention, intervention components and alternate interventions including effectiveness in promoting healthier choices	Exiting customers at all five intervention sites	Mixed effects logistic regression examined responses by age, gender, socio-economic position by area and shopping patterns.
Staff surveys To (i) investigate staff involvement with and attitudes towards the intervention and (ii) assess perceptions of customer response to the intervention	Anonymous self-completed surveys asked questions on staff demographics, interactions with customers, attitudes towards the overall initiative and specific components of *Eat Well @ IGA* (measured on 7-point Likert scales).	(i) Staff demographics; (ii) interactions with customers; (iii) perceptions of the overall intervention, intervention components and alternate or additional interventions and (iv) perceptions of the intervention and individual component effectiveness in promoting healthier choices	Managers, floor and checkout staff within all the intervention and control stores	Descriptive statistics

(continued)

Table 24.1 (continued)

Data source; aim	Brief methods	Outcomes	Participants	Analysis
Stakeholder interviews To explore (i) stakeholder perceptions of the intervention and (ii) factors that enabled or inhibited implementation and may affect maintenance and scalability	Semi-structured interviews with 19 stakeholders 2–3 months after the official end of the trial. Interviews asked participants to reflect on their role in *Eat Well @ IGA*, its advantages and disadvantages, sustainability, project partnerships and potential improvements.	Programme advantages and disadvantages, sustainability, project partnerships and potential improvements	Purposive sampling of stakeholders given the likely knowledge of different intervention components, including supermarket managers, store staff council employees and research staff	Inductive analysis to identify the key themes
Cost-effectiveness analysis To determine the cost-effectiveness of the intervention package	Cost-effectiveness assessed from a societal perspective including a "trial-based evaluation" (costs and outcomes exactly as per the trial) and a "modelled economic evaluation", which extended the target population (total Australian population), time horizon (lifetime of the cohort) and decision context (all Australian supermarkets).	Changes in the percentage sales of healthy and unhealthy foods converted to changes in energy balance, weight and body mass index (BMI). BMI units saved were converted to disability-adjusted life years (DALYs) saved. Incremental cost-effectiveness was expressed as net costs per DALY saved.	N/A	Simulation modelling was used to calculate 95% uncertainty intervals around the probabilities and cost estimates.

24.4.4.2 Process Evaluation Outcomes

The mixed methods process evaluation effectively captured the perspectives of a range of stakeholders. The evaluation demonstrated high acceptability for the initiative among the store staff, managers and customers and revealed important considerations for long-term maintenance and scale-up of the initiative (Blake et al., 2021). Of the 500 customers surveyed, 97% agreed that the supermarket chain should continue its efforts to encourage healthy purchasing. Similarly, the 82 staff surveys and in-depth stakeholder interviews revealed highly favourable impressions of the intervention components including trolley signs, floor signs and HSR shelf tags. Some concerns were raised by the retailer about the relatively high staff time needed to maintain shelf tags. In addition, the retailer identified that if the initiative were to be continued, they had concerns around the cost of refreshing intervention materials in order to maintain salience for customers.

Interviews with 19 stakeholders demonstrated that the co-design collaborative process was central to intervention design and implementation. The collaborative process was supported by the strong partnership between the academics, retailer and local government. Importantly, the programme was executed within the context of traditional industry operations focused around sales and profitability. The underlying focus on profitability sometimes competed with the health promotion objectives of the project. It was acknowledged that a sustainable and scalable healthy supermarket intervention needed to be at least profit-neutral and preferably profit-generating for the retailer.

24.5 Lessons Learnt

24.5.1 General Reflections

The story of the *Eat Well @ IGA* collaboration demonstrated the value of a multi-partner approach to healthy food retail change, particularly in a commercial retail setting. Each of the partners brought different and critical skills and capacities to the project and ensured its long-term viability and success. The thorough process evaluation that considered the perspectives of a wide range of stakeholders demonstrated the varying motivations for engaging with the project and the importance of outcomes beyond just change in customer purchasing behaviour.

From a health promotion perspective, a key lesson from this project was the value of fostering and maintaining longer-term relationships. The strength of the partnership and what it had achieved by the end of this project could not have been envisioned at the start. Confidence in the partnership and a growing understanding of each partner's motivations and perspectives was central to its growth and longevity. The structure of the project, involving multiple pilot studies prior to the larger *Eat Well @ IGA* RCT, allowed time for learning and refinement of ideas and methods. All parties integrated lessons from the initiative into their practice, with the retailer now heavily focused on fresh food in their most recent major store renovations, which represents a major shift for their brand.

24.5.2 Reflections on Partnership

The principles of collective impact guided the partnership approach of the project (Kania & Kramer, 2013). Table 24.2 summarizes our reflections on the way in which the project embodied the five principles of collective impact, reflections on

Table 24.2 Application of the collective impact framework to the *Eat Well @ IGA* partnership

Collective impact principle	How the project addressed the principle	Reflections on usefulness and potential improvements
Collaboration between multiple actors from different sectors	Partnership between health promotion, local government, academia and retail	Partnership engagement was time consuming but was crucial to project feasibility and longevity. Partnership reach could have been strengthened by engaging suppliers, Australian retailer head office and customer representatives.
Solutions developed in real-world conditions of complexity	Co-design approach explicitly incorporated retailer experience with research evidence. Short-term real-world Phase 1 pilot trials informed the larger Phase 2 trial.	This was core to ensuring the feasibility of selected interventions. A multicomponent intervention was still not as complex as the usual retail practices. However, this was a necessary compromise to simplify the intervention for a well-defined research trial.
Continuous learning based on feedback	Learning from Phase 1 pilot trials informed the larger Phase 2 trial. Long-term nature of the partnership provided opportunities for adaptation and learning over time. In the Phase 2 trial, additional promotional material was added halfway through the 12-month project.	Regular evaluation updates from the researchers to retailers were practically challenging given the difficulty in extracting sales data from a point-of-sale system. Retailers were more able to give researchers updates on sales insights. Promotional materials were refreshed much less regularly than usual retail practices, which may have reduced salience for customers. The ability to regularly refresh materials was restricted by the high cost of materials and limited resources.
Multiple organizations looking through the same lens to see change	Partner organizations agreed on a shared agenda of promoting healthy food sales.	The shared agenda was achieved. However, the need to maintain sales for retailers limits the ability to address the significant problem of unhealthy processed food sales.
A "backbone" coordinating organization	The City of Greater Bendigo liaison role coordinated communication and action between the retailer and research team.	This was essential to project success and supported longevity. The single key contact in the liaison role for the entire project duration enhanced continuity.

usefulness of the actions and potential ways to strengthen project design and co-ordination to further align the approach with the collective impact principles.

The key leaders of the retail and local government partners were strong champions of the initiative since its inception, which was central to its success and longevity. The relationships between these individuals in a small regional community and the fact that the key individuals involved in the project remained in their roles for its duration were the glue that bound the partnership. The role of the local government partner (with the lead positioned in a research evaluation capacity) was also critical to facilitating the relationship between the academic and retail partners. The local government partner shared the local focus of the retailer and the public health focus of the academic partners and was thus an ideal conduit between the two parties. Notably, the relationships formed through *Eat Well @ IGA* created a range of other opportunities locally, including partnerships between a food relief organization (Bendigo Foodshare) and Champions IGA. The initiative formed part of the successful application for Bendigo to become a UNESCO City of Gastronomy (City of Greater Bendigo, 2022). Finally, funding provided by VicHealth and the National Health and Medical Research Council (NHMRC) supported the purchase of materials and maintenance of in-store changes and a thorough research evaluation while maintaining academic financial independence.

Despite the strengths of the partnership, there were several potential threats. Below, we outline these potential threats and how they were managed during the project.

- Changes in staff/management personnel:
  - We were fortunate that the core team of retail, local government and academic partners remained stable during the project – that was not through good design.
  - Having the academic and local government partners both driving the aspects of the project meant that both had a motivation to see it succeed.
  - Dealing with several key staff at the retailer head office (Executive Chair, CEO, marketing manager, data manager) meant that changes to store manager roles and even a change in the Executive Chair had minimal impact. Despite this, it was acknowledged by the research and local government partners that there was always a chance that the retailer would decide to cease their involvement in the project to focus on other promotions or because their business direction changed – fortunately this has not happened to date.
- Research versus retail timelines:
  - The time taken to apply for grants and to accurately match product data to nutrition data, and analyzing data was a source of tension at times, with the retailer used to extremely quick turnaround times. Despite this, all partners could see that independent grant funding, which meant a rigorous approach to evaluation, was essential for the project to proceed and would ultimately mean that the work was acknowledged as high quality and trustworthy by other researchers, the public, health promoters and other retailers.
- Public health versus retail perspectives:
  - All preliminary planning meetings involved a robust negotiation between the public health and corporate perspectives. Ultimately, we arrived at a project emphasizing the promotion of healthy and fresh food, which was a win-win.
- Conflicts of Interest:
  - Early in the partnership, it was acknowledged that we had differing perspectives. While the retailer would continue to promote and sell unhealthy food, alcohol and tobacco, the researchers were clear that they would also continue

other research, holding retailers and other food industry actors to account, and that the partnership did not mean an exclusive relationship that prevented them from working on unrelated projects with other retailers.

- Tensions between public health and retailer ownership of the initiative:
  - The ability of the research team and local government partners to both secure funding for the interventions from competitive research grants and implement most components of the interventions was central to the success of the project. On the other hand, the highly active role of the research team as part of the implementation of the initiative somewhat removed the ownership and responsibility for the implementation of the initiative from the retailer.
  - In order for the initiative to be scaled up and embedded into the usual retail practice, the pendulum would need to swing towards greater ownership by the retailer, with the partners providing an advice and evaluation function, rather than being central to the implementation of the project. However, from a public health perspective, there is a risk that as ownership of the initiative shifts, the public health impact could be diluted by other priorities. It is likely to take substantial time for public health objectives to be embedded within the retailer's operations, and ongoing involvement of all partners (in some form) is likely to be required if a health promotion focus is to be maintained.

24.5.3 Research Translation

Research translation outcomes for partners included regular reports to all retail stakeholders, a social media campaign and local media exposure for the initiative. A growing supermarket health promotion community of practice involving more than 15 health promotion workers throughout Australia was established as a result of the initiative, and an international supermarket researcher network is currently being developed. Numerous interventions in supermarkets and other settings (including stores in remote Indigenous Australian communities) are drawing upon the experience of *Eat Well @ IGA* to support the research design and implementation of their own work. The example of the *Eat Well @ IGA* project has been central to the success of several major competitive research grants[1] and several research fellowships. The *Eat Well @ IGA* project has also received three research awards[2].

[1]Australian National Health and Medical Research Council (NHMRC) Centre of Research Excellence in Food Retail Environments for Health (RE-FRESH) (2019-2023).

[2]The Konrad Jamrozik Prize from the Australian Population Health Congress (2015), VicHealth Award for Promoting Healthy Eating (2016) and the Council of Academic Public Health Institutions of Australia Team Research Award (2017).

24.5.4 Implications for Research and Policy

The next phase of *Eat Well @ IGA* will involve working with supermarket retailers to identify if and how the project can be adapted and implemented at scale. The rigorous evaluation means that the *Eat Well @ IGA* multicomponent approach is thoroughly evidence-based. The challenge will be to transition the project from the context of a research project to an embedded, sustainable and adaptive programme that provides the retailer with a credible programme and brand upon which to build its healthy purchasing credentials. By positioning their brands as socially responsible and making support for the health and well-being of their customers a priority, supermarkets and their suppliers can play a major role in the efforts to improve the healthiness of population diets.

24.6 Conclusions

This project demonstrated the value of multi-sector collaboration (retail, academic and government) to all parties. The co-design approach assisted in the creation of retail interventions that are effective, feasible and acceptable to all partners. The project also revealed the challenges and benefits of working with commercial partners. Practitioners partnering with commercial organizational structures should be aware of the different commercial priorities and timelines. A formal conflict of interest management approach is recommended including a clear delineation of partner roles, the provision of external funding to maintain researcher financial independence, the inclusion of local government in a liaison role, and acknowledging multiple stakeholder priorities and outcomes. Our mixed methods approach to evaluation, underpinned by a strong theoretical basis and programme logic with a controlled study design, allowed the capture of a holistic range of outcomes relevant to each partner. A considered research translation approach ensured dissemination of research findings and progress in this important field of health promotion.

Financial Support

This work was supported by the National Health and Medical Research Council, Australia (Partnership Project Grant No. 1133090), the Victorian Health Promotion Foundation (VicHealth) and Deakin University. MRB, GS, JM and AJC are researchers within the NHMRC-funded Centre of Research Excellence in Food Retail Environments for Health (RE-FRESH) (APP1152968). The opinions, analysis and conclusions of this chapter are those of the authors and should not be attributed to the NHMRC. AJC and GS are recipients of Future Leader Fellowships from the National Heart Foundation of Australia (Project Numbers 102611 and 102035).

Acknowledgements The *Eat Well @ IGA* project is the result of the joint efforts of the retail, government, academic and funding partners. IGA staff: store managers, executive chairman and staff of the participating IGAs. City of Greater Bendigo: Rebecca Huddy, Alicia O'Brien and Nerida Firman. VicHealth: Anthea Gregoriou and Tara Heneghan. Research team: Cliona Ni Mhurchu, Boyd Swinburn, Marj Moodie, Fabrice Etile, Liliana Orellana, Helena Romaniuk, Jaithri Ananthapavan, Bruce Neale, Tom Steele, Emma Charlton, Winnie Ngan, Ella Robinson, Michelle Crino, Fraser Taylor, Jane Martin, Bruce Neal, Anna Peeters, Rob Carter, Steven Allender, Marjin Stok, Crystie Ballard, Kristy Bolton, Sandra Canning, Sarah Dean, Lee Duffin, Rachael Else, Victoria Giantsios, Hollie Hildebrandt, Melissa Klein, Josh Lee, Jasmine Lindsay, Jessie Little, Linda Maat, Abbe Moriarty, Jasmine Noske, Chris Russo, Rhiannon Speechley, Christine Spencer, Trish Stuart, Bethany Takakis, Christine Spencer, Christine Walters and Sarah Wittick.

References

Ajzen, I. (1991). The theory of planned behavior. *Organizational Behavior and Human Decision Processes, 50*(2), 179–211. https://doi.org/10.1016/0749-5978(91)90020-T

Australian Bureau of Statistics (2017). 2016 Census QuickStats: Greater Bendigo (C). ABS. https://www.abs.gov.au/websitedbs/D3310114.nsf/Home/2016%20QuickStats. Accessed 16 Sep 2020.

Blake, M.R., Sacks, G., Zorbas, C., Marshall, J., Orellana, L., Brown, A.K., Moodie, M., Mhurchu, C.N., Ananthapavan, J., Etilé, F. & Cameron, A.J. (2021). The 'Eat Well@ IGA' healthy supermarket randomised controlled trial: process evaluation. *International Journal of Behavioral Nutrition and Physical Activity, 18*(1), 1-13. https://doi.org/10.1186/s12966-021-01104-z

Cameron, A. J., Thornton, L. E., McNaughton, S. A., & Crawford, D. (2013). Variation in supermarket exposure to energy-dense snack foods by socio-economic position. *Public Health Nutrition, 16*(7), 1178–1185. https://doi.org/10.1017/S1368980012002649

Cameron, A. J., Charlton, E., Ngan, W., & Sacks, G. (2016). A systematic review of the effectiveness of supermarket-based interventions involving product, promotion or place, on the healthiness of consumer purchases. *Current Nutrition Reports, 5*(3), 129–138. https://doi.org/10.1007/s13668-016-0172-8

Chandon, P., & Wansink, B. (2012). Does food marketing need to make us fat? A review and solutions. *Nutrition Reviews, 70*(10), 571–593. https://doi.org/10.1111/j.1753-4887.2012.00518.x

Charlton, E. L., Kahkonen, L. A., Sacks, G., & Cameron, A. J. (2015). Supermarkets and unhealthy food marketing: An international comparison of the content of supermarket catalogues/circulars. *Preventive Medicine, 81*, 168–173. https://doi.org/10.1016/j.ypmed.2015.08.023

City of Greater Bendigo. (2022). City of Gastronomy. City of Greater Bendigo. https://www.bendigo.vic.gov.au/About/City-of-Gastronomy. Accessed 11 Mar 2022.

Dahlgren, G., & Whitehead, M. (1991). *Policies and strategies to promote social equity in health.* Institute for Future Studies.

Dawson, J. (2013). Retailer activity in shaping food choice. *Food Quality and Preference, 28*(1), 339–347. https://doi.org/10.1016/j.foodqual.2012.09.012

Department of Health. (2019). *Health Star Rating System.* Australian Department of Health. http://healthstarrating.gov.au/. Accessed Jan 10 2019

Department of Health and Human Services. (2018). *Victorian Population Health Survey 2014.* State of Victoria. Available at: https://www2.health.vic.gov.au/

Euromonitor International. (2020). Retailing in Australia. Available at: https://www.portal.euromonitor.com/

Glasgow, R. E., Vogt, T. M., & Boles, S. M. (1999). Evaluating the public health impact of health promotion interventions: the RE-AIM framework. *American Journal of Public Health, 89*(9), 1322–1327. https://doi.org/10.2105/AJPH.89.9.1322

Greenhalgh, T., Hinton, L., Finlay, T., Macfarlane, A., Fahy, N., Clyde, B., et al. (2019). Frameworks for supporting patient and public involvement in research: systematic review and co-design pilot. *Health Expectations, 22*(4), 785–801. https://doi.org/10.1111/hex.12888

Grigsby-Duffy, L., Schultz, S., Orellana, L., Robinson, E., Cameron, A. J., Marshall, J., et al. (2020). The healthiness of food and beverages on price promotion at promotional displays: A cross-sectional audit of Australian supermarkets. *International Journal of Environmental Research and Public Health, 17*(23), 9026. https://doi.org/10.3390/ijerph17239026

Hawkes, C. (2009). Sales promotions and food consumption. *Nutrition Reviews, 67*(6), 333–342. https://doi.org/10.1111/j.1753-4887.2009.00206.x

Kania, J., & Kramer, M. (2013). Embracing emergence: How collective impact addresses complexity. *Stanford Social Innovation Review*.

Nakamura, R., Pechey, R., Suhrcke, M., Jebb, S. A., & Marteau, T. M. (2014). Sales impact of displaying alcoholic and non-alcoholic beverages in end-of-aisle locations: an observational study. *Social Science & Medicine, 108*(100), 68–73. https://doi.org/10.1016/j.socscimed.2014.02.032

National Health and Medical Research Council. (2013). *Australian Dietary Guidelines*. NHMRC.

Payne, C. R., Niculescu, M., Just, D. R., & Kelly, M. P. (2015). Shopper marketing nutrition interventions: Social norms on grocery carts increase produce spending without increasing shopper budgets. *Preventive Medicine Reports, 2*, 287–291. https://doi.org/10.1016/j.pmedr.2015.04.007

Strugnell, C., Millar, L., Churchill, A., Jacka, F., Bell, C., Malakellis, M., et al. (2016). Healthy together Victoria and childhood obesity—a methodology for measuring changes in childhood obesity in response to a community-based, whole of system cluster randomized control trial. *Archives of Public Health, 74*(1), 16. https://doi.org/10.1186/s13690-016-0127-y

Swinburn, B. A., Sacks, G., Hall, K. D., McPherson, K., Finegood, D. T., Moodie, M. L., et al. (2011). The global obesity pandemic: shaped by global drivers and local environments. *The Lancet, 378*(9793), 804–814. https://doi.org/10.1016/S0140-6736(11)60813-1

Thornton, L. E., Cameron, A. J., McNaughton, S. A., Waterlander, W. E., Sodergren, M., Svastisalee, C., et al. (2013). Does the availability of snack foods in supermarkets vary internationally? *International Journal of Behavioral Nutrition and Physical Activity, 10*, 56. https://doi.org/10.1186/1479-5868-10-56

Chapter 25
Participatory Approaches to Researching Intersectoral Actions in Local Communities: Using Theory of Change, Systems Thinking and Qualitative Research to Engage Different Stakeholders and to Foster Transformative Research Processes

Viola Cassetti and Joan J. Paredes-Carbonell

25.1 Introduction

Over the past two decades, health inequalities, defined as the unfair, avoidable and systematic differences in health between and within places (Kawachi et al., 2002), have been at the core of public health discourse, research and practice in high-income countries (Cassetti, 2020; WHO Europe, 2013). However, despite over two decades of policies and actions to tackle these unfair differences in health, inequalities have remained high (WHO Europe, 2019), and the public health community has been urging for innovative approaches to tackle them (Cassetti, 2020; WHO Europe, 2011).

In such a scenario, a resurgence of interest has been seen in some countries in Europe towards the role that community-based initiatives to promote health can have in reducing – or at least in mitigating – the impact of health inequalities in local

This chapter is based on the work of Dr. Paredes-Carbonell in La Ribera Health Department (Valencia, Spain) (Egea-Ronda et al., 2022, in press) and draws upon the work of Dr. Cassetti carried out during her PhD in Public Health at the University of Sheffield (Cassetti 2020)

V. Cassetti (✉)
Independent researcher in health promotion, affiliated researcher to the UNESCO Chair in Global Health and Education, València, Spain

J. J. Paredes-Carbonell
La Ribera Health District, Alzira-València, Spain

Fundación FISABIO, València, Spain

Universitat de València, València, Spain

L. Potvin, D. Jourdan (eds.), *Global Handbook of Health Promotion Research, Vol. 1*,
https://doi.org/10.1007/978-3-030-97212-7_25

areas. More specifically, in countries like Spain and the UK, emphasis has been placed on the importance of working collaboratively across different sectors, to support people in increasing control over their own health and its determinants. Significantly, intersectoral actions to tackle health inequalities in local communities have been at the core of the health promotion paradigm since the beginning, as stated in the Ottawa Charter for Health Promotion (WHO, 1986), and were reinforced as a key priority to promote health during the Fourth International Conference on Health Promotion held in Jakarta in 1997 (WHO, 1997).

However, researching intersectoral actions in local communities has posed a variety of challenges to researchers and practitioners. This is because local communities are better understood as complex systems (Hawe et al., 2009; South et al., 2020; Trickett et al., 2011), i.e. systems characterized by being non-linear, unpredictable and adaptable (Quinn-Patton, 2011; Rickles et al., 2007), making it challenging to study using more traditional research paradigms because of the dynamics and evolving interactions that can occur at the local level (Cassetti, 2020). This view on communities can also be applied to the relationships that make up these communities, understood as a network of social relations, which are at the same time structured but dynamic, where information travels within these relationships and where the contexts containing these relationships are shaped by internal and external events and are subjected to continuous change (May 2013; Cassetti, 2020). Intersectoral actions can thus be seen as "events" interacting with the dynamics of the local contexts and evolving according to how the different components of those initiatives interact with the local contexts (Hawe et al., 2009), becoming research objectives themselves. Similarly, intersectoral health partnerships can be an example of those complex networks of relationships, connecting people and institutions under a common purpose.

This chapter will describe a novel approach to researching community-based intersectoral actions, with a specific focus on the development and functioning of local partnerships, using participatory methods informed by systems thinking, theory-based evaluation and qualitative research paradigms. Participatory approaches are central to health promotion research, as community engagement per se can promote health, and health promotion research and practice should be action-oriented, to produce knowledge while fostering social changes. In addition to that, considering the complexity of the research topic as introduced above, systems thinking approaches are helpful when studying complex interventions, such as health promotion initiatives, implemented in complex settings. A systems thinking approach refers to an approach underpinning the research process that aims to account for the complexity of the phenomenon under study, both at the data collection stage (thus fostering the collection of different types of data from different types of stakeholders and using multiple methods) and at the data analysis stage (through accounting for contextual factors that can either favour or hinder changes to be achieved when synthesizing the different types of data collected). To further such understanding, theory-based evaluation can shed light on how these complex interventions work, what assumptions interventions are based upon and what factors can favour or hinder the achievement of expected outcomes. Finally, qualitative research can better capture the complexity of both communities and intersectoral actions because it allows exploring the phenomenon under study from a variety of perspectives, supporting researchers and engaged stakeholders to synthesize these data into a shared new knowledge, thus making health promotion research a transformative research process. A transformative research process can be defined as an empowering research for all stakeholders taking part in it, namely, the researchers and the participants. It is also a research linked to practice as it aims to produce knowledge while at the same time fostering social change, which should be oriented towards promoting the health of the people participating in it.

This combination of underpinning research strategies presents a novel approach to researching community-based intersectoral actions, as this chapter will further illustrate using a case study of a local intersectoral partnership to promote health in a region of eastern Spain as an example of practice-based evidence.

25.2 Local Partnerships to Promote Health: An Introduction

Since the mid-1980s, one of the strategies to tackle health inequalities in places, as proposed by the health promotion community, has been the settings approach (Dooris, 2006), which recognizes the role played by contexts and social relationships in the lives of people living in specific communities (Whitelaw et al., 2001) and encourages health promotion initiatives to be implemented in those "settings" where people live and work (Poland et al., 2009), such as place-based communities. In fact, as stated above, communities are complex settings, where people from different sectors and backgrounds continuously interact with each other, and these interactions influence how different social determinants can affect the health of the people living there, for instance, by impacting local networks, service availability and delivery. Working across sectors thus becomes the key to addressing health inequalities, as it is the combination of different social determinants that affect health in place-based communities, and tackling these through single-sector initiatives does not account for the complexity of place-based communities and their dynamics and its effectiveness would be limited (WHO Europe, 2019).

It is important to note that the emphasis on intersectoral work has been central to some of the latest European policies proposed to tackle place-based health inequalities (Donkin et al., 2017). For instance, as early as 2006, the European Commission initiated the Health in All Policies Approach, a strategy to tackle the social determinants of health from the macro political level across different sectors (Puska, 2007). However, a recent scoping review of the European policies on health inequalities has found that the focus has highly remained on changing health behaviours rather than on tackling the wider determinants of health inequalities (Pons-Vigués et al., 2014), thus suggesting that the development and support of intersectoral partnerships to tackle health inequalities remains a pending issue. Significantly, a recent report of the WHO (Mcdaid et al., 2018) has identified the lack of intersectoral funding schemes and the lack of trust among organizations as the main barriers to intersectoral work, issues that have also been found central to the case study on which this chapter is centred.

Nonetheless, although efforts to foster intersectoral work at the national level appear to have resulted in limited actions at more regional and local levels, in some areas of Spain and the UK, local policies and practices have been developed to encourage the uptake of new approaches to promote health in small municipalities or neighbourhoods. The case of the Valencian region, located along the east cost of Spain, is an example of such implementation and will be the case study of this chapter, as sub-heading 2.2 will further illustrate.

25.2.1 Local Partnerships to Promote Health: Who Can Participate and Why It Matters?

As introduced above, partnership work has been central to the health promotion paradigm and has recently been emphasized by public health researchers and policymakers. Over the decades, there have been many examples of local partnerships to promote health, where different stakeholders living and working in a local area come together with the purpose of achieving a common goal (Jones & Barry, 2011). Moreover, partnerships are based on relationships between different stakeholders, and, thus, developing trustworthy relationships between the different parts becomes the key to the successful organization and development of a partnership (Corbin, 2017). Nonetheless, Woulfe et al. (2010) commented that for a partnership to be successful, besides having developed trustworthy relationships and a common vision, it is also important to include the communities that should benefit from the partnerships' actions in defining the vision and goals, to ensure that the local residents can also feel ownership of the strategies implemented by the partnership. This is when community engagement becomes the key when talking about local partnerships to promote health.

Over the past few decades, involving citizens in decision-making has become an issue of fundamental interest as a way to promote health and reduce inequalities, both nationally and internationally. There is a growing body of literature on the role of participation and engagement in the promotion of health and well-being in communities (Marmot, 2013; NICE, 2016; O'Mara-Eves et al., 2013). Sometimes used interchangeably with participation, community engagement is considered as an overarching term (O'Mara-Eves et al., 2013; NICE, 2008, 2016), as it moves beyond the idea of taking part in an event to take an active role in the proposed action. O'Mara-Eves et al. (2013), p.6) define it as "a direct or indirect process of involving communities in decision-making and/or in the planning, design, governance and delivery of services, using methods of consultation, collaboration and/or community control." Although there are different definitions of engagement, the idea of active involvement remains central.

Importantly, community engagement in health has been at the core of the health promotion paradigm since its inception in 1986, but it can also be traced back a few years to the Alma-Ata Declaration, where participation in health was defined as a right and a duty of the people. Significantly, engaging people in decision-making processes supports them in increasing control over their health and its determinants (Whitehead et al., 2016), which reflects the core value of health promotion (WHO, 1986). In fact, recent emphasis has been placed on the importance of co-creating initiatives (Leask et al., 2019) as a way to ensure that a health promotion programme reflects and embeds the context in which it is implemented and the perspectives of those who should benefit more from its implementation. In addition, having an inclusive partnership is more likely to represent the diversity of the community members whose health the partnership aims to improve. This, in turn, could support the partnership in developing interventions, which reflect the social contexts in which they are to be implemented (Woulfe et al., 2010).

Nonetheless, engaging people and communities in decision-making processes, and in the implementation and evaluation of community-based health promotion initiatives, has shown to be challenging for many public health and health promotion practitioners, especially in Spain (Cassetti et al., 2018, 2020). This chapter presents a case study whereby researchers and policymakers have come together with the local communities to design, implement and evaluate a local health promotion initiative called La Ribera Camina (literally, La Ribera goes walking), an initiative where primary healthcare professionals together with local government representatives and community members started a health promotion programme aimed at promoting physical activity, active ageing and reducing social isolation in the adult population living in a regional district near Valencia (Spain) called La Ribera (Egea-Ronda et al., 2022, in press). It is a case study that embeds the complexity of intersectoral health actions and presents a novel approach to research this area of health promotion practice, which has been widely theorized but not properly researched, resulting in the availability of limited practice-based evidence.

25.2.2 *"La Ribera Camina": An Example of a Local Partnership Initiative to Promote Health Where Engagement Is the Key*

In 2016, in a small town of the regional district of La Ribera, near Valencia (Spain), a group of primary healthcare professionals organized a walking group to support their patients in increasing their levels of physical activity. An initial evaluation found that patients not only increased their weekly hours of physical activities and their flexibility but also developed new relationships with other community members and were eager to engage in more activities. Following this, the primary healthcare team contacted the local government and local sports organizations, and, together, they decided to join forces and scale up the initiative to 19 health centres across 11 health districts in the La Ribera region. After joint planning using theory of change methods, the program "La Ribera Camina" (La Ribera goes walking) was launched. Primary healthcare professionals can now prescribe the walking group to their patients. Some walking groups are led by health professionals, others are led by lay volunteers and, in some cases, the local government supports the initiative through providing a physical activity trainer. A few years after its inception, the coordinating team decided to adopt more participatory approaches to plan, implement and evaluate the health promotion initiative, thus setting the basis for innovative and transformative research in intersectoral work.

25.2.2.1 The Purpose of the Research Project

The aim of the research was to plan and evaluate the program "La Ribera Camina" through a participatory approach using theory of change methods (Egea-Ronda et al., 2022, in press).

The specific objectives of the research were to:

1. Identify the medium- and long-term changes, which the program aims to achieve according to the stakeholders involved (primary care and public health professionals, local government representatives and walking participants) through organizing three theory of change sessions and direct observations;
2. Identify the activities to be carried out to achieve the expected changes;
3. Identify the contextual facilitators and barriers, which can either support or hinder the achievement of the expected changes;
4. Identify process and outcome indicators and define how to evaluate their achievement;
5. Analyze the differences or similarities between genders in the different elements of the program to propose appropriate solutions should these differences generate inequities;
6. Develop a final evaluation plan.

The research was developed in 2019–2020 by the primary healthcare team. These aims and objectives were defined through two theory of change sessions carried out with health professionals and local government representatives. It is an example of an applied research in health promotion, which aims to engage different stakeholders (practitioners, policymakers and community members) to produce knowledge so that they can explore how a program works, define what changes can be achieved and how to evaluate them.

25.3 Producing Data for the Processes of Planning, Implementing and Evaluating Intersectoral Actions to Promote Health in Communities: A Research Challenge

As introduced above, place-based communities are complex settings where health is affected by the interactions of people and relationships with their contexts (Vaandrager & Kennedy, 2017). In addition to that, a variety of social determinants can affect health in local places, making the planning, implementation and evaluation of community-based health promotion initiatives a challenge for many researchers and practitioners.

This view of communities as complex and open social systems (Dooris, 2006; Hawe, 2015; Shareck et al., 2013), and as networks of people interacting with their own contexts, becomes even more important when researching local intersectoral partnerships and actions.

25.3.1 The Underpinning Research Paradigm

Two major approaches to methodology, quantitative and qualitative, have traditionally been found in research paradigms, linked to two ontological positions, namely, realism and idealism. However, realism and idealism can be seen as the two opposites of a continuum where other research paradigms can be situated (Ormston et al., 2014). This is the case of subtle realism, an ontological position, which becomes helpful when studying complex issues such as community-based initiatives. In subtle realism, "an external reality exists, but is only known through the human mind and socially constructed meanings" (Ormston et al., 2014, p.5). Brought forward by Hammersley in 1992, researchers who align themselves with subtle realism believe that although an independent reality may exist, our knowledge of it is always mediated by researchers' and participants' own social and cultural values. In summary, looking at reality through the lens of subtle realism implies that this reality is complex and that there can be a variety of ways to perceive and understand it (Cassetti, 2020). This is why it is important to involve a variety of stakeholders in the research process, to account for the different perspectives they may have on the same topic, thus providing a holistic picture of the topic researched.

As introduced at the beginning of this chapter, this research adopted a participatory approach, informed by systems thinking approaches, theory-based evaluation and qualitative research. The following paragraphs will further describe each of these approaches and discuss how they can contribute to knowledge production in the context of health promotion research in local communities.

First, adopting a participatory approach to the planning, implementation and evaluation of a community-based health promotion initiative is the key to enhancing its success and can be considered as a health promotion strategy itself (Nitsch et al.,

2013). In fact, research has shown that engaging stakeholders during the planning and implementation processes can enhance its acceptability and its sustainability in the long term (NICE, 2016). Moreover, participatory approaches can foster the empowerment of engaged stakeholders through supporting an increased understanding and control of the results of the evaluation (Nitsch et al., 2013). Involving stakeholders in the planning of an evaluation can also help identify collaboratively which areas of the initiative need improvements and which need to be further explored, to focus the evaluation on the specific aspects of the initiatives, which are decided together.

Second, systems thinking approaches can provide a helpful perspective to understand changes in place-based communities because of their emphasis on taking a holistic and complex approach to study place-based initiatives (Cassetti, 2020; Hawe et al., 2009; South et al., 2020; Trickett et al., 2011) For example, Foster-Fishman and Behrens (2007) discuss systems as made of parts, and it is the interaction between the parts that makes the system behave in one way or another. According to these authors, a change in one part of a system may not necessarily lead to change in the other parts – and consequently nor to changes in the whole system, as it all depends on the leverage that one part may have on the others, as to its capacity to influence more long-term changes (Foster-Fishman & Behrens, 2007). Systems thinking thus supports stakeholders to understand initiatives as embedded within their contexts rather than considering these as an isolated set of activities. Additionally, Hawe et al. (2009) have drawn attention to the challenges associated with researching community-based initiatives. According to these authors, it is important to understand that both the initiative and the community where it is implemented are complex. A complex system is characterized by being non-linear, unpredictable and adaptable (Quinn-Patton, 2011; Rickles et al., 2007). Therefore, when an initiative leads to changes in some parts of the system, the system itself needs to adapt to this new configuration, and this adaptation may be hard to anticipate. This is why it is important to discuss with the key stakeholders how changes are expected to be achieved, a discussion that forms the basis of theory-based evaluation.

Third, theory-based evaluation has recently been increasingly adopted when evaluating public health initiatives (Breuer et al., 2016). One of its main methods has been the development of a theory of change (Weiss, 1995). A theory of change is a model, most often a visual map, of how an initiative is expected to work; in other words, it is a visual representation of the theory underpinning the initiative under study. It includes the initiatives' outcomes, activities, key stakeholders and inputs, as traditional logic models do. However, a theory of change also includes the assumptions that stakeholders may have regarding how and why the initiative should work and the processes through which expected changes can be achieved. When it comes to evaluating the initiatives, these assumptions are the key to understanding whether an initiative is working as expected or whether the underlying assumptions may have been based on external factors or conditions, which could have negatively affected the successful achievement of the anticipated results (Cassetti & Paredes-Carbonell, 2020). Moreover, a theory of change can support researchers and stakeholders in identifying the variety of desired and unexpected changes, which an initiative can generate, and thus support the planning of an evaluation by taking into account multiple outcomes and avoiding limiting the evaluation to a set of predefined outcomes. In fact, previous researches on community engagement initiatives have highlighted that evaluation research has often focussed on short-term predefined outcomes, which are generally restricted to individual-level achievements, as these are easier to measure (South & Phillips, 2014).

Finally, drawing on qualitative research paradigms and methods can support the data production in a way that reflects the complexity of the phenomenon under study (Cassetti, 2020). For instance, developing a theory of change reflects a form of a more interactive interview, which as a qualitative research method allows the researcher to further explore topics as they emerge throughout the interview process (Legard et al., 2003). Moreover, interviews represent a form of dialogue, thus creating a space for respondents to express themselves in an open and discursive way while at the same time allowing different interviewees to discuss and contrast different points of view on the same phenomenon (Lewis & McNaughton Nicholls, 2014). Additionally, qualitative research offers approaches to the data analysis process, which can embed the complexity discussed throughout this chapter, thus supporting health promotion researchers in both the production of new knowledge (epistemology) and the fostering of research, which can act as a change process itself (transformative research).

This is why combining participatory research, systems thinking approaches, theory-based evaluation and qualitative research has provided a helpful framework for this study. As the initiatives and changes that can be generated result from the interactions between people, relationships and contexts, understanding the contexts and how their pre-existing socio-cultural structures and dynamics may impact the processes and changes, which are expected to be achieved, becomes a fundamental part of the research process (Cassetti, 2020).

25.3.2 *The Research Process: Data Collection*

As introduced above, the La Ribera Camina initiative started as a small-scale pilot project carried out by a team of primary healthcare professionals. When the project team decided to scale up the initiative to the rest of the health district, three theory of change workshops were carried out to plan the new program. Through shared dialogues between primary healthcare professionals, local government representatives and community members already participating in the pilot project, the program was designed and adapted according to the specificities of each local area. This resulted, for instance, in some areas having locally trained volunteers to guide the walking groups, whereas in other areas, these were guided by a fitness trainer or a member of the primary healthcare team.

At the beginning of 2020, the coordinating team planned a series of theory of change workshops to be carried out with three groups of stakeholders: health professionals, local government representatives and community members. The theory of change workshops were aimed at collecting data on the underlying program theory by asking specific questions to identify the main goals of the initiative and working backwards to identify short- and mid-term changes, together with current activities being carried out. During each session, the aim was also to engage participants to discuss which factors could either favour or hinder the achievement of the expected changes and to gain information regarding the key stakeholders' roles and responsibilities within the initiative. To make the research process as participatory and empowering as possible, a training session was organized with an external consultant so that team members could gain specific skills on how to conduct theory of change workshops and become actively involved in the data collection process (Egea-Ronda et al., 2022, in press).

Following this, research participants were invited to attend the theory of change workshops for this study using purposive samples. Each session was audio-recorded after obtaining written consent from each participant and transcribed verbatim for analysis. Two workshops were carried out before the COVID-19 pandemic outbreak: one with health professionals and the other with local government representatives. Two additional workshops were organized with walking participants during the autumn of 2020, even though the La Ribera Camina initiative is currently suspended given the restrictions in group activities during the COVID-19 pandemic. A participatory workshop will be organized when safety measures can be guaranteed, to share the results of the research project with all stakeholders and thus to receive feedback for the evaluation plan (Egea-Ronda et al., 2022, in press) (Fig. 25.1).

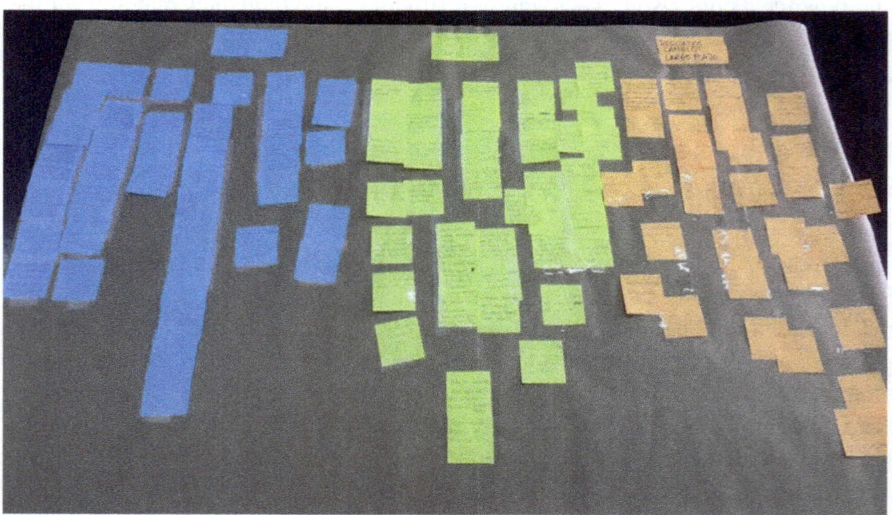

Fig. 25.1 An example of the theory of change model developed for La Ribera Camina

25.3.3 The Research Process: Data Analysis and Preliminary Results

With the aim to develop a comprehensive theory of change of the program, including a synthesis of discussed contextual facilitators and barriers as well as the underlying assumptions, an initial analysis was carried out using an iterative approach between the coding process and the comparison with the theory of change diagrams developed during the four sessions (Egea-Ronda et al., 2022, in press). It soon became clear that although the three participant groups represented stakeholders from different backgrounds and roles, their views on the program, and more importantly on the challenges that the program was facing, shared a lot of similarities. The analysis also allowed merging the contributions of all four workshops in a single theory of change diagram, which was organized through synthesizing the data presented by participants in the workshops into the following four main blocks of change:

1. Changes in physical and social health, ranging from an increased sense of belonging to reduced cardiovascular risks;
2. Organizational and relational changes, such as improved coordination between institutions, or improved relationships between end users and professionals;
3. Environmental changes, identified as, for example, improved urban infrastructures like walking trails or green gyms;
4. Program activities (currently being undertaken or needed), ranging from increasing the weekly walks schedule to ensuring support from line managers to allow health professionals and local government workers to dedicate time to the program (Egea-Ronda et al., 2022, in press).

In addition to developing a final theory of change that synthesized and embedded the perspectives of all three types of participants, the transcription of the four workshop sessions has been analyzed using thematic analysis approaches (Egea-Ronda et al., 2022, in press). Thematic analysis is an analytical method frequently adopted in qualitative research to analyze the narrative data taking an inductive approach. It aims to assign codes to fragments of the transcription and then group these codes based on similarities into more high-level and abstract themes (Charmaz, 2006; Ritchie et al., 2003).

The aim of this more explorative analysis was to identify the ongoing changes and potential explanations as to why some changes can be hard to achieve as well as to identify suggestions to redesign and improve the initiative itself.

After familiarizing with the transcripts, the researcher assigned codes to the texts, which were then organized into three main themes:

1. Expected changes
2. Perceived changes
3. Contexts

Expected changes refer to those changes that are intended to be achieved through the program, and each of the sub-topics in this section can help redesign the programme, taking into account these expected changes as if they were objectives to be achieved and/or to prepare the evaluation plan prioritizing the evaluation of the aspects identified in this topic.

Perceived changes refer to changes that have already occurred, according to workshop participants. This is important, as it allows the use of the data generated during the theory of change workshops as data to inform the process evaluation of the initiative. In fact, this theme includes either changes that stakeholders see in themselves, in other people around them and/or in the organization of the programme itself or changes that the program has generated in their environments. For instance, both walking participant groups have highlighted how their social life has improved after meeting new people in the walking group as well as how their relationship with the health professionals have changed, making them feel closer to their healthcare providers because of spending time with them outside the health centre. As for health professionals and local government representatives, one of the most significant perceived changes was identified as the opportunity to work intersectorally through this initiative, having developed collaborative relationships across the two institutions to work together for a common purpose and sharing resources to achieve this change in work relationships, which none of them had experienced before (Egea-Ronda et al., 2022, in press).

Finally, the third theme, contexts, refers to those elements of the context that can act as barriers and/or facilitators when implementing the initiative and achieving the expected changes. This topic can be used as a reference to understand the reason for certain perceived changes and, at the same time, as the key elements to take into account when redesigning the La Ribera Camina initiative.

The final step to conclude the research process refers to the organization of the participatory feedback session, where all stakeholders will be able to meet and discuss the findings collaboratively and plan both changes in the current program organization and define the evaluation plan accordingly. Due to the continuous pandemic of COVID-19, it has not yet been possible to organize this session, but it is hoped that it will be done as soon as safety measures can be guaranteed.

25.3.4 The Research Process: Novel Contribution of Adopting a Combined Research Approach

As introduced earlier in the chapter, the aim of the research was to plan and evaluate the program "La Ribera Camina". The research had six specific objectives, which were mostly achieved as anticipated, as shown in Table 25.1.

However, the novelty of using this combined approach in the research has resulted in achieving more than the anticipated and expected results. Looking at both the theory of change diagram and the thematic analysis of the transcripts, it can

Table 25.1 Examples of the specific objectives and results obtained during the research process[a]

Specific objectives	Example of results
1. Identify the medium- and long-term changes, which the program aims to achieve according to the stakeholders involved (primary care and public health professionals, local government representatives and walking participants)	As mentioned earlier in the text, the synthesized theory of change diagram includes medium- and long-term changes, synthesized as changes in physical and social health, organizational and relational changes and environmental changes.
2. Identify the activities to be carried out to achieve the expected changes	As above, the final theory of change includes a specific section with actions to be undertaken (ranging from making T-shirts to fostering a sense of belonging to the group, to develop additional side activities and health promotion and education workshops for walking participants).
3. Identify the contextual facilitators and barriers, which can either support or hinder the achievement of the expected changes	Contextual barriers and facilitators can be identified in the theory of change diagram but have also emerged throughout the workshops and have been identified through thematic analysis. This included, for instance, the importance of engaging more health professionals and local government representatives, to increase shared ownerships of the initiative or to ensure that walking trails can be adapted to the different needs of participants.
5. Analyze the differences or similarities between genders in the different elements of the program to propose appropriate solutions should these differences generate inequities	Gender differences emerged throughout the workshops in terms of limited participation of men in the walking groups. Research participants commented that this may be due to historical cultural differences, such as associating group activities with women. However, discussing these challenges also allowed research participants to propose solutions, such as fostering the prescription of the walking group by health professionals.

More examples are described in Egea-Ronda et al., (2022, in press)

[a]The data generated will be used as the starting point to co-create an evaluation plan (as stated in specific objectives 4 and 6), which can take into account the perspectives of all stakeholders involved. However, due to the current COVID-19 pandemic, this research is still ongoing and the final session to elaborate the evaluation plan will be organized when safety measures can be guaranteed

be argued that this research process has allowed knowledge production in a variety of forms. First, during the process itself, participants in each session were able to co-create knowledge about the initiative and their roles within it, making this research process transformative for those taking part in it. Second, by synthesizing the different theory of change diagrams, the final version represents a new understanding of the La Ribera Camina initiative, embedding the perspectives of different stakeholders and sectors, which not only have a role in its development as a health promotion action but can also benefit from its implementation. Third, throughout the research, knowledge has been produced about the ongoing changes, both expected and unexpected, thus acting as a process evaluation research itself

(Egea-Ronda et al., 2022, in press). Finally, the data generated can now be used as an evidence base to redesign the initiative for its improvement, following suggestions that emerged during the four workshops, thus becoming a form of co-creating the planning and the implementation of the intersectoral action itself.

To conclude, this research has shown that taking a participatory approach by combining theory of change tools, informed by systems thinking with qualitative methods, has enhanced the knowledge of the production process in relation to the planning, implementation and evaluation of intersectoral actions to promote health in communities. It has shown how research can become a process where the stakeholders involved not only produce research data but also generate meaningful learning through engaging in the research process itself.

25.4 Conclusions

Researching community-based intersectoral partnerships and actions has always been challenging because of the complexity of these initiatives, which makes it difficult to research them using traditional study designs. Although participatory approaches to health promotion research have been increasingly advocated for by a growing community of health promotion researchers in the past few decades, participation (when occurring) has tended to take the form of consulting end users to inform the planning or delivery of interventions, but it is quite limited in terms of fostering a shared decision-making process in the planning, implementation and evaluation of local actions. This research used systems thinking and qualitative methods to analyze data produced in theory of change workshops, which has resulted in the development of a visual map synthesizing the perspectives of different stakeholders and sectors involved in a local intersectoral partnership (Egea-Ronda et al., (2022, in press). At the same time, the research process has allowed stakeholders and researchers to better understand the local health action and the variety of contextual factors that can influence its development, and it has set the basis to inform the planning, implementation and evaluation of the local intersectoral partnership and action.

This study contributes to advancing health promotion research as it has shown that taking this participatory approach, by combining different methods and paradigms, to researching community-based intersectoral actions can enhance the production of practice-based evidence. Moreover, through supporting stakeholders of all backgrounds to engage in the study, this research process can be seen both as "epistemic" (producing knowledge), and "transformative" (empowering those participating in it) while contributing to improving the decision-making process for the planning and evaluation of local intersectoral actions to promote health.

References

Breuer, E., Lee, L., De Silva, M., et al. (2016). Using theory of change to design and evaluate public health interventions: a systematic review. *Implementation science: IS, 11*(63). Available at: https://doi.org/10.1186/s13012-016-0422-6

Cassetti, V. (2020). *Asset-based approaches to promote health and reduce inequalities in neighbourhoods. A qualitative theory-based investigation of two cases.* PhD Thesis. University of Sheffield. Available at: http://etheses.whiterose.ac.uk/27890/

Cassetti, V., & Paredes-Carbonell, J. J. (2020). La teoría del cambio: una herramienta para la planificación y la evaluación participativa en salud comunitaria. *Gaceta Sanitaria, 34*(3), 305–307. https://doi.org/10.1016/j.gaceta.2019.06.002

Cassetti, V., León García, M., López-Villar, S., et al. (2020). Community engagement to promote health and reduce inequalities in Spain: a narrative systematic review. *International Journal of Public Health, 65*, 313–322. https://doi.org/10.1007/s00038-020-01344-z

Cassetti, V., Paredes-Carbonell, J. J., López Ruiz, V., et al. (2018). Evidencia sobre la participación comunitaria en salud en el contexto español: reflexiones y propuestas. Informe SESPAS 2018 [Evidence of community engagement in health in Spain: Thoughts and proposals. SESPAS Report 2018]. *Gaceta Sanitaria, 32*(S1), 41–47. https://doi.org/10.1016/j.gaceta.2018.07.008

Charmaz, K. (2006). *Constructing grounded theory: A practical guide through qualitative analysis*. Sage Publications Inc.. https://doi.org/10.1016/j.lisr.2007.11.003

Corbin, J. H. (2017). Health promotion, partnership and intersectoral action. *Health Promotion International, 32*(6), 923–929. https://doi.org/10.1093/heapro/dax084

Donkin, A., Goldblatt, P., Allen, J., et al. (2017). Global action on the social determinants of health. *BMJ Global Health, 3*. BMJ Publishing Group. https://doi.org/10.1136/bmjgh-2017-000603

Dooris, M. (2006). Healthy settings: challenges to generating evidence of effectiveness. *Health Promotion International 21*(1), 55–65. https://doi.org/10.1093/heapro/dai030

Egea-Ronda, A., Niclós Esteve, M., Ródenas, A., et al. (2022, in press). Teoría del cambio aplicada al programa de promoción de la actividad física "La Ribera Camina". *Gaceta Sanitaria (in press).*

Foster-Fishman, P. G., & Behrens, T. R. (2007). Systems change reborn: rethinking our theories, methods, and efforts in human services reform and community-based change. *American Journal of Community Psychology, 39*(3–4) Blackwell Science Ltd., 191–196. https://doi.org/10.1007/s10464-007-9104-5

Hawe, P., Shiell, A., & Riley, T. (2009). Theorising interventions as events in systems. *American Journal of Community Psychology, 43*, 267–276. https://doi.org/10.1007/s10464-009-9229-9

Hawe, P. (2015). Lessons from Complex Interventions to Improve Health. *Annual Review of Public Health 36*(1), 307–323. https://doi.org/10.1146/annurev-publhealth-031912-114421

Jones, J., & Barry, M. M. (2011). Exploring the relationship between synergy and partnership functioning factors in health promotion partnerships. *Health Promotion International, 26*(4), 408–420. https://doi.org/10.1093/heapro/dar002

Kawachi, I., Subramanian, S. V., & Almeida-Filho, N. (2002). A glossary for health inequalities. *Journal of Epidemiology & Community Health, 56*, 647–652. https://doi.org/10.1136/jech.56.9.647

Leask, C. F., Sandlund, M., Skelton, D. A., et al. (2019). Framework, principles and recommendations for utilising participatory methodologies in the co-creation and evaluation of public health interventions. *Research Involvement and Engagement, 5*(2) Research Involvement and Engagement, 1–16.

Legard, R., Keegan, J., & Ward, K. (2003). In depth interviews. In J. Ritchie, J. Lewis, C. McNaughton Nicholls, & R. Ormston (Eds.), *Qualitative research practice: A guide for social science students and researchers*. Sage.

Lewis, J., & McNaughton Nicholls, C. (2014). Design issues. In J. Ritchie, J. Lewis, C. McNaughton Nicholls, & R. Ormston (Eds.), *Qualitative research practice: A guide for social science students and researchers* (pp. 47–76). Sage.

Marmot, M. (2013). *Report on social determinants of health and the health divide in the WHO European Region. World Health Organization*. Available at: http://www.euro.who.int/__data/assets/pdf_file/0004/251878/Review-of-social-determinants-and-the-health-divide-in-the-WHO-European-Region-FINAL-REPORT.pdf?ua=1

May, C. (2013). Towards a general theory of implementation. *Implementation Science, 8*:18. https://doi.org/10.1186/1748-5908-8-18

Mcdaid, D., Kluge, H. & Figueras, J. (2018). Using economic evidence to help make the case for investing in health promotion and disease prevention. *WHO Policy Brief, Health Systems for Prosperity and Solidarity*. Available at: http://www.euro.who.int/en/about-us/partners/

NICE. (2008). Community engagement. NICE-National Institute for Health and Clinical Excellence Guideline.

NICE. (2016). *Community engagement: Improving health and wellbeing and reducing health inequalities*. Available at: https://www.nice.org.uk/guidance/ng44

Nitsch, M., Waldherr, K., Denk, E., et al. (2013). Participation by different stakeholders in participatory evaluation of health promotion: A literature review. *Evaluation and Program Planning, 40*, 42–54. https://doi.org/10.1016/j.evalprogplan.2013.04.006

O'Mara-Eves, A., Brunton, G., McDaid, D., et al. (2013). Community engagement to reduce inequalities in health: A systematic review, meta-analysis and economic analysis. *Public Health Research, 1*(4), 1–526. https://doi.org/10.3310/phr01040

Ormston, R., Spencer, L., Barnard, M., et al. (2014). The foundations of qualitative research. In J. Ritchie, J. Lewis, C. McNaughton Nicholls, et al. (Eds.), *Qualitative research practice: A guide for social science students and researchers* (2nd ed., pp. 1–26). Sage.

Poland, B., Krupa, G., & McCall, D. (2009). Settings for health promotion: An analytic framework to guide intervention design and implementation. *Health Promotion Practice, 10*(4), 505–516. Available at: http://ovidsp.ovid.com/ovidweb.cgi?T=JS&PAGE=reference&D=med5&NEWS=N&AN=19809004

Pons-Vigués, M., Diez, È., Morrison, J., et al. (2014). Social and health policies or interventions to tackle health inequalities in European cities: A scoping review. *BMC Public Health, 14*(1), 198. https://doi.org/10.1186/1471-2458-14-198

Puska, P. (2007). Health in all policies. *European Journal of Public Health, 17*(4), 328. https://doi.org/10.1093/eurpub/ckm048

Quinn-Patton, M. (2011). *Developmental evaluation: Applying complexity concepts to enhance innovation and use*. Guilford Press.

Rickles, D., Hawe, P., & Shiell, A. (2007). A simple guide to chaos and complexity. *Journal of Epidemiology & Community Health, 61*(11), 933–937. https://doi.org/10.1136/jech.2006.054254

Ritchie, J., Spencer, L., & O'Connor, W. (2003). Carrying out qualitative analysis. In J. Ritchie & J. Lewis (Eds.), *Qualitative research practice: A guide for social science students and researchers* (1st ed.). Sage.

Shareck, M., Frohlich, K. L., & Poland, B. (2013). Reducing social inequities in health through settings-related interventions — a conceptual framework. *Global Health Promotion 20*, 39–52. https://doi.org/10.1177/1757975913486686

South, J., & Phillips, G. (2014). Evaluating community engagement as part of the public health system. *Journal of epidemiology and community health, 68*, 692–696. https://doi.org/10.1136/jech-2013-203742

South, J., Button, D., Quick, A., et al. (2020). Complexity and community context: Learning from the evaluation design of a national community empowerment programme. *International Journal of Environment and Public Health, 17*(1), 91. https://doi.org/10.3390/ijerph17010091

Trickett, E., Beehler, S., Deutsch, C., et al. (2011). Advancing the science of community-level interventions. *Am J Public Health, 101*(8), 1410–1419. https://doi.org/10.2105/AJPH.2010.300113

Vaandrager, L., & Kennedy, L. (2017). The application of salutogenesis in communities and neighborhoods. In M. B. Mittelmark, S. Sagy, M. Eriksson, et al. (Eds.), *The handbook of salutogenesis* (pp. 159–170). Springer. https://doi.org/10.1007/978-3-319-04600-6

Weiss, C. H. (1995). Nothing as practical as good theory: Exploring theory-based evaluation for comprehensive community initiatives for children and families. In: J. P. Connell, A. C. Kubisch, L. Schorr, & C. H. Weiss eds. *New Approaches to Evaluating Community Initiatives: Concepts, Methods, and Contexts.* The Aspen Institute, pp. 65–92.

Whitehead, M., Pennington, A., Orton, L., et al. (2016). How could differences in 'control over destiny' lead to socio-economic inequalities in health? A synthesis of theories and pathways in the living environment. *Health & Place 39*, 51–61. https://doi.org/10.1016/j.healthplace.2016.02.002

Whitelaw, S., Baxendale, A., Bryce, C., et al. (2001). 'Settings' based health promotion: A review. *Health Promotion International, 16*(4), 339–353. https://doi.org/10.1093/heapro/16.4.339

WHO – World Health Organization. (1986). *WHO | The Ottawa charter for health promotion.* World Health Organization. [online]. [Viewed 8 October 2016] Available from: <http://www.who.int/healthpromotion/conferences/previous/ottawa/en/> [Viewed 1 December 2015].

WHO – World Health Organization. (1997). *The Jakarta declaration on leading health promotion into the 21st century.* WHO. [online] [Viewed 22 March 2017] Available from:. https://doi.org/10.1093/heapro/12.4.261

WHO Europe. (2011). Promoting health and reducing health inequities by addressing the social determinants of health. [Strategic objective 7].: 1–22. Available at: http://www.euro.who.int/__data/assets/pdf_file/0016/141226/Brochure_promoting_health.pdf

WHO Europe. (2013). *Health 2020: A European policy framework and strategy for the 21st century.* Available at: https://www.euro.who.int/__data/assets/pdf_file/0011/199532/Health2020-Long.pdf

WHO Europe. (2019). *Healthy, prosperous lives for all: The european health equity status report.* WHO Regional Office for Europe. Available at: https://www.euro.who.int/en/health-topics/health-determinants/social-determinants/health-equity-status-report-initiative/health-equity-status-report-2019

Woulfe, J., Oliver, T. R., Zahner, S. J., et al. (2010). Multisector partnerships in population health improvement. *Preventing Chronic Disease, 7*(6), A119. Available at: http://www.ncbi.nlm.nih.gov/pubmed/20950526

Chapter 26
A Salutogenic, Participatory and Settings-Based Model of Research for the Development and Evaluation of Complex Interventions: The Trøndelag Model for Public Health Work

Monica Lillefjell, Kirsti Sarheim Anthun, Ruca Elisa Katrin Maass, Siw Tone Innstrand, and Geir Arild Espnes

26.1 Introduction

To achieve international and national objectives for promoting population health, quality of life and health equity, the adoption of knowledge-based strategies as well as the involvement of citizens, stakeholders and multi-sectoral governance are highly recommended (WHO, 1986, 2013, 2016; Fosse, 2012; Tones & Green, 2004). Questions regarding evidence of effect are, however, challenging because the implementation and evaluation of complex health promotion (HP) interventions do not follow a simple linear cause–effect relationship. Additionally, the processes of implementation do not always correspond with the demands of evidence-based practice. Participation from citizens is emphasized as being particularly important to improve the transparency of decisions and the efficacy of health-promoting

M. Lillefjell (✉) · R. E. K. Maass
Department of Neuromedicine and Movement Science, Faculty of Medicine and Health Sciences, Norwegian University of Science and Technology, Trondheim, Norway
e-mail: monica.lillefjell@ntnu.no

K. S. Anthun
Department of Neuromedicine and Movement Science, Faculty of Medicine and Health Sciences, Norwegian University of Science and Technology, Trondheim, Norway

Department of Health Research, SINTEF Digital, Trondheim, Norway

S. T. Innstrand
Department of Psychology, Faculty of Social and Educational Sciences, Norwegian University of Science and Technology, Trondheim, Norway

G. A. Espnes
Department of Public Health and Nursing, Faculty of Medicine and Health Sciences, Norwegian University of Science and Technology, Trondheim, Norway

L. Potvin, D. Jourdan (eds.), *Global Handbook of Health Promotion Research, Vol. 1*,
https://doi.org/10.1007/978-3-030-97212-7_26

actions (Weiss et al., 2016; Brown et al., 2014; Lillefjell et al., 2013; Brownson et al., 2009). Governance of health and coordination of activities do, however, demand new skills and changes in the implementation of multilevel, multi-sectoral, participatory actions; it requires the development of trust and the establishment of shared ethics and goals among those involved. These principles are crucial not only for health promotion activities but also for health promotion research (Lillefjell et al., 2013; Kickbusch & Gleicher, 2012; Raphael, 2000).

A focus on evidence-based public health actions implies that local communities are required to actively adopt evidence-based strategies in selecting, implementing and evaluating health-promoting actions. This includes employing the best available scientific- and experience-based knowledge, using data and information systematically, applying programme-planning frameworks, engaging the community in decision-making, conducting sound evaluations and disseminating the resulting knowledge (Lillefjell et al., 2013). According to the new public healthPublic health act in Norway, county and local municipal governments are required to move towards a proactive approach that incorporates the effective use of scientific- and experience-based knowledge (Norwegian Public Health Act, 2012). As a response to the public health act, the Trøndelag model for public health work (Lillefjell et al., 2018) was developed in a 4-year multi-sectoral innovation and research project (2012–2016). The model has since been accepted as the main policy for implementing health-promoting measures in several municipalities in Norway.

The model development process followed the key principles of health promotion (WHO, 1986, 2016; Grabowski, 2017) such as (1) a broad and positive health concept, (2) participation and involvement of the key stakeholders, (3) build action and action competence by involving and empowering target groups, (4) a setting perspective and (5) equity in health as well as the principles of Health in All Policies (HiAP) (WHO, 2013; McQueen et al., 2012). In line with these principles, the model emphasizes the promotion of knowledge-based, systematic, multi-sectoral public health work as well as joint ownership of local resources, initiatives and policies; it offers a step-by-step process that strengthens the development, implementation and evaluation of research-based measures aimed at promoting health, quality of life and health equity in, for and with municipalities.

In this chapter, we outline the Trøndelag model for public health work (Lillefjell et al., 2018), with the main emphasis on the research elements in the model. Furthermore, we introduce the Malvik path intervention (Anthun et al., 2019a, b) and others as examples of practices that characterize the working model. In the concluding chapter, attention is paid to how and why the practices presented contribute to shaping health promotion research.

26.2 Trøndelag Model for Public Health Work

The development of the Trøndelag model for public heath work, a working model for health promotion efforts in municipalities, was partly motivated by the Norwegian Public Health Act's demand that public health work must be knowledge-based, multi-sectoral and characterized by the widespread involvement of stakeholders and the population. Additionally, the development of the model was guided by three main theoretical and strategic approaches, namely, salutogenesis (Antonovsky, 1987), participatory research (Baum et al., 2006; Minary et al., 2018; Conner, 2005) and a settings approach (Green et al., 2015; Poland et al., 2009).

Salutogenesis provides a theoretical framework linking societal matters and resources to health outcomes, and it enables researchers and practitioners to focus on "the positive side of health" and examines factors and processes linked to resources, coping and individual health outcomes (Maass et al., 2017; Antonovsky, 1987). In salutogenesis theory, individual conditions for good health are linked to experiences of comprehensibility, manageability, meaningfulness and overcoming challenges. It thereby provides a strong argument for participatory approaches that offer experiences for gaining knowledge and understanding, contribute to the design and distribution of resources and enhance meaningfulness through participation in decision-making.

A participatory approach was applied while developing, implementing and planning the evaluation of complex public health initiatives in three municipalities (Israel et al., 1998, 2008; Conner, 2005). A range of different methods, such as observations, interviews, document analyses, public meetings, knowledge from the local municipality administration and international and national public health and health promotion research, were used to identify vital elements that support legal requests for knowledge-based, systematic, multi-sectoral public health actions. Elements identified during this process informed the development of the Trøndelag model for public health work (Lillefjell et al., 2018).

The settings approach (Green et al., 2015; Dooris, 2009; Poland et al., 2009) is a relevant and useful conceptual framework for developing intervention-based initiatives aimed at sustainable impacts on community health promotion. In this approach, a "setting" is defined as a systemic whole, and the focus is on how the different parts of this setting are related to and affect each other (Green et al., 2015; Hodgins & Griffiths, 2012; Hodgins & Scriven, 2012; Scriven, 2012a, b). The settings approach is characterized by community participation, partnership, empowerment and equity. Thus, integrated and coordinated actions together with a participatory approach are emphasized to achieve synergistic effects and sustainable impacts through setting initiatives (Green et al., 2015; Hodgins & Griffiths, 2012). Research in line with a settings approach should thereby ensure that the research process itself contributes to empowerment and locally grounded solutions (Hodgins & Griffiths, 2012; Dooris, 2009).

The model is characterized by broad user involvement and offers a seven-step guide for developing, implementing and evaluating complex public health measures. This is a dynamic working model. Decisions are made at each step, providing the basis for the next step, sometimes making it necessary to revisit a previous step to verify the correctness of the information. This means that none of the seven steps should be bypassed. In the Malvik path example to be presented, emphasis is placed on Steps 2 and 6 in the working model as they constitute important research elements.

26.2.1 Step 1: Governments' Legislative and Social Responsibility

The overall responsibility of the municipalities in public health work is to develop local communities that promote health, reduce social inequality in health and participation and promote safe social and environmental conditions as well as sustainable welfare services. The work required of the municipality in Step 1 subsequently includes:

- Obtaining a general view of health conditions and the factors that could influence them
- Anchoring, following up and reporting public health issues in accordance with governing systems
- Identifying and using strategies, arenas and forums for involvement and participation
- Identifying and using strategies, arenas and forums that promote multi-sectoral interaction and knowledge sharing

26.2.2 Step 2: Establishing a Knowledge Base

Knowledge-based and systematic public health work presupposes a compilation of knowledge and evidence. Knowledge should be drawn from existing legislation, professionals, policymakers, citizens, businesses, non-governmental organizations (NGOs) and local authorities as well as from research including different types of population data. This knowledge should provide the basis for multi-sectoral collaboration and decision-making processes in terms of selecting, implementing and evaluating relevant measures. As our health is affected by factors and conditions from all sectors of society, the collection of knowledge cannot be limited to the health sector. We need knowledge about the positive and negative factors that influence our health in general, and we must also identify resources among individuals, groups and local communities. Defining who is responsible for collecting the knowledge, how the knowledge is discovered and what sources of information are used are therefore seen as crucial to ensuring the required scope and extent. The municipality should determine what knowledge it requires. As soon as this knowledge has been obtained, a comprehensive analysis of the accumulated knowledge takes place, leading to a common understanding of the challenges, which is a precondition for decisions and implementation of targeted measures that ensure broad involvement among actors involved in public health work. Thus, the work required in Step 2 includes (1) collecting and analyzing the best possible data/evidence available and (2) establishing a common understanding of the challenges.

26.2.3 Step 3: Involve and Develop

Based on Step 2 (the best possible data/evidence available and a common understanding of the challenges), Step 3 moves on to identify and prioritize sustainable local actions that promote health and quality of life and reduce social inequalities in health. A concrete plan for interventions is developed using the participative planning method "search conference" (Emery & Purser, 1996; Emery, 1982). This method, a mixed strategy using both bottom-up and top-down approaches (Green et al., 2015), is useful for setting new policy directions, strategies and actions in any sector, public or private.

26.2.4 Step 4: Plan for Action

In this step, the results from the search conference (Step 3) are followed up. Overall, the responsibility lies with the municipal authorities, who must clarify who will be responsible for multi-sectoral planning and see to it that the ideas and plans for initiatives generated at the search conference are developed further and that the selected initiative(s) are implemented. It is vital that mutual responsibilities are clarified and that strategies for anchoring, communication, information and evaluation are developed.

26.2.5 Step 5. Implementation

During this step, the initiatives are implemented. The process must be monitored, described and documented. Adjustments should be made for eventual changes related to, e.g. financial issues, political situation, need of competences, etc. Possible repercussions must be considered: the chosen initiatives might influence other health-promoting initiatives.

26.2.6 Step 6. Evaluation

Sustainable, knowledge-driven public health work requires systematic evaluation of implemented measures. It is crucial to assess whether certain objectives and measures have led to intended/unintended consequences and/or positive/negative effects. Information regarding the experiences of users, how the measures have been implemented and who has participated is also important in the evaluation of health-promoting measures. Even measures that have not had the desired effect could yield important information for future initiatives. Evaluations can be carried out by the municipality itself, in cooperation with others or as an external assignment. It is, however, important that planning of the evaluation is included in the planning of the measure itself. Important key points to clarify are:

- What is to be evaluated (objectives of the evaluation)?
- How should it be evaluated (methods and data sources)?
- When should the evaluation take place (before, midway through or after the initiative)?
- How and when should the target group(s) become involved?
- Budget, time schedule, human resources and management responsibilities;
- Plan for reporting.

There are several methods of evaluation. An appropriate evaluation forms based on the aim of the initiatives, and evaluations (e.g. output, outcome, process evaluation, cost–benefit analyses) must be identified. However, it is important to be aware that the evaluation of public health work involves several challenges (Koelen et al., 2001). What one tries to achieve can often be affected by conditions beyond one's scope of action. In many cases, local measures can also be influenced by other local or national public health initiatives. This could make it trickier to isolate consequences and select criteria for the evaluation work. It can also take time before the effects of public health work become evident. Although these challenges are difficult to resolve, this should not be used as an argument against evaluation.

26.2.7 Step 7: From Action to Knowledge

Based on the data from the evaluations, it is essential to clarify central knowledge and experiences. The new knowledge obtained should influence future public health decisions and policymaking, resulting in the continuous improvement of public health work. Identifying and participating in important arenas for dissemination is therefore crucial. Here, central political, administrative and academic arenas as well as others for local stakeholders, enterprises, NGOs and inhabitants should be considered.

26.3 The Malvik Path: An Example of an Intervention that Characterizes the Working Model

The overarching aim of the Malvik path intervention was to promote health and well-being, environmental sustainability, social inclusion and health equity. The entry point involved changing the outdoor environment for the local inhabitants by constructing a universally designed path and a green space area that can be accessed and used by all people regardless of age, size, ability or disability. The Malvik path is a 3-kilometre-long walking and biking path built on an old railway track connecting two residential areas. Along the path are designated spots for social interaction, fishing, playing and barbecuing. Benches invite people to rest and admire the scenery, and information boards on historical events and the area's wildlife and historical artefacts are displayed to provide a sense of place in a wider context (Anthun et al., 2019a; Lillefjell et al., 2018). In this way, the inhabitants' exposure to activity-friendly, pleasant green spaces could increase, and they can be offered improved possibilities for social interaction, physical activity, nature contact and tension reduction.

The path development is characterized by the following processes:

26.3.1 Step 1. Governments' Legislative and Social Responsibilities

In order to fulfil the governments' legislative and social responsibilities for promoting health, reducing social inequality in health and participation and promoting safe social and environmental conditions as well as sustainable welfare services, the municipality initiated a formal collaborative partnership. The partnership aimed to ensure knowledge-based work in which scientific evidence and values, resources and contextual factors would be taken into account in decision-making and implementation processes (Lillefjell et al., 2013; McQueen et al., 2012; Raphael, 2000). An agreement was established between the research group, regional authorities and the project group at the municipal level (representing sectors of health, culture, planning, education and environment) as to which tasks were to be handled by whom. Citizens and politicians as well as public administration, voluntary (NGOs), corporate and research sectors were all designated with shared responsibilities. The agreement regarding knowledge-based work required the development of a knowledge base that could inform the process and ensure a shared understanding of the local resources and challenges related to population health.

26.3.2 Step 2: Establishing a Knowledge Base

In collaboration with researchers, the municipality of Malvik defined, collected and analyzed data from various sources to provide the information required. They initiated their own population survey, used data from Statistics Norway and the County Council and collected experiences from professionals, experts, policymakers, inhabitants, businesses and NGOs. In addition, the researchers provided a compilation of research-based knowledge by several means (methods and data sources, e.g. literature reviews, document analyses and population surveys).

The researchers developed the population survey questionnaire and collected and analyzed data in close collaboration with the municipal project group. In Norway, municipalities have access to various types of national health registers and official statistics. These provide a good overview of disease rates and the risk of disease in the population, but they have very little information about what promotes health. To provide an overview of the local living conditions and the factors that residents of the municipality deemed significant for the promotion of well-being, quality of life and good health, the municipality initiated their own population survey (to be conducted every 4 years), focusing on health-promoting factors and quality of life in the local community. The questionnaire contained measures of satisfaction with a number of local resources with respect to accessibility, quality and frequency of use that provided valuable information about how the existing resources work and are applied in everyday life.

The overall results from the data analyses showed a need for low-threshold arenas that could facilitate physical activity and social interaction for all population groups. Specifically, the population survey clearly communicated that the inhabitants wanted better access to green areas along the coast. These findings were compiled with relevant knowledge generated from international and national public health and health promotion research indicating, for example, that the lack of local green areas for social interaction and physical activity designed to be accessed and used by all people regardless of age, size or abilities contributes to local pressures linked to health, equity and sustainability (Maas et al., 2006). Ensuring that public green spaces are accessible to all population groups has been shown to promote social interaction and more active behaviours (walking, running and cycling), therefore helping to improve both health and well-being. Knowledge related to urban green spaces and reduction of air pollution and noise levels (Whitmee et al., 2015) were also included in the knowledge base. Taken together, the broad knowledge base established laid the foundation for the further process of selecting, implementing and evaluating the Malvik path intervention.

26.3.3 Step 3: Involve and Develop

Results from the population survey were disseminated to the inhabitants of Malvik at a public meeting and followed up in a search conference (Emery & Purser, 1996; Emery, 1982). In line with approaches described as important for accomplishing evidence-based health promotion (Brownson et al., 2009), the search conference methodology involves participation aimed at increasing responsibility within the local community. By involving local stakeholders, citizens, politicians, administrative staff, non-governmental organizations (NGOs) and private and public enterprises, knowledge-based public health initiatives and joint ownership of local resources were developed (Magnus et al., 2016). The search conference methodology is an innovative way to disseminate research results and discuss implications and implementation with practitioners in the field. Whilst various ideas to positively influence inhabitants' health and well-being were discussed during the conference, the decision to establish a low-threshold walking path was considered to be the top initiative worthy of carrying to fruition. As the latest population survey had clearly communicated that the inhabitants wanted to have access to the coast, it was decided to solicit the Norwegian Railway Agency to establish a walking and cycling path on the old abandoned railway trail along the coast of Malvik. This would create a green space area right next to the city centre and along the seaside, which would make it easily accessible to many people in the area and support both active and social lifestyles. Another important input from the public was that such a path should be open to the public and free of charge, permitting access to all citizens.

26.3.4 Step 4: Plan for Actions/Step 5: Implementation

The project group was responsible for planning and implementing the Malvik path, and it did so over a period of 4 years. The initiative was anchored amongst property owners in the nearby residential area, local politicians, local businesses and inhabitants as well as in the long-term governance plan, as this ensured support politically, administratively and across sectors (health, education, environment planning and culture), despite political shifts. Early on, a communication plan was designed by the project group, where the messages, target groups, communication channels and the timing of various communication events were specified. An association of local history enthusiasts was engaged to design informative boards along the path, and other groups created boards with information about the local flora and fauna. Children at the local school were asked to make a quiz to go along the path, and a local group of senior men volunteered to contribute to the deforestation along the path.

26.3.5 Step 6: Evaluation

Planning of the evaluation coincided with planning of the initiative, and appropriate evaluation forms based on the aims of the initiatives and the evaluations were identified in a collaboration between research partners, the municipal project group and other partners. Process evaluation as well as an outcome and cost–benefit evaluation were carried out.

The overarching aim of the Malvik path evaluation was to investigate who uses the path, what types of activities the path stimulates and whether and how green spaces are beneficial to providing health, social inclusion and physical activities for all citizens in the communities.

A mixed methods research design (Johnson and Onwuegbuzie 2004), combining a quantitative component consisting of counting data, questionnaire surveys and registry data with a qualitative component of observations and structured interviews, was applied to fulfil the aims of the outcome evaluations. The use of a diverse range of data and information sources provided relevant and sensitive evidence of effects, including types of activities afforded by the path and possible social and health benefits. The data were collected before, during and after the opening of the path.

The methods used to measure outcomes include (1) a digital counter that registers the number of people using the path each day; (2) iSOPARC, an observational tool used to obtain direct information on people's use of open spaces (McKenzie et al., 2006); (3) a population survey conducted on-site among inhabitants in the municipality of Malvik; (4) structured, on-site interviews with users of the path; (5) a short survey given to users of the path; (6) photovoice, a process by which people can identify, represent and enhance their community through a specific photographic technique (Wang & Burris, 1997) and (7) cost–benefit analyses.

Research in line with a setting and participatory approach ensured that the research process itself contributed to empowerment and locally grounded solutions (Dooris, 2009; Conner, 2005). Empowering the municipality in self-evaluation processes and in engaging local people in dialogue and participation in implementing the path was thus significantly emphasized by the researchers (Brown et al., 2014). The research process facilitated, for example, mechanisms that fostered participation and engagement by citizens and different vulnerable groups in developing the path by making use of the photovoice methodology (Wang & Burris, 1997). In this way, ongoing participatory analysis of community strengths, resources, structure and dynamics informed the implementation and evaluation of the path. The municipality was empowered through guidance on various matters critical to the implementation process. Self-evaluation processes were facilitated using a setting approach in planning as well as in integrating and coordinating the work. Different communication methods and arenas for knowledge sharing were established in order to ensure a high degree of accountability and transparency. Moreover, the continuous compilation of context-sensitive knowledge during the implementation process empowered the municipality in decision-making. Thus, attention to context is vital since the effectiveness of similar interventions can vary accordingly (Oliver et al., 2014).

Regular meetings were held between the research group and the multi-sectoral project group, as well as between formal collaborating partners and stakeholders, to discuss and obtain feedback on the HP initiative's relevance, progress, obstacles and results throughout the implementation period in order to improve the validity and reliability of the process evaluation. A close collaboration between researchers and county and municipal authorities was emphasized to promote ownership in the process, which was crucial to ensuring continuous improvement of practice.

26.3.6 Step 7: From Action to Knowledge

New knowledge obtained during the implementation and evaluation process continuously informed municipal public health planning, decisions and policymaking, ensuring continuous improvements in public health work in the municipality. Central political, administrative and academic arenas, as well as other arenas for local stakeholders, enterprises, NGOs and inhabitants, were systematically used to disseminate new knowledge.

Taken together, strengthening the capacities of municipalities on the basis of how to work more systematically, in a knowledge-based and multi-sectoral manner, for promoting health and health equity in the population seems closely related to success in engaging comprehensively with all stakeholders. A close collaboration between researchers and county and municipal authorities truly facilitated ownership in the implementation and evaluation process. This recognition is also emphasized in other practices characterizing the working model; the INHERIT project (https://www.inherit.eu) emphasizes the use of the suggested framework in various contexts and for various social groups, arguing that this provides valuable insights into processes and factors that can optimize the research as well as the effectiveness of health-promoting measures (Anthun et al., 2019b; Bell et al., 2019). This is also in line with a study by Horghagen et al. (2017) showing how knowledge from citizens can strengthen the quality of public health planning and the successful local implementation of health promotion policy.

26.4 Contribution to Health Promotion Research and Practice

The working model presented here enables health promoters to systematically work towards wide-ranging health goals in a specific setting in line with the WHO's key principles of health promotion (WHO, 1986, 2016). The Malvik path intervention, as one example of an intervention that characterizes the model, specifies crucial research elements that should be considered when implementing and evaluating complex health-promoting initiatives.

The Trøndelag model for public health Work contributes to shaping health promotion research, while differing from earlier models in four ways. First, it ensures a balance between bottom-up and top-down decision-making throughout the work process. Second, it differs from the existing models in emphasizing the use of a broader knowledge base, including not only research evidence but also professional and lay knowledge, throughout the process that will potentially shape health promotion research. Third, it assigns dedicated roles to various participants during all steps, and it goes beyond the health sector to find these (including commercial actors, voluntary associations, NGOs, research institutions and citizens). Fourth, the Trøndelag model provides specific directions on how to obtain feedback loops between action and knowledge to ensure that experiences and knowledge gained from implemented initiatives inform and improve later decisions. Thus, the Trøndelag model seeks to contribute to the continuous improvement of public health work and provides specific measures for active dissemination of results. Moreover, the working model is an operationalization of the HiAP approach and the settings approach (WHO, 2013; Dooris, 2009). Using the proposed model in various contexts and for various social groups will provide valuable insights into processes and factors that can optimize the effectiveness of public health measures and potentially shape health promotion research.

The model and interventions presented demonstrate how the applied frameworks can be useful in optimizing the systematic planning, implementation and evaluation of health promotion interventions. A settings approach focuses on the physical, organizational and social contexts in which people are found (Dooris, 2009). Thus, a better understanding of settings will heighten the possibility of fostering successful implementation of knowledge-based public health interventions. This type of framework goes beyond the notion of simply tweaking a standard intervention protocol to "fit" a particular setting (Dooris, 2009; Poland et al., 2009). Instead, as shown in the example of the Malvik path, it involves a detailed analysis of the context involving who is there; how they think or operate; implicit social norms; hierarchies of power; accountability mechanisms; the local moral, political and organizational culture; the physical and psychosocial environments and the broader socio-political and economic contexts.

As implementing and evaluating complex health promotion interventions in local community settings are highly context-dependent (Minary et al., 2018; Pfadenhauer et al., 2015), continuous work with processes in and between the various settings that make up the arenas of everyday life (Bloch et al., 2014) is required. By making use of a participatory process evaluation, the interpretation of effects and results was done more precisely while simultaneously offering the opportunity to conduct continuous quality improvement (Minkler et al., 2006; Conner, 2005). This is, perhaps, one of the most important, yet overlooked, strategies in public health practice to guide implementation of plans into effective public health initiatives (Conner, 2005). By making use of integrated and coordinated actions in line with a participatory settings approach, the research process itself contributed to empowerment and locally grounded solutions (Isreal et al., 1998, 2008). Moreover, an analysis of the setting at an early stage was helpful in organizing for action and optimizing the likelihood of a sustainable HP solution, and it created valuable opportunities for capacity building within the setting.

Close track was kept of all research activities, thus increasing the transparency of the research process. Involvement of community members in research activities as well as in ongoing analyses of community strengths, resources, structure and dynamics improved access to context-sensitive knowledge and enabled researchers to grasp the lived reality of the implementers, thereby revealing the complex challenges and possible solutions corresponding to experiences in their day-to-day work. It is essential to note here that the results of each research step were immediately fed back into the process. However, rich data and different sources of information crave different means of analysis, and a balance between rich data and deep analysis must be handled with caution.

26.5 Conclusions

Taken together, the research elements and key steps related to the Trøndelag model development underscore the advantages of combining new paradigms in research methods with an orientation towards the democratic processes of social and organizational change. In addition, developing extensive knowledge on health and well-being in the municipality and combining this with inhabitants' feedback on what needed improvement in the municipality turned out to constitute an important facilitating factor that secured the anchoring of the initiative with evidence and inhabitants' wishes, something that led to strong commitment from all the involved stakeholders.

Acknowledgements The Trøndelag model for public health work was developed in close collaboration with the Trøndelag county and the municipalities of Malvik, Steinkjer and Vikna and is funded by Regionalt Forskningsfond (RFF). Ongoing research, in the context of "Program for Public Health Work in Municipalities", in which we make use of the model, is funded by The Research Council of Norway ref. 302705.

References

Anthun, K. S., Maass, R. E. K., Hope, S., Espnes, G. A., Bell, R., Khan, M., & Lillefjell, M. (2019a). Addressing inequity: Evaluation of an intervention to improve accessibility and quality of a green space. *International Journal of Environmental Research and Public Health, 16*(24).

Anthun, K. S., Lillefjell, M., Espnes, G.A., Hope, S., Maass, R., Nguyen, C., Sætermo, T. F., & Morris, G. (2019b) *INHERIT: Implementing triple-win case studies for living, moving and consuming that encourage behavioural change, protect the environment, and promote health and health equity; EuroHealthNet: Brussels, Belgium.* https://www.inherit.eu/implementing-triple-win-case-studies/. Accessed July 2020.

Antonovsky, A. (1987). *Unraveling the mystery of health—How people manage stress and stay well.* Jossey-Bass.

Baum, F., MacDougall, C., & Smith, D. (2006). Participatory action research. *Journal of Epidemiology and Community Health, 60*(10), 854.

Bell, R., Khan, M., Romeo-Velilla, M., Stegeman, I., Godfrey, A., Taylor, T., Morris, G. A., et al. (2019). Ten lessons for good practice for the INHERIT triple win: Health, equity, and environmental sustainability. *International Journal of Environmental Research and Public Health, 16*(22), 4546.

Bloch, P., Toft, U., Reinbach, H. C., Clausen, L. T., Mikkelsen, B. E., Poulsen, K., & Jensen, B. B. (2014). Revitalizing the setting approach–supersettings for sustainable impact in community health promotion. *International Journal of Behavioral Nutrition and Physical Activity, 11*(1), 1–15.

Brown, C., Harrison, D., Burns, H., & Ziglio, E. (2014). *Governance for health equity: Taking forward the equity values and goals of health 2020 in the WHO European region.* Final report. World Health Organization. Updated reprint.

Brownson, R. C., Fielding, J. E., & Maylahn, C. M. (2009). Evidence-based public health: A fundamental concept for public health practice. *Annual Review of Public Health, 30*, 175–201.

Conner, R. (2005). Community-based evaluation. In S. Mathison (Ed.), *Encyclopedia of evaluation*. Sage.

Dooris, M. (2009). Holistic and sustainable health improvement: The contribution of the settings-based approach to health promotion. *Perspectives in Public Health, 129*(1), 29–36.

Emery, M. (1982). *Searching: For new directions, in new ways, for new times*. Centre for Continuing Education, Australian National University.

Emery, M., & Purser, R. E. (1996). *The search conference: A powerful method for planning organizational change and community action*. Jossey-Bass.

Fosse, E. (2012). National objectives – local practice. Implementation of health promotion policies. In B. Wold & O. Samdal (Eds.), *An ecological perspective on health promotion: Settings, systems and social processes*. University of Bergen/Bentham e-Books.

Grabowski, D., Aagaard-Hansen, J., Willaing, I., & Bruun Jensen, B. (2017). Principled promotion of health: Implementing five guiding health promotion principles for research-based prevention and management of diabetes. *Societies, 7*, 10.

Green, J., Tones, K., Cross, R., & Woodall, J. (2015). *Health promotion: Planning and strategies* (3rd ed.). Sage.

Hodgins, M., & Griffiths, J. (2012). A whole systems approach to working in settings. In A. Scriven & M. Hodgins (Eds.), *Health promotions settings: Principles and practice*. Sage.

Hodgins, M., & Scriven, A. (2012). Health promotion settings: Introduction to part 2: Healthy settings. In Scriven & M. Hodgins (Eds.), *Health promotion settings: Principles and practice*. Sage.

Horghagen, S., Magnus, E., Anthun, K. S., Knudtsen, M. S., Wist, G., & Lillefjell, M. (2017). Involving citizens' occupation-based knowledge in public health planning: Why and how. *Journal of Occupational Science*, 1–12.

Isreal, B. A., Schulz, A. J., Parker, E. A., et al. (1998). Review of community-based research: Assessing partnership approaches to improve public health. *Annual Review of Public Health, 19*, 173–202.

Isreal, B. A., Schultz, A. J., Parker, E. A., Becker, A. B., Allen, A. J., Guzman, R., Wallerstein, N., et al. (2008). Critical issues in developing and following CBPR principles. In *Community-based participatory research for health: From process to outcomes* (pp. 47–66). Jossey-Bass.

Johnson, R. B., & Onwuegbuzie, A. J. (2004). Mixed methods research: A research paradigm whose time has come. *Educational Researcher, 33*(7), 14–26.

Kickbusch, I., & Gleicher, D. (2012). *Governance for health in the 21st century*. World Health Organization.

Koelen, M. A., Vaandrager, L., & Colomér, C. (2001). Health promotion research: Dilemmas and challenges. *Journal of Epidemiology and Community Health, 55*, 257–262.

Lillefjell, M., Knudtsen, M. S., Wist, G., & Ihlebæk, C. (2013). From knowledge to action in public health management. Experiences from a Norwegian context. *Scandinavian Journal of Public Health, 41*, 771–777.

Lillefjell, M., Magnus, E., Knudtsen, M. S., Wist, G., Horghagen, S., Espnes, G. A., Maass, R., & Anthun, K. S. (2018). Governance for public health and health equity—The Tröndelag model for public health work. *Scandinavian Journal of Public Health, 46*(Suppl. 22), 37–47.

Maas, J., Verheij, R. A., Groenewegen, P. P., de Vries, S., & Spreeuwenberg, P. (2006). Green space, urbanity, and health: how strong is the relation? *Journal of Epidemiology and Community Health, 60*(7), 587–592.

Maass, R., Espnes, G. A., & Lillefjell, M. (2017). Cities and towns. In M. B. Mittelmark (Ed.), *Handbook of Salutogenesis- Past, present, future*. Springer.

Magnus, E., Knudtsen, M. S., Wist, G., Weiss, D., & Lillefjell, M. (2016). The search conference as a method in planning community health promotion actions. *Journal of Public Health Research, 5*(621), 60–67. https://doi.org/10.4081/jphr.2016.621

McKenzie, T. L., Cohen, D. A., Sehgal, A., Williamson, S., & Golinelli, D. (2006). System for observing play and recreation in communities (SOPARC): Reliability and feasibility measures. *Journal of Physical Activity & Health, 3*(Suppl. 1), 5208–5222.

McQueen, D., Wismar, M., Lin, V., et al. (Eds.). (2012). *Intersectoral governance for health in all policies. Structures, actions and experiences* (Observatory studies series 26). World Health Organization.
Minary, L., Alla, F., Cambon, L., Kivits, J., & Potvin, L. (2018). Addressing complexity in population health intervention research: The context/intervention interface. *Journal of Epidemiology and Community Health, 72*, 319–323. https://doi.org/10.1136/jech-2017-209921
Minkler, M., Vásquez, V. B., Warner, J. R., Steussey, H., & Facente, S. (2006). Sowing the seeds for sustainable change: A community-based participatory research partnership for health promotion in Indiana, USA and its aftermath. *Health Promotion International, 21*(4), 293–300.
Oliver, K., Lorenc, T., & Innvær, S. (2014). New directions in evidence-based policy research: A critical analysis of the literature. *Health Research Policy and Systems, 12*(1), 34.
Pfadenhauer, L. M., Mozygemba, K., Gerhardus, A., et al. (2015). Context and implementation: A concept analysis towards conceptual maturity. *Z Evid Fortbild Qual Gesundhwes, 109*, 103–114.
Poland, B., Krupa, G., & McCall, D. (2009). Settings for health promotion: An analytic framework to guide intervention design and implementation health promotion practice. *Society for Public Health Education, 10*(4), 505–516. https://doi.org/10.1177/1524839909341025
Raphael, D. (2000). The question of evidence in health promotion. *Health Promotion International, 15*, 355–367.
Scriven, A. (2012a). Health promotion principles and the settings approach: Introduction to part 1: Principles and practice in a settings approach. In A. Scriven & M. Hodgins (Eds.), *Health promotion settings: Principles and practice*. Sage.
Scriven, A. (2012b). Health promotion settings: An overview. In A. Scriven & M. Hodgins (Eds.), *Health promotion settings. Principles and practice*. Sage.
The Norwegian Public Health Act. (2012). *Oslo: Helse- og omsorgsdepartementet.*
Tones, K., & Green, J. (2004). *Health promotion: Planning and Strategies*. Sage.
Wang, C. C., & Burris, M. (1997). Photovoice: Concept, methodology, and use for participatory needs assessment. *Health Education & Behavior, 24*, 369–387.
Weiss, D., Lillefjell, M., & Magnus, E. (2016). Facilitators for the development and implementation of health promoting policy and programs–A scoping review at the local community level. *BMC Public Health, 16*(1), 140. https://doi.org/10.1186/s12889-016-2811-9
Whitmee, S., Haines, A., Beyrer, C., Boltz, F., Capon, A. G., de Souza Dias, B. F., et al. (2015). Safeguarding human health in the Anthropocene epoch: Report of The Rockefeller Foundation – Lancet Commission on planetary health. *Lancet, 386*(10007), 1973–2028.
World Health Organization (WHO). (1986). *The Ottawa Charter for health promotion.* Available at: www.who.int/healthpromotion conferences/previous/ottawa/en/index1.html. Consulted July 2020.
World Health Organization (WHO). (2013, June 10–14). *The Helsinki statement on health in all policies*. In The 8th global conference on health promotion, Helsinki, Finland, Consulted July 2020.
World Health Organization (WHO). (2016, October 15–31). *The Shanghai declaration on health promotion*. In The 9th global conference on health promotion, Shanghai, China, Consulted July 2020.

Chapter 27
The Contribution of Health Promotion Research to Advancing Local Policies: New Knowledge, Lexicon and Practice–Research Network

Eric Breton, Yann Le Bodo, Dieinaba Diallo, William Sherlaw, Cyrille Harpet, and Hervé Hudebine

27.1 Introduction

The health promotion movement was heralded by the work surrounding the Alma-Ata Declaration on primary health care (WHO, 1978), which brought a new perspective on what a health system should deliver at the local level (primary care, health education, health promotion, prevention, sanitation, etc.). This new vision of the realm of actions to improve population health was further developed a few years later by defining the concept of health promotion (WHO, 1986).

Health promotion research features a number of characteristics that reflect its grounding in the social and public health movements that led to the Alma-Ata Declaration and the Ottawa Charter. The most obvious are its strong focus on the structural upstream determinants of health (i.e. the so-called prerequisites for health) and its positive perspective on health (not just the absence of disease), which was the subject of theoretical work with the development of the salutogenic orientation by Antonovsky (1996) and others (Eriksson & Lindström, 2008; Mittelmark & Bauer, 2017). Last but not least is the strong social justice agenda underpinning health promotion research. In other words, health promotion research is not just research, it is research framed by a set of values (equity, people's engagement and empowerment).

E. Breton (✉) · Y. Le Bodo · C. Harpet
EHESP School of Public Health, Rennes, France

Arènes Research Unit, UMR CNRS 6051, Rennes, France
e-mail: eric.breton@ehesp.fr

D. Diallo · W. Sherlaw
EHESP School of Public Health, Rennes, France

H. Hudebine
LABERS Research Unit, Université de Bretagne Occidentale (UBO), Brest, France

L. Potvin, D. Jourdan (eds.), *Global Handbook of Health Promotion Research, Vol. 1*,
https://doi.org/10.1007/978-3-030-97212-7_27

As stated by Potvin and McQueen (2008, p. 28),

> to the extent that health promotion is also based on a set of values and principles in addition to scientific knowledge about the production of health, it should be expected that any activity linked to health promotion, such as health promotion evaluation, should also relate to its general goals, or at least not interfere with their pursuit.

Besides inheriting a set of values and a specific perspective on population health action, health promotion research also has strong and historical connections with community health, understood here in its broadest sense as health-promoting action constructed and implemented at the local level. Given the prominence of salutogenic processes and health determinants that one can find nested at the local level, health promotion research ought to cater to the needs of community health action and policies. This is where our contribution to this handbook fits in by providing elements of answer to the question: How can health promotion research produce evidence informing local health policies – evidence that will find its way into practice?

In this chapter, we present an account of the ongoing research undertaken on local health contracts (LHCs: *Contrats locaux de santé*), a policy implemented in France's continental and overseas territories. Through this account, we illustrate how health promotion principles and the knowledge developed in this field can shape a research endeavour and how health promotion research can contribute to knowledge production and uptake by raising the legitimacy of an object, enriching the lexicon of practitioners and policymakers and improving connections between the two worlds of practice and research. Let us begin by reflecting on the different forms that knowledge takes.

27.2 The Three Forms of Knowledge

In the field of public policy analysis, Freeman and Sturdy (2014) have put forward a phenomenology to describe how different forms or phases of knowledge may contribute to policy. Three forms are postulated: embodied, inscribed and enacted. Embodied knowledge is the knowledge associated with individuals. It is often tacit and built up through experience. It is also the stuff of lay and academic/professional personal expertise, in many ways the essence of "unwritten" practice. Inscribed knowledge may be found in texts, documents and plans as well as in tools. For instance, we suggest that local health contracts and associated documents are good examples of inscribed knowledge. They may be considered as being both documents and tools for guiding and influencing policy. Enacted knowledge is knowledge in action. For instance, one may consider that embodied and inscribed knowledge may be enacted in a working group or at a public meeting through interaction and sharing of ideas between participants. Enacted knowledge allows emergence and creativity, though it is unstable. It is related to both of the other forms of knowledge but is underdetermined by them. According to this conceptual framework, knowledge can be translated back and forth between these different phases. We suggest that our research is constituted by and relies on all three phases of knowledge and that each of these phases has importance in its own right. Furthermore, many insights may be gained by pinpointing and understanding how knowledge is translated through its different phases, which actors are involved and by identifying the role of research and researchers in this process.

We will now move on to explore how the research object was born/emerged and to present further insights and findings.

27.3 Local Intersectoral Mobilization Devices as an Object of Research

Researching on policies often means investigating an object that has not been informed by scientific evidence – an object that follows its own rationality. This is definitely the case when one looks at the provisions of the 2009 Health Act (République Française, 2009) describing the local health contract (LHC) as a tool that regional health agencies (RHAs) (one for each of the 17 regions across mainland and overseas France) can use to locally implement their regional health policies. In contrast to the other provisions of the law that created the regional health agencies, and aimed at improving access to healthcare services, the provisions pertaining to the LHC made for an extremely minor piece of legislation that went almost unnoticed for a few years. LHCs were intended to improve coordination within the multitude of actions that are implemented in cities, towns, villages and neighbourhoods by hundreds (if not thousands) of large and small NGOs. The provisions were first thought of as an instrument of planning and coordination at the local level aimed at reducing inequities in health. In practice, a local health contract takes the form of a multi-year action programme detailed in a set of thematic action forms (see Box 27.1 for an illustration). Interestingly, and in contrast to the many pieces of legislations and application decrees in France, it was largely left with few guidelines on what it should cover and through which processes it should deliver on its promises.

Box 27.1 The 2016–2019 Local Health Contract of Quimperlé Communauté

Located in the Finistère Department (Brittany region), Quimperlé Communauté has 57,291 inhabitants spread over 16 communes. The first local health contract (LHC) was signed with a regional health agency (RHA) in 2016 for a period of 3 years. Besides the local government and the RHA, the contract also bears the signatures of the heads of the central government authority for the department (Prefecture), the regional government of Brittany, the Departmental Council of Finistère, the Retirement and Occupational Health Insurance Fund and the local branches of the State Health Insurance Fund and of the Agricultural Social Mutual Insurance Fund. In addition to the

(continued)

Box 27.1 (continued)

signatories, the contract successfully mobilized a large set of partners, namely, family allowance funds, social services, the education board, labour/employment, hospitals, mental health centres and self-employed health professionals. The partners contributed to its drafting and some agreed to implement one or another action listed in the contract. Several NGOs were also involved in developing and implementing the actions.

The LHC was supervised by a steering committee on which sat three elected officials and three heads of service of Quimperlé Communauté (the elected officials in charge of health and solidarity, children and youth and of the Intercommunal Social Action Centre), the representatives of the regional health agency and the manager of the LHC.

The first LHC (2016–2019) aimed to:

- Improve interconnections among the local actors working to improve health;
- Promote cooperation and bridges across actions developed over the territory by addressing organizational silos;
- Implement, over several years, a collective health strategy.

Its action programme covered four main areas, each with several sub-objectives:

1. Improving access to care (12 actions listed in the contract);
2. Strengthening prevention and health promotion (12);
3. Adapting to and supporting healthy ageing (9);
4. Coordinating and communicating to reduce health inequalities (9).

The contract was developed over a period of 18 months. The process involved numerous actors from the territory who were invited to contribute through a number of working groups. These groups used a comprehensive diagnosis of the territory's needs, resources, strengths and weaknesses, which was drawn up on available socio-economic and health data and on more than 50 interviews conducted "with professionals and volunteers in the territory working in the health, social care and social fields".

The actions were mainly resourced through in-kind contributions from various state organizations and grant applications submitted to the regional health agency and other state agencies. The LHC coordination team played a key role in the search for funding.

Following the positive results of the final evaluation of the LHC, and in order to benefit from the momentum, a second contract was signed in September 2021 for a period of 5 years. While the first health contract has mainly contributed to facilitating interconnection and establishing a partnership dynamic among the actors, the second one will take advantage of this same dynamic to lead preventive actions towards the general public. The new

(continued)

Box 27.1 (continued)

LHC will also strive to involve citizens, notably with the creation of a citizen steering committee and the setting up of a participatory budgeting project.

Sources: Quimperlé Communauté local health contract, appendix to the contract and territorial diagnosis (www.quimperle-communaute.bzh). We are most grateful to Imane BENAICH, coordinator of the LHC, for her much-valued comments and suggestions.

Looking at the key features of the LHC, our research team saw in it a health-in-all-policy device that could potentially improve population health by mobilizing a whole range of local agencies, NGOs, inhabitants and elected officials in order to address a large spectrum of the social determinants of health conducive to improved daily living circumstances and reduced inequities in health. A review of the academic and grey literatures on the topic conducted in 2017 stressed the absence of a public health perspective on this instrument (Le Ru, 2017). Drawing on the scientific literature on community-based intervention, the idea of an interventional research project emerged from this vision.

27.3.1 *Health Promotion in France: A Marginal Function of the Health System Poorly Supported by the Research Infrastructure*

Consequently, a research programme was developed in a way reflective of a set of contextual parameters. In France, national and regional decision-makers of the health system pay little more than lip service to health promotion, and, when showing interest, they mostly subsume it into behaviour change programmes (Breton et al., 2011; Porcherie et al., 2020). Health promotion and community health hardly feature in the organizational charts of public health agencies, and the same holds true for the national public health institute (Public Health France). With regard to the latter, it is worth noting that, following major cuts in its budgets, most of its programmes aimed at fostering mobilization of the local actors who were outsourced to other organizations, scaled down or terminated. Public Health France still has no professionals dedicated to the LHCs, and there is no coordination of an LHC network at the national level.

Even though the key concepts brought forth by the World Health Organization (WHO)'s statements on health promotion were acknowledged by national public health institutions, it is unlikely that they play much of a role in shaping practice. Such inscribed knowledge may be easily ignored unless it becomes enacted and woven into practice, policy and, indeed, concrete tools. Initial appraisal of the local policy and practice suggested that actions on the ground hinting at the influence of the health promotion movement were more an outcome of ad hoc mobilization of regional/local administrations and a diversity of local health and social service professionals and NGOs who could tap into the training they received and the experiences (including experiences abroad) that shaped their perspectives (Clavier, 2013).

The same holds true with regard to the positioning of health promotion in the academic system. Public health research is dominated by epidemiologists trained in medicine, and professorships are out of reach for most would-be public health researchers with no medical training. This means that health promotion strategies receive very little attention from research as most studies focus on risk factors or health care.

There is also little collaboration between researchers and regional health agencies. The fact that researchers, especially social scientists, have not invested much in interventional research may explain this situation. A few joint initiatives of university–public health agency partnerships have developed over the last few years. These may have somehow contributed to changing the views of public health practitioners and decision-makers, but overall, regional health agencies staff do not bear much expectation towards the contribution of research to programme and policy improvement. It is worth noting that even with regard to the evaluation of programmes and policies driven or funded by the regional health agencies, there are very few instances of impact and outcome evaluations. Most evaluative activities revolve around process evaluations and, even in this case, rarely go beyond audit operations to ensure the proper and legitimate use of funds. Furthermore, few professionals are trained in the diverse skills necessary for evaluation of health promotion programmes. It is worth noting that within the Ministry of Health and regional health agencies, few professionals occupying public health positions are trained in this discipline. Such a situation reflects a general dearth of public health culture, a complaint one hears regularly in French public health circles.

It is within this general context that, in 2010, LHCs started to be signed across France. One or two Ministry of Health professionals were responsible for helping the regional health agencies implementing this policy instrument. As our results would later show (see Table 27.1), commitment and investment in local health contracts varied greatly across regions. Regardless of promoting LHCs or not, we found instances of Lord Mayors being the ones who knocked at the regional agencies' door to initiate talks with a view to develop and sign such a contract.

27.4 Researching Local Policies: The CLoterreS Study

Five years on from the emergence of the first local health contract, our consortium of researchers submitted a research grant application to the interventional research funding axis of the national public health research institute (IReSP). A dual opportunity was sought to investigate local health contract initiatives with respect to their commitment to health promotion, social determinants of health and health inequities while at the same time permitting reflection on the underlying public health

Table 27.1 Distribution of the local health contracts as per the French region

French region	Total number of LHCs signed in France up to Mar 2018	LHCs signed between Jan 2015 and Mar 2018 and from which CLoterreS draws its sample of 53 LHCs
Auvergne-Rhône-Alpes	28	12
Bourgogne-Franche-Comté	34	15
Bretagne	18	10
Centre-Val de Loire	28	17
Corse	10	3
Grand Est	22	12
Guadeloupe	9	4
Guyane	3	2
Hauts-de-France	26	7
Île-de-France	96	30
Martinique	3	2
Normandie	15	5
Nouvelle-Aquitaine	40	15
Occitanie	32	16
Océan Indien	8	3
Provence Alpes Côte d'Azur	6	2
Pays de la Loire	19	10
TOTAL	**397**	**165**

principles embodied implicitly or explicitly within them. In particular, this was to be achieved through three main means: 1) the analysis of the texts of the contract and associated documents, 2) the conduct of semi-structured interviews with local and regional stakeholders and 3) the creation of a steering committee (known as the strategic committee). On the committee sat representatives from the Ministry of Health, Public Health France, regional public health agencies, national NGOs and two coordinators of an LHC.

In order to get funding, the case was made to the granting body that researching a local policy was indeed investigating an intervention. This was not well understood, even by some fellow public health researchers sitting on the grant application evaluation panel, who saw the array of interventions amenable to investigation in this research call as restricted to interventions that are custom-made by researchers conducting the study. Hawe (2015) warned against this restricted view on intervention research. Indeed, in many cases, more helpful lessons can be learned from the existing interventions than from new ones cooked up in a laboratory. The fact that they are already functioning in real-world settings means that a number of implementation issues have been previously resolved, for instance, those related to the marshalling of the resources needed for the project such as funding, staff, volunteers, legitimacy, etc. Research-led interventions are often implemented through the levelling of resources that can only be dreamed of in real-life situations.

The call for grant applications was framed mostly in terms of risk factors. Therefore to get funded, we built a rationale prioritizing analyses of preventive actions over actions on daily living conditions. Our research protocol included five main objectives, i.e. to document and analyze:

- The objectives of the LHCs related to the prevention of chronic diseases
- The strategies selected to prevent them
- The capacity-building strategies associated with actions on the social determinants of health
- The strategies implemented by the regional public health agencies to foster the local implementation of their health policies
- The factors associated with the LHCs featuring strategies targeting the structural and environmental determinants of health

Early on in the development stage of the grant application, we agreed that the first step of the project was to raise its profile and relevance within the very circles of those who were most likely to benefit from our results. We felt that to be taken seriously, we needed an identity for the project that would, to some extent, compensate for the modest means we had in expertise and research capacities. We gave our project a name, CLoterreS, which proved catchy and easy to remember. With this name, and besides the acronym conveyed by the capital letters (CLS for *Contrat Local de Santé*), the notion of territory (terre) is put at the forefront and set as a critical component of our research object. We also mandated a freelancer to develop a logo and a website. We used the website as our business card when writing to request documents for our database or participation in a research interview. This proved to be an effective way to enhance our visibility and to foster a sense of identity within our own ranks. Fellow researchers who later joined our consortium – to initiate a new research arm on primary health care – quickly adopted and referred to "CLoterreS" when communicating on it. This illustrates the strong sense of identity we achieved.

Borrowing from Callon (Bilodeau & Potvin, 2016; Callon, 1984), we devised an *intéressement* strategy that included visits to the Ministry of Health staff whose briefs included the LHCs and the creation of the above-mentioned strategic committee. The steering committee was instrumental in adjusting our objectives and outcomes to the needs of the users, in securing access to the data and in opening up different channels for the dissemination of the results.

As only a few exploratory studies had been carried out on LHCs, and none from a prevention and health promotion standpoint, our first task was to characterize the action plans of a sample of contracts. This was done after completing a laborious census of all local health contracts ever signed between a regional health agency and a local government (see Table 27.1).

The instrument (Le Bodo et al., 2020) we developed to analyze the contracts drew from the WHO's *Conceptual Framework for Action on the Social Determinants of Health* (2010) and *Self-Assessment Tool for the Evaluation of Essential Public*

Health Operations in the WHO European Region (WHO Regional Office for Europe, 2015). In order to more precisely characterize the actions addressing the four risk factors of particular interest in our study (tobacco, alcohol, diet and physical activity), we also integrated categories of actions borrowed from the World Cancer Research Fund's typology (WCRF, 2018). Finally, to reflect the strong interest of the local stakeholders for environmental health, sub-themes drew on a WHO report on environmental risks (Prüss-Üstün et al., 2016) as well as on other pieces of research related to the risk factors. These reports enabled us to identify the types of actions relevant at the local level.

Our tool for the analyses of the LHCs also enabled us to consider how actions to prevent tobacco and alcohol use, to promote a healthy diet and to advocate physical activity fared in terms of addressing the environmental/structural determinants of health. It was important for us to not only assess whether the local health contracts were instruments geared for preventing four of the most important behaviour-related chronic disease risk factors but also to consider ground gained by the socio-ecological perspective in this process (Richard et al., 2004).

27.5 Shedding New Light on Local Health Contracts and Advocating for Improved Practice

Today, as we just concluded the first funding phase of this research project, there are still many analyses that can be performed on the large body of data we collected. It is nevertheless possible to highlight some of the results/outcome derived from this research so far.

First, our project yielded a portrait of practices and policies. Interestingly, the regional distribution of the local health contracts that we produced on the basis of our census of 397 LHCs signed up to March 2018 (see Table 27.1) stood out as new inscribed knowledge in the eyes of the RHAs, which have little opportunities to inquire about health promotion policies and practices in other regions. Although an LHC database was maintained within the Ministry of Health, it was outdated. As mentioned above, the census shed light on the significant discrepancies in the adoption of this policy instrument. There is no evidence establishing a causal link between the dissemination of our study results and an increased interest for LHCs in some regions. However, we noted at least one example of a regional health agency lagging far behind in terms of implementation of LHCs deciding to devote new staff time promoting this device.

Looking at the accounts on the development process that we found in the texts of the contracts of a regionally stratified random sample of LHCs (n=53), we systematically coded and analyzed a broad range of factors susceptible to influence health promotion planning. It included variables such as the type of local government signing the contract, the local public health culture and experience in community-based health actions, the socio-demographic characteristics of the territory or the health needs assessment conducted over the territory. For this last point, we took a close look at the participation of the population and highlighted that slightly less than half of the contracts were mentioning it. Among those, roughly only half of the contracts briefly alluded to population participation, whereas the other half reported using tools such as focus groups, interviews, questionnaires, walk-in interviews, public meetings, conferences, etc. Only three contracts stood out for a more active participatory approach, whether through needs assessment workshops, the involvement of a "citizen committee" or a participatory action research approach. This result reflects a recurrent observation voiced by the regional/local stakeholders that we interviewed on the willingness of the elected officials to see inhabitants more engaged in the elaboration and implementation of LHCs (and more broadly in community-based health and social or urban planning initiatives). However, interviewees continued to stress the multiple barriers they face in improving people's participation such as lack of time, capacities and skills.

The pictures we generated on the thematic categories of actions planned in our sample of LHCs (n=53), in particular with regard to health promotion, protection and disease prevention (see Fig. 27.1), also brought a new perspective of public health action to both the regional health agencies and local governments and their partners involved in an LHC. Whereas the regional health agencies planned actions using broad and ill-defined categories such as prevention/health promotion (both terms being used interchangeably), medical and social care and environmental health, we came up with much finer descriptions of the actions featuring in the contracts. For example, we found that actions on psychosocial life circumstances (e.g. access to services) and primary prevention of diseases (e.g. patient education by health professionals) feature in almost all LHCs. Alcohol, smoking, diet and physical activity are factors frequently targeted. It is also the case of mental health and,

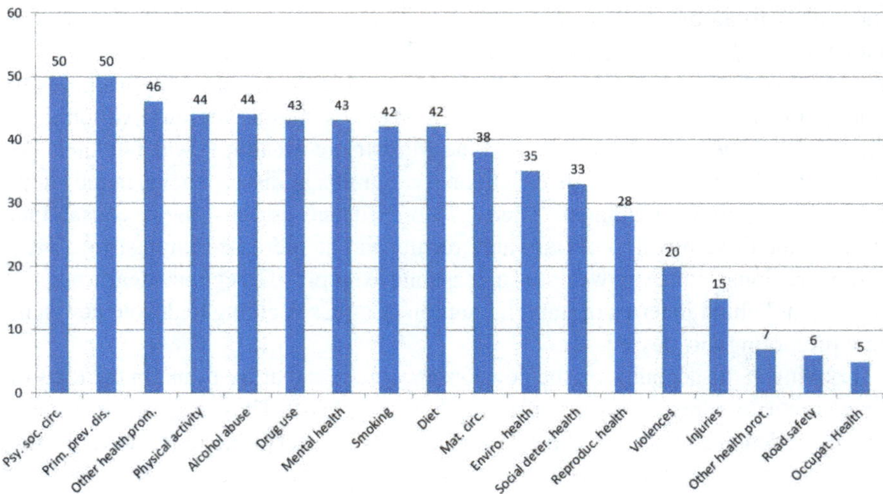

Fig. 27.1 Number of LHCs (n=53) addressing the themes related to the social determinants of health, health promotion and protection or primary prevention in at least one action form

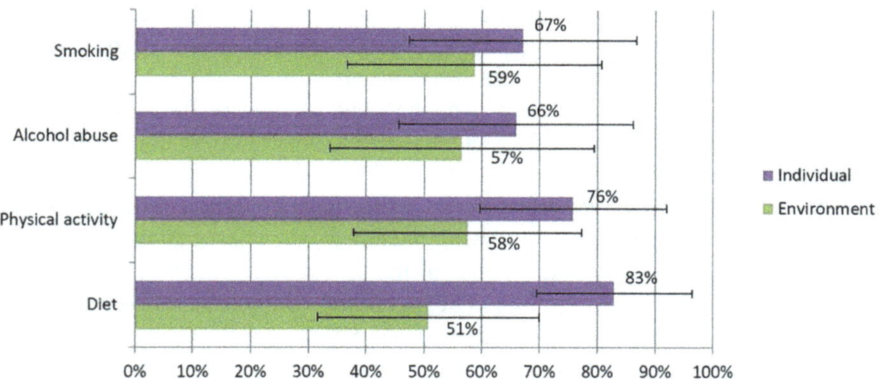

Fig. 27.2 Average proportion of the action forms/LHC targeting individual factors and/or environmental/ structural ones when smoking, alcohol, physical activity or diet was addressed

to a lesser extent, material life circumstances and environmental health (e.g. housing condition, air quality).

Having postulated that most actions described in the contracts would be restricted to health education strategies targeting improvement of knowledge, skills, motivation and changing attitudes towards a given behaviour, our results (see Fig. 27.2) turned out to present a slightly more optimistic picture of the state of practice than foreseen. Looking closely at the actions targeting key factors such as smoking, alcohol, physical activity and diet, those do tend to focus more often on changing the individuals identified as the ultimate beneficiaries but also include components focusing on their environments. It concerns most often not only the interpersonal environment to which the individuals are exposed (family, carers, educators, health professionals) but also encompasses organizational, community and political environments. For example, with regard to physical activity, most health contracts directly target individuals through awareness events, capacity-building workshops or the intervention of health professionals (e.g. physical activity as a therapy). However, a few innovative measures requiring the collaboration of other sectors such as leisure and sports, land use planning and transportation or parks and green spaces are sometimes planned to produce changes in the living environments. Such results underline the fundamental difference in the nature of preventive actions that can be implemented at the local level. Therefore, invitations to present these results to practitioners and decision-makers were used as teachable moments to further advocate the socio-ecological and health-in-all-policy approach to health promotion and prevention. We also gained deeper insights into the conditions of practice from the ensuing discussions we had with practitioners and decision-makers.

One striking observation we made of this policy instrument is on its broad diversity of forms and contents. There are no two contracts alike in terms of content and ambitions. This reflects the fact that the legislator only set a general aim for the policy instrument and kept from dictating the way to achieve it. All the legislation said was that contracts were to be co-signed by a RHA and a local government; this is an ordinance that does not preclude other institutional partners to be included in the list of signatories, something that we regularly felt across our sample of contracts. It also restricted the realm of actions to the areas of prevention, health promotion and measures to improve access to medical and social care, thus leaving much leeway on what could be planned. Even the extent to which the contracts had to fall in line with the regional health policies was left to the signatories. While some regional health agencies were found to remind the local governments of their main regional priority areas, others hardly mentioned them when negotiating the terms of the contract. The likelihood of this policy instrument to be adjustable to the population needs and to the resources that can be mobilized locally is therefore important. Interviews conducted with the coordinators of LHCs and local elected officials involved in the negotiation further evidenced this key characteristic.

27.6 What We Learned for Health Promotion Research

Through our account of the genesis and construction of local health contracts, we saw how they became objects of research and how we implemented a strategy of "intéressement" (Akrich et al., 2002), a means aiming to translate interdisciplinary health promotion theory into local health policy, planning and practice.

We suggest that our research has involved different forms of knowledge and its translation. First, we have drawn upon both inscribed knowledge from the literature and our embodied and "embrained" experience as social scientists to construct our object of research. This involved classifying and drawing up an inventory of health-related actions through consultation of drafted local health contracts; at times this also involved calling upon informants with personal experience concerning particular contracts. These different actions were classified and related to broader well-recognized frameworks formulated/championed by the WHO. Crucially, it depended on carrying out a series of semi-structured interviews with key personnel in local health administrations to draw out personal embodied knowledge and insights concerning local health contracts, their formulation and management. Through this process, embodied knowledge became crystalized into inscribed knowledge. Furthermore, innovative work drawing on the literature in qualitative research methodology provided a realistic means for interview analysis. These different translations led to preliminary research findings and the possibility for senior members of the French health administration to make comments and suggestions, which had the effect of reorienting or enriching the research process. During the enactment of the research findings through presentation and interaction with participants, opportunities of learning were offered to all. We suggest that potential insights were gained by senior officials, which may be incorporated into new practice in the future. Undoubted questions were raised, and the research was improved by providing such a forum. As the research progressed through these different processes and publications (further inscribed knowledge), we feel we have contributed to rendering latent and invisible policy streams visible to health administration actors. This offers the possibility of learning through policy (Freeman, 2008). We suggest applying Freeman and Sturdy's framework will further crystalize what is at stake in this health promotion policy research.

One interesting, albeit expected, fallout of CLoterreS was that it has improved the access of our research consortium to regional and local policy fora. Repeated contacts with the members of our steering committee to present intermediate results snowballed into a number of invitations to present them at meetings organized by the regional health agencies and local ones held by city councils[1]. It is also worth mentioning that our results and perspectives on these types of health promotion strategies were disseminated among professionals within the framework of continuing education programmes and to postgraduate students.

We were also mandated by two regional health agencies to study their LHCs in order to address questions raised by their upper managements with regard to the added value of these contracts and the nature of the support they should provide to the local communities. Acting as experts is a way for us to secure the future of CLoterreS while we define the next phase of our research agenda. The upcoming release of our results regarding the different regional health agencies' approaches to supporting and shaping LHCs in line with their regional health policies is likely to further enhance the reach of our research results within policy circles.

Health promotion research is an essential instrument to improve practice and policy. As we have shown, researchers investigating a policy can play a central role in fostering new expectations and practices towards the existing ones. They can also enrich the lexicon through which actions and strategies can be described and appraised. However, and no matter how enlightening they are, this does not happen only at the results' face value. Recasting the research in terms of Freeman and Sturdy's schema has allowed us to consider how such health promotion research knowledge can potentially influence practice and policy. This allows consideration of the actors involved and clearer thinking in terms of research–practice networks or systems. This is valuable as it enables to better account for the complexity of the context in which a policy is grounded and to device more adapted strategies to improve the impact of research. Our strategic committee may be considered as the forum for the enaction of many of our findings and has proved most valuable in many ways as it got us in sync with the discussions currently taking place among practitioners and policymakers (who were not expecting much from research), to secure access to data and to find forms and outlets for the dissemination of our results.

[1] For example, the CLoterreS team was invited to present intermediary results during (sub-)regional meetings on healthcare management, health promotion, local health contracts and sometimes on a specific public health issue (e.g. on nutrition, addictions).

27.7 Conclusions

If public health is a science of solution (Hawe & Potvin, 2009), so is health promotion research with its focus on practices and policies as they happen in the real world. A unique contribution of health promotion research lies in the way it embraces the broad array of health determinants in order to advance population health. This stands in contrast to the premise of prevention research, which always relates to a specific pathology/injury or a risk factor. The main focus of health promotion is on how the actors of a system, taken as a whole, can improve the control a population has over its own health.

However, and as we have stressed, due to their marginal position in health and academic systems, health promotion researchers are facing many challenges; the lack of funding and secure research positions are significant examples of the challenges they face in France and in many countries. Lack of flexibility in the use of research funding can also limit the capacity a researcher–practitioner partnership to adopt a system-wide perspective and to make the most of opportunities to inform and impact policies that may arise over the course of the project.

Health promotion research cannot be carried out without accounting for its institutional context. Typically, research activities for the analysis of a local health-in-all-policy device come down to applying the body of knowledge and values that characterize health promotion in order to shed new light on this object of research and see how it fares in terms of evidence-based practice. While we scrupulously adopted this approach, the context also dictated to invest energies and resources in the building and strengthening of the visibility, relevance and legitimacy of our contribution. To this end, a key strategic component of CLoterreS was the research–practitioner network we developed.

Clearly, health promotion research is primarily a social enterprise, and health promotion researchers would be well advised to cast their scientific objectives within practitioner–policy networks that will facilitate access to data, improve the relevance of their objectives and open up channels through which they can influence policymaking.

CLoterreS can be credited for illustrating how by combining scientific and networking activities, researchers can inform the development of local policy devices and strengthen their legitimacy. In our case, this was achieved by making more visible their potential and identifying paths to improving their capacity to impact population health. This was underpinned by the efforts to boost the interaction between the embodied, inscribed and enacted forms of knowledge.

For health promotion researchers, informing local policies should be considered a priority. Let us not forget that the most common pathway for the adoption of innovative practices is from local experiments to national guidelines and policies. This, in itself, should convince anyone on the value of health promotion research on the local policies.

References

Akrich, M., Callon, M., Latour, B., & Monaghan, A. (2002). The key to success in innovation part I: The art of interessement. *International Journal of Innovation Management, 06*(02), 187–206. https://doi.org/10.1142/S1363919602000550

Antonovsky, A. (1996). The salutogenic model as a theory to guide health promotion. *Health Promotion International, 11*(1), 11–18. https://doi.org/10.1093/heapro/11.1.11

Bilodeau, A., & Potvin, L. (2016). Unpacking complexity in public health interventions with the Actor–Network Theory. *Health Promotion International, 33*(1), 173–181. https://doi.org/10.1093/heapro/daw062

Breton, E., Pommier, J., Porcherie, M., Lima, E., Gindt-Ducros, A., & Diop, N. (2011). The state of health promotion practice, research and training in France : Better days ahead? In *Twenty Years of Capacity Building in Health Promotion. Evolution of Salutogenic Training : The ETC « Healthy Learning » Process* (p. 159-162). The European Training Consortium in Public Health and Health Promotion (ETC-PHHP) and the Andrija Štampar School of Public Health, School of Medicine, University of Zagreb.

Callon, M. (1984). Some Elements of a Sociology of Translation: Domestication of the Scallops and the Fishermen of St Brieuc Bay. *The Sociological Review, 32*(1_suppl), 196–233. https://doi.org/10.1111/j.1467-954X.1984.tb00113.x

Clavier, C. (2013). Les causes locales de la convergence. *Gouvernement et action publique, 2*(3), 395–413.

CSDH. (2008). *Closing the gap in a generation : Health equity through action on the social determinants of health. Final Report of the Commission on Social Determinants of Health (Executive summary).* World Health Organization.

Eriksson, M., & Lindström, B. (2008). A salutogenic interpretation of the Ottawa Charter. *Health Promotion International, 23*(2), 190–199. https://doi.org/10.1093/heapro/dan014

Freeman, R. (2008). Learning in Public Policy. In R. E. Goodin, M. Moran, & M. Rein (Eds.), *The Oxford Handbook of Public Policy*. Oxford University Press. https://doi.org/10.1093/oxfordhb/9780199548453.003.0017

Freeman, R. T., & Sturdy, S. (2014). Introduction: knowledge in policy: embodied, inscribed, enacted. In R. T. Freeman & S. Sturdy (Eds.), *Knowledge in policy: embodied, inscribed, enacted* (pp. 1–18). Policy Press.

Hawe, P. (2015). Lessons from Complex Interventions to Improve Health. *Annual Review of Public Health, 36*(1), 307–323. https://doi.org/10.1146/annurev-publhealth-031912-114421

Hawe, P., & Potvin, L. (2009). What is population health intervention research? *Canadian Journal of Public Health, 100*(1), I8–I14.

Le Bodo, Y., Fonteneau, R., Harpet, C., Hudebine, H., Jabot, F., Sherlaw, W., Kendir, C., Bourgueil, Y., & Breton, E. (2020). Analysing disease prevention and health promotion action plans at the local level : Development of the CLoterreS instrument. *Revue d'Épidémiologie et de Santé Publique*.

Le Ru, A. (2017). *Les contrats locaux de santé : une recension systématique de la littérature scientifique* (p. 52). Ecole des Hautes Etudes en Santé Publique et Consortium CLoterreS.

Maass, R., Lillefjell, M., & Espnes, G. A. (2017). The application of salutogenesis in cities and towns. In M. B. Mittelmark, S. Sagy, M. Eriksson, G. F. Bauer, J. M. Pelikan, B. Lindström, & G. A. Espnes (Eds.), *The handbook of salutogenesis* (pp. 171–179). Springer. https://link.springer.com/content/pdf/10.1007%2F978-3-319-04600-6_17.pdf. Accessed 12 Sept 2016

Mittelmark, M. B., & Bauer, G. F. (2017). The meanings of salutogenesis. In M. B. Mittelmark, S. Sagy, M. Eriksson, G. F. Bauer, J. M. Pelikan, B. Lindström, & G. A. Espnes (Eds.), *The handbook of salutogenesis* (pp. 7–13). Springer. http://link.springer.com/10.1007/978-3-319-04600-6. Accessed 12 Sept 2016

Porcherie, M., Pommier, J., Ferron, C., & Jabot, F. (2020). Promotion de la santé en France. In E. Breton, F. Jabot, J. Pommier, & W. Sherlaw (Eds.), *La promotion de la santé. Comprendre pour agir dans le monde francophone* (2nd ed., pp. 341–352). Presses de l'EHESP. www.presses.ehesp.fr.

Potvin, L., & McQueen, D. V. (2008). Practical dilemmas for health promotion evaluation. In L. Potvin, D. V. McQueen, M. Hall, L. de Salazar, L. M. Anderson, & Z. M. A. Hartz (Eds.), *Health promotion evaluation practices in the Americas* (pp. 25–45). Springer New York. https://doi.org/10.1007/978-0-387-79733-5_3

Prüss-Üstün, A., Wolf, J. de, Corvalán, C. F., Bos, R., & Neira, M. P. (2016). *Preventing disease through healthy environments: a global assessment of the burden of disease from environmental risks.* : World Health Organization.

Raphael, D., & Bryant, T. (2002). The limitations of population health as a model for a new public health. *Health Promotion International, 17*(2), 189–199.

République Française. (2009). *LOI n° 2009-879 du 21 juillet 2009 portant réforme de l'hôpital et relative aux patients, à la santé et aux territoires.*

Richard, L., Lehoux, P., Breton, E., Denis, J.-L., Labrie, L., & Léonard, C. (2004). Implementing the ecological approach in tobacco control programs: Results of a case study. *Evaluation and Program Planning, 27*(4), 409–421.

WCRF. (2018). *Driving action to prevent cancer and other non-communicable diseases : A new policy framework for promoting healthy diets, physical activity, breastfeeding and reducing alcohol consumption*. World Cancer Research Fund.

WHO. (1978). *The Declaration of Alma-Ata : International Conference on Primary Health Care.* World Health Organization.

WHO. (1986). *First International Conference on Health Promotion.* World Health Organization.

WHO. (2010). *A conceptual framework for action on the social determinants of health.*

WHO Regional Office for Europe. (2015). *Self-assessment tool for the evaluation of essential public health operations in the WHO European Region*. WHO Regional Office for Europe.

Chapter 28
Implementation Research on Comprehensive Sexuality Education in Ghana: Lessons for Health Promotion Research

Joshua Amo-Adjei and Eric Y. Tenkorang

28.1 Introduction

Comprehensive sexuality education (CSE) is a "curriculum-based process of teaching and learning about the cognitive, emotional, physical and social aspects of sexuality. It aims to equip children and young people with knowledge, skills, attitudes, and values that will empower them to realize their health, well-being, and dignity, develop respectful social and sexual relationships, consider how their choices affect their own well-being and that of others, and understand and ensure the protection of their rights throughout their lives". (UNESCO et al., 2018, p. 16) Classroom implementation of a CSE curriculum faces diverse challenges, ranging from teacher preparedness to community and parental acceptance of some topics. While there is some evidence of acceptance of CSE at the student, teacher and community levels, we know less about what actually happens in the classroom.

In 2014, we developed a research programme in Ghana to investigate CSE curriculum content in relation to what and how classroom implementation occurs. To legitimize the findings and make them relevant to the context, we set up an advisory panel of experts as collaborators and co-creators of knowledge and as promoters and end users of the evidence. The collaborative learning platforms established at the start of the study resulted in immediate application of the evidence to develop new national guidelines to make CSE teaching effective.

This chapter reflects on the research trail and draws lessons for implementing similar research programmes in related contexts. This chapter situates our narrative of CSE through three critical lenses, comprising the three main sections of this

J. Amo-Adjei
Department of Population and Health, University of Cape Coast, Cape Coast, Ghana

E. Y. Tenkorang (✉)
Department of Sociology, Memorial University of Newfoundland, St. John's, NF, Canada
e-mail: eytenkorang@mun.ca

L. Potvin, D. Jourdan (eds.), *Global Handbook of Health Promotion Research, Vol. 1*,
https://doi.org/10.1007/978-3-030-97212-7_28

chapter: ontological, epistemological and methodological issues. An ontological question focuses on the form and nature of social reality and answers the question, "what is" (Guba & Lincoln, 1994). Some critics conceive ontology as questioning whether a social reality exists and is independent of the individual's conceptions of commonly accepted realities (Marsh & Furlong, 2002; Ormston et al., 2014). Epistemological questions focus on the relationship between the knower (the researcher), what can be known (Guba & Lincoln, 1994) and how we (the researchers) make sense of the world around us. Crotty (1998) argues that epistemology is more concerned with the nature of knowledge and its constituents. Cohen et al., (2013) say epistemology comprises the "very basis of knowledge – its nature and form, how it can be acquired, and how it is communicated to other human beings" (p. 7). Methodological questions are answered by documenting the processes of knowing and discovering what we seek to know (Guba & Lincoln, 1994), bearing in mind issues of ethics, appropriateness, legitimacy and acceptability. This chapter applies these critical lenses to the various practices/activities pursued in the research project on CSE implementation in Ghana.

28.2 CSE in the Ghana Context

Ghana became an independent state in 1957 after 113 years of indirect and direct British rule (Hanson, 2017). The 1960 post-independence census enumerated 6.6 million people, with around 1.2 million aged 10–24 years (Ghana Census Office, 1962). In 2020, the population was estimated at 31 million with about 9.5 million (~30%) aged 10–24 years (United Nations Department of Economic and Social Affairs, 2020). To protect and promote the sexual and reproductive health of the population, the Government of Ghana has formulated a number of population policies. The first appeared in 1969 and was revised in 1994 and 2015 (Kwankye & Cofie, 2015). This policy provided a broad national framework for addressing sexual and reproductive health and rights (SRHR). In addition, the government promulgated an Adolescent Sexual and Reproductive Health policy in 2000 to provide political leadership in tackling the sexual health challenges of adolescents and young people.

Within this space, sexual and reproductive health and rights (SRHR) interventions, programmes and research have flourished. Yet, some enduring problems are noted among adolescents. For example, adolescent pregnancy remains a public health concern, with virtually no decrease in prevalence over time (Ghana Statistical Service et al., 2018). Although a high number of older (15–19 years) adolescents are sexually active (43% of females and 27% of males), less than half use contraceptives (Ghana Statistical Service, Ghana Health Service and ICF, 2015). Similarly, a high proportion of adolescents endorse myths and misconceptions of HIV, and there is high prevalence of gender-based violence (Tenkorang, 2013; Darteh et al., 2020).

CSE provides an important starting point for providing school-going and out-of-school youth with information that can transform unfavourable gender/cultural norms and challenge misconceptions – that is, if implemented correctly. Therefore, we developed a research programme to generate evidence about and strengthen the classroom implementation of sexuality education curriculum and policies.

28.3 Ontological Lens

This section focuses on the historical and conceptual notions of CSE and explains why the programme is important. We situate this in what was/is known (CSE impacts and debates) and what needs to be known (knowledge gaps).

28.4 Historical and Conceptual Formulations: Why Does Classroom Implementation of CSE Matter?

CSE provides an important entry point to reach adolescents with timely, age-appropriate and culturally relevant information on sexual and reproductive functioning, choices and consequences (UNESCO et al., 2018). The benefits of CSE to young people are well documented. It is known to help delay the timing of sexual debut (Vasilenko et al., 2016; Tenkorang et al., 2020a), improve the use of contraceptives and promote safer sex among adolescents (Bodnar & Tornello, 2019). These benefits may lead to reduced incidence of unintended pregnancies, unsafe abortions, sexually transmitted infections (STIs), HIV infections (Li et al., 2017; Richards et al., 2019) and coercive and violent sexual practices (Haberland & Rogow, 2015). CSE equips young people with decision-making skills and competencies to develop safer sexual practices and behaviours, including abstinence (Braeken & Cardinal, 2008; Green et al., 2017; Kershner et al., 2017).

In sexuality education, facilitator/teacher fidelity is an important determinant of success (Kirby & Laris, 2009) and curriculum implementation. Fidelity is defined as the degree to which teachers and other providers implement programmes as intended by the programme developers (Dusenbury et al., 2003). Fidelity to implementation is shaped by competent planning receptive to the needs of learners/participants, contextualized training, supportive environments for implementation and creation, and adaptation of resources that appeal to the intended audience. Other important drivers of fidelity are teacher training, programme characteristics, teacher characteristics and organizational characteristics (Dusenbury et al., 2003; James-Traore et al., 2004; Harn et al., 2013; Andreou et al., 2015; Wang et al., 2015).

The uniqueness of sexuality education presents a substantive challenge to teacher fidelity. The intimate and personal nature of some sexuality education contents can make it impossible for teachers and learners to separate the personal from the objective. Indeed, experts of pedagogical content knowledge (PCK) argue that instructors' teaching philosophies directly or indirectly shape the content delivered. PCK is the knowledge that teachers develop over time and through experience about how to teach a particular content in ways that enhance students' understanding (Loughran et al., 2012). The implication for sexuality education is that instructors need contextualized guidelines to guarantee fidelity (Wagner et al., 2017).

28.5 Problematizing the Knowledge Gap

Comprehensive and timely provision of information and skills building on sexual and reproductive health and rights is essential if young people are to be prepared to achieve sexual health and rights and to prevent negative health outcomes (UNESCO et al., 2018). In developing countries, young people continue to be vulnerable to STIs and HIV infections, unintended pregnancies (that may lead to unplanned births or unsafe abortions), pressure to engage in sexual intercourse and violence (Quarshie et al., 2020; Izugbara et al., 2017; Tenkorang et al., 2020b). These outcomes raise questions about the provision, coverage and quality of comprehensive sex education for schools in developing countries.

The research programme described in this study aimed at understanding the degree of implementation of sexuality education policies and curricula, the mode and quality of the teaching, programme monitoring and evaluation tools and the adequacy and quality of teacher training. Other objectives included understanding the level of support for or the opposition to the subject among students, teachers and the wider community and the effectiveness of the existing programmes in achieving the desired knowledge and behavioural outcomes.

28.6 Theoretical Positioning

The theoretical framing of our research programme followed Anderson et al.,' (2001) reconceptualization of Bloom's taxonomy of educational objectives. Originally, Bloom and his collaborators formulated the constituents of educational enterprises as follows: knowledge (recall), comprehension (understanding), application (use of abstractions), analysis (breakdown of a subject into its parts), synthesis (putting parts together to form a whole) and evaluation (judgements about the value of a material) (Bloom et al., 1984). Anderson et al., (2001, p. 236) overhauled the seemingly static levels of educational objectives and proposed a modified version that facilitates a shared understanding of knowledge by asking such questions as: "What is worth learning? How will teaching and learning take place? What is to be examined?" These questions basically translate into objectives, structure and processes, cognition, knowledge and assessment.

To answer the first question on what is worth learning, we asked multiple stakeholders – pupils/students, parents, teachers, school administrators, community leaders (traditional and religious) and education policymakers at regional and national levels and non-governmental actors – whether sexuality topics are worth teaching and learning and, if so, what is important to learn at various points in the lives of adolescents. To complement this, we explored the current curriculum contents on sexuality. To answer the second question, we examined the quality of methods and activities used in the teaching of sexuality and the availability of teaching and learning materials. The final question sought to understand whether sexuality education is taken as an extracurricular intervention or as part of formal school activity. While the former will not be examinable, the latter lends itself to graded assessment. We were particularly keen on understanding this, as the interest and commitment of both learners and educators to a particular course of study may be influenced by the extent to which it is examinable or otherwise (see Gerritsen-van Leeuwenkamp et al., 2019). This framework has received support in educational psychology as an efficacious model for disseminating health information. It has guided teaching and learning objectives for youth, including the framing of survey and interview questions.

28.7 Epistemological Perspective

Empiricism (knowledge as human experience) and instrumentalism (knowledge that recognizes perceptions as important tools to dissect human experiences) are two broad perspectives that shape research and inquiry into social phenomena. Whilst empiricism leads to positivist interpretations, instrumentalism leans towards constructivist epistemology in knowledge creation (Sumner & Tribe, 2004). Orthodox allegiance to these perspectives tends to create tensions and conflicts. A third strand, the pragmatic perspective, provides a dialectical bridge connecting positivist and social constructivist views to encourage meaningful methods of discovery (Greene, 2007; Johnson et al., 2007). The pragmatic paradigm values the logic of justification over an entrenched attachment to research (Johnson & Onwuegbuzie, 2004).

We found the pragmatic worldview appealing because it allows the generation of evidence from multiple perspectives and different relational pathways, leading to multiple types of outcomes (Peters et al., 2013a), and, as such, is eminently suitable for implementation research, defined as a scientific process deployed to understand the implementation of proven initiatives and the contextual factors that underlie meaningful/effective implementation (Peters et al., 2013b). Implementation research also draws on pragmatic trials, effectiveness–implementation hybrid trials, quality improvement studies and participatory action research. For a comprehensive review, see Peters et al., (2013b). In the next section, we deliberate on some implementation research obligations that significantly shaped and contributed to our research on CSE in Ghana.

28.8 Partnerships to Define a Research Agenda

As Peters, Tran, and Adams contend, "Successful implementation begins and ends with successful collaborations" (Peters et al., 2013b, p. 35). The end game of implementation research – understanding implementation needs and concerns in a naturalistic setting – implies that study participants are consciously brought into a study in their applicable contexts. In essence, we needed to work on both direct and indirect beneficiaries of the research outcomes. This pursuit speaks to the question of research legitimacy, which is an important research concern, especially in the context of our research. Research legitimacy describes the ability of research findings to account for the concerns, insights and interests of relevant stakeholders. The production of knowledge needs to be localized to minimize the mistrust between researchers and prospective users of research evidence (Lebel & McLean, 2020). Conceptions of reality as an instrumental epistemological question are embedded in contexts where varying levels of interpretations converge and diverge (Ormston et al., 2014). The implications of these for the success of our project meant that we sought to build strong partnerships, first among researchers and then between researchers, research users and beneficiaries of interventions and programmes/policies based on the research findings (Peters et al., 2013b).

The initial partnership comprised adolescent reproductive health researchers based at the Department of Population and Health, University of Cape Coast (UCC) and The Guttmacher Institute. The partnership was based on equity and autonomy. The partnering was seamless as it was built on a previous partnership between the same institutions on an earlier research programme, *Protecting the Next Generation: Understanding HIV Risk Among Youth*, between 2003 and 2007 (see Biddlecom et al., 2007).

The study described in this chapter was a multi-country project involving Ghana, Kenya, Peru and Guatemala but focused on classroom implementation of CSE in Ghana between 2014 and 2017. Although the practices and the corresponding justifications discussed here are exclusive to Ghana, there were major similarities across countries. For insights into the multi-country studies, see Keogh et al., (2018) and Panchaud et al., (2019).

The next level of partnerships and collaborations included policymakers, some of whom were also research participants ("upstream stakeholders") as well as adolescents/young people and direct/primary beneficiaries of an improved learning environment for CSE ("downstream stakeholders"). These partnerships were crucial to the success of the research agenda, as our conception of success went beyond novel findings and publication in high-impact journals. Success to us meant a transparent research trail, replicability, legitimacy and contextually relevant evidence/findings/conclusions.

Although these benchmarks were important, probably the most crucial was dealing with the controversies surrounding the implementation of CSE within the school setting. As elsewhere in the world, discourse on the SRHR of adolescents is divisive and contentious in Ghana (Clark & Stitzlein, 2018; Bialystok & Wright, 2019; Chandra-Mouli et al., 2018; Santelli et al., 2017; 2018). On the one hand, adolescent sexuality is viewed as a moral issue, and adolescents' innocence must be guarded by adult gatekeepers (Shannon, 2016). If considered acceptable at all, CSE content is largely confined to sexual abstinence (Awusabo-Asare et al., 2017). Socio-cultural and religious values continue to suppress adolescent sexual rights and freedoms whilst hindering access to quality information and education (McCarty-Caplan, 2013). On the other hand, many view SRHR as a public health issue, a human right and an educational need (McCarty-Caplan, 2013; Shannon, 2016) to be promoted and protected nationally.

Considering these tensions and opportunities, we prioritized drawing important stakeholders into the policy and programme spaces. These partners/collaborators were drawn from local and international organizations and included state and non-state actors whose acceptance, participation and involvement were important markers of success. We considered the process of assembling individuals and institutions to create an epistemic community (Haas, 1992) to be a useful research legitimatization activity because these constituencies possess varying rights, privileges, power and influence across different scales and levels. Such engagements provide a strong collective identity in defining and refining impactful research (Lebel & McLean, 2020).

To this end, we set up an advisory panel at the national level when we started the research. The group included people in policy formulation and programme implementation – both governmental and non-governmental. At the national level, our key collaborators were the National Population Council, the School Health and Education Programme (SHEP), the Curriculum Research and Development Division (CRDD) of the Ghana Education Service (GES) (now the National Council for Curriculum and Assessment (NaCCA) and the Family and Reproductive Health Directorate of the Ghana Health Service. A representative of Palladium International (a UK-based management and advisory organization) was on the panel as well. These various actors contribute to different dimensions of any CSE content taught in schools or in out-of-school settings. For instance, the mandate of the National Population Council is to advise the government on all matters of population, under the authority of Act 485, 1994. The NaCCA and its predecessor, the Curriculum Research and Development Division, Ministry of Education, has the mandate to review and assess the curriculum of all subjects taught at pre-tertiary levels to ensure that the subject contents are relevant to national aspirations and will produce students who can compete globally. SHEP coordinates all curricular and extracurricular health-related programmes/activities in pre-tertiary schools (Grades 1–12). Other members of the advisory committee were drawn from the United Nations Population Fund (UNFPA) country office, Planned Parenthood Association of Ghana and Curious Minds, parent–teacher association representatives and students.

This advisory group was established at the outset of the project and provided critical and useful input to the questions explored in the entire programme of work. These important stakeholders contributed in diverse and complementary ways. First, they helped us refine the conceptualization of the study, particularly with respect to the research questions and the relevant target for each question. Second, they provided an extensive review of data collection tools in terms of context appropriateness. For example, some advisory panel members believed that "sexuality education" should be replaced with a terminology that is more familiar and common in the SRHR space. Accordingly, "sexuality education" was replaced with "adolescent reproductive health education". This resonated with all the major stakeholders. As mentioned previously, sexuality education raises suspicion in conservative societies (Chandra-Mouli et al., 2018) and did so here, but the need to assess teacher preparedness and capacity needs, the overall school environment and the content delivered remained unchanged. Finally, the advisory group facilitated and solicited the support of the primary gatekeepers for the study settings.

The early involvement of the above institutions in the planning gave us almost universal and unimpeded access to all research participants at both the community and institutional levels. For instance, ahead of the field study, all the regional education directors had been engaged in the study subject. These directors, in turn, connected the study teams to the various district directors of education and, subsequently, to the school heads. This facilitated timely execution of the project and enhanced cooperation during the fieldwork. The continuous engagement of the key constituencies in the formulation and refinement of the study set the stage for later acceptance of the findings.

For an advisory group in implementation research to work effectively, the group's composition and timing of formation deserves important consideration. In our case, we ensured that the group comprised experts representing different institutions. The group was heavily government sector-oriented, but this minimized the tensions that may arise in such processes when non-government actors dominate (Roodsaz, 2018). Moreover, in Ghana, in-school programmes are largely run by government agencies – the GES and the Ghana Health Service (GHS) – making it important to ensure that they had a major stake in the advisory process.

28.9 Involvement of the Primary Beneficiaries (Adolescents) in Defining and Refining Research Questions

One of the dimensions of research quality is research relevance. Others include integrity, legitimacy and positioning for use (Ofir et al., 2016). Relevant research prioritizes the needs of the prospective users – not only policymakers and programme implementers but also programme beneficiaries. Guided by this idea, we considered co-creation with participants (adolescents) to be an important and legitimate step. We consequently undertook a heuristic assessment of adolescents' concerns about the teaching of CSE. This helped us reframe and streamline the key research questions in order to contribute to both knowledge generation and policy change. To achieve this, we engaged a small group of adolescents in two secondary schools within the precincts of the University of Cape Coast where the local researchers were based. This meeting was to test the adolescents' knowledge of sexuality education and gauge the areas in which they needed additional information and knowledge.

A secondary school in Cape Coast was a great resource to gain a preliminary understanding of the entire country, as schools attract students from across Ghana. This helped us develop a heuristic appreciation of the sexuality education landscape in the country. However, we deliberately selected one school whose students have average performance to avoid privileging the best secondary school students. The essence of this process is the current paradigm in curriculum development and revision: it moves away from privileging expert opinions to seeing the views and needs of learners as equally profound. One of the goals of our research was to inform policy changes in CSE. The incorporation of students into the process allowed us to gauge how our work would contribute to the local priorities or to the needs of the primary beneficiaries. The practical value of this step was reflected in the development and finalization of the research instruments, the timeliness of the fieldwork and the clarity of the tools administered to students (noted in the response rate of ~95%).

28.10 Methodological Approach

Our pragmatic research philosophy meant that we collected both quantitative and qualitative data. We collected quantitative data to measure some elements of CSE and the quality of teaching (time, resources, teaching methods, etc.), students' expectations of what is worth learning and how learning should occur. Qualitative data included the participants' notions of the relevance of sexuality education and the contextual opportunities and challenges to teaching CSE. Both quantitative and qualitative data were collected concurrently (Creswell et al., 2003).

We analyzed the data using a sequential approach. Our aim was to highlight the unique perspectives of each approach. The first step involved a data analysis workshop with project team members to identify the items that adequately answered the research questions. This exercise resulted in an analytical framework that we used to shape the results. We then developed dummy tables and reviewed them repeatedly to ensure that all relevant items were captured. The qualitative analysis was both deductive and inductive. Two expert qualitative researchers double-coded the narratives. Inconsistencies in codes were resolved by the entire project team (five members) in a majority vote. The findings from both quantitative and qualitative data were integrated or merged. The quantitative data were presented under each theme, followed by the addition of qualitative extracts/texts. Whilst both datasets were valued equally, the quantitative data dominated the reporting.

28.11 Evidence Dissemination and Communication

Research findings can be the key to thinking big and broadening the range of policy options (Uzochukwu et al., 2016). Yet, policymakers may question the credibility of research, whilst researchers may question the commitments of the policymakers to use evidence in decision-making (Gollust et al., 2017). As implementation researchers whose main objective was to generate evidence to improve policy, we aimed to make evidence available to diverse interest groups: policymakers, advocacy groups, media, CSE implementers and other researchers. We attempted to use mutually inclusive tools, even though the peculiarity of certain groups required deliberate targeting.

The first attempt to make the evidence available to the key stakeholders was the organization of two report-launching activities. The study team and the Communications and Publications Administrative Operations of The Guttmacher Institute worked with a Ghanaian public relations consultant to develop modalities to launch the study report, with activities planned for the Greater Accra and Brong Ahafo regions. Greater Accra, one of the study sites, was selected because it hosts the national capital – Accra. It is also the headquarters of several state and non-state institutions that advocate for sexuality education for adolescents and young people. This was important to gain immediate traction and generate publicity via the many media outlets in Accra. The second dissemination site, the Brong Ahafo region, was chosen because of the study's findings. The adolescent participants surveyed in this region reported unfavourable SRHR outcomes (e.g. girls in the region were more likely to initiate sex earlier). The choice of Brong Ahafo was also strategic because the Palladium Group, in partnership with the Ghana Health Service, was implementing the Ghana Adolescent Sexual and Reproductive Health Project in the region. The choice stood to promote the interest of regional- and district-level policymakers in providing and expanding ongoing reproductive health programmes for adolescents. The Ghana Education Service (GES), the primary implementing agency of the Ministry of Education, was integral to the dissemination of our findings; the co-ownership of the evidence by the GES was crucial in that it attracted attention in national conversations on in-school sexuality education. One of the main precursors to making the evidence relevant was our deliberate decision to produce non-academic and technical papers. By complementing the report with a policy brief, stakeholders in a position to influence policies and programmes had easy access to evidence fit for their needs.

28.12 Lessons for Researching Sensitive SRHR

For health promotion research to be effective and to deliver the evidence needed to change specific health outcomes, intersectoral collaboration and public participation in the research process are appropriate. The fundamental principle of health promotion research, according to McQueen (1991), is a conscious effort to create a collaborative learning experience for researchers and their beneficiary communities. Israel et al., (1998) argue that health promotion research ought to recognize communities as units of identity and proceed to build on their strengths and resources (human, material, etc.) to facilitate collaborative partnerships from the inception to the completion of research projects/programmes.

Importantly, the partnerships with different interest groups facilitated a seamless execution of the study. The partners from the GES negotiated school entry access for the research team, particularly in the public schools (some are managed by religious bodies even though infrastructure and staff emoluments are provided by the state). The national headquarters of the GES worked with the regional and district directors of education who, in turn, encouraged the research team's access to schools and students. Even though we were granted access to most schools, there were pockets of resistance from some private religious schools on the grounds that they had zero tolerance for any discussion of sexuality with students.

The co-creation and co-ownership modalities established at the outset built a strong platform for buy-in of the findings for policy. Our non-academic collaborators played a significant role in disseminating findings to high-level stakeholders both within and outside the government. One of the outstanding findings – the general lack of guidelines for the teaching of CSE – resulted in a collaborative initiative between some of Ghana's international partners, the GES and the researchers to create guidelines for teaching CSE in pre-tertiary institutions (Ghana Education Service, 2019).

As researchers, we learned that recognizing the research users, together with their local contexts, needs and knowledge systems in mutually respectful ways, was important before, during and after research activities. We appreciated their wealth of knowledge on critical concerns and their ability to put the study findings to use. Researching on and with high-level decision-makers requires significant investment in behind-the-scenes preparations to yield results. Many had extremely tight and busy schedules, and we needed to be methodical when planning meetings and interviews. Even so, in some instances, appointments were rescheduled or postponed due to impromptu official meetings. With hindsight, we wonder if some of the high-level meetings and interviews could have been conducted online to save time and financial resources.

28.13 Positionality and Ethical Reflections

A common research dilemma is balancing biases and positionalities on topics of interest. It is noteworthy that all the team members had been involved in research and advocacy on diverse aspects of adolescent sexual and reproductive health, including safe abortion, contraception and family planning. Moreover, some of the Ghanaian researchers had been involved in the development of important national government policies that emphasize the need for in-school and out-of-school

CSE. In essence, our team comprised long-standing advocates for CSE. This was both a challenge and an opportunity.

It was a challenge because it was difficult to be objective and neutral. Yet, the multi-country nature of the study helped minimize bias. We used a tool with a core content, reviewed and discussed comprehensively by all in-country teams, thus reducing threats to "objectivity". Moreover, our long-standing engagement in adolescent sexual and reproductive health was strategic to gaining the attention and interest of the key stakeholders.

We also benefited from and leveraged on the original mission of the UCC in training teachers and principals for secondary schools. In the majority of the schools, we profited from the goodwill of the UCC, as several of the teachers and principals had completed a BA or postgraduate degree at the university. Although this was important in many respects (e.g. ease of access to participants/respondents, including students), it raised some ethical concerns. The line between willing participation and "enforced/compelled" participation was always blurry. Therefore, at each step of the field operations, we were mindful of the consenting process, especially for students. To provide the adolescent participants with a non-intimidating environment, we relied on young researchers (~23–25 years). Whilst school heads/principals consented to students' participation, we also secured students' individual assent. Finally, we ensured teachers were not present at the venues where students completed the questionnaire. A few students declined to participate in the survey, but the majority were excited to respond to the questionnaire, given the subject of inquiry.

28.14 Conclusions

This chapter has provided an overview of implementation research conducted to assess the effectiveness of comprehensive sexuality education taught in Ghanaian secondary schools. The inquiry was driven by a shared understanding between international and local researchers, on the one hand, and a group of policymakers and programme implementers, including teachers and beneficiaries, on the other hand. As part of the collaborative learning process, all stakeholders acknowledged the instrumental value of CSE for children and adolescents and the importance of teachers' fidelity to developed curricula. This provided a strong platform to guide the development of research questions considered appropriate for the creation of knowledge with practical relevance to the teaching and learning realities of policymakers, teachers (implementers) and students (beneficiaries).

In executing research projects in school settings on delicate subjects like sexuality, the usability of findings must be contemplated at the start of the project design and not simply added as an appendage to the knowledge generation process. As is widely known in research for development circles, the uptake and utilization of research evidence are important. This demands significant outlay in appreciating the contexts, the user-friendliness of research products (e.g. policy briefs) and timely dissemination. As we see it, the wide acceptance and efforts to put the findings to immediate use can be largely attributed to the collaborations and partnerships formed at the conceptual stage of the study.

References

Anderson, L. W., Krathwohl, D. R., Airasian, P., Cruikshank, K., Mayer, R., Pintrich, P., et al. (2001). *A taxonomy for learning, teaching and assessing: A revision of Bloom's taxonomy*. Longman Publishing.

Andreou, T. E., McIntosh, K., Ross, S. W., & Kahn, J. D. (2015). Critical incidents in sustaining school-wide positive behavioral interventions and supports. *The Journal of Special Education, 49*(3), 157–167.

Awusabo-Asare, K., Stillman, M., Keogh, S., Doku, D. T., Kumi-Kyereme, A., Esia-Donkoh, K., et al. (2017). *From paper to practice: Sexuality education policies and their implementation in Ghana*. Guttmacher Institute.

Bialystok, L., & Wright, J. (2019). 'Just say no': Public dissent over sexuality education and the Canadian national imaginary. *Discourse: Studies in the Cultural Politics of Education, 40*(3), 343–357.

Biddlecom, A. E., Hessburg, L., Singh, S., Bankole, A., & Darabi, L. (2007). *Protecting the next generation in sub-Saharan Africa: Learning from adolescents to prevent HIV and unintended pregnancy*. Guttmacher Institute.

Bloom, B. S., Krathwohl, D. R., & Masia, B. B. (1984). *Bloom taxonomy of educational objectives*. Allyn and Bacon.

Bodnar, K., & Tornello, S. L. (2019). Does sex education help everyone?: Sex education exposure and timing as predictors of sexual health among lesbian, bisexual, and heterosexual young Women. *Journal of Educational and Psychological Consultation, 29*(1), 8–26.

Braeken, D., & Cardinal, M. (2008). Comprehensive sexuality education as a means of promoting sexual health. *International Journal of Sexual Health, 20*(1–2), 50–62.

Chandra-Mouli, V., Garbero, L. G., Plesons, M., Lang, I., & Vargas, E. C. (2018). Evolution and resistance to sexuality education in Mexico. *Global Health: Science and Practice, 6*(1), 137–149.

Clark, L., & Stitzlein, S. M. (2018). Neoliberal narratives and the logic of abstinence only education: Why are we still having this conversation? *Gender and Education, 30*(3), 322–340.

Cohen, L., Manion, L., & Morrison, K. (2013). *Research methods in education*. Routledge.

Creswell, J. W., Plano Clark, V. L., Gutmann, M. L., & Hanson, W. E. (2003). Advanced mixed methods research designs. In *Handbook of mixed methods in social and behavioral research* (pp. 209–240).

Crotty, M. (1998). *The foundations of social research: Meaning and perspective in the research process*. Sage.

Darteh, E. K. M., Dickson, K. S., Rominski, S. D., & Moyer, C. A. (2020). Justification of physical intimate partner violence among men in sub-Saharan Africa: A multinational analysis of demographic and health survey data. *Journal of Public Health*, 1–9.

Dusenbury, L., Brannigan, R., Falco, M., & Hansen, W. B. (2003). A review of research on fidelity of implementation: Implications for drug abuse prevention in school settings. *Health Education Research, 18*(2), 237–256.

Gerritsen-van Leeuwenkamp, K. J., Joosten-ten Brinke, D., & Kester, L. (2019). Students' perceptions of assessment quality related to their learning approaches and learning outcomes. *Studies in Educational Evaluation, 63*, 72–82.

Ghana Census Office. (1962). *The 1960 population census of Ghana*. Ghana Census Office.

Ghana Education Service. (2019). *Guidelines for comprehensive sexuality education in Ghana*. M. o. Education.

Ghana Statistical Service, Ghana Health Service & ICF. (2015). *Ghana demographic and health survey 2014*. GSS, GHS, and ICF International.

Ghana Statistical Service, Ghana Health Service, & ICF International GSS, GHS, and ICF (2018) *Ghana maternal health survey 2017*. Accra, Ghana.

Gollust, S. E., Seymour, J. W., Pany, M. J., Goss, A., Meisel, Z. F., & Grande, D. (2017). Mutual distrust: Perspectives from researchers and policy makers on the research to policy gap in 2013 and recommendations for the future. *INQUIRY: The Journal of Health Care Organization, Provision, and Financing, 54*, 0046958017705465.

Green, J., Oman, R. F., Vesely, S. K., Cheney, M., & Carroll, L. (2017). Beyond the effects of comprehensive sexuality education: The significant prospective effects of youth assets on contraceptive behaviors. *Journal of Adolescent Health, 61*(6), 678–684.

Greene, J. C. (2007). *Mixed methods in social inquiry*. Wiley.

Guba, E. G., & Lincoln, Y. S. (1994). Competing paradigms in qualitative research. *Handbook of Qualitative Research, 2*(163–194), 105.

Haas, P. M. (1992). Introduction: Epistemic communities and international policy coordination. *International Organization, 46*(1), 1–35.

Haberland, N., & Rogow, D. (2015). Sexuality education: Emerging trends in evidence and practice. *Journal of Adolescent Health, 56*(1), S15–S21.

Hanson, J. H. (2017). *The Ahmadiyya in the Gold Coast: Muslim cosmopolitans in the British empire*. Indiana University Press.

Harn, B., Parisi, D., & Stoolmiller, M. (2013). Balancing Fidelity with flexibility and fit: What do we really know about Fidelity of implementation in schools? *Exceptional Children, 79*(2), 181–193. https://doi.org/10.1177/001440291307900204

Israel, B. A., Schulz, A. J., Parker, E. A., & Becker, A. B. (1998). Review of community-based research: Assessing partnership approaches to improve public health. *Annual Review of Public Health, 19*(1), 173–202.

Izugbara, C., Wekesah, F., Amo-Adjei, J., Kabiru, C., Dimbuene, Z. T., & Emina, J. (2017). *Young people in west and Central Africa: Health, demographic, education and socioeconomic indicators*. African Population and Health Research Center.

James-Traore, T. A., Finger, W., Ruland, C. D., & Savariaud, S. (2004). Teacher training: Essential for school-based reproductive health and HIV/AIDS education. *Youth Issues Paper, 3*.

Johnson, R. B., & Onwuegbuzie, A. J. (2004). Mixed methods research: A research paradigm whose time has come. *Educational Researcher, 33*(7), 14–26.

Johnson, R. B., Onwuegbuzie, A. J., & Turner, L. A. (2007). Toward a definition of mixed methods research. *Journal of Mixed Methods Research, 1*(2), 112–133.

Keogh, S. C., Stillman, M., Awusabo-Asare, K., Sidze, E., Monzón, A. S., Motta, A., et al. (2018). Challenges to implementing national comprehensive sexuality education curricula in low-and middle-income countries: Case studies of Ghana, Kenya, Peru and Guatemala. *PloS One, 13*(7).

Kershner, S. H., Corwin, S. J., Prince, M. S., Robillard, A. G., & Oldendick, R. W. (2017). Support for comprehensive sexuality education and adolescent access to condoms and contraception in South Carolina. *American Journal of Sexuality Education, 12*(3), 297–314.

Kirby, D., & Laris, B. (2009). Effective curriculum-based sex and STD/HIV education programs for adolescents. *Child Development Perspectives, 3*(1), 21–29.

Kwankye, S. O., & Cofie, E. (2015). Ghana's population policy implementation: Past, present and future. *African Population Studies, 29*(2).

Lebel, J., & McLean, R. (2020). Research quality plus: Another way is possible. *Transforming Research Excellence*.

Li, C., Cheng, Z., Wu, T., Liang, X., Gaoshan, J., Li, L., et al. (2017). The relationships of school-based sexuality education, sexual knowledge and sexual behaviors—A study of 18,000 Chinese college students. *Reproductive Health, 14*(1), 103. https://doi.org/10.1186/s12978-017-0368-4

Loughran, J., Berry, A., & Mulhall, P. (2012). Pedagogical content knowledge. In J. Loughran, A. Berry, & P. Mulhall (Eds.), *Understanding and developing science teachers' pedagogical content knowledge* (pp. 7–14). SensePublishers. https://doi.org/10.1007/978-94-6091-821-6_2

Marsh, D., & Furlong, P. (2002). A skin not a sweater: Ontology and epistemology in political science. *Theory and methods in political science, 2*, 17–41.

McCarty-Caplan, D. M. (2013). Schools, sex education, and support for sexual minorities: Exploring historic marginalization and future potential. *American Journal of Sexuality Education, 8*(4), 246–273.

McQueen, D. V. (1991). The contribution of health promotion research to public health. *The European Journal of Public Health, 1*(1), 22–28.

Ofir, Z., Schwandt, T., Duggan, C., & McLean, R. (2016). Research quality plus (RQ+): A holistic approach to evaluating research.

Ormston, R., Spencer, L., Barnard, M., & Snape, D. (2014). The foundations of qualitative research. *Qualitative Research Practice: A Guide for Social Science Students and Researchers, 2*, 52–55.

Panchaud, C., Keogh, S. C., Stillman, M., Awusabo-Asare, K., Motta, A., Sidze, E., et al. (2019). Towards comprehensive sexuality education: A comparative analysis of the policy environment surrounding school-based sexuality education in Ghana, Peru, Kenya and Guatemala. *Sex Education, 19*(3), 277–296.

Peters, D. H., Adam, T., Alonge, O., Agyepong, I. A., & Tran, N. (2013a). Implementation research: What it is and how to do it. *BMJ, 347*, f6753.

Peters, D. H., Tran, N. T., & Adam, T. (2013b). *Implementation research in health: A practical guide*. World Health Organization.

Quarshie, E. N., Waterman, M. G., & House, A. O. (2020). Self-harm with suicidal and non-suicidal intent in young people in sub-Saharan Africa: A systematic review. *BMC Psychiatry, 20*, 1–26.

Richards, S. D., Mendelson, E., Flynn, G., Messina, L., Bushley, D., Halpern, M., et al. (2019). Evaluation of a comprehensive sexuality education program in La Romana, Dominican Republic. *International Journal of Adolescent Medicine and Health.*

Roodsaz, R. (2018). Probing the politics of comprehensive sexuality education: 'Universality' versus 'cultural sensitivity': A Dutch–Bangladeshi collaboration on adolescent sexuality education. *Sex Education, 18*(1), 107–121.

Santelli, J. S., Kantor, L. M., Grilo, S. A., Speizer, I. S., Lindberg, L. D., Heitel, J., et al. (2017). Abstinence-only-until-marriage: An updated review of US policies and programs and their impact. *Journal of Adolescent Health, 61*(3), 273–280.

Santelli, J. S., Grilo, S. A., Choo, T.-H., Diaz, G., Walsh, K., Wall, M., et al. (2018). Does sex education before college protect students from sexual assault in college? *PLoS One, 13*(11), e0205951. https://doi.org/10.1371/journal.pone.0205951

Shannon, B. (2016). Comprehensive for who? Neoliberal directives in Australian 'comprehensive' sexuality education and the erasure of GLBTIQ identity. *Sex Education, 16*(6), 573–585.

Sumner, A., & Tribe, M. (2004). 'The nature of epistemology and methodology in development studies: What do we mean by 'rigour'' *Development Studies Association Annual Conference.*

Tenkorang, E. Y. (2013). Myths and misconceptions about HIV transmission in Ghana: What are the drivers? *Culture, Health & Sexuality, 15*(3), 296–310.

Tenkorang, E. Y., Amo-Adjei, J., & Kumi-Kyereme, A. (2020a). Assessing components of Ghana's comprehensive sexuality education on the timing of sexual debut among in-school youth. *Youth & Society, 0044118X20930891.*

Tenkorang, E. Y., Amo-Adjei, J., Kumi-Kyereme, A., & Kundhi, G. (2020b). Determinants of sexual violence at sexual debut against in-school adolescents in Ghana. *Journal of Family Violence*, 1–12.

UNESCO, UNAIDS, UNFPA, UNICEF, UN Women, & WHO. (2018). *International technical guidance on sexuality education: An evidence-informed approach*. Paris UNESCO Publishing.

United Nations Department of Economic and Social Affairs. (2020). *World population prospects, 2020*. Accessed: 18th June 2020.

Uzochukwu, B., Onwujekwe, O., Mbachu, C., Okwuosa, C., Etiaba, E., Nyström, M. E., et al. (2016). The challenge of bridging the gap between researchers and policy makers: Experiences of a health policy research group in engaging policy makers to support evidence informed policy making in Nigeria. *Globalization and Health, 12*(1), 67.

Vasilenko, S. A., Kugler, K. C., & Rice, C. E. (2016). Timing of first sexual intercourse and young adult health outcomes. *Journal of Adolescent Health, 59*(3), 291–297.

Wagner, L. M., Eastman-Mueller, H. P., Oswalt, S. B., & Nevers, J. M. (2017). Teaching philosophies guiding sexuality instruction in US colleges and universities. *Teaching in Higher Education, 22*(1), 44–61. https://doi.org/10.1080/13562517.2016.1213231

Wang, B., Stanton, B., Deveaux, L., Poitier, M., Lunn, S., Koci, V., et al. (2015). Factors influencing implementation dose and fidelity thereof and related student outcomes of an evidence-based national HIV prevention program. *Implementation Science, 10*(1), 44.

Chapter 29
Oral Health Promotion Intervention Research: A Pathway to Social Justice Applied to the Context of New Caledonia

Stephanie Tubert-Jeannin, Helene Pichot, Amal Skandrani, Nada El Osta, and Estelle Pegon-Machat

29.1 Introduction

The WHO (World Health Organization, s.d.) defines equity as "the absence of avoidable or remediable differences among groups of people, whether those groups are defined socially, economically, demographically, or geographically. Health inequities therefore involve more than inequality. They also entail a failure to avoid or overcome inequalities that infringe on fairness and human rights norms" (Rochaix & Tubeuf, 2009). The concept of health inequities then considers the measures against health inequalities as a requirement to be integrated into health policies with the underlying objective of making fundamental human rights effective. The absence of recognition of health inequalities as being unfair and/or the inability to deal with them are, in themselves, factors that both increase health inequalities and generate a lack of health equity. Therefore, health equity goes beyond observing health inequalities or unequal access to health resources: it also means putting in place health promotion (HP) interventions that are aimed at avoiding or overcoming injustices and thus respecting human rights.

S. Tubert-Jeannin (✉) · E. Pegon-Machat
Université Clermont Auvergne, laboratoire CROC, Clermont-Ferrand, France

CHU Clermont-Ferrand, Service d'Odontologie, Clermont-Ferrand, France
e-mail: stephanie.tubert@uca.fr

H. Pichot
Health and Social Agency of New Caledonia, Nouméa, New Caledonia

A. Skandrani
Université Clermont Auvergne, laboratoire CROC, Clermont-Ferrand, France

N. El Osta
Université Clermont Auvergne, laboratoire CROC, Clermont-Ferrand, France

Department of Public Health, Saint-Joseph University, Beirut, Lebanon

L. Potvin, D. Jourdan (eds.), *Global Handbook of Health Promotion Research, Vol. 1*,
https://doi.org/10.1007/978-3-030-97212-7_29

From the point of view of an approach to research that is based on a pragmatic worldview, the process that leads to the implementation of effective HP interventions in terms of health equity has to go through some key steps (Potvin et al., 2008). The reality of health inequalities has to be measured and pointed out, and information must be disseminated to the community and all stakeholders. Following this, inequalities have to be interpreted as unfair, and the responsibility to act needs to be identified as a political and collective imperative. This should lead to the implementation of interventions that are adapted to the population's needs. Finally, the impacts of the HP interventions on health outcomes and on health inequalities have to be evaluated. Within this process, implementation and knowledge production are simultaneously undertaken.

Indeed, there are different ways to implement HP interventions and to produce data on how to improve health for all and reduce inequities (Cambon et al., 2010). From the perspective of intervention research, implantation and research are closely intertwined. Research brings about information and allows for complex analyses and deep understanding at each stage of the search process for equity. Researchers can thus provide both support for political decisions and people's participation and be actors involved in the implementation and evaluation of HP interventions. One-shot interventions are rarely relevant to inequality reduction, so there is a need to implement long-term research frameworks. Since the origin of health inequalities is complex and multidimensional, HP programmes have to be intersectoral and comprehensive.

In this chapter, we will describe an oral health promotion intervention and research programme conducted in New Caledonia (NC), an archipelago in the south-western Pacific Ocean. While remaining focused on the issue of equity, the aim of this intervention and research programme is the production of knowledge in the field of health promotion applied to oral health. In particular, the research is aimed at evaluating the relevance, scope and effect of the interventions implemented within the New Caledonian oral health promotion programme. The general orientation of the research that guides our activities relates to empirical science, which is a traditional form of research in HP. Epidemiological or intermediate data on intervention processes are collected to evaluate the effects of an oral health promotion (OHP) programme and then to enable us to make the necessary revisions to better improve oral health. Our underlying hypothesis is that causes (the interventions of the programme) determine measurable effects such as positive health outcomes. Within this orientation, the research aims at measuring the reality with objective data and rational considerations that shape knowledge. The information collected is based on questionnaires completed by participants and on clinical observations made by the researchers. While taking into account the influence of behavioural risk factors and social determinants on oral health and general health, conducting two successive epidemiological studies and their associated multidimensional analyses makes it possible to measure the changes produced after the development of the programme.

Since the beginning, researchers have been extremely careful about their positioning that is both internal (they have been involved from the outset in the design and development of the interventions) and external (they also work on the programme as a separate entity). Then, research allows to verify whether the interventions were actually implemented, whether the target public benefited from them or participated in them, whether they had a positive impact on children's health and, at the very least, whether they did not lead to an increase in health inequalities.

Our research approach is slightly participative as the people involved (stakeholders, families, etc.) were consulted in the development of prevention tools and as qualitative research methodologies were used to better integrate their representations. This participatory approach has been maintained throughout both the implementation and evaluation processes in order to not only better understand the social actors' representations of oral health and dental care or prevention but also identify the barriers and solutions needed for improving the compatibility of the interventions with the representations of the different actors.

It should be noted that the research here is also intertwined with NC's political agenda. The stakeholders involved in the programme lent a voice to the participants, took into account the needs of the local population and focused on the issue of health inequalities within the local context. The research tries to be transformative in that it links research to political agenda in order to advocate for better oral health and to promote social justice through the reduction of health inequalities.

Finally, the research methodology is largely pragmatic, with the use of mixed methods (qualitative and quantitative) brought together to ensure that the health needs of the local population, within the context of NC, are met. The research approach is intended to help identify vulnerable populations (already affected by diseases or at risk of being so) to highlight social injustices and to enable relevant HP interventions to be combined in a coherent manner in responding to the complexity of health inequalities previously described and understood. The programme and its evaluation processes are thus open to many different approaches for generating, collecting and analyzing data to arrive at the best understanding of the complexity of health issues in NC and to help the promotion of health (Creswell & Creswell, 2018).

In this chapter, we will describe the oral health promotion intervention and research programme conducted in New Caledonia (NC). After describing the context of New Caledonia, we will explore how the different stages for the search of equity are followed to allow oral health to be recognized as an issue for health promotion, to ensure stakeholder participation, integrate it into a general health promotion approach and undergo quality research in oral health promotion.

29.2 The "My Teeth, My Health" Intervention and Research Programme

29.2.1 The Context of New Caledonia

New Caledonia is a French territory with broad autonomy since the 1980s that, since then, has been following a political process to decide its future potential independency. New Caledonia is divided into three provinces (North, South and Loyalty

Islands). The population of New Caledonia (n = 271,407 in 2019) is multi-ethnic with 39% of the population declaring belonging to the Kanak community, 27% being Europeans and 8% Polynesians. The distribution of the population is extremely uneven between provinces with strong social, economic and cultural interprovincial gaps. The geographic and socio-economic inequalities are superimposed on ethnic disparities. As an example, in the Loyalty Islands, 94% of the inhabitants belong to the Kanak community compared to 26% in the Southern Province where the capital Noumea is situated. In 2008, the relative poverty rate was estimated at 22% in NC varying from 9% in the South Province, 35% in the Northern Province and 52% in the Loyalty Islands (INSEE Première, 2015). In NC, non-communicable diseases (NCDs) tend to be highly prevalent among the New Caledonian population (67.3% of adults had a body mass index (BMI) >25, of which 37.7% were obese in 2018 (BMI >30)). The prevalence of diabetes was estimated at 5% of the population in 2017, and the NC Congress has made diabetes a priority public health issue (« documents, rapports, études | Direction des Affaires Sanitaires et Sociales de Nouvelle-Calédonie », s. d.).

29.2.2 *Oral Health Inequalities: Recognized as a Social Injustice in NC*

Those patterns in non-communicable diseases such as oral diseases have been considered to be of particular concern in NC for a number of decades but until recently had not be completely objectivized. Since oral diseases have been listed amongst the leading causes of chronic disorders worldwide (GBD 2017 Oral Disorders Collaborators et al., 2020) and have been shown to impact general health and quality of life in many ways (Petersen et al., 2005), the New Caledonian Health Agency (Agence sanitaire et sociale de la Nouvelle-Calédonie, ASS-NC) conducted an epidemiological survey in 2011–2012 among a representative sample of 2734 children (744 6 year olds, 789 9 year olds and 1201 12 year olds) (Pichot et al., 2014). The study described the oral health status of New Caledonian children and investigated the related environmental and behavioural risk factors. It found that most of the children had untreated oral diseases: more than 50% had gingivitis and 60% of 6 and 9 year olds had at least one deciduous or permanent tooth with untreated caries. The mean number of decayed, missing and filled teeth (DMFT) was 2.09 ± 2.82 for 12-years-old children with 25% declaring that they had recently experienced dental pain.

Oral diseases such as other NCDs are linked to common socio-environmental determinants along with behavioural risk factors (Watt & Sheiham, 2012). Low-income, socially or even medically disadvantaged populations experience higher levels of chronic diseases, and this gradient is particularly evident for oral diseases, which affect populations from early childhood (Marmot, 2003; Watt et al., 2018). Difficulties in accessing oral health services for underprivileged populations increase health inequalities and worsen the impairments caused by oral diseases (Harris, 2016). In NC, the number of carious lesions was related to unfavourable health behaviours, deprived social status and no access to preventive care. Kanak, Polynesians and Caledonians were more affected by oral diseases than were metropolitan French and Asian children. Children with many untreated carious lesions complained of chewing difficulty and had higher scores for dental anxiety, which in turn reduces accessibility to dental care (Pichot et al., 2014).

In the same way as for other chronic diseases, oral diseases and their impacts have to be positioned within a broader concept of health. In the same approach as for the definition of health, oral health has recently been defined as "the ability to speak, smile, smell, taste, touch, chew, swallow and convey a range of emotions through facial expressions with confidence and without pain, discomfort and disease of the craniofacial complex". This definition integrates functional and psychosocial dimensions and insists on the fact that oral health cannot be considered separately from general health. Thus, throughout life, oral health is seen as part of a continuum that is shaped by many individual, commercial and socio-environmental determinants and that has an impact on and interacts with general health (Glick et al., 2017). Therefore, the assessment of oral health in NC has taken into account dimensions that go beyond the presence or absence of oral diseases or its related symptoms. The Caledonian study also integrated the evaluation of oral health-related quality of life (OHrQOL) among 12-year-old children ($n = 311$) from diverse ethnic groups. The Child Oral Health Impact Profile (French COHIP-36) questionnaire was used to evaluate functional well-being, social and emotional well-being, school environment and self-image linked to oral health as well as overall OHrQOL. According to COHIP, 96.2% of the children had experienced oral health problems in the previous 3 months, 72.9% had functional difficulties, 60.2% had socio-emotional impacts, 31.8% had school or environmental impacts and 92.2% had self-image impacts. Lower COHIP scores were significantly associated with the self-perception of poor general or oral health, having dental problems, needs for dental treatment and chewing difficulties. The COHIP scores also varied between participants according to gender, ethnic group, oral hygiene, dental attendance and dental fear. The COHIP scores were related to the presence of oral diseases, acute pain, dental trauma or urgent needs for care (El Osta et al., 2015).

Among these results, the impact of oral diseases on children's lives, especially socially, reflects a loss of opportunity for some children compared to others. More than an epidemiological description of the oral health status, this kind of study brings to light for decision-makers the associated injustice: children, whose autonomy must be acquired as a matter of principle, are hindered very early on by a combination of negative impacts, particularly at school (Ruff et al., 2019).

29.2.3 Oral Health Promotion: Integrated into a General Health Promotion Approach in NC

The most frequently used definition of health promotion (HP) comes from the Ottawa Charter (World Health Organisation, 1986). This classical approach to HP includes health education (increased knowledge and skills to improve health), health protection (policies to promote healthy environments) and disease prevention. This vision is still being largely adhered to, particularly in oral health promotion (OHP) (Fraihat et al., 2019). Preventive school-based (or even nursery-based) programmes in particular have been shown to be effective vehicles for advancing oral health promotion by facilitating the impact of OHP interventions among vulnerable populations (Gargano et al., 2019). However, recent trends have considered that health promotion should not be restricted to the health sector nor to the promotion of healthy lifestyles with hierarchically built, linear and "top-down" interventions. Indeed, the concept of HP has evolved since the Ottawa Charter, with strategies that now place greater emphasis on empowerment, inter-professionality and multiple partnerships. Interventions that are more directed towards changing social and environmental conditions are now preferred. This trend is also being developed in the field of oral health promotion, where some recent publications have suggested the need for context paradigms and the potential for participatory research and systems thinking in oral health (Brocklehurst et al., 2021). Thus, the development of co-designed interventions, with multiple stakeholders and with the community is becoming a prerequisite to effective HP including OHP (Singh, 2012), with this being crucial for the development of culturally appropriate health promotion initiatives (Jamieson et al., 2008).

In practice, opposing those two approaches is not relevant since they are complementary in promoting health and effectively prevent and manage chronic diseases. This is particularly true in the field of oral health, where awareness about oral disease challenges is extremely low for all, including decision-makers. Thus, the bottom-up process alone in the field of oral health would result in missing oral health challenges as, paradoxically, oral health is seen as an important matter but either does not or only rarely emerges in the context of HP priorities being set. Therefore, the third vision that is based on intersectoral collaboration and the use of mixed approaches should be explored particularly in the field of oral health.

In addition, health promotion is increasingly concerned with the issue of health-related quality of life and the reduction of health inequalities. Chronic diseases such as oral diseases are, in theory, easily preventable, but the real question for health promotion is how to prevent them effectively and in good time in the most socially vulnerable groups and how to avoid exacerbating health inequalities with inequitable interventions. Oral diseases thus represent very early markers of social inequalities in health, justifying the implementation of early OHP interventions that can both have measurable impacts on health inequalities and influence children's health in the longer term (Pussinen et al., 2019).

Since oral health inequalities come across the whole social body according to a gradient, the challenge is also to take that gradient into account when implementing and evaluating public health interventions. An efficient intervention might have no effect on health inequalities if all socio-economic groups benefit equally. In addition, it may even increase health inequalities if the wealthiest groups benefit more (Lee & Divaris, 2014). Indeed, the more affluent communities are often in a better position to implement health promotion programmes not only for financial reasons but also because of environmental factors or being in possession of greater manpower resources. Unfortunately, there is very little evidence concerning the equity effects of health-related interventions. There is therefore a need to better develop interventions that could ensure equity (World Health Organisation, 2020). Moreover, the knowledge of the mechanisms to be taken into account for ensuring proportionate universalism in HP interventions is the responsibility of those experts who are capable of positioning a specific problem such as oral health inequities within a specific local context such as NC.

29.2.4 The Development of the Oral Health Promotion Intervention Research, "My Teeth, My Health"

The data from the NC 2012 study highlighted the need for new strategies aimed at improving children's oral and general health and at reducing inequalities. An alternative approach to the traditional health care and preventive interventions was chosen in collaboration with NC's local populations and government, based on the principles of health promotion (HP). The programme is multi-sectoral and involves multiple actors such as health professionals, social welfare organizations, political actors, education institutions and teachers who were involved in the design of the intervention along with the local communities. The programme is coordinated by the ASS-NC in connection with regional educational and health authorities, health-fund bodies and the dental profession.

The OHP programme was developed in connection with health programmes related to the prevention of other chronic diseases such as rheumatic heart disease and obesity. Indeed, the 2012 NC study also evaluated the children's weight status with results showing high prevalence of overweight and obese individuals; 22% of the 12 year olds were overweight, 20% obese and one-third had an excess of abdominal adiposity (Tubert-Jeannin et al., 2018). High-risk groups were identified with children affected by both oral diseases and obesity, showing the need for health promotion programmes specifically addressed to native populations who are particularly exposed to oral diseases and obesity, integrating a multiple risk factor approach, in order to prevent the onset of chronic diseases in adulthood. The common risk factor approach was thus privileged in order to address risk factors common to those chronic conditions within the context of the local environment (Watt

& Sheiham, 2012). As an example, the promotion of healthy oral health habits is related to the promotion of a healthy diet or physical activity.

The programme targets the entire New Caledonian population with more emphasis on promoting children's health. However, health professionals as well as the educational community, teachers, school staff, parents and pregnant women are also the targets of some interventions. The programme has three overarching axes (Fry & Zask, 2017), with the development of (1) oral health promotion in schools for better educational achievement (Langford et al., 2015); (2) the promotion of healthy lifestyles (oral hygiene or nutrition) such as the implementation of tooth brushing in primary schools and (3) the reorientation of oral health services towards providing more effective and preventive interventions (a dental sealant programme). The dental sealant programme, which has existed since 2009, was renewed in order to ensure its quality and that all 6-year-old schoolchildren can benefit from it. Indeed, dental sealants have been shown to be an effective preventive intervention when evaluated in real-life school conditions (Ahovuo-Saloranta et al., 2017; Muller-Bolla et al., 2013). The aim was to reduce the number of untreated oral diseases by 20% in children aged 6–12 years within a period of 5 years, with a special focus on ensuring that trend in the more deprived areas. Thus, a great part of the programme's interventions is carried out in schools (primary, secondary) or kindergartens. Primary schools offer an adequate infrastructure for the implementation of the health promotion programmes in NC with almost all children being integrated into the education system from the age of 6.

The OHP programme was developed by first generating a strategic plan with a vision, three overarching aims, associated with operational objectives. This plan was coordinated by the NC health agency and openly discussed with the community, the health professionals and the education sector, all in accordance with NC's government health policies. Interprofessional, intersectoral collaboration as well as the involvement of the local stakeholders were searched all along the development, implementation and evaluation phases. In the area of oral health promotion, it is particularly important to help multiple actors – such as public health personnel, oral health professionals, educators, the public and politicians – work together and understand how oral health inequalities emerge, impact people's life and can be effectively prevented and managed. In dentistry, there is a specific need for development of partnerships between health professionals and academics as research in OHP is still poorly developed. For this reason, since the beginning of the programme, the NC health agency has signed partnership agreements with universities and research teams that had been identified as having adequate expertise.

Many oral health practitioners are daunted at the prospect of participating in a public health intervention or evaluation of community-based programmes. Practitioners' knowledge, skills and confidence need to be developed to facilitate progress in this area (Tubert-Jeannin & Jourdan, 2018). This is particularly true in countries such as France where the vast majority of dentists are private practitioners and where apart from dentists there are almost no associated oral health professionals such as dental hygienists (Pegon-Machat et al., 2016). In the OHP programme, the oral health professionals have thus been involved through their participation in the dental sealant programme. The sealant programme has been put in place within the context of routine local practices. Existing clinical practices were identified and improvements were facilitated. The sealant programme has been supported within the OHP programme, first because it is an effective, evidence-based intervention with a solid rationale and, second, because oral health providers had already been involved in a similar programme in the past. The likelihood of adoption and effective implementation by health professionals was therefore high. Indeed, the dental sealants programme is offered to all Caledonian children at the age of 6. Sealants are applied either at school in a mobile dental surgery or in public dental offices. In 2016, for example, 30 general dental practitioners (of approximately 126 in NC) performed dental examinations and applied the fissure sealants. They were recruited by the NC health agency within public regional health services and through the council of private dentists. The practitioners were assigned to one or several schools, depending on the feasibility criteria that were mostly dependent on geographical locations. Prior to the start of the programme, all the practitioners underwent a training course consisting of a presentation of the NC OHP programme, the sealant application protocol, illustrations with clinical situations and training about the data collection process. A retrospective study of the quality and impact of the fissure sealant programme showed a high participation rate and acceptable effectiveness – as measured with the 1-year retention rates – for a fissure sealant intervention conducted in real-life conditions and integrated into a large health promotion programme. Nevertheless, the results pointed out some issues of generalizing well-proven, effective preventive procedures within specific real-life contexts (Pichot et al., 2020). The results emphasized the need for continuous and targeted training programmes for the programme actors to help optimize effectiveness.

29.3 Research Approaches for Evaluating the NC OHP Programme

In the field of oral health, systematic reviews and randomized clinical trials (RCTs) have brought about the efficacy of preventive interventions such as tooth brushing with fluoridated toothpastes or dental fissure sealing for preventing tooth decay (Ahovuo-Saloranta et al., 2017; Walsh et al., 2019). However, using this type of study to inform public health decisions has its limitations, because health promotion interventions are complex and depend heavily on the local context. HP programmes combine different actions that have often been evaluated independently and have usually already shown their value. What is sought in the evaluation of HP programmes is rather to understand how interventions that are known to be effective under ideal implementation conditions can work in the field with different local conditions and actors. However, it appears that research on programmes' modalities of implementation is limited with regard to HP and particularly OHP (Leeman et al., 2017). In a context where little evidence exists, it is important to critically evaluate what is working well and what is not in real-life conditions in order to achieve oral health equity. This is the reason why the evaluation of OHP interventions in NC is being conducted with a pragmatic strategy, using pluralistic and mixed research approaches and combined research designs (Wolfenden et al., 2017).

Participatory designs, which include the community at each stage of HP development, implementation and evaluation, are gaining increasing emphasis. In HP research, it is integral to address the concerns of policymakers as well as those of the people in the community. From the research perspective, there is a need to evaluate health outcomes that are important to people and to be able to translate them in terms that everybody can understand. This is why it is important that the evaluation task is shared between the key players and participants; it should be a shared work with researchers, health professionals and the public actively cooperating together in the evaluation process. The consultation and involvement of the local community is a key aspect: the results of evaluations must be accessible and clear to them. If we consider oral health, this aspect is crucial because the criteria used in oral health research are often incomprehensible to the uninitiated. To succeed in publishing in international high-quality journals, it would, for example, be recommended to measure the DMFT/S indices with precise diagnostic criteria such as with the International Caries Detection and Assessment System (ICDAS). For patients and policymakers, these indicators are both too complex and meaningless. A decision-maker will be far more interested in the reduction in the percentage of children with untreated caries so that they value a reduction in dental needs from the HP intervention. Parents, particularly those in deprived populations, will prefer the decrease in the number of children with acute pain or an improvement in their ability to eat, smile, sleep or to go to school (Ahonen et al., 2020; Ni Riordain et al., 2020). This is what has been done in NC with the use of different indicators of oral health that each can be meaningful to the different groups of people involved. In addition, obesity and oral diseases have been linked within the initial epidemiological survey, the development of the OHP programme and during the evaluation process. This inter-relation between those two health issues also made it possible to consider the functional, health and psychosocial impacts of oral diseases. Taking into account OHrQOL helps objectify the reality of the OHP programme impacts and their relationship with broader issues such as nutrition (El Osta et al., 2015; Pichot et al., 2014; Tubert-Jeannin et al., 2018).

With OHP programmes, a wide diversity of intervention approaches can be combined. The methodologies selected for research need to be relevant to the nature and timescale of the interventions (Petersen & Kwan, 2004). The choice of methods depends on the nature of the intervention, the purpose of the evaluation and the resources available. Evaluation of OPH interventions requires both process and outcome data. Process evaluation seeks data on how the intervention was implemented and may uncover information on unexpected activities and results. As seen before, in 2017, a retrospective study evaluated the dental sealant programme conducted among 6-year-old children after 1 year (Pichot et al., 2020). This type of information is a valuable form of feedback in reviewing the development and delivery of the intervention. However, health outcome measures are also essential indicators assessing the effects of the intervention, in the short, intermediate or longer term. In 2019, therefore, further epidemiological studies were conducted in NC in order to chart the evolution of oral health, dental status and weight status after 5 years of programme development.

Moreover, if oral health inequalities are seen as unfair and avoidable, then equity in HP interventions represents a highly important issue. HP research has to focus on both how HP programmes are equitable and what the barriers or facilitating factors are that influence equity (de Silva et al., 2016; Lorenc et al., 2013). In the NC OPH programme, the risk is that more affluent communities (in the South region) might be in a better position to implement or participate in the programme, not only for financial reasons but also because of cultural and environmental factors and greater manpower resources. The research methods privileged in NC aim to be thorough in taking into account the extent of the impacts of the OHP programme depending on the children's social situation, their participation in the programme or their area of residence by integrating complex, multidimensional statistical analyses.

If experimental designs and epidemiological surveys allow us to appreciate the effects of a programme on health outcomes, the contextual knowledge of the local conditions helps us understand the complexity of the conditions for change. In this field, qualitative research has an important role to play in the evaluation of OHP programmes (Gupta & Keuskamp, 2018). A qualitative study was conducted to evaluate the determinants of the use of oral health services in New Caledonia (Agence sanitaire et sociale de la Nouvelle-Calédonie, 2015). The 2012 NC study showed a high prevalence of oral diseases marked by major social inequalities. It also illustrated that there was an insufficient use of oral health services; at age 6, only 50% of children had ever visited a dental practice and 22% declared themselves to be afraid of the dentist. It therefore appeared necessary within the OHP programme to ensure that oral health services would be more accessible and to give priority access to preventive services to children at high risk of dental caries. The barriers to using oral health services thus needed to be identified before implementing incentive measures. A qualitative survey was therefore conducted to better understand Caledonian families' impressions of oral health and oral diseases and the ways in which parents considered and accessed prevention and dental care for themselves and their children.

29.3.1 The Impact of the "My Teeth, My Health" Programme

This qualitative study first allowed to evaluate the determinants of the use of oral health services in New Caledonia (Agence sanitaire et sociale de la Nouvelle-Calédonie, 2015). Semi-structured interviews were conducted with 26 families (10 Southern Province, 7 Island Province and 9 Northern Province) whose children needed dental care (≥1 decayed tooth). Results showed that parents defined oral health through three dimensions, namely, oral health is seen, felt and can be influenced by them. Parents also clearly mentioned a link to general health, but they stated that their expectations of oral health care were mainly that it was designed to administer curative dental care when oral health was impaired. These opinions about the oral healthcare system, the usefulness of attending and the perceived and attributed field of competence of oral health professionals were believed to be the key determinants for the health promotion programme's success in developing efficient interventions. Although the lack of pain in dental care argued against many expectations, deconstructing the representations that led to the non-use of preventive oral health care was set as one of the overarching objectives of the OHP interventions.

In the survey, a number of attitudes were identified, with some families attending dental practices on a regular basis, whereas others only attended for emergency treatments and the last group in which parents attended only for emergency dental treatments but were regular attendees for their children. The existence of this last group, which was not expected, changed the project leaders' impressions of parents' real expectations for their children's oral health. The opinion that consisted in assuming from the outset that children whose parents are not regular dental care users would not be able to participate in regular preventive activities or to benefit from comprehensive dental treatments, was then discussed once again with oral health professionals.

Barriers to dental care accessibility were identified at different stages: upstream at the time of the perception of the dental needs, when the decision to seek care is taken; at the first contact with the oral healthcare system and later for the continuation of dental care after the first contact with the oral healthcare system. Numerous barriers were identified, particularly at the time at which the decision was made to seek care: fear of the dentist; supposed high costs; limited offers; lack of an emergency structure; and negative impressions of dentists. These findings were extremely useful for the development, implementation and evaluation of the OHP programme. They helped identify solutions that could change the families' perception of the role of the oral healthcare system, i.e. the need to value regular and preventive oral healthcare for children. This study also showed that parents had a positive view concerning oral health promotion for their children. However, it was demonstrated that a better use of oral health services could be obtained only by ensuring better accessibility to adequate, sufficient, child-friendly oral health services. Based on those results, it was believed that changing oral health professionals' views about vulnerable populations and high-risk children in NC could also be useful in facilitating the accessibility of oral health care, if other barriers were simultaneously removed.

As seen above, a retrospective study conducted in 2017 evaluated the dental sealant programme conducted among 6-year-old children after 1 year. Findings showed that the participation rate was extremely high and that, on average, children had approximately 80% of their dental sealants present after 1 year but caries increment (i.e. caries incidence) varied depending on the sealant retention rates as well as on the region. A mediation analysis showed that living in a more deprived area was a strong determinant for high caries increment, particularly when the retention rates were low. A good balance of participation and quality of intervention has been obtained by focusing efforts on ensuring accessibility to the intervention in every location, even those that are more deprived and isolated. Yet, having a high retention rate was particularly important for the children in the Islands. Hence, the retention rate was a good intermediate indicator of the effect of the preventive intervention on oral health inequalities, showing that accessible and high-quality interventions are crucial for deprived populations. These results justify the need for more proportionate universalism in oral health promotion interventions in NC with reinforced resources adapted to the needs of the populations in deprived sectors (Pichot et al., 2020).

An epidemiological study was conducted in 2019 in order to assess the evolution of oral health, dental status and weight status since 2012 and after 5 years of programme development. A sample of children aged 6, 9 and 12 years was randomly selected using a computerized cluster sampling method with a probability proportional to size. The pool of NC schools was stratified according to the area (South/North/Island) and the type of school (public/private). The total sample size was 369 6 year olds, 412 9 year olds and 693 12 year olds. Pertinent indicators to be recorded were identified through a literature review, after interviews with professionals, experts in epidemiology and paediatric dentistry and local actors. Indicators similar to the ones used in 2012 were privileged in order to enable us to draw comparisons. Dental status was clinically evaluated by calibrated dentists along with the weight status, as in 2012. Socio-demographic variables were recorded, and children and/or parents responded to questions relating to lifestyle, self-perceptions of oral health and conditions of life. Results are being analyzed and have not yet been published, but some trends appear from initial analyses in 12-year-old children. The prevalence of dental caries and experience of caries decreased significantly between 2012 and 2019, with higher improvements in the North and South regions as compared to the Islands. These positive trends, even if not completely attributable to the OHP programme, are in line with the local situation with better implementation of the programme in the North and South regions and a lower social status in the Islands.

29.4 Conclusions

Conducting HP research does not purely consist of gathering successive epidemiological data; it must allow to build a holistic and comprehensive approach to the determinants of health including the effects of HP interventions such as the effects on the accessibility of health services or on populations' capacity building. As such, the research conducted in NC has used epidemiological data to better describe and then help understand the determinants of children's oral health within the local context. Using the OHP programme in NC as an example, it is possible to appreciate how the reality of oral health inequalities can be measured and taken into consideration by the community and local stakeholders. In NC, oral health inequalities have been interpreted as being unfair and the responsibility to act has been accepted by local political and community stakeholders. This has led to the implementation of

OHP interventions that are adapted to the population's needs. Research provided support to local political decisions, and researchers were active actors involved in the implementation of OHP interventions. It was possible to identify vulnerable populations (already affected by diseases or at risk of being so), to highlight social injustices and to enable relevant HP interventions to be combined in a coherent manner to respond to the complexity of health inequalities previously described and understood. Nevertheless, many limits can be found in the NC example, such as the lack of evaluation of its cost-effectiveness; and these limitations are especially important to policymakers, along with a need for greater emphasis on implementation science and community-based participatory research. However, in view of the complexity of conducting HP research in OHP, the example of the OHP programme in NC is almost unique and has the merit of existing in a field of oral health still too little explored.

References

Agence sanitaire et sociale de la Nouvelle-Calédonie. (2015). *Evaluation des freins et des leviers du recours aux soins dentaires en Nouvelle-Calédonie. Programme Mes Dents Ma Santé*. https://www.santepourtous.nc/les-thematiques/mes-dents-ma-sante/presentation. Accessed 18 Jan 2021.

Ahonen, H., Kvarnvik, C., Norderyd, O., Broström, A., Fransson, E. I., & Lindmark, U. (2020, August 12). Clinical and self-reported measurements to be included in the core elements of the World Dental Federation's theoretical framework of oral health. *International Dental Journal*. https://doi.org/10.1111/idj.12614

Ahovuo-Saloranta, A., Forss, H., Walsh, T., Nordblad, A., Mäkelä, M., & Worthington, H. V. (2017). Pit and fissure sealants for preventing dental decay in permanent teeth. *The Cochrane Database of Systematic Reviews, 7*, CD001830. https://doi.org/10.1002/14651858.CD001830.pub5

Brocklehurst, P. R., Baker, S. R., & Langley, J. (2021). Context and the evidence-based paradigm: The potential for participatory research and systems thinking in oral health. *Community Dentistry and Oral Epidemiology, 49*(1), 1–9. https://doi.org/10.1111/cdoe.12570

Cambon, L., Ridde, V., & Alla, F. (2010). Reflections and perspectives on evidence-based health promotion in the French environment. *Revue D'epidemiologie Et De Sante Publique, 58*(4), 277–283. https://doi.org/10.1016/j.respe.2010.05.001

Creswell, J. W., & Creswell, J. D. (2018). *Research design: Qualitative, quantitative, and mixed methods approaches* (5th ed.). Sage.

de Silva, A. M., Hegde, S., Akudo Nwagbara, B., Calache, H., Gussy, M. G., Nasser, M., et al. (2016). Community-based population-level interventions for promoting child oral health. *The Cochrane Database of Systematic Reviews, 9*, CD009837. https://doi.org/10.1002/14651858.CD009837.pub2

Documents, rapports, études | Direction des Affaires Sanitaires et Sociales de Nouvelle-Calédonie. (s.d.). https://dass.gouv.nc/votre-sante/documents-rapports-etudes. Accessed 18 Jan 2021.

El Osta, N., Pichot, H., Soulier-Peigue, D., Hennequin, M., & Tubert-Jeannin, S. (2015). Validation of the child oral health impact profile (COHIP) French questionnaire among 12 years-old children in New Caledonia. *Health and Quality of Life Outcomes, 13*, 176. https://doi.org/10.1186/s12955-015-0371-9

Fraihat, N., Madae'en, S., Bencze, Z., Herczeg, A., & Varga, O. (2019). Clinical effectiveness and cost-effectiveness of oral-health promotion in dental caries prevention among children:

Systematic review and meta-analysis. *International Journal of Environmental Research and Public Health, 16*(15), 2668. https://doi.org/10.3390/ijerph16152668

Fry, D., & Zask, A. (2017). Applying the Ottawa Charter to inform health promotion programme design. *Health Promotion International, 32*(5), 901–912. https://doi.org/10.1093/heapro/daw022

Gargano, L., Mason, M. K., & Northridge, M. E. (2019). Advancing oral health equity through school-based oral health programs: An ecological model and review. *Frontiers in Public Health, 7*, 359. https://doi.org/10.3389/fpubh.2019.00359

GBD 2017 Oral Disorders Collaborators, Bernabe, E., Marcenes, W., Hernandez, C. R., Bailey, J., Abreu, L. G., et al. (2020). Global, regional, and national levels and trends in burden of oral conditions from 1990 to 2017: A systematic analysis for the global burden of disease 2017 study. *Journal of Dental Research, 99*(4), 362–373. https://doi.org/10.1177/0022034520908533

Glick, M., Williams, D. M., Kleinman, D. V., Vujicic, M., Watt, R. G., & Weyant, R. J. (2017). A new definition for oral health developed by the FDI World Dental Federation opens the door to a universal definition of oral health. *Journal of Public Health Dentistry, 77*(1), 3–5. https://doi.org/10.1111/jphd.12213

Gupta, A., & Keuskamp, D. (2018). Use and misuse of mixed methods in population oral health research: A scoping review. *Community Dental Health, 35*(2), 109–118. https://doi.org/10.1922/CDH_4250Gupta10

Harris, R. V. (2016). Do « poor areas » get the services they deserve? The role of dental services in structural inequalities in oral health. *Community Dental Health, 33*(2), 164–167.

INSEE Première. (2015). *Recensement de la population en Nouvelle-Calédonie en 2014* (No. 1572). https://www.insee.fr/fr/statistiques/1560282. Accessed 18 Jan 2021.

Jamieson, L. M., Parker, E. J., & Richards, L. (2008). Using qualitative methodology to inform an Indigenous-owned oral health promotion initiative in Australia. *Health Promotion International, 23*(1), 52–59. https://doi.org/10.1093/heapro/dam042

Langford, R., Bonell, C., Jones, H., Pouliou, T., Murphy, S., Waters, E., et al. (2015). The World Health Organization's health promoting schools framework: A Cochrane systematic review and meta-analysis. *BMC Public Health, 15*, 130. https://doi.org/10.1186/s12889-015-1360-y

Lee, J. Y., & Divaris, K. (2014). The ethical imperative of addressing oral health disparities: A unifying framework. *Journal of Dental Research, 93*(3), 224–230. https://doi.org/10.1177/0022034513511821

Leeman, J., Birken, S. A., Powell, B. J., Rohweder, C., & Shea, C. M. (2017). Beyond « implementation strategies »: Classifying the full range of strategies used in implementation science and practice. *Implementation Science, 12*(1), 125. https://doi.org/10.1186/s13012-017-0657-x

Lorenc, T., Petticrew, M., Welch, V., & Tugwell, P. (2013). What types of interventions generate inequalities? Evidence from systematic reviews. *Journal of Epidemiology and Community Health, 67*(2), 190–193. https://doi.org/10.1136/jech-2012-201257

Marmot, M. G. (2003). Understanding social inequalities in health. *Perspectives in Biology and Medicine, 46*(3 Suppl), S9–S23.

Muller-Bolla, M., Lupi-Pégurier, L., Bardakjian, H., & Velly, A. M. (2013). Effectiveness of school-based dental sealant programs among children from low-income backgrounds in France: A pragmatic randomized clinical trial. *Community Dentistry and Oral Epidemiology, 41*(3), 232–241. https://doi.org/10.1111/cdoe.12011

Ni Riordain, R., Glick, M., Al Mashhadani, S. S. A., Aravamudhan, K., Barrow, J., Cole, D., et al. (2020, July 5). Developing a standard set of patient-centred outcomes for adult oral health – An international, cross-disciplinary consensus. *International Dental Journal*. https://doi.org/10.1111/idj.12604

Pegon-Machat, E., Faulks, D., Eaton, K. A., Widström, E., Hugues, P., & Tubert-Jeannin, S. (2016). The healthcare system and the provision of oral healthcare in EU Member States: France. *British Dental Journal, 220*(4), 197–203. https://doi.org/10.1038/sj.bdj.2016.138

Petersen, P. E., & Kwan, S. (2004). Evaluation of community-based oral health promotion and oral disease prevention – WHO recommendations for improved evidence in public health practice. *Community Dental Health, 21*(4 Suppl), 319–329.

Petersen, P. E., Bourgeois, D., Ogawa, H., Estupinan-Day, S., & Ndiaye, C. (2005). The global burden of oral diseases and risks to oral health. *Bulletin of the World Health Organization, 83*(9), 661–669. S0042-96862005000900011.

Pichot, H., Hennequin, M., Rouchon, B., Pereira, B., & Tubert-Jeannin, S. (2014). Dental status of New Caledonian children: Is there a need for a new oral health promotion programme? *PloS One, 9*(11), e112452. https://doi.org/10.1371/journal.pone.0112452

Pichot, H., Pereira, B., Magnat, E., Hennequin, M., & Tubert-Jeannin, S. (2020). Implementation and impact of a dental preventive intervention conducted within a health promotion program on health inequalities: A retrospective study. *PloS One, 15*(3), e0230639. https://doi.org/10.1371/journal.pone.0230639

Potvin, L., Bilodeau, A., & Gendron, S. (2008). Trois défis pour l'évaluation en promotion de la santé. *Promotion & Education, 15*(suppl 1), 17–21. https://doi.org/10.1177/1025382308093991

Pussinen, P. J., Paju, S., Koponen, J., Viikari, J. S. A., Taittonen, L., Laitinen, T., et al. (2019). Association of childhood oral infections with cardiovascular risk factors and subclinical atherosclerosis in adulthood. *JAMA Network Open, 2*(4), e192523. https://doi.org/10.1001/jamanetworkopen.2019.2523

Rochaix, L., & Tubeuf, S. (2009). Mesures de l'équité en santé. Fondements éthiques et implications. *Revue economique, 60*(2), 325–344.

Ruff, R. R., Senthi, S., Susser, S. R., & Tsutsui, A. (2019). Oral health, academic performance, and school absenteeism in children and adolescents: A systematic review and meta-analysis. *Journal of the American Dental Association (1939), 150*(2), 111–121.e4. https://doi.org/10.1016/j.adaj.2018.09.023

Singh, S. (2012). Evidence in oral health promotion-implications for oral health planning. *American Journal of Public Health, 102*(9), e15–e18. https://doi.org/10.2105/AJPH.2012.300893

Tubert-Jeannin, S., & Jourdan, D. (2018). Renovating dental education: A public health issue. *European Journal of Dental Education, 22*(3), e644–e647. https://doi.org/10.1111/eje.12347

Tubert-Jeannin, S., Pichot, H., Rouchon, B., Pereira, B., & Hennequin, M. (2018). Common risk indicators for oral diseases and obesity in 12-year-olds: A South Pacific cross sectional study. *BMC Public Health, 18*(1), 112. https://doi.org/10.1186/s12889-017-4996-y

Walsh, T., Worthington, H. V., Glenny, A.-M., Marinho, V. C., & Jeroncic, A. (2019). Fluoride toothpastes of different concentrations for preventing dental caries. *The Cochrane Database of Systematic Reviews, 3*, CD007868. https://doi.org/10.1002/14651858.CD007868.pub3

Watt, R. G., & Sheiham, A. (2012). Integrating the common risk factor approach into a social determinants framework. *Community Dentistry and Oral Epidemiology, 40*(4), 289–296. https://doi.org/10.1111/j.1600-0528.2012.00680.x

Watt, R. G., Mathur, M. R., Aida, J., Bönecker, M., Venturelli, R., & Gansky, S. A. (2018). Oral health disparities in children: A canary in the coalmine? *Pediatric Clinics of North America, 65*(5), 965–979. https://doi.org/10.1016/j.pcl.2018.05.006

Wolfenden, L., Nathan, N. K., Sutherland, R., Yoong, S. L., Hodder, R. K., Wyse, R. J., et al. (2017). Strategies for enhancing the implementation of school-based policies or practices targeting risk factors for chronic disease. *The Cochrane Database of Systematic Reviews, 11*, CD011677. https://doi.org/10.1002/14651858.CD011677.pub2

World Health Organisation. (1986). *The Ottawa Charter for health promotion.* In Ottawa: First international conference on health Promotion. https://www.who.int/publications/i/item/ottawa-charter-for-health-promotion. Accessed 18 Jan 2021.

World Health Organisation. (2020). *Oral health: Achieving better oral health as part of the universal health coverage and noncommunicable disease agendas towards 2030* (EXECUTIVE BOARD EB148/8 148th session). https://apps.who.int/gb/ebwha/pdf_files/EB148/B148_8-en.pdf. Accessed 18 Jan 2021.

World Health Organization. (s. d.). *Definition of equity*. World Health Organization. https://www.who.int/healthsystems/topics/equity/fr/. Accessed 18 Jan 2021.

Chapter 30
Methodological Reflections on the "SMART Eating" Trial: Lessons for Developing Health Promotion Practices

Jasvir Kaur, Manmeet Kaur, Venkatesan Chakrapani, and Rajesh Kumar

30.1 Introduction

Health promotion is fundamental in the drive to reduce the growing chronic disease burden across the globe (WHO, 2008). The prevention of chronic diseases requires behaviour modifications. Health promotion interventions aim to engage and empower individuals and communities to choose healthy behaviours and make changes that reduce the risk of developing chronic diseases and other morbidities. "SMART Eating" is an example of such a health promotion intervention aimed at optimizing the consumption of fat, sugar, salt and fruits and vegetables among urban North Indian adults from diverse socio-economic backgrounds, i.e. low-income group (LIG), middle-income group (MIG) and high-income group (HIG) (Kaur et al., 2018). **SMART** stands for **S**mall, **M**easurable and **A**chievable dietary changes by **R**educing fat, sugar and salt consumption and **T**rying different vegetables and fruits.

Health promotion interventions like "SMART Eating", being contextual and community-based, are often complex (Tremblay & Richard, 2014). Considering the complexity of this intervention trial, following the pragmatic worldview (Creswell, 2014), a mixed methods approach applying both deductive and inductive logics

J. Kaur · M. Kaur (✉)
Postgraduate Institute of Medical Education and Research, Chandigarh, India
e-mail: Kaur.manmeet@pgimer.edu.in

V. Chakrapani
Centre for Sexuality and Health Research and Policy (C-SHaRP), Chennai, TN, India

R. Kumar
State Health Systems Resource Center, Department of Health and Family Welfare, Government of Punjab, Chandigarh, India

L. Potvin, D. Jourdan (eds.), *Global Handbook of Health Promotion Research, Vol. 1*,
https://doi.org/10.1007/978-3-030-97212-7_30

combining both quantitative and qualitative approaches was used to better understand unhealthy dietary behaviours. The intervention design was based on a healthy and productive combination of theory-based (top-down) approach and active involvement of end-user communities (Kaur et al., 2020a).

The research objectives were identified and refined based on our personal experiences, interactions and discussions with the community, the literature reviews and discussions with public health and nutrition experts. Based on the work experience in this community setting, we realized that the high prevalence of chronic diseases is one of the major health issues. Discussions with the community people to explore their understanding of the causes of chronic diseases revealed that the majority were not even aware of the link between unhealthy diet and chronic diseases and, even more, what constitutes a healthy diet as a preventive measure. These discussions motivated us to work on exploring innovative ways to deal with unhealthy dietary behaviour – a major risk factor for chronic diseases. This chapter describes the epistemological analysis of the research framework, paradigms, approaches and methods used in the planning, implementation and evaluation of the "SMART Eating" health promotion intervention that used a cluster randomized trial design.

30.2 The "SMART Eating" Research Framework

Evidence of theoretical use for developing methodology and deciding on analyses can guide navigating the intervention process. The transtheoretical model, the theory of planned behaviour and the health belief model are the common behaviour change theories attempting to understand dietary behaviours at the individual level (Davis et al., 2015). These have been used less in collectivistic cultures like India, where dietary decision-making occurs at the family level (Daivadanam et al., 2015). Furthermore, there is seldom a "one-size-fits-all" solution to address an issue adequately. No single theory can account for all the complexities of dietary behaviour change as health behaviour, culture and context differ widely (Darnton, 2008).

A potential solution could be the use of planning models such as the PRECEDE–PROCEED model (PPM) (Glanz et al., 2008) or the intervention mapping (IM) approach (Bartholomew et al., 1998), both of which provide specific guidance for systematically developing theory-based interventions through the selection of appropriate micro-, meso- and macro-level behaviour change theories. The PRECEDE–PROCEED model is one of the most comprehensive and most used approaches in ecological and ethical health promotion practice (Porter, 2015) and has been found useful to researchers in conducting health behaviour change trials (Aldiabat, 2013). Both the PPM and IM share similar characteristics in applying a social-ecological framework and behaviour theories for intervention building, emphasizing multilevel multiple interventions and involving stakeholders and the existing resources in intervention development (Yoo & Kim, 2010). However, IM employs PRECEDE assessments based on the PPM and calls for logic models, while the PPM itself is an example of a logic model, in that it links the causal assessment and the intervention planning and evaluation to one overarching planning framework (Glanz et al., 2008).

Therefore, we chose to use the PPM to plan the "SMART Eating" trial. The model was a road map for the entire research work and specific theories and models (the social-ecological model (SEM), the transtheoretical model, the attitude–social influence–self-efficacy model (ASE) and the UK Medical Research Council (MRC)'s framework) directed towards the goal through different phases of the project. Hence, the research framework for "SMART Eating" was guided by a combination of compatible theories, models and frameworks (Fig. 30.1).

The PRECEDE–PROCEED model's "Educational Diagnosis" PRECEDE (Predisposing, Reinforcing and Enabling Constructs in Educational Diagnosis and Evaluation) guided the intervention development and the "Ecological Diagnosis" PROCEED (Policy, Regulatory and Organizational Constructs in Educational and Environmental Development) guided intervention alignment, implementation and evaluation (Glanz et al., 2008). Designing effective interventions for achieving the desired dietary behaviour changes requires an in-depth study of people's behaviours situated in their socio-cultural and interpersonal contexts. The social-ecological model (SEM) is pertinent to understanding behaviour in terms of interactions among various multilevel influences (Bronfenbrenner, 1977). In the first phase (qualitative formative research), we explored stakeholders' perspectives to understand the multilevel influences on dietary behaviours, the barriers and facilitators to dietary behaviour change and intervention preferences (Kaur et al., 2020a). The formative research findings helped in understanding the local contexts and tailoring the design

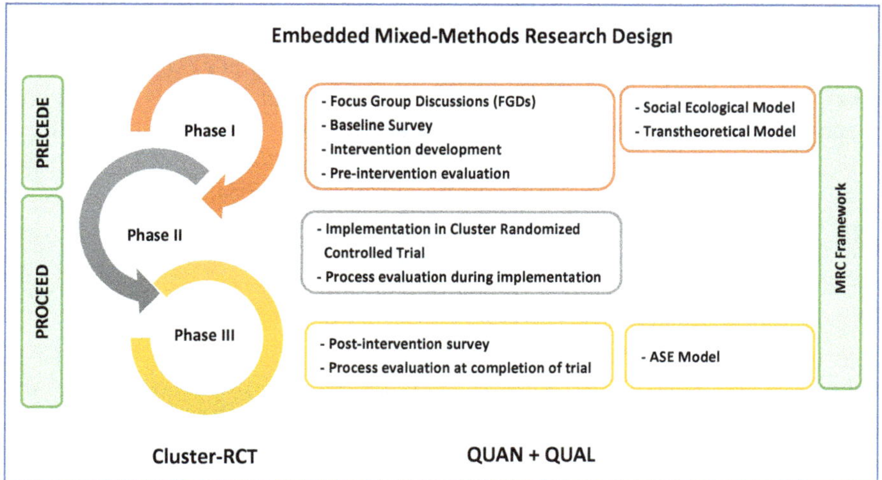

Fig. 30.1 Research framework for 'SMART Eating' intervention. *MRC* Medical Research Council, *ASE* Attitude–Social-influence–Self-efficacy, *QUAN* Quantitative, *QUAL* Qualitative

and conduct of the "SMART Eating" intervention for enhancing its efficacy (Darlington et al., 2020).

During the next phase, we used the transtheoretical model to identify the stage of readiness for fat, sugar, salt, fruit and vegetable consumption of the participants. However, we realized that applying the stages of change to dietary behaviour poses difficulties because of the complexity of dietary behaviours and the lack of stage stability over time even before intervention (Brug et al., 2004). As dietary behaviours may be different for a different set of diets, people may hold different self-efficacy beliefs and may be in different stages of change for each of the desired behaviours (Adams & White, 2004). The lack of knowledge about the recommended dietary intake among the participants (98%) (baseline survey) could have led to misconceptions about their consumption, and the majority were categorized in the maintenance stage (Lechner et al., 1998; Bogers et al., 2004). Their intention to change based on subjective qualitative assessment (whether they think their consumption is sufficient/low/high? yes/no) of the adequacy of their dietary intake did not match the dietary consumption estimated quantitatively using a food frequency questionnaire (FFQ) (Lechner et al., 1998), which is regarded as the pre-contemplation stage (Greene et al., 1999). Hence, considering the participants' pre-contemplation stage, a common intervention was developed based on the qualitative formative research (Kaur et al. 2020a), the empirical literature on interventions and the dietary guidelines by the National Institute of Nutrition, India (ICMR, 2011).

The UK Medical Research Council (MRC)'s framework for designing and evaluating complex interventions guided the process evaluation (Moore et al., 2015). The attitude–social influence–self-efficacy (ASE) model (Engbers et al., 2006) and the SEM-based formative research findings (Kaur et al., 2020a) informed an a priori identification of the potential mediators, namely, attitude, social influence, self-efficacy, monthly household purchase and consumption, and guided the mediation analyses for understanding the mechanisms of the intervention's effect on the outcomes. The ASE model, a social cognition model that integrates concepts from the theory of planned behaviour and social cognitive theory, is commonly used to predict and explain dietary behaviours (Sandvik et al., 2007; de Vries et al., 1988).

30.3 Methods

30.3.1 Community Involvement

Community involvement is a fundamental principle of health promotion. We involved the stakeholders during all trial phases, i.e. intervention development, implementation and evaluation. Given that an ecological approach is central to the concepts and methods of health promotion, involving participants as co-researchers rather than as just data sources as in conventional biomedical approaches – being our priority – and the lack of prior empirical evidence from India on understanding multilevel influences on multiple dietary behaviours among urban North Indian adults, we conducted formative research to develop a context-specific culturally acceptable intervention. We chose a qualitative approach to explore the diverse experiences and perspectives related to the consumption of fat, sugar, salt, fruits and vegetables (Brink & Wood, 1998). Focus group discussions (FGDs) were conducted with adults. The participants were recruited with the help of influential people from local communities who provided immense support and cooperation. The FGDs were held at venues suggested by the participants as per their convenience. As our department has been working in the study areas to strengthen healthcare services, its strong rapport with the communities over several years has resulted in openness in responses. The key findings are presented in Box 30.1 (Kaur et al., 2020a).

Box 30.1 Multilevel Influences on Dietary Behaviours

Individual level: Lack of knowledge about the recommended dietary intake; lack of food measurement skills; low-risk perception for chronic diseases; frequent consumption of packaged food; frequent reporting of eating out; low self-efficacy in adapting to healthy eating related to the inability to influence family cooking habits.

Family level: The role of women as the "main chef" of the family, family norms and preferences of family members.

Structural level: Societal norms, high cost of fruits and vegetables and use of pesticides/harmful injections on fruits and vegetables.

The participants' narratives indicated that individuals alone may not be able to adapt healthy dietary behaviours without family support, given that food cooked at home is consumed by all members of the family and family food habits are strongly influenced by the prevalent social norms and cultural practices regarding food consumption. Hence, family or community approach could be more likely to be effective in settings where collectivistic cultures exist. Furthermore, the lack of knowledge about the recommended dietary intake suggested that efforts should be made to translate written documents on these guidelines into practical applications. Given that provision of knowledge alone may be insufficient to motivate people to initiate the desired changes, considering multilevel influences on dietary behaviours (Box 30.1), we decided that, alongside knowledge provision, the intervention should focus on increasing awareness about the benefits of adapting healthy dietary behaviours, improving risk perceptions related to chronic diseases, developing food measurement skills and enhancing self-efficacy. These qualitative findings may be applicable to other similar settings in India (transferability or analytical generalizability). We discuss the involvement of the stakeholders in intervention implementation and evaluation in the forthcoming sections.

30.3.2 Multi-Channel Communication Approach

Identifying appropriate communication channels is crucial for successful intervention implementation. Face-to-face individual counselling or group education, being effective methods of education, have been often used for promoting healthy dietary behaviours; however, they may be expensive to scale up in resource-constrained settings (Pomerleau et al. 2005). As unhealthy dietary behaviours are prevalent in most populations, nutrition interventions should reach large numbers of people at a low cost. mHealth (mobile health) could be a potential solution to this problem as IT has penetrated across different socio-economic strata. However, in developing countries, mHealth is still at an early stage of development, and the effectiveness of such interventions to improve dietary behaviours has not yet been explored adequately (Marcolino et al., 2018). Furthermore, the exclusive use of a single technology alone may be insufficient to alter complex, multifactorial, multiple dietary risk behaviours (Svetkey et al., 2015).

Therefore, in the qualitative formative research, we also explored the participants' preferences for the intervention content, messages, channels and modes of communication, duration of the intervention and the target audience for implementing the intervention (Box 30.2). Qualitative information on preferences for the use of IT tools was supplemented by a rapid feasibility survey of the study area and the baseline survey, which revealed extensive use of mobile phones (100%), including smartphones (91%) and the Internet (92%), among all families, including those from the low-income group. Thus, considering the participants' intervention preferences (Box 30.2), the intervention was implemented for a period of 6 months using a multi-channel communication approach (Figs. 30.2 and 30.3) including information technology (short message service – SMS, email, WhatsApp and a project website) and interpersonal communication along with the provision of innovative educational tools ("SMART Eating" kit) (Kaur et al., 2020b). Based on the participants' language preferences and literacy levels, the contents were made available in the local languages (Hindi and Punjabi) and in English. Content validation was done by eight experts from related fields. The website design was validated by three experts. The intervention aids were pre-tested, and modifications were made.

Box 30.2 Participants' Intervention Preferences: Findings from the Qualitative Formative Research

Content of the intervention: Provision of knowledge on the recommended quantity of fat, sugar, salt, fruits and vegetables; how to measure the quantity; benefits of eating the recommended quantity; risks of eating more or less.

Methods of communication: Telephone calls, SMS, educational videos, Internet, social media (WhatsApp), mass media (TV and radio) and face-to-face individual or group education. In addition, low-income group participants preferred innovative printed materials (pamphlets/posters/banners).

Duration of the intervention: Preferences ranged from 1 month to 1 year, and the majority preferred at least 6 months.

Frequency of message delivery: Weekly, fortnightly.

Language preferences: Hindi, Punjabi, English.

Target audience for intervention implementation: The majority suggested that the person responsible for cooking should be the primary target audience for implementing the intervention. Some participants indicated the need to involve other family members to help the target audience (Kaur et al., 2020b).

Given the importance of the family's role in dietary behaviours, we used the family champions approach for implementing the intervention, adapted from the health champions approach (Warwick-Booth et al., 2013). One family champion (an adult in the family who usually cooks food) was selected as the target audience from each family to motivate other family members to adapt healthy eating behaviours. Considering the potential challenge that not all family champions will be using IT tools, a co-champion to assist the family champion was identified by the family champion. Guidance was provided on the use of different components of the intervention. The trial had no provision for any kind of monetary incentives for participation in the trial.

Components of IT-enabled Intervention	**Implementation**
Interpersonal component	**1 month**
• Guidance	• Single home visit to guide families (family champions and co-champions) regarding the use of intervention components.
• 'SMART Eating' kit - Dining table mat - Kitchen calendar - Measuring spoons	• 'SMART Eating' kit provided to all intervention group families
• Pamphlet	• Provided to all comparison group families
Information technology	**6 months**
• 'SMART Eating' website	• Content delivery in parts over three months in English, Hindi and Punjabi; Fortnightly addition of new content
• SMS/Email	• Weekly in English
• Social networking app (WhatsApp)	• Text messages, images and videos weekly in English, Hindi, and Punjabi • Prompt responses to participants' queries by the experts in the field of nutrition

Fig. 30.2 Description of the 'SMART Eating' intervention

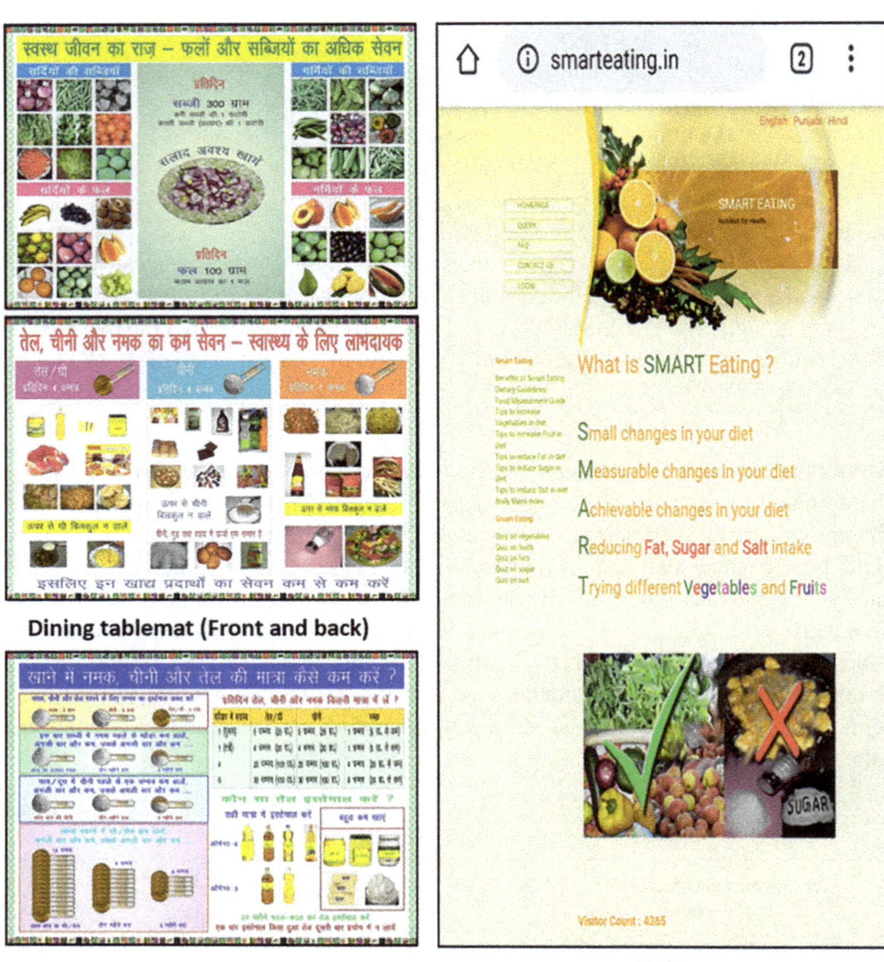

Fig. 30.3 Educational aids. *Dining tablemat, kitchen calendar* © Kaur et al. CC BY 4.0; *project website* by authors, in School of Public Health, PGIMER, Chandigarh. (Open from 2016 to 2020)

30.3.3 The Cluster Randomized Controlled Trial Design

The randomized controlled trial (RCT) design is a widely accepted "gold standard" experimental design for evaluating health interventions (The Lancet, 2019). We opted for a two-arm cluster randomized controlled trial design to test the proposed intervention's effectiveness, as, in an individual-level RCT, there is a threat of contamination (Campbell et al., 2012). Compared with individually randomized trials, cluster RCTs are more complex to design. They require a greater number of participants for equal statistical power and an estimate of between-cluster variance or intraclass correlation (often not available from the published literature) and entail more complex analysis due to clustered observations – all of which are important for internal validity in pragmatic trials measuring effectiveness (Kerry & Bland 1998a, b). Cluster RCTs involve randomization of clusters (groups of individuals) to intervention conditions, and participants' recruitment often takes place post randomization. Thus, the lack of blinding to allocation status to those recruiting the participants can result in poor internal validity. However, due to the nature of interventions, blinding is not always feasible, especially in behavioural interventions (Campbell et al., 2012), like "SMART Eating". However, the random selection of the families and individuals from clusters can minimize that bias.

Based on the type of housing, a total of 12 clusters (i.e. 4 each from the LIG, MIG and HIG) were recruited before randomization. Similar socio-economic group clusters were paired based on the clusters' geographical distance to form six pairs to avoid a possible spillover effect. Then, from each of the six pairs, clusters were randomly allocated to the intervention and comparison arms in a 1:1 ratio using computer-generated simple randomization by a researcher not involved in the study. While accounting for clustering in sample size estimations, across 12 clusters, a total of 732 families were recruited with equal numbers of families from each cluster using systematic random sampling. One adult per family was randomly selected as an index case to measure the change in the outcomes.

Given that most intervention studies target high-risk groups or vulnerable populations, we aimed to focus on the general population in a real-world setting as unhealthy dietary behaviours and related chronic conditions are common. Furthermore, we believe that, although chronic diseases are relatively well managed within the government healthcare systems, government healthcare services lack the resources to focus on health promotion or to facilitate behaviour changes among otherwise healthy people. For example, for a focus group participant, a low-salt diet meant not adding extra salt. Additionally, we believe that reinforcement is an essential aspect of health promotion. Hence, to enable all people to achieve their fullest health potential – "equity in health", a basic principle of health promotion (Grabowski et al., 2017) and the mission of the International Union for Health Promotion and Education (IUHPE) – we included all participants, except pregnant women and those with critical health problems.

Furthermore, to ensure equal representation of all socio-economic groups in the project, the sample was stratified by the type of housing as assigned by the Chandigarh Administration – i.e. low-income group (LIG), middle-income group (MIG) and high-income group (HIG). The type of housing thus served as a proxy for socio-economic status (SES). Formative research indicated that participants from all SESs perceived themselves at greater risk of nutrition-related diseases and all, even those from the LIG, were supportive of the dietary change intervention. Therefore, the LIG was also included in the project, despite the fact that affordability could be a barrier to "SMART Eating" in this group (John & Ziebland, 2004). In recognition of the high price of fruits and vegetables, we emphasized the use of seasonal fruits and vegetables available at low price and explicitly pointed out that money spent on junk foods could be used to purchase fruits and vegetables.

30.3.4 Mixed Methods Design

Mixed methods research (MMR) is becoming increasingly used and recognized as a major research paradigm, along with quantitative and qualitative approaches (Johnson et al., 2007). Mixed methods approach based on the pragmatic worldview (using pluralistic approaches based on the complexity of the problem) involves a combination or integration of quantitative (post-positivism philosophy) and qualitative (constructivist worldview) approaches (Creswell, 2014). It provides a more comprehensive understanding of the problem under study rather than using either of these (Creswell & Plano Clark, 2007). MMR is unique and superior to the single approach as it improves inference quality (internal validity in QUAN and credibility in QUAL) and inference transferability (external validity in QUAN and transferability in QUAL) (Tashakkori & Teddlie, 2003).

Mixed methods research is increasingly used in the health promotion field (Nutbeam, 1998), and the experts emphasize that the use of mixed methods is most appropriate for evaluating complex health promotion interventions (Pommier et al., 2010). As health promotion is concerned with producing generalizable knowledge and transforming reality, qualitative and quantitative methods should be viewed as complementary in health promotion research (Rootman et al., 2001). Choosing the most appropriate design for a particular study, i.e. whether purely mixed with equal status to both QUAN and QUAL or dominant design, is pivotal to MMR (Almalki, 2016). We used an embedded mixed methods research design, which sees one method of inquiry being used in a supportive secondary role to another primary method of inquiry, which enables making sense of the study in its entirety. This method is used in quantitative experimental designs (Creswell, 2014). Our approach is a quantitative dominant mixed methods research, with the QUAN component in the dominant role (cluster RCT) and the QUAL component in the supporting role in the overall design (formative research and process evaluation) (Johnson et al., 2007). The intervention was informed by the qualitative formative research (QUAL data), the effectiveness of the intervention was evaluated using a cluster RCT design (QUAN data) and the participants' perceptions regarding the effect of the intervention (process evaluation) were explored using post-intervention extreme case interviews (QUAL data).

30.3.5 Measurements

Measurement of outcomes needs to be accurate to check whether an intervention is effective or not. An accurate estimation of diet requires a complete and unbiased assessment of foods consumed and a comprehensive database of the nutrient content of foods. We used food frequency questionnaires (FFQs) to capture information on 113 food items that had been validated in an urban North Indian setting (Mahajan et al., 2013). The reported intakes were converted into food and nutrient data using

Indian food composition tables. However, errors inherent in subjective dietary assessment may lead to biases towards or away from the null hypothesis (Naska et al., 2017). FFQs, being highly comprehensive, are prone to overestimation compared to other methods (Steinemann et al., 2017). On the other hand, recall bias in self-reported dietary intake could underestimate the actual intake. Similarly, the possibility of social desirability bias could lead to overestimation of the effect size. Hence, objective assessment, where possible, needs to complement self-reported measures.

Nutritional biomarkers provide an objective assessment of dietary outcomes; however, they are often expensive (Bingham, 2002). Although 24-h urinary sodium excretion, a nutritional biochemical biomarker, is the gold standard for estimating salt intake, spot urine samples can also be used to estimate the mean change in the population salt intake (Petersen et al., 2017b). The equations to estimate 24-h salt from spot urine samples have been previously tested in different Indian populations (Petersen et al., 2017a). Hence, in addition to subjective assessment based on FFQs, we chose spot urine samples to estimate salt intake objectively. Changes in the body mass index, blood pressure, haemoglobin, fasting plasma glucose and serum lipid levels were the other anthropometric, physiological and biochemical biomarkers (Dragsted et al., 2017). The significant net changes observed in some of these biomarkers indicated that the aforementioned biases in self-reported measures did not bias the study results.

30.3.6 Data Analysis Methods

Besides robust measurements, careful selection of robust analysis methods for both quantitative and qualitative data analyses is imperative for unbiased estimates of the intervention's effect and correct interpretation and generalizability of the findings. Randomized trials present special requirements for analysis, including the use of the intention-to-treat (ITT) principle, accounting for unobserved causes of the outcome and multiple comparisons and understanding the causal mechanisms. The loss to follow-up is often hard to avoid in randomized trials. We used ITT analysis by the inclusion of all participants in data analysis to reduce selection bias. ITT is strongly recommended in RCTs to minimize type-I error and produce an unbiased estimate of the treatment effect (Campbell et al., 2012). It ensures comparability between groups and maintains sample size as the original randomization, and the number of participants remains unchanged.

The difference-in-differences (DiD) method was used to determine the net mean change in the outcomes in the intervention group relative to the comparison group. This approach removes the biases from comparisons over time in the intervention, which could be due to other unobserved causes of the outcome (Zhou et al., 2016). The analyses were adjusted to account for the clustering in the data using multilevel mixed effects linear regression models to reduce type-I error (Hayes & Moulton, 2017).

Furthermore, multiple comparisons are common in experimental studies due to logistic issues. The statistical inference in experimental research is always drawn from the statistical testing of hypotheses, in which an acceptable cut-off of probability (0.05 or 0.01) is used for decision-making. However, the probability of committing false statistical inferences would considerably increase when more than one hypothesis is simultaneously tested, i.e. in multiple comparisons (Smith et al., 1987). For multiple confirmatory hypotheses testing, there needs to be a proper adjustment to the alpha level to preserve the overall family-wise type-I error rate, which is mandatory. To this end, Holm's adjustment was made for the four primary outcomes, i.e. fat, sugar, salt and fruit and vegetable intake (Chen et al., 2017). However, several statistical tests conducted for secondary outcomes and subgroups as exploratory analyses could serve as a guide to developing confirmatory hypothesis in future studies.

Mediation analysis is a recommended statistical tool for understanding the mechanisms of impact in RCT interventions (Moore et al., 2015). Multiple mediation analyses assessed whether, and to what extent, attitude, social influence, self-efficacy, monthly household purchase and consumption mediated the intervention's effect on dietary behaviour outcomes. As in RCTs, it is the intervention that is randomized, not the mediators; we used the "ANCOVA approach for mediation", which is strongly recommended to reduce confounding in mediation analysis in RCTs (Landau et al., 2018). Hence, the mediation analyses were adjusted for baseline measures of the mediators and outcomes and the baseline covariates.

The focus group data were audio-recorded and transcribed verbatim. The data were analyzed using narrative thematic analysis informed by the framework analysis approach (Ritchie & Lewis, 2003) and techniques derived from the grounded theory approach (Holton, 2010). Guided by the social-ecological model, two analysts, the first and the second author, developed the coding framework based on "a priori" codes derived from the topic guide and the empirical literature and emergent codes. The coding framework was discussed with the third author, an expert in qualitative data analyses with years of qualitative research experience. Differences in coding were resolved by discussions and consensus.

30.3.7 Comprehensive Evaluation

Guided by the PRECEDE–PROCEED model, we undertook a comprehensive evaluation that was participatory, continuous and theory-driven, as shown in Fig. 30.1. To ensure a comprehensive evaluation, a mixed methods approach was used, which is the recommended design for evaluations within the trials, including cluster RCTs (Grant et al., 2013). The effectiveness evaluation using a cluster RCT showed significant net improvements in all dietary behaviours (i.e. reduction in fat, sugar and salt consumption and an increase in fruit and vegetable intake) in the intervention group relative to the comparison group (Kaur et al., 2020b) – an indication that it is feasible to change multiple risk behaviours. A significant net beneficial effect on body mass index, diastolic blood pressure, fasting plasma glucose, triglycerides and urinary salt excretion observed from the exploratory analysis supported the above-presented findings of the confirmatory hypothesis testing.

Subgroup comparisons showed significant improvements in all dietary behaviours among all socio-economic groups, except for salt consumption in the HIG. Further, the effect of the intervention was significant for fat, sugar and fruit and vegetable intake irrespective of age and gender. However, the effect on salt intake was significant in the younger age group and in women. These findings indicated that for fat, sugar and salt behaviours, the LIG performed better than did the MIG and HIG. However, for fruit and vegetable consumption, the increase observed in the LIG, though significant, was of much lower magnitude compared to those observed in the MIG and HIG. The lesson learned from these findings is that reducing fat, sugar and salt consumption (activities that do not involve money) is feasible even among low-income groups. However, achieving a higher effect on fruit and vegetable behaviour among the LIG would require supportive government policies. Lack of the intervention effect on salt intake in the HIG group warrants exploration of design-suitable interventions for improving salt consumption among this group – another learning.

Besides effect evaluation, process evaluation (Table 30.1) of complex interventions is an indispensable component of the comprehensive evaluation. Guided by the MRC framework (Moore et al., 2015), the process evaluation documented high fidelity and reach (91%) in both the groups, adequate dose for SMS (93%), WhatsApp (89%) and "SMART Eating" kit (100%) with low website usage (50%) in the intervention group and inadequate use of pamphlets (46%) in the comparison group. The participants reported no unintended adverse effects. The mediation analysis adjusted for the covariates indicated that the improvements in attitude, social influence, self-efficacy, household purchase and consumption behaviours mediated the effect of the intervention on dietary behaviour outcomes. These findings suggest that health promotion interventions that target these components will be more likely to be effective in optimizing the intake of fat, sugar, salt and fruits and vegetables. Post-intervention feedback from the participants indicated that the intervention was well-liked by the participants across all socio-economic groups, with some of them demanding programme extension. We found the evidence for adherence to the intervention from the participants' responses to the social networking app messages, their queries and interactions with the intervention implementer and home observations on the use of the "SMART Eating" kit provided to them.

Besides, it is important to understand that not everyone treated or intervened will change. Deviant cases always lie on a continuum indicating two extremes, i.e. poor performers exhibiting no change in their behaviour and excellent performers. From the extreme case interviews with poor performers, we learned that no perceived effect of the intervention on fruit and vegetable behaviour among the LIG was related to high cost and among the MIG and HIG to poor quality (use of pesticides/harmful hormonal injections for enhancing the production). These findings highlight the need for government policies for promoting healthy dietary behaviours. Similarly, no effect of the intervention on fat, sugar and salt behaviours among

Table 30.1 Process evaluation components of the "SMART Eating" intervention

Process evaluation components	Data sources	Methods	Timing of data collection
1. Context			
Local context	Evaluator and participants	Focus groups	Beginning of the intervention
Multilevel influences on dietary behaviour			
Barriers/facilitators			
Implementation preferences			
Content validation	Experts	Experts' opinion	
Pre-testing the intervention	Participants	Participants' opinion	
2. Implementation			
Fidelity	Evaluator	Log book	Beginning of the intervention
Dose delivered		Log book Home observations on the use of the "SMART Eating" kit	During the intervention
Adaptations		Log book	During the intervention
3. Mechanisms of impact			
Reach	Evaluator	Dropout rate	During and after the intervention
Dose received (exposure/interaction/response to the intervention)	Evaluator and participants	Website login/visitor count Participants' responses to the social networking app messages Participants' queries Open-ended questions on barriers	During the intervention
		Attitude, social influence and self-efficacy questionnaire Monthly household food purchase and consumption questionnaire	Before and after the intervention
Dose received (satisfaction)		Feedback from participants (social networking app) Questionnaire on usefulness of intervention components Extreme case interviews regarding the perceived effect of the intervention	After the intervention

deviant cases across all socio-economic groups was found to be related to the lack of family support and perceived adequacy of personal intake. These findings point to the need to explore more effective strategies to enhance family support and improve perceptions about the adequacy of personal intake in future interventions.

Further, an important issue in evaluating behaviour change interventions is the evaluation of the maintenance of behaviour change or positive gains following the intervention, which could be defined as a significant between-group difference for the outcomes at post-intervention and at follow-up (Fjeldsoe et al., 2011). The importance of maintenance of outcomes to inform the translation of evidence-based health behaviour interventions into practice is often overlooked, and only a few interventions include evaluation of the maintenance of dietary behaviour change. Our initial protocol, approved by the institute ethics committee, included a plan to assess the maintenance of behaviour change through between-group differences at the end of the 6-month intervention (post-intervention) and at 12 months (follow-up). However, this project, being a doctoral project (of the first author) with limited time and resources, could not be continued beyond 5 months.

We believe that the positive effect gained would have been maintained over time as our intervention was well received by the participants and used practical strategies, such as emphasis on small gradual changes, enhancing self-efficacy through family support, development of food measurement skills, interactive help to allow interactions with the intervention implementer, timely replies to their queries by the experts and provision of innovative material to meet their preferences, which they would retain for a long time and use to reinforcing desired behaviours in the family – the enabling, empowering and relapse prevention strategies. Given that behaviour change is a challenging and complex process, further work is needed to determine the maintenance of the intervention effect along with exploratory research on understanding the facilitators of and the barriers to long-term maintenance.

30.4 Implementation Challenges and Remedies

Through formative research, we identified certain issues that might affect implementation and took steps to address them in the intervention (e.g., developing the intervention based on the participants’ preferences, identifying the target audience for intervention implementation at the family level and the provision of interactive help to discuss difficulties in using the intervention). Despite the best efforts and careful implementation planning, we faced some unforeseen challenges. The intervention implementation through different components was easiest, except the use of the social networking app in the beginning.

First, retaining participants in WhatsApp groups was the most challenging task. Although while obtaining informed consent, they were explained that group messaging will be used for WhatsApp messages, many users left the groups immediately saying “we are not familiar with other group members”, “we do not want to be in any group (especially girl co-champions)”, and others left without specifying any reason. Very few participants continued with the group messages. Second, as an alternative to group messaging, an individual message to a larger audience (91% WhatsApp users) was not allowed by the WhatsApp service. The broadcast list, an alternative to these problems (allowing an individual message to 256 recipients in one go with a single click), requires the recipients to save the sender's contact number in their phone books – again a tedious exercise in a community-based nutrition intervention. Despite these challenges, we could manage these difficulties, and WhatsApp proved to be one of the most useful, successful and interactive methods of education in this project. Therefore, a solution to these problems needs to be explored for efficient use of WhatsApp or similar social media in future public health interventions.

Another unanticipated implementation challenge was the minimal use of the project website. At 1 month of intervention implementation, the project website was reported to be least used for being password-protected, causing difficulty for the participants to login. Therefore, the password was removed, and the visitor count was added as an indicator of the website usage. Although remedial measures improved the website usage from 7% at 1 month to 50% by post-intervention, the website was still the least used component. The majority of the participants in this project reported using the Internet just for using social networking apps. Despite extensive mobile Internet penetration and timely remedial measures, low website usage indicates the need to explore strategies for improving website usage for planning future web-based interventions (Blackford et al., 2017).

30.5 Epistemological Issues in Health Promotion Intervention Research

Evidence-based health promotion practice needs to focus on the appropriate measurement of effectiveness using theories (Green, 2000). The "SMART Eating" intervention designed based on a theory-based (top-down) approach and qualitative research evidence through community consultations, evaluated using a cluster RCT, was successful in achieving the desired behaviour changes. The intervention implementation based on users' preferences using the family approach made the intervention acceptable to the users across diverse socio-economic groups. Further, the intervention posed no additional burden on the families as it used the available community resources. It focused on capacity building and facilitating change at the individual and family levels through enabling the home environment.

One of the major epistemological issues in health promotion intervention research is understanding which paradigm or a set of paradigms is the most appropriate for health promotion intervention research. The complexity in health promotion practice needs to be dealt with simple, cost-effective, innovative, culturally and geographically appropriate models, ensuring community participation. Therefore, we used a transdisciplinary approach, which accommodated diverse perspectives and contributed to enhancing the understanding of unhealthy dietary behaviours (Soskolin, 2000), resulting in a common conceptual framework (Albrecht et al., 1998). Experts from different disciplines (sociologists, epidemiologists, an anthropologist, nutrition experts and other community health professionals) agreed on the methodological pluralism required in answering the research questions of the "SMART Eating" project. Hence, the selection of the research approach was based on the pragmatic worldview that allows pluralistic approaches based on the complexity of the health issues (Creswell, 2014). Using a dialectic method to resolve the differences, a mixed methods approach combining both quantitative and qualitative methods to data collection, analysis and evaluation was deemed appropriate. Furthermore, the experts reached a consensus on the need to use multiple compatible theories to practise evidence-based health promotion.

Another important epistemological issue is the external validity, which refers to the extent to which study results can be applied to other settings. The "SMART Eating" experiences showed that evaluated using a cluster RCT, the intervention showed the evidence of effectiveness in improving dietary behaviour among urban Indian adults from diverse socio-economic backgrounds. Hence, the findings of this research could be used to plan and implement interventions in different settings with modifications to account for the contextual factors. The use of IT as a health promotion strategy for future interventions in different settings may prove successful because it removes the limitations of resources and geographical distances.

Further, growing evidence supports the need for interventions to target factors that influence health behaviours at multiple levels (Paskett et al., 2016). However, it is not always feasible to intervene at all levels due to the challenges in designing, implementing and evaluating multilevel interventions, such as the need for teams with diverse expertise, managing complex teams over extended periods and unpredictability of timelines (Sallis, 2018) – another important issue. Using qualitative formative research, we learned that intervening at the individual, interpersonal and structural levels would be appropriate for "SMART Eating". However, the "SMART eating" intervention was restricted to individual and interpersonal levels. Although, to address structural influences, namely, high cost and poor quality of fruits and vegetables (due to rampant use of pesticides) and media influence (misleading advertisements portraying the usefulness of packaged food often high in fat/sugar/salt), we devised strategies such as an emphasis on substituting snacks with seasonal low-cost fruits and vegetables, altering the home environment (making healthy food more visible) and food label reading; intervening at the structural level was beyond the scope of this project due to logistic reasons, being a time-consuming activity.

However, we acknowledge that intervening at social-structural levels (increasing tax on unhealthy food, access to unprocessed food, making healthy food available at grocery stores or provision of packaged food containing low fat/sugar/salt) would certainly add to the effectiveness of and complement interventions at the individual and interpersonal levels, leading to more effective and sustainable behaviour changes. Hence, through the dissemination of our study findings, we try to influence the "structure" by the "agent" as our participants demanded supportive policies for promoting healthy eating behaviours (fruits and vegetables) and restrictive policies to facilitate healthy food production and wanted their voice to reach the government, as evident from these quotes from our published study (Kaur et al., 2020a):

> These days, media is affecting our thinking very badly. Advertisements are showing usefulness of ready-to-eat food products, not even a single advertisement tells how harmful are they?" (MIG); "Fruits are too expensive to be consumed; same is the scenario for vegetables. Government should open such stores where poor people get commodities [fruits and vegetables] at subsidized rates" (LIG); "Government should do something…vegetables are grown with medicines…ghiya [gourd] is grown to 1 kg with injection…this is all wrong…it is happening everywhere across the globe…corrective measures should be taken…" (LIG); "Can you convey our message to the government that food adulteration [with injections] and use of pesticides/fertilizers should be reduced (MIG).

30.6 Conclusions

The "SMART Eating" project was guided by the PRECEDE–PROCEED – a community-oriented ecological health promotion model, which guided the selection of compatible theories. A transdisciplinary approach was used, which accommodated diverse perspectives and contributed to the holistic understanding of dealing with unhealthy dietary behaviour. Based on the pragmatic worldview, a mixed methods approach was used combining quantitative and qualitative methods applying deductive and inductive logics. An embedded mixed methods design was used with the QUAN component in the dominant role and the QUAL component in the supporting role in the cluster RCT. Community involvement, empowerment and equity were the other distinctive features of this health promotion intervention research.

From the implementation of the "SMART Eating" health promotion intervention, we learned how different worldviews can be integrated into health promotion research. Furthermore, we illustrated that instead of following only one major research tradition (quantitative or qualitative), philosophy or school of thought and working in watertight compartments, health promotion research needs to be open and flexible and different traditions should learn from each other and collaborate to meet the community's needs while taking contexts into consideration. Such openness and flexibility will help capture the nuances of the research problems and thus design and implement appropriate solutions for complex health problems. From this project, we learned that several ingredients are crucial for the successful implementation of complex health promotion interventions: actively involving stakeholders in the formative research (intervention development), selecting appropriate enabling and empowering intervention strategies based on their needs, intervening at multiple levels of influences and having a complete theory-driven evaluation strategy from the inception to the end.

References

Adams, J., & White, M. (2004). Why don't stage-based activity promotion interventions work? *Health Education Research, 20*(2), 237–243. https://doi.org/10.1093/her/cyg105

Albrecht, G., Freeman, S., & Higginbotham, N. (1998). Complexity and human health: the case for atransdisciplinary paradigm. *Culture, Medicine and Psychiatry, 22*(1), 55–92. https://doi.org/10.1023/a:1005328821675

Aldiabat, K. (2013). developing smoking cessation program for older Canadian people: An application of precede-proceed model. *American Journal of Nursing Science, 2*, 33. https://doi.org/10.11648/j.ajns.20130203.13

Almalki, S. (2016). Integrating quantitative and qualitative data in mixed methods research—Challenges and benefits. *Journal of Education and Learning, 5*, 288. https://doi.org/10.5539/jel.v5n3p288

Bartholomew, L. K., Parcel, G. S., & Kok, G. (1998). Intervention mapping: A process for developing theory- and evidence-based health education programs. *Health Education & Behavior, 25*(5), 545–563. https://doi.org/10.1177/109019819802500502

Bingham, S. A. (2002). Biomarkers in nutritional epidemiology. *Public Health Nutrition, 5*(6a), 821–827. https://doi.org/10.1079/phn2002368

Blackford, K., Lee, A., James, A. P., Waddell, T., Hills, A. P., Anderson, A. S., et al. (2017). Process evaluation of the Albany Physical Activity and Nutrition (APAN) program, a home-based intervention for metabolic syndrome and associated chronic disease risk in rural Australian adults. *Health Promotion Journal of Australia, 28*(1), 8–14. https://doi.org/10.1071/he16027

Bogers, R. P., Brug, J., van Assema, P., & Dagnelie, P. C. (2004). Explaining fruit and vegetable consumption: The theory of planned behaviour and misconception of personal intake levels. *Appetite, 42*(2), 157–166. https://doi.org/10.1016/j.appet.2003.08.015

Brink, P. J., & Wood, M. J. (1998). *Advanced design in nursing research* (2nd ed.). Sage.

Bronfenbrenner, U. (1977). Toward an experimental ecology of human development. *American Psychologist, 32*, 513–531.

Brug, J., Conner, M., Harré, N., Kremers, S., McKellar, S., & Whitelaw, S. (2004). The Transtheoretical Model and stages of change: A critique: Observations by five commentators on the paper by Adams, J. and White, M. (2004) Why don't stage-based activity promotion interventions work? *Health Education Research, 20*(2), 244–258. https://doi.org/10.1093/her/cyh005

Campbell, M. K., Piaggio, G., Elbourne, D. R., & Altman, D. G. (2012). Consort 2010 statement: Extension to cluster randomised trials. *BMJ, 345*. https://doi.org/10.1136/bmj.e5661

Chen, S.-Y., Feng, Z., & Yi, X. (2017). A general introduction to adjustment for multiple comparisons. *Journal of Thoracic Disease, 9*(6), 1725–1729. https://doi.org/10.21037/jtd.2017.05.34

Creswell, J. W. (2014). *Research design: Qualitative, quantitative, and mixed methods approaches* (4th ed.). Sage.

Creswell, J. W., & Plano Clark, V. L. (2007). *Designing and conducting mixed methods research*. Sage.

de Vries, H., Dijkstra, M., & Kuhlman, P. (1988). Self-efficacy: The third factor besides attitude and subjective norm as a predictor of behavioural intentions. *Health Education Research, 3*(3), 273–282. https://doi.org/10.1093/her/3.3.273

Daivadanam, M., Wahlstrom, R., Thankappan, K. R., & Ravindran, T. K. (2015). Balancing expectations amidst limitations: The dynamics of food decision-making in rural Kerala. *BMC Public Health, 15*, 644. https://doi.org/10.1186/s12889-015-1880-5

Darlington, E., Namara, P., & Jourdan, D. (2020). Enhancing the efficacy of health promotion interventions: A focus on the context. *Public Health in Practice, 1*, 100002. https://doi.org/10.1016/j.puhip.2020.100002

Darnton, A. (2008). *Practical guide: An overview of behaviour change models and their uses*. Government Social Research Unit/University of Westminster: Centre for Sustainable Development.

Davis, R., Campbell, R., Hildon, Z., Hobbs, L., & Michie, S. (2015). Theories of behaviour and behaviour change across the social and behavioural sciences: A scoping review. *Health Psychology Review, 9*(3), 323–344. https://doi.org/10.1080/17437199.2014.941722

Dragsted, L. O., Gao, Q., Praticò, G., Manach, C., Wishart, D. S., Scalbert, A., et al. (2017). Dietary and health biomarkers-time for an update. *Genes & Nutrition, 12*, 24–24. https://doi.org/10.1186/s12263-017-0578-y

Engbers, L. H., van Poppel, M. N., Chin, A. P. M., & van Mechelen, W. (2006). The effects of a controlled worksite environmental intervention on determinants of dietary behavior and self-reported fruit, vegetable and fat intake. *BMC Public Health, 6*, 253. https://doi.org/10.1186/1471-2458-6-253

Fjeldsoe, B., Neuhaus, M., Winkler, E., & Eakin, E. (2011). Systematic review of maintenance of behavior change following physical activity and dietary interventions. *Health Psychology, 30*, 99–109. https://doi.org/10.1037/a0021974

Glanz, K., Rimer, B. K., & Viswanath, K. (2008). *Health behavior and health education: Theory, research, and practice* (4th ed.). Jossey-Bass.

Grabowski, D., Aagaard-Hansen, J., Willaing, I., & Jensen, B. B. (2017). Principled promotion of health: Implementing five guiding health promotion principles for research-based prevention and management of diabetes. *Societies, 7*(2). https://doi.org/10.3390/soc7020010

Grant, A., Treweek, S., Dreischulte, T., Foy, R., & Guthrie, B. (2013). Process evaluations for cluster-randomised trials of complex interventions: A proposed framework for design and reporting. *Trials, 14*, 15–15. https://doi.org/10.1186/1745-6215-14-15

Green, J. (2000). The role of theory in evidence-based health promotion practice. *Health Education Research, 15*(2), 125–129. https://doi.org/10.1093/her/15.2.125

Greene, G. W., Rossi, S. R., Rossi, J. S., Velicer, W. F., Fava, J. L., & Prochaska, J. O. (1999). Dietary applications of the stages of change model. *Journal of the American Dietetic Association, 99*(6), 673–678. https://doi.org/10.1016/s0002-8223(99)00164-9

Hayes, R. J., & Moulton, L. H. (2017). *Cluster randomised trials* (2nd ed.). Chapman & Hall/CRC Biostatistics Series.

Holton, J. (2010). The coding process and its challenges. *The Grounded Theory Review, 9*(1), 21–40. https://doi.org/10.4135/9781848607941.n13

John, J. H., & Ziebland, S. (2004). Reported barriers to eating more fruit and vegetables before and after participation in a randomized controlled trial: A qualitative study. *Health Education Research, 19*(2), 165–174. https://doi.org/10.1093/her/cyg016

Johnson, R. B., Onwuegbuzie, A. J., & Turner, L. A. (2007). Toward a definition of mixed methods research. *Journal of Mixed Methods Research, 1*(2), 112–133. https://doi.org/10.1177/1558689806298224

Kaur, J., Kaur, M., Webster, J., & Kumar, R. (2018). Protocol for a cluster randomised controlled trial on information technology-enabled nutrition intervention among urban adults in Chandigarh (India): SMART eating trial. *Global Health Action, 11*(1), 1419738. https://doi.org/10.1080/16549716.2017.1419738

Kaur, J., Kaur, M., Chakrapani, V., & Kumar, R. (2020a). Multilevel influences on fat, sugar, salt, fruit, and vegetable consumption behaviors among urban indians: Application of the social ecological model. *SAGE Open, 10*(2), 2158244020919526. https://doi.org/10.1177/2158244020919526

Kaur, J., Kaur, M., Chakrapani, V., Webster, J., Santos, J. A., & Kumar, R. (2020b). Effectiveness of information technology–enabled 'SMART Eating' health promotion intervention: A cluster randomized controlled trial. *Plos One, 15*(1), e0225892. https://doi.org/10.1371/journal.pone.0225892

Kerry, S. M., & Bland, J. M. (1998a). The intracluster correlation coefficient in cluster randomisation. *BMJ, 316*(7142), 1455–1455. https://doi.org/10.1136/bmj.316.7142.1455

Kerry, S. M., & Bland, J. M. (1998b). Statistics notes: Sample size in cluster randomisation. *BMJ, 316*(7130), 549. https://doi.org/10.1136/bmj.316.7130.549

Landau, S., Emsley, R., & Dunn, G. (2018). Beyond total treatment effects in randomised controlled trials: Baseline measurement of intermediate outcomes needed to reduce confounding in mediation investigations. *Clinical Trials (London, England), 15*(3), 247–256. https://doi.org/10.1177/1740774518760300

Lechner, L., Brug, J., De Vries, H., van Assema, P., & Mudde, A. (1998). Stages of change for fruit, vegetable and fat intake: Consequences of misconception. *Health Education Research, 13*(1), 1–11.

Mahajan, R., Malik, M., Bharathi, A. V., Lakshmi, P. V., Patro, B. K., Rana, S. K., et al. (2013). Reproducibility and validity of a quantitative food frequency questionnaire in an urban and rural area of northern India. *National Medical Journal of India, 26*(5), 266–272.

Marcolino, M. S., Oliveira, J. A. Q., D'Agostino, M., Ribeiro, A. L., Alkmim, M. B. M., & Novillo-Ortiz, D. (2018). The impact of mhealth interventions: Systematic review of systematic reviews. *JMIR mHealth and uHealth, 6*(1), e23. https://doi.org/10.2196/mhealth.8873

Moore, G. F., Audrey, S., Barker, M., Bond, L., Bonell, C., Hardeman, W., et al. (2015). Process evaluation of complex interventions: Medical Research Council guidance. *BMJ, 350*, h1258. https://doi.org/10.1136/bmj.h1258

Naska, A., Lagiou, A., & Lagiou, P. (2017). Dietary assessment methods in epidemiological research: Current state of the art and future prospects. *F1000Research, 6*, 926–926. https://doi.org/10.12688/f1000research.10703.1

National Institute of Nutrition. Indian Council of Medical Research. (2011). *Dietary guidelines for Indians: A manual* (Vol. 20 Sept 2017). ICMR.

Nutbeam, D. (1998). Evaluating health promotion: Progress, problems and solutions. *Health Promotion International, 13*(1), 27–44. https://doi.org/10.1093/heapro/13.1.27

Paskett, E., Thompson, B., Ammerman, A. S., Ortega, A. N., Marsteller, J., & Richardson, D. (2016). Multilevel interventions to address health disparities show promise in improving population health. *Health Affairs (Project Hope), 35*(8), 1429–1434. https://doi.org/10.1377/hlthaff.2015.1360

Petersen, K. S., Johnson, C., Mohan, S., Rogers, K., Shivashankar, R., Thout, S. R., et al. (2017a). Estimating population salt intake in India using spot urine samples. *Journal of Hypertension, 35*(11), 2207–2213. https://doi.org/10.1097/HJH.0000000000001464

Petersen, K. S., Wu, J. H. Y., Webster, J., Grimes, C., Woodward, M., Nowson, C. A., et al. (2017b). Estimating mean change in population salt intake using spot urine samples. *International Journal of Epidemiology, 46*(5), 1542–1550. https://doi.org/10.1093/ije/dyw239

Pomerleau, J., Lock, K., Knai, C., & McKee, M. (2005). Interventions designed to increase adult fruit and vegetable intake can be effective: A systematic review of the literature. *Journal of Nutrition, 135*(10), 2486–2495.

Pommier, J., Guével, M.-R., & Jourdan, D. (2010). Evaluation of health promotion in schools: A realistic evaluation approach using mixed methods. *BMC Public Health, 10*, 43–43. https://doi.org/10.1186/1471-2458-10-43

Porter, C. (2015). Revisiting Precede-Proceed: A leading model for ecological and ethical health promotion. *Health Education Journal, 75*(6), 753-764. https://doi.org/10.1177/0017896915619645

Ritchie, J., & Lewis, J. (2003). *Qualitative research practice: A guide for social science students and researchers*. Sage.

Rootman, I., Goodstadt, M., Potvin, L., & Springett, J. (2001). A framework for health promotion evaluation. In I. Rootman, M. Goodstadt, B. Hyndman, D. V. McQueen, L. Potvin, & J. Springett (Eds.), *Evaluation in health promotion* (pp. 7–38). WHO Regional Publications.

Sallis, J. F. (2018). Needs and challenges related to multilevel interventions: Physical activity examples. *Health Education & Behavior, 45*(5), 661–667. https://doi.org/10.1177/1090198118796458

Sandvik, C., Gjestad, R., Brug, J., Rasmussen, M., Wind, M., Wolf, A., et al. (2007). The application of a social cognition model in explaining fruit intake in Austrian, Norwegian and Spanish schoolchildren using structural equation modelling. *International Journal of Behavioral Nutrition and Physical Activity, 4*, 57. https://doi.org/10.1186/1479-5868-4-57

Smith, D. G., Clemens, J., Crede, W., Harvey, M., & Gracely, E. J. (1987). Impact of multiple comparisons in randomized clinical trials. *American Journal of Medicine, 83*(3), 545–550. https://doi.org/10.1016/0002-9343(87)90768-6

Soskolin, C. (2000). Transdisciplinary approaches for public health. *Epidemiology, 11*(4), S122.
Steinemann, N., Grize, L., Ziesemer, K., Kauf, P., Probst-Hensch, N., & Brombach, C. (2017). Relative validation of a food frequency questionnaire to estimate food intake in an adult population. *Food & Nutrition Research, 61*(1), 1305193. https://doi.org/10.1080/16546628.2017.1305193
Svetkey, L. P., Batch, B. C., Lin, P. H., Intille, S. S., Corsino, L., Tyson, C. C., et al. (2015). Cell phone intervention for you (CITY): A randomized, controlled trial of behavioral weight loss intervention for young adults using mobile technology. *Obesity, 23*(11), 2133–2141. https://doi.org/10.1002/oby.21226
Tashakkori, A., & Teddlie, C. (2003). *Handbook of mixed methods in social and behavioral research*. Sage.
The Lancet. (2019). Where next for randomised controlled trials in global health? *Lancet, 394*, 1481.
Tremblay, M. C., & Richard, L. (2014). Complexity: a potential paradigm for a health promotion discipline. HealthPromot Int, 29(2), 378–388. https://doi.org/10.1093/heapro/dar054. (Advance Access published 8 September, 2011)
Warwick-Booth, L., Cross, R., Woodall, J., Day, R., & South, J. (2013). Health champions and their circles of influence as a communication mechanism for health promotion. *International Review of Social Research, 3*(2), 113–129.
World Health Organization. (2008). *2008–2013 Action plan for the global strategy for the prevention and control of noncommunicable diseases*. World Health Organization.
Yoo, S.-H., & Kim, H.-K. (2010). Intervention development stages in health promotion planning models: PRECEDE-PROCEED and intervention mapping. *Korean Journal of Health Education and Promotion, 27*.
Zhou, H., Taber, C., Arcona, S., & Li, Y. (2016). Difference-in-differences method in comparative effectiveness research: Utility with unbalanced groups. *Applied Health Economics and Health Policy, 14*(4), 419–429. https://doi.org/10.1007/s40258-016-0249-y

Chapter 31
Researching the Practices of Policymakers in Implementing a Social Policy Intervention in Ghana

Ebenezer Owusu-Addo

31.1 Introduction

This chapter presents a case study of a research project focused upon understanding how a social policy intervention called the Livelihood Empowerment Against Poverty (LEAP) works to influence the social determinants of health (SDH) in Ghana and examining the factors that influence health sector involvement in the programme. It highlights the epistemological and ethical framework within which this health promotion research was structured. The aim of this work was to analyse the practices of policymakers and actors in the design and implementation of the LEAP programme. In doing so, the chapter examines how the practices of policy actors and policy entrepreneurs advance or fail to advance action on the SDH. It also outlines the contribution of this case study to advancing health promotion research.

Health promotion (HP) is conceived of as an action-oriented field (Lahtinen et al., 2005) and a field of social practice (Potvin et al., 2008) focused upon 'enabling people to increase control over and improve their health' (WHO, 1986). As such, one of the ontological underpinnings of HP is that the practices and actions of policymakers and other institutional actors have wider implications for health. For instance, it has been acknowledged that to reduce health inequities, there is the need to take action on the social determinants of health (SDH) through the development of culturally appropriate public policies and programmes (Marmot et al., 2012). In view of this, repeated calls have been made on the need for policymakers and other policy actors to have an SDH lens to the development and implementation of public policies.

E. Owusu-Addo (✉)
Bureau of Integrated Rural Development, Kwame Nkrumah University of Science and Technology, Kumasi, Ghana
e-mail: eowusu-addo.canr@knust.edu.gh

L. Potvin, D. Jourdan (eds.), *Global Handbook of Health Promotion Research, Vol. 1*,
https://doi.org/10.1007/978-3-030-97212-7_31

As HP is grounded on humanist values such as equity, empowerment and participation (Mantoura & Potvin, 2013), a collaborative approach was used in both the design and implementation of the research to optimise HP values. The adoption of such a participatory approach to this research and the evidence that it derives, called for different epistemological attitudes to knowledge production and to reject traditional models of evidence, which considers study participants as object to be studied. Epistemologically, therefore, the evaluation research reported in this chapter hinged on the assumption that HP as a field of social practice considers both the symbolic and subjective dimensions of social practices including those of policymakers in the pursuit of valued goals. In line with this epistemic position, the realist evaluation approach (Pawson, 2013) offered the best fit for studying how and under what circumstances the LEAP programme works to influence the SDH.

31.2 Programme Under Investigation

The Commission on the Social Determinants of Health (CSDH) through its publication: *Closing the gap in a generation: health equity through action on the social determinants of health* made a passionate call for governments across the globe to design and implement policies and interventions focused upon addressing the social determinants of health (SDH) (Commission on Social Determinants of Health, 2008). A foundational element of contemporary HP, therefore, has been the central role of public policy in improving the health of populations (Marmot et al., 2012; World Health Organization, 2011). It is widely acknowledged that without appropriate social interventions that address the SDH, the health of most people, particularly in low- and middle-income countries, will continue to deteriorate (de Leeuw, 2017; Marmot et al., 2012).

31.2.1 The Livelihood Empowerment Against Poverty (LEAP) Programme

LEAP is a social cash transfer programme introduced in 2008 as the flagship program of Ghana's Social Protection Strategy. Aside from the cash payments, LEAP provides free health insurance to beneficiaries through a National Health Insurance Scheme (NHIS) (Owusu-Addo et al., 2020a). The aim of the programme is to reduce poverty by increasing consumption and promoting access to social services and opportunities among beneficiary households. The programme is implemented by the Department of Social Welfare in the Ministry of Gender, Children and Social Protection (Ministry of Gender Children and Social Protection [MoGCSP], 2020). As a cash transfer programme, LEAP combines both conditional cash transfer

Table 31.1 Key characteristics of the LEAP Program

Program attribute	Description
Type of CT	UCT & CCT
Beneficiaries/ target groups	LEAP targets extremely poor and vulnerable households which have the following four categories of eligible members: Orphaned and vulnerable children (OVC) or, Persons with severe disability without any productive capacity and Elderly persons who are 65 years and above Extremely poor or vulnerable households with pregnant women and mothers with infants
Programme conditions	LEAP conditions for households with OVC are enrolment of children in school; school attendance; birth registration; utilisation of antenatal and post-natal services; complete immunization of babies; protection of children against child labour; and enrolment in the National Health Insurance Scheme
Programme benefits	Cash grant plus National Health Insurance
Transfer size	The amounts paid to beneficiaries have increased from GH¢ 8 -GH¢ 15 (about USD 8–15) per month in 2008 to GH¢ 64–GH¢ 106 (about USD 11–18) in 2020
Frequency of transfer	Bi-monthly
Mode of cash grant payment	Electronic payment
Coverage	LEAP covers all 216 administrative districts in Ghana with 213,044 beneficiary households, which translates to about 937,904 individuals
Program partners	World Bank, United Nations Children's Fund, World Food Program, United States Development Agency, United Nations Population Fund, European Union, and United Nations Development Program
Management structure	The LEAP management structure consists of the National Program Management Secretariat, which is responsible for overall program implementation and monitoring and evaluation; the District LEAP Implementation Committee (DLIC) led by the District Social Welfare Officers (DSWOs), responsible for program implementation at the district and community levels, and the community LEAP implementation committees (CLICs), which support program implementation at the community level

(CCT) and unconditional cash transfer (UCT). Table 31.1 summarises the programme characteristics.

With the focus of LEAP upon poverty reduction and human capital development, they constitute a healthy public policy, and have direct linkages to health and well-being by addressing the SDH (Owusu-Addo, 2016; Owusu-Addo et al., 2019a, 2020a).

31.2.2 LEAP Linkages to Health Promotion Values and Theory

The LEAP programme aligns with HP values of empowerment, participation, equity, social justice and inter-sectoral collaboration. Active community participation is at the centre of LEAP from the targeting stage to the implementation stage. The programme relies on participation and mobilisation of the community structures, and community experiences and knowledge for programme delivery. For example, as a matter of principle, community implementing committees (CLIC) must engage with community members in the selection of programme beneficiaries before forwarding eligible beneficiaries to the district programme office for onward submission to the national level. The national programme unit reviews the list from the community, check for eligibility, and then sends the list back to the community for approval before beneficiaries are finally enrolled unto the program. Community empowerment in the programme is further achieved through the recognition and use of community structures, and capacity building for community programme implementation committees.

With a focus on the poor and the vulnerable in society, LEAP works to tackle the root causes of poor health, injustice in society and the health gradient. For instance, LEAP emphasis on child education has led to improved enrolment and schooling for children (Owusu-Addo, 2016; Owusu-Addo et al., 2020a), which could potentially increase employment opportunities in adulthood, and ultimately raise socio-economic status. This in a way would help in addressing social and health inequities to promote health across the lifespan.

Similarly, LEAP aligns with HP principle of inter-sectoral collaboration. By its nature, LEAP promotes inter-sectoral action on SDH and therefore, aligns with the concept of "health in all policies.". LEAP's cross-sectoral objectives (e.g., improving health, education, nutrition and poverty reduction) thus call for the active involvement of the health sector (Owusu-Addo et al., 2019a, 2020b).

31.3 The Research Process and Implications for Health Promotion Research

31.3.1 The Research on the LEAP Programme

31.3.1.1 Framing the Research Aims

The overall aim of the research was to understand how LEAP works to influence the SDH, and to examine the factors that influence health sector involvement in the programme. The project was informed by the fact that while LEAP could potentially influence a broad range of SDH and as result promote health equity, past evaluations of the programme have not taken an SDH lens to produce evidence that would inform programme design and adaptation. Further, with the potential of LEAP for achieving health sector objectives, there is a growing concern that the health sector and health promoters have not been actively involved in the programme.

31.3.2 The Research Framework

HP research moves beyond the question of what works to include how and why health promotion programmes work. This research was thus underpinned by the realist evaluation approach (Pawson, 2013; Pawson et al., 1997). The choice of realist evaluation framework, which is a theory-driven approach, was informed by the aims of the study which is focused upon understanding how and why LEAP works to influence the SDH. Because of the inherent complexities within the LEAP programme (Owusu-Addo et al., 2020a) and the possibility that their operations are context dependent, it was important to identify a methodological approach that could elucidate the causal process by which changes and impacts are achieved, and to address questions relating to how and why the programme works, and the factors influencing health sector involvement in the programme, which are all of high relevance to policy and practice.

The role of theory in HP research has been widely acknowledged (Crosby & Noar, 2010; DiClemente et al., 2002; Green, 2000). LEAP operates at the macro, meso and micro levels of a system. Therefore, to understand the programme's mechanisms of change and the context within which they operate to influence the SDH, a number of formal theories were drawn upon in this research, including Kingdon (2011) 'multiple streams' theory of policy action, partnership synergy theory (Lasker et al., 2001), Sen's capability theory (Sen, 2001), empowerment theory (Friedmann, 1992), self-determination theory (Ryan & Deci, 2000), and self-efficacy theory (Bandura, 1982).

Kingdon argues that the convergence of three streams, namely, the problem (in this case, how CTs are perceived as an action on the SDH), policy (here, the nature of government and the CT policy-making process) and politics (changes in government and public opinion), create a window of opportunity for a policy action. In Kingdon's view, prospective policies are developed from a 'primeval soup' where ideas are constantly being discussed and developed. He emphasised the importance of 'policy entrepreneurs' who make use of available windows to instigate policy change. In this research, Kingdon's framework provided a useful analytical tool for understanding the windows of opportunity that LEAP opens for health sector involvement, and the factors that may facilitate or inhibit the role of the health sector and health promoters as policy entrepreneurs in the LEAP programme. In line with critical realist thinking, the findings of this study show that CTs' cross-cutting goals (poverty reduction, health, nutrition, etc.) and a health sector mandate for health promotion constitute the key structures and powers with the potential to trigger a more substantive involvement of health sector and health promoters in the programme. Kingdon argues that policy entrepreneurs exert influence through their advocacy efforts, which necessitates leadership and commitment to a policy agenda. The application of this framework, however, showed that while LEAP opens a window of opportunity for a more substantive role to be played by the health sector, it appears the Ministry of Health and the Ghana Health Service did not have input into the formulation and design of the LEAP policy. In the language of the participants, without these national-level actors 'showing a clear commitment to the LEAP as well as acknowledging its implications for the SDH, there will be low involvement of local health units in the programme. In the Ghanaian context, it appears that the dominance of curative health services has 'crowded' (Kingdon, 2011) the health policy agenda, leaving little room for health sector involvement in the CT policy. Factors found to influence health sector involvement in the LEAP included understanding of the SDH, legitimisation of health promotion in the health policy portfolio, national health sector commitment to SDH agenda, evidence linking the LEAP programme to SDH, intersectoral collaboration, and health promoters' knowledge of the policy-making process.

Sens' capability theory (Sen, 2001), which focuses on an agent's capability to make 'valued choices' offered a valuable explanation of the operation and impact of LEAP at the micro level. In the words of the programme beneficiary households interviewed, the LEAP gives them 'power' and makes them feel 'empowered' (both economically and psychologically), 'motivated' and that they have 'a new sense of hope' upon receipt of the cash grant (Owusu-Addo et al., 2020a). This aligns with the capability theory which acknowledges the need to focus on agency and empowerment in poverty reduction programmes. Partnership synergy theory (Lasker et al., 2001) posits that leveraging of resources and skills of various stakeholders enhances programme design, implementation processes, and realisation of outcomes. Using this theory, it was found that building partnership and collaboration for LEAP would mean the government first showing clear leadership and commitment to LEAP, providing the relevant policy frameworks and fostering intersectoral working at the ministerial level. Building partnerships also meant training key programme partners about the programme, creating a shared vision around the programme across sectors and nurturing trust and transparency amongst stakeholders to enhance their participation and embedding of LEAP activities into their work schedules. According to Kabeer (1999), empowerment theory has two inter-related dimensions, namely, resources and agency. In relation to LEAP, this highlights the resources offered by the programme to households, and how these resources enable choices and decision making (agency) under different conditions (Owusu-Addo et al., 2019b). Self-efficacy theory also posits that if the LEAP social grant serves as incentives to boost household and/or caregiver confidence, then they can trigger intrinsic motivation. Applying this theory to LEAP in this research proved very useful as it helped explore the circumstances under which LEAP promotes households' self-efficacy, and how the programme can be better designed to optimise this.

31.3.3 Involvement of Research Participants in the Planning and Conduct of the Research

Stakeholder involvement has been identified as one of the critical components of HP research and evaluation planning in ensuring the uptake of findings (Fetterman et al., 2017; Owusu-Addo et al., 2015; Patton, 2011). Further, HP research is done with people and not on people (Owusu-Addo et al., 2015). In view of this, and to optimise HP value of participation, at the design stage of the research, meetings were held with LEAP policymakers and development partners who fund and support the programme to establish the aims and relevance of the research to their work. This approach was taken to ensure co-design and production of knowledge that would be useful for both HP policy and practice. This was found to be a useful strategy in getting the findings of the study to inform the practices of policymakers and other national level actors. While a participatory approach to HP research often results in the researcher relinquishing control over the research process (Woodall et al., 2018), this does not necessarily result in loss of 'scientific' rigour of HP research (Allison & Rootman, 1996).

The findings of the research were shared with key stakeholders involved in the LEAP programme, including policymakers, development partners, national programme managers, local-level programme implementers and local health directorates. The purpose of the research dissemination was to make known to the stakeholders that while LEAP might not have been designed with an SDH lens, the programme constitutes a healthy public policy with significant impacts on the SDH and the potential to reduce health inequities. This means that to optimise LEAP impact on the SDH and reduce health inequities, health promoters and the health sector should be actively engaged in terms of the programme design, implementation and evaluation. Engagement with health promoters during data collection and in the dissemination of the findings revealed that nearly all of them had never thought of the linkages between the LEAP programme and the SDH, and thus described the sessions as an 'eye opener'. In this way, the research process became empowering and emancipatory for study participants and thus produced positive, and transformative effects.

Additionally, participants observed that LEAP policymakers' knowledge of the SDH and their appreciation of the linkages between the programme and health determinants were important in fostering collaboration with the health sector. These suggest that knowledge of the evidence linking LEAP to the SDH can be an activating factor for health sector and health promoters' involvement in the programme design and implementation. The health promoters further noted that while the need to address the SDH requires political action, politicisation of the LEAP closes the window that would have allowed policy entrepreneurs such as health promoters to contribute to the programme design and implementation. The active engagement with the policymakers and development partners revealed that while they had a common understanding of the influences of social factors upon health, there was a limited recognition and uptake of the SDH concept in LEAP design and implementation, and the need to engage with the health sector.

31.3.4 Design and Methods Used

Addressing the question of how LEAP works implies making an inquiry into the mechanisms by which change is produced by the programme. This makes the realist framework appropriate for researching the LEAP programme, which is inherently complex. Realist research and evaluation is method neutral (Pawson et al., 1997). This research thus followed four sequential phases, as outlined in Fig. 31.1. In phase 1, rather than starting with a middle-range theory about programme mechanisms, the study commenced with identifying the programme's patterns of outcomes through a systematic review (Owusu-Addo et al., 2018b) and looked for the contexts and mechanisms that might explain them. The systematic review was complemented by a methodological review to further establish the applicability and relevance of a realist approach to this research (Owusu-Addo et al., 2018a).

To make sense of the linkages between LEAP and the SDH, in Phase 2, a conceptual framework was developed conceptualising the potential linkages between cash transfer programmes, SDH and health equity (Owusu-Addo et al., 2019a). The framework aided the design of the empirical phase of the study, including the identification of relevant key stakeholders for initial programme theory development. Phase 3 had two components. The first was a realist qualitative study to develop initial hypotheses regarding how the LEAP programme was expected to influence the SDH (Owusu-Addo et al., 2019b). The theories were then tested and refined using a realist qualitative case study design (methods included interviews, focus groups and observations) (Owusu-Addo et al., 2020a). As the health sector has been called upon to take leadership role in actions on the SDH, Phase 4 of the study entailed an exploration of the factors affecting health sector involvement in the LEAP using a critical realist case study design (methods included interviews and document analysis) (Owusu-Addo et al., 2020b).

31.3.4.1 Study Participants and Sampling

This research studied the practices of development partners (i.e., The World Bank, Department for International Development and United Nations Children's Fund), policymakers and programme managers in relation to the design and implementation of the LEAP programme and the programme's impact on the beneficiaries. A maximum variation purposive sampling technique (Patton, 2015) was used to select information-rich cases across a broad range of programme stakeholders who have had lived experiences of the programme. Program stakeholders were drawn across the policy, management, implementation and community levels of the programme.

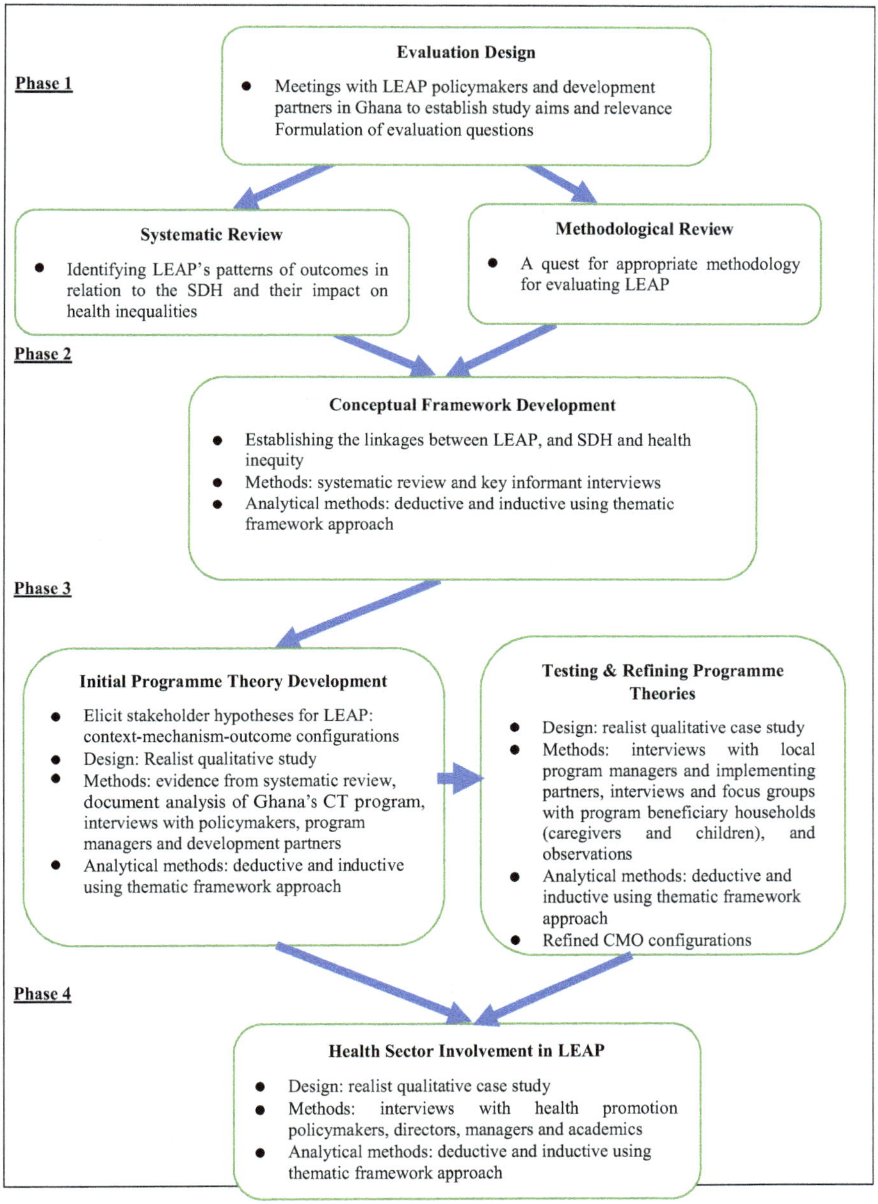

Phase 1

Evaluation Design

- Meetings with LEAP policymakers and development partners in Ghana to establish study aims and relevance Formulation of evaluation questions

Systematic Review

- Identifying LEAP's patterns of outcomes in relation to the SDH and their impact on health inequalities

Methodological Review

- A quest for appropriate methodology for evaluating LEAP

Phase 2

Conceptual Framework Development

- Establishing the linkages between LEAP, and SDH and health inequity
- Methods: systematic review and key informant interviews
- Analytical methods: deductive and inductive using thematic framework approach

Phase 3

Initial Programme Theory Development

- Elicit stakeholder hypotheses for LEAP: context-mechanism-outcome configurations
- Design: Realist qualitative study
- Methods: evidence from systematic review, document analysis of Ghana's CT program, interviews with policymakers, program managers and development partners
- Analytical methods: deductive and inductive using thematic framework approach

Testing & Refining Programme Theories

- Design: realist qualitative case study
- Methods: interviews with local program managers and implementing partners, interviews and focus groups with program beneficiary households (caregivers and children), and observations
- Analytical methods: deductive and inductive using thematic framework approach
- Refined CMO configurations

Phase 4

Health Sector Involvement in LEAP

- Design: realist qualitative case study
- Methods: interviews with health promotion policymakers, directors, managers and academics
- Analytical methods: deductive and inductive using thematic framework approach

Fig. 31.1 Research process flow chart

31.3.4.2 Data Collection and Analysis

Data collection entailed in-depth interviews with policy-, management- and implementation-level stakeholders and programme beneficiaries, and focus groups with programme beneficiaries and field observations. The use of method triangulation (interviews, focus groups, observations and document analysis), and data triangulation (collecting data from various stakeholders) strengthened the dependability and credibility of the findings (Hesse-Biber, 2011; Liamputtong, 2013; Patton, 2015).

Using a realist analytical 'lens', the data generated in this research were analysed following the five steps of the thematic approach (familiarisation, identifying of a thematic framework, indexing, charting, mapping and interpretation) described by Ritchie et al. (2008). As noted by Maxwell (2012), in realist research, "data collected through qualitative means are not considered constructions. Data are instead considered evidence for real phenomena and processes (p. 103)". This aligns with the participation value of HP, which requires researchers to take a collaborative research–practice relationship in developing knowledge about HP practices by attending to and privileging stakeholders' views as the lens by which to understand and place value on policies and programmes. This implies that in HP research, participants' experiences and understandings can complement or challenge existing scientific knowledge and theory. Data analysis in this study therefore, moved from constructions to explanation of causal mechanisms.

31.3.5 Specific Challenges of Health Promotion Research Enlightened by the Programme

While the application of realist approaches seems to be well established in health services research with exemplary case studies (Marchal et al., 2012), this is not the case in the HP field. The absence of clear guidelines for using realist approaches in researching HP practices like LEAP, which are not only complex but operate in complex cultural and collectivist environments, compounded the operational challenges that were encountered in this research.

Another limitation of the realist approach in HP research is the difficulty of defining and distinguishing mechanisms from contexts. While Pawson and Manzano-Santaella (2012) argue that distinguishing between contexts, mechanisms and outcomes is determined by their explanatory role, and Dalkin et al. (2015) have developed guidelines clarifying how mechanisms can be operationalised in practice, distinguishing mechanisms from contexts in this realist evaluation was still a challenge. What proved to be helpful in this study was clarifying the outcome patterns of LEAP first through the systematic review. This clarification pointed to the mechanisms that explain how and why LEAP worked or failed to work.

31.4 Conclusions

Theoretically, using an SDH lens in studying the practices of policymakers and other institutional actors is of value. By using such a lens, this research was able to examine how LEAP works to influence the SDH and the factors affecting health sector involvement in the programme. The findings provided useful insights to policymakers, programme designers and managers, evaluators and the health sector regarding how the LEAP programme can be used as an HP strategy to tackle the SDH and contribute to reducing health inequities. In terms of HP research methods, it is clear from this study that a single qualitative research method may give limited insight, but combinations (i.e., interviews, focus groups, observations and document analysis) give a rich picture of intervention processes, impacts and conditions for improvement. What is also clear from this research is that HP research should lay emphasis on working with people collaboratively by adopting study designs that value the dignity of all participants rather than adopting an approach that detaches the researcher from the participants (i.e., the experts-know-best approach). This research has shown that both theory development and realist evaluation are feasible and valuable for advancing HP research in relation to how non-health sector interventions like LEAP work or fail to work.

Conceptually, the findings point to the need to consider an SDH perspective in LEAP policy-making, design and implementation, and to foster strong inter-sectoral collaboration and partnerships across sectors. The evidence from this research indicates that there is limited recognition, knowledge and application of the SDH concept in LEAP policy-making, implementation and evaluation. A number of factors could explain this, including the limited involvement of the health sector in the programme as well as the limited recognition of the SDH in non-health sectors (Lawless et al., 2017). Due to LEAP's cross-cutting objectives (e.g., poverty reduction, education, health and nutrition), the programme should concomitantly be underpinned by inter-sectoral collaboration among sectors, including but not limited to education, health, agriculture and social development. This calls for a participatory approach to LEAP policy formulation, design and implementation involving key programme sectors as well as ensuring policy complementarity.

This research also highlights the need to give a due recognition to the role of the health sector in taking action on the SDH, and the opportunity that social policy interventions like LEAP offer the health sector in tackling health inequities. The research suggests that national health sector leadership of the SDH and commitment to the LEAP programme are critical to health sector involvement in the programme design and implementation. This means that unless the health sector in Ghana makes addressing the SDH part of the health policy portfolio and legitimises HP, there will be minimal or no involvement of the health sector and health promoters in non-health sector programmes such as the LEAP. This would result in missing out on the opportunities that such programmes offer in addressing health inequities. The implication here is that while LEAP sits outside of the health sector, health policymakers and practitioners can still facilitate collaborative work across the sectors to help optimise programme impacts on SDH. For this to occur, however, the health sector must first show leadership and a clear commitment to the SDH agenda to build its own legitimacy.

Lastly, for HP theory and practice to make a difference, realist approach to research and evaluation is critical. By using the realist approach, this research was able to show that LEAP can be one of the most effective means for addressing the SDH in Ghana, particularly among the poor and the vulnerable, suggesting the need to make them a formal part of public policies and health policy portfolios in the country.

References

Allison, K. R., & Rootman, I. (1996). Scientific rigor and community participation in health promotion research: Are they compatible? *Health Promotion International, 11*(4), 333–340.

Bandura, A. (1982). Self-efficacy mechanism in human agency. *American Psychologist, 37*(2), 122.

Commission on Social Determinants of Health. (2008). *Closing the gap in a generation: Health equity through action on the social determinants of health: Final report of the Commission on Social Determinants of Health*. World Health Organization.

Crosby, R., & Noar, S. M. (2010). Theory development in health promotion: Are we there yet? *Journal of Behavioral Medicine, 33*(4), 259–263.

Dalkin, S., Greenhalgh, J., Jones, D., Cunningham, B., & Lhussier, M. (2015). What's in a mechanism? Development of a key concept in realist evaluation. *Implementation Science, 10*(1), 1–7.

de Leeuw, E. (2017). Engagement of sectors other than health in integrated health governance, policy, and action. *Annual Review of Public Health, 38*, 329–349.

DiClemente, R. J., Crosby, R. A., & Kegler, M. C. (2002). *Emerging theories in health promotion practice and research: Strategies for improving public health* (Vol. 15). Wiley.

Fetterman, D. M., Rodríguez-Campos, L., & Zukoski, A. P. (2017). *Collaborative, participatory, and empowerment evaluation: Stakeholder involvement approaches*. Guilford Publications.

Friedmann, J. (1992). *Empowerment: The politics of alternative development*. Blackwell.

Green, J. (2000). *The role of theory in evidence-based health promotion practice*. Oxford University Press.

Hesse-Biber, S. N. (2011). *The practice of qualitative research* (2nd ed.). SAGE.

Kabeer, N. (1999). Resources, agency, achievements: Reflections on the measurement of women's empowerment. *Development and Change, 30*(3), 435–464.

Kingdon, J. W. (2011). *Agendas, alternatives, and public policies (updated)* (Vol. 128, pp. 251–257). Pearson.

Lahtinen, E., Koskinen-Ollonqvist, P., Rouvinen-Wilenius, P., Tuominen, P., & Mittelmark, M. B. (2005). The development of quality criteria for research: A Finnish approach. *Health Promotion International, 20*(3), 306–315.

Lasker, R. D., Weiss, E. S., & Miller, R. (2001). Partnership synergy: A practical framework for studying and strengthening the collaborative advantage. *The Milbank Quarterly, 79*(2), 179–205.

Lawless, A., Lane, A., Lewis, F. A., Baum, F., & Harris, P. (2017). Social determinants of health and local government: Understanding and uptake of ideas in two Australian states. *Australian and New Zealand Journal of Public Health, 41*(2), 204–209.

Liamputtong, P. (2013). *Qualitative research methods* (4th ed.). Oxford University Press.

Mantoura, P., & Potvin, L. (2013). A realist–constructionist perspective on participatory research in health promotion. *Health Promotion International, 28*(1), 61–72.

Marchal, B., Van Belle, S., Van Olmen, J., Hoerée, T., & Kegels, G. (2012). Is realist evaluation keeping its promise? A review of published empirical studies in the field of health systems research. *Evaluation, 18*(2), 192–212.
Marmot, M., Allen, J., Bell, R., Bloomer, E., Goldblatt, P., & Consortium for the European Review of Social Determinants of Health. (2012). WHO European review of social determinants of health and the health divide. *Lancet, 380*(9846), 1011–1029.
Maxwell, J. A. (2012). *A realist approach for qualitative research*. Sage.
Ministry of Gender Children and Social Protection [MoGCSP]. (2020). *Livelihood empowerment against poverty*. Available at http://leap.gov.gh/. Accessed 16 Nov 2020.
Owusu-Addo, E. (2016). Perceived impact of Ghana's conditional cash transfer on child health. *Health Promotion International, 31*(1), 33–43.
Owusu-Addo, E., Edusah, S. E., & Sarfo-Mensah, P. (2015). The utility of stakeholder involvement in the evaluation of community-based health promotion programmes. *International Journal of Health Promotion and Education, 53*(6), 291–302.
Owusu-Addo, E., Renzaho, A., & Smith, B. (2019a). Cash transfers and the social determinants of health: A conceptual framework. *Health Promotion International, 34*(6), e106–e118.
Owusu-Addo, E., Renzaho, A., & Smith, B. (2019b). Cash transfers and the social determinants of health: Towards an initial realist program theory. *Evaluation, 25*(2), 224–244.
Owusu-Addo, E., Renzaho, A. M., & Smith, B. J. (2018a). Evaluation of cash transfer programs in sub-Saharan Africa: A methodological review. *Evaluation and Program Planning, 68*, 47–56.
Owusu-Addo, E., Renzaho, A. M., & Smith, B. J. (2018b). The impact of cash transfers on social determinants of health and health inequalities in sub-Saharan Africa: A systematic review. *Health Policy and Planning, 33*(5), 675–696.
Owusu-Addo, E., Renzaho, A. M., & Smith, B. J. (2020a). Developing a middle-range theory to explain how cash transfers work to tackle the social determinants of health: A realist case study. *World Development, 130*, 104920.
Owusu-Addo, E., Renzaho, A. M., & Smith, B. J. (2020b). Factors affecting health sector involvement in public policies addressing the social determinants of health: A critical realist case study of cash transfers in Ghana. *International Journal of Health Promotion and Education, 58*, 1–19.
Patton, M. Q. (2011). *Essentials of utilization-focused evaluation*. Sage.
Patton, M. Q. A. (2015). *Qualitative research & evaluation methods: Integrating theory and practice* (4th ed.). SAGE.
Pawson, R. (2013). *The science of evaluation: A realist manifesto*. Sage.
Pawson, R., & Manzano-Santaella, A. (2012). A realist diagnostic workshop. *Evaluation, 18*(2), 176–191.
Pawson, R., Tilley, N., & Tilley, N. (1997). *Realistic evaluation*. Sage.
Potvin, L., Mcqueen, D. V., & Hall, M. (2008). Introduction. Aligning evaluation research and health promotion values: Practices from the Americas. In *Health promotion evaluation practices in the Americas* (pp. 1–9). Springer.
Ritchie, J., Spencer, L., & O'Connor, W. (2008). Carrying out qualitative analysis. In J. Ritchie & J. Lewis (Eds.), *Qualitative research practice* (pp. 219–262). Sage.
Ryan, R. M., & Deci, E. L. (2000). Self-determination theory and the facilitation of intrinsic motivation, social development, and well-being. *American Psychologist, 55*(1), 68.
Sen, A. (2001). *Development as freedom* (Oxford Paperbacks). Oxford University.
WHO. (1986). *Ottawa charter for health promotion*. Retrieved from https://www.euro.who.int/__data/assets/pdf_file/0004/129532/Ottawa_Charter.pdf. Accessed 4 June 2021.
World Health Organization. (2011). *Closing the gap: Policy into practice on social determinants of health*. Discussion paper.
Woodall, J., Warwick-Booth, L., South, J., & Cross, R. (2018). What makes health promotion research distinct? *Scandinavian Journal of Public Health, 46*(20_suppl), 118–122.

Chapter 32
Capturing Complexity in Health Promotion Intervention Research: Conducting Critical Realist Evaluation

Katherine L. Frohlich, Kate St-Arneault, and Mikael St-Pierre

32.1 Introduction

Since the inception of the Ottawa Charter (WHO, 1986), health promotion has championed the idea that health is inextricably linked to the conditions in which daily life takes place (WHO, 1986); being able to make healthy choices and live a healthy life depend on the opportunities and constraints offered by the environment. More recently, concerns about how to understand the role of the environment in producing health have led to fruitful and abundant discussions about context (Craig et al., 2018; Frohlich et al., 2001), or "the circumstances or events that form the environment within which something exists or takes place" (Encarta, 1999). This more sophisticated understanding of the environment invites us to study everyday settings such as schools, neighbourhoods and cities not just as containers of individuals, units of analysis or captive audiences but as systems of relationships.

Despite this more refined understanding of context, health promotion evaluation research and practice continues to treat context as a source of potential confounding that needs to be either "factored in" (as variables that apply across cases) or "factored out" (as variables to be controlled for) (Poland et al., 2008). Context is thus still often considered a nuisance or a compromise to implementation fidelity and programme outcomes. This limits our ability to understand the fit and responsiveness of our interventions to situational context.

K. L. Frohlich (✉) · K. St-Arneault
Département de médecine sociale et préventive, École de Santé Publique et Centre de Recherche en Santé Publique, Université de Montréal (ESPUM & CReSP), Montréal, Québec, Canada
e-mail: katherine.frohlich@umontreal.ca

M. St-Pierre
Montreal Urban Ecology Center (MUEC), Montréal, Québec, Canada

L. Potvin, D. Jourdan (eds.), *Global Handbook of Health Promotion Research, Vol. 1*,
https://doi.org/10.1007/978-3-030-97212-7_32

We situate our work amongst those who more recently are attempting to systematically "unpack" those aspects of settings experienced by programme participants during, and due to, health promotion interventions. Aligned with a critical realist epistemology, we understand the world to be *real*, existing and operating independently of our awareness or knowledge of it (Bhaskar, 2013; Sayer, 2000). According to this perspective, the world comprises three things: objects, structures and generative mechanisms, all of them existing in the realm of the *real*. When diverse objects are assembled in varying configurations, or networks, through existing structures, they trigger certain generative mechanisms leading to *actual* events (e.g. health problems or behaviours, racism, social inequalities). But since many *real* elements and *actual* events are not visible, it is impossible for us to *empirically* measure, observe, or even be aware of all of them. This is especially the case for many of the objects within the social sphere (Sayer, 2000). Our understanding as to what might have led to an event (an outcome) is therefore an inference about its cause – what *real* elements were present, how they were structured together and what mechanism this configuration triggered.

We view critical realism as being particularly helpful in understanding how the various intersecting, interacting and inter-influencing complex systems (Byrne & Callaghan, 2014) that we study in health promotion influence our health. For example, communities comprise smaller-scale complex systems (e.g. families, individuals, nervous or cardiovascular systems, cells), but are also part of higher-level systems (e.g. cities, countries). Whatever happens in one complex system – a health problem in one individual for instance – will impact other systems to which it is related and with which it interacts, e.g. an individual's family, neighbourhood or workplace, even though the impact might be relatively small. Since each one of these complex systems has the capacity to adapt to its continuously changing environment (i.e. other systems) to try to gain a certain equilibrium, complex systems are thereby dynamic, ever-changing and evolving. Change, however, does not happen in a linear way (an increase in input does not necessarily proportionally lead to an increase in output) (Byrne & Callaghan, 2014). Moreover, how a system evolves over time, i.e. its trajectory is unpredictable.

Understanding the world as a complex system has substantial implications for health promotion research. First, in our research, we understand health promotion interventions to be complex social interventions: they are intentional change efforts inserted into pre-existing social relations (Poland et al., 2008). These change efforts create the opportunity for systems to deviate from their current trajectories (Hawe et al., 2009). The capacity of an intervention to change a system's dynamics relies on the interaction between the resources it offers and the pre-existing configuration of the system. By coupling and embedding with the pre-existing configuration, therefore changing it, health promotion interventions create opportunities to trigger new mechanisms and generate different events (outcomes). Designing and implementing interventions able to couple with and embed in a system's pre-existing configuration requires deep knowledge about the system. Accessing and mobilising such knowledge can only be achieved through intense engagement with the system, using participatory methods for instance. During the development and evaluation of health promotion interventions, researchers must develop a relationship with a variety of professionals, practitioners, bureaucrats, politicians, members of special interest groups (e.g. teachers, non-profit organisations, recreation workers, community members, parents). This also means that health promotion interventions need to and will differ from one system to another, leaving no place for standardisation.

Now, if systems' trajectories systems are unpredictable and interventions need to differ from one system to another, how can we know which way to go if we would like to see specific changes happen in another system? Learnings from traditional and repeated efficacy evaluation of interventions (i.e. is the intervention able to produce the desired effects over and over again) seem to offer very little guidance here. On the other hand, focussing on a system's trajectory, i.e. on how a system's dynamic has changed over time following the introduction of an intervention, helps us understand "how things have come to be what they are" (Byrne & Callaghan, 2014, p. 154). Since we cannot predict change, we must work on explaining it, on opening its black box. Realist evaluation aims precisely at this – developing, testing and refining such explanations (Pawson & Tilley, 1997). It is only with such explanations in hand that we will eventually be able to understand how to adapt our interventions to other systems.

Our positionality with regard to the importance of critical realist evaluation stems, in part, from our object of study; change in human activities in urban centres. Cities are themselves complex systems, a part of higher-level complex systems (regional, provincial or national governments), but also comprise smaller scale complex systems (various departments or neighbourhoods, elected officials, employees or citizens). Cities are therefore composed, as well as parts, of various intersecting, interacting and interinfluencing complex systems. In other words, cities' policies and practices act as a major structural determinant of population health through their formal and informal institutions, micro and macro politics, and how these intersect with the day-to-day activities of citizens. Understanding and trying to change citizens' health-related practices without understanding and working on how cities' policies and practices shape them is unrealistic.

Finally, such a worldview implies that it is utopian to think that research focussing solely on outcomes can generate transferable knowledge from one city to another. Outcomes stemming from the interaction of complex systems such as cities and their citizens are unpredictable since each system continuously adapts to micro and macro changes happening in other systems with which they interact (e.g. families, workplaces, healthcare systems, etc., hence each system's unique environment or structure). To be able to produce useful knowledge, the primary focus of health promotion research should be less about outcomes per se and more about the processes, and their underlying conditions, leading to stability or change in outcomes. The real burning question for health promotion research about how cities' policies and practices interact with health then is not "does change happen?" but rather "how and why does it, or does it not, happen?". Such questions cannot be answered by randomised control trials, often considered the gold standard method for evaluating interventions. Epistemologies, such as critical realism, and realist evaluations using mixed methods, prove more appropriate here.

Using our research project, *Levelling the Playing Fields* as an example, this chapter aims to illustrate how we translate this research framework into our research practices. In doing so, we aim to highlight the interest and relevance of the critical realism paradigm for studying complex systems from a health promotion research perspective.

32.1.1 Levelling the Playing Fields*: An Urban Health Intervention to Enable Free-Play to Arise in Cities*

Children and youth in a growing number of countries, but particularly in the Global North, have become excluded, or are excluding themselves (with the help of their parents and other adults) from playing and otherwise being in previously used public spaces such as streets, back-lanes, empty vacant lots, and even parks and playgrounds. Indeed, this exclusion has become endemic. In addition, by-laws have been passed in cities around the world leading to a reduction in children's ability to play in streets, sometimes making noise (such as happy shouting of children while playing) punishable through fines. In sum, children and youth have increasingly lost the right to the city, with their activities confined to few "acceptable" places to play outdoors, such as private property, playgrounds and/or in scheduled, organised activities.

This turned our attention to the critical role that urban environments and governance were playing in the well-being and health opportunities for children and youth. City planning helps structure the distribution of social, physical, and economic "goods and bads" that influence human health and explain persistent urban health inequities (de Leeuw & Simos, 2017). In other words, city planning acts as a structural determinant of health through: its formal and informal institutions, its micro and macro politics, and how these intersect with the day-to-day activities of children and youth. To be health promoting, cities need to enable children and youth to both play and interact in public spaces (physically and socially) and encourage the experience of active citizenship. In other words, a healthy city for children and youth is a place where they are able to be, play and interact in public spaces, but also where they can experience that their voice matters (Winge & Lamm, 2019).

The extent to which cities support children's outdoor play – i.e. their *playability* – can be directly linked not only to children's health, levels of obesity and psychological well being but also to the population's well-being as a whole. While we now have important documentation regarding the dearth of outdoor free-play in Canadian cities (ParticipACTION, 2018), we have nearly no intervention research knowledge about how feasible it is to intervene on our cities in order to change their practices in relation to children's free-play and independent mobility.

From these concerns, we developed the population-intervention research project entitled *Levelling the Playing Fields*. Our project is a participatory, inter-sectoral and interdisciplinary health promotion intervention. The intervention aims to orient social change not by changing the health-related behaviours traditionally associated with health promotion but by addressing and bringing to the fore the right to the city that citizens, and children in particular, have lost through the dominance of the automobile and other societal factors. *Levelling the Playing Fields* aims in the long-term to make urban centres across Canada more conducive to outdoor free-play for children and youth and increase physical activity levels, independent mobility, active transport, social cohesion and mental health amongst children, youth and city residents in general.

With *Levelling the Playing Fields,* we are proposing to test the effects of School Streets and Play Streets in neighbourhoods of contrasting levels of social and material deprivation, in two Canadian cities. The School Street part of our intervention will run during the entire school year and will close off between 50 and 200 m of streets to car traffic, 15–60 min prior to and after school, during the entire school year. School streets are new in Canada and have never been fully evaluated for their health effects. The Play Street interventions will involve the closing of circumscribed residential streets to through-traffic at least twice a week, for at least one hour, also over the course of an entire year.

32.1.2 The Montreal Urban Ecology Center as a Critical Partner for Participatory Planning

The paradigm shift required in municipal policymaking and priorities to advance the ideas mobilised by *Levelling the Playing Fields* can, however, be difficult to initiate due to regulation constraints maladapted to innovation. Indeed, the implementation of pilot projects to transform the built environment using innovative ideas such as Play and School Streets, in two entirely different cities, is complex. It requires a clear articulation of the idea and the development of collaborative relationships with municipal decision-makers, professionals and local community members. It also requires the adoption of a language of operationalisation already mastered by urban planning professionals, something that researchers do not always have within their skill set. Our research team at the *École de Santé Publique, Université de Montréal* (ESPUM) turned to a non-governmental organisation, the *Montreal Urban Ecology Center* (MUEC), to accompany us in the development, implementation and research process we foresaw as being critical to success. This organisation, in existence since 1996, has as its mission to contribute to the building of ecological, democratic and healthy cities in Quebec and Canada. Its focus and expertise include urban planning, participatory processes and mobility issues.

Over the course of its history, the MUEC has contributed to developing and disseminating knowledge about participatory urban planning approaches. Participatory urban planning is the "effective participation of residents and users in the programming and design of a project" (Montreal Urban Ecology Center, 2015). Participatory urban planning requires broad stakeholder participation as well as the delegation of decision-making. The premise behind the approach is that collaboration between urban planning professionals and different users of the city make it possible to best meet the needs of the community.

Considering that *Levelling the Playing Fields* wishes to offer citizens leverage for transforming their local streets in favour of free-play and independent mobility for children, the participatory urban planning approach developed by MUEC was considered ideal for helping the research team achieve change. First, for School Streets, it will be necessary to find tools that promote dialogue and concertation between all the actors involved, whether they are school related (management, school boards), parents whose children attend the school, the city and residents, as well as businesses and other institutional neighbours to the school. This work of dialogue and concertation should be carried out while keeping children's right to the city at the heart of the discussion. Similar plans exist for Play Streets. The various stages leading to decision-making must take place in dialogue and concertation between affected residents, involving other stakeholders, starting with the city.

The toolkit of participatory urban planning is perfectly suited to empower residents to act and promote the transformation of the built environment in favour of free-play in the city. This is achievable, first, by promoting the involvement of a multitude of stakeholders in decision-making processes in order to promote the understanding and consideration of multiple points of view. Second, the approach offers tools to develop a common and concerted vision, identify implementation milestones, decide on some of the characteristics and modalities of transformation projects and evaluation strategies, all in concert with the authorities who are engaged in the process. Third, the approach also encourages the participation of children in the process in order to foster the development of cities that meet their needs and aspirations.

During the first two years of collaboration, several benefits of this concerted work have become apparent. First, numerous joint presentations of the research project to influential actors (including municipally elected officials, municipal bureaucrats, school officials, community organisations and others), targeted upstream, made it possible to reach certain milestones, in particular with regard to the authorisations required for the implementation of the pilot project. By including both the scientific and implementation sides to the equation at all of these meetings, stakeholders were provided information, and able to exchange about both the science and the concrete urban planning advantages and issues involved in the project. This clearly reassured the stakeholders and amplified the importance of the interventions. Indeed, following several meetings with key elected officials, the pilot project approval process ended up being initiated by the local administration, a clear sign of buy-in. Consequently, the research team was put in touch with various municipal bureaucrats (town planners, engineers, recreation workers, communications experts) to assess the potential for the project to be carried out. Multiple meetings have ensued in which we have tackled various tests of realism – legal, logistical, political, physical – with local administrations. The complementarity of the experiences available within the overall team clearly helped to obtain all the necessary authorisations and to inspire confidence with the municipal bureaucrats that there was a clear advantage for them to engage in the intervention and research process.

32.2 Evaluating Complex Processes: Applying a Critical Realist View of Causality to Our Intervention

As mentioned above, *Levelling the Playing Fields* engages stakeholders and local citizens in a participatory urban planning approach to be able to develop a concerted vision of the problem, but also of the possible solution. Throughout this participatory process, children, parents, neighbours, municipally elected officials and staff, as well as school principals and staff are contributing to the interventions' development. Indeed, the exact locations of Play and School Streets, their frequency and duration, their rules of operation, the activities that will be offered (or not), the expected level of supervision from adults, etc., will result from collective discussions ensuring that interventions are relevant to local needs, concerns and preferences.

Some health promotion researchers might consider such interventions to be too *out of control* to be rigorously evaluated because they cannot be entirely standardised across sites. How could the results of such an evaluation ever be useful? To date, the few Play Street interventions that have been evaluated, have used pre-test-post-test designs with control groups and have largely investigated the intervention effects alone (Cortinez-O'Ryan et al., 2017; D'Haese et al., 2015; Zieff et al., 2016). While some demonstrated change due to the interventions were found in these studies regarding the number of steps taken or minutes of time spent outdoors for children, we have no information as to *how* or *why* this happened. We argue that it is not helpful to place primacy on the standardisation of the intervention's package if we are concerned with local participation and buy-in. We will describe here how the evaluations of such interventions can produce rigorous and transferable results, particularly for interventions seeking to follow health promotion principles of involving community stakeholders.

As mentioned in our introduction, according to the critical realist ontology, social actors are *real* (Byrne & Uprichard, 2012). Each social actor is an individual complex system comprising her own social objects, structures and generative mechanisms, able to produce her own *actual* events. Each social actor is also an object of higher-level complex systems, such as his family or community. These *real* higher-level systems also have their own structure and generative mechanisms able to produce *actual* events (Byrne & Uprichard, 2012; Houston, 2010). For example, most children love to play outdoors because it is fun and exciting (Brockman et al., 2011; Lee et al., 2015). By perceiving outdoor free-play to be enjoyable (mechanism), children tend to engage in it (actual). But parents also impose time and space constrains, i.e. rules about when and where they can play, due to safety concerns (Brockman et al., 2011) or prioritise activities deemed more productive and useful, such as organised sports (Lee et al., 2015). By perceiving outdoor free-play as risky or futile (different mechanism), parents limit their children's play opportunities, hence contributing to lowering outdoor play levels (actual).

This critical realist ontology has important consequences for our understanding of what shapes health-related problems and solutions. First, it is fair to say that problematic events should be understood as resulting from the interaction between multiple systems, hence from the interaction between their multiple generative mechanisms. For instance, the meanings parents place on outdoor free-play (risky, trivial) have been identified as mechanisms that play a role in diminishing outdoor free-play. But neighbourhood-level reinforcing or countervailing mechanisms also seem to be at play. Indeed, parents are sensitive to the judgment of others; no parent wishes to be labelled a *bad parent* (Allin et al., 2014; Francis et al., 2017). What is considered good parenting, however, differs according to local norms. In middle-class neighbourhoods, parents might be expected to impose strict rules about outdoor play and constantly supervise their children, while in working-class neighbourhoods, granting children more freedom about how they play and move around is more acceptable (Valentine & McKendrck, 1997). Individually, parents may wish to grant their children more or less freedom than what is expected of them, but still choose to, at least partially, comply with local norms so they are not seen to be inappropriate (Allin et al., 2014; Francis et al., 2017; Valentine & McKendrck, 1997). This means that understanding *what* causes an outcome is not about discovering what was *the* activated mechanism, but rather exploring the constellations of activated mechanisms per intervention site.

This also means that different groupings of mechanisms can produce the same type of event. Albeit at different intensities, low levels of children's outdoor play seem to be generated by parental fear of strangers in both high-SES and low-SES neighbourhoods. Being a common mechanism of low levels of outdoor play in a diversity of contexts, addressing parental fear of strangers would then seem to be a key feature of an eventual intervention. But even if addressing parental fear of strangers appears to be essential, it might be, and in fact it probably is, insufficient for outdoor play levels to increase substantially in every context. For instance, as mentioned above, parents from high-SES neighbourhoods often perceive outdoor free-play as a fun, but nevertheless wasteful, way for their children to use their free time (Pynn et al., 2019; Clark & Dumas, 2020). This interpretation of outdoor free play leads them to prioritise "useful" pursuits such as organised activities, leaving less time to play freely. On the other hand, families living in low-SES neighbourhoods have less access to safe and attractive outdoor play spaces (Rigolon, 2016; Ridge, 2011), which could lead them, to turn, to engage in other types of activities than outdoor play, perhaps indoors. This means that *what* causes an event cannot be entirely generalised from one context to another, even though different contexts might nevertheless share common mechanisms that apparently play key roles in the production of the event.

Moreover, since the activation of specific mechanisms is contingent on their configurations of objects and structures, understanding *what* causes an outcome is not only about uncovering what were the activated mechanisms, but also determining what activated them. For instance, the idea that parents should be fearful that their child might be injured or kidnapped if not in their presence at all times is contextually constructed. Many parents relate media coverage of kidnappings or other types of crime committed against children as their primary source of fear (Francis et al., 2017; Crawford et al., 2017). Not knowing neighbours also exacerbates this fear, especially if parents cannot count on familiar faces to intervene and help their child in case of need (Crawford et al., 2017; Witten et al., 2013). Assessing commonalities across contexts (e.g. media coverage, neighbourhood relations) and which specific mechanisms were activated (parental fear of strangers) then allows for the identification of essential assemblages of contextual elements that appear to be necessary to their activation.

So, what does this all mean with regard to our intervention *Levelling the Playing Fields?* As previously mentioned, for critical realists, an intervention is an attempt to disrupt pre-existing configurations of objects and structures, to activate new mechanisms and change the course of expected events. In this sense, an intervention is the incarnation of a theory about what is able to cause the desired outcome (Pawson & Tilley, 1997). The aim of a realist evaluation is to uncover how an intervention couples and embeds itself with the pre-existing configuration of a system (the context), what new interpretations (mechanisms) this new remodelling triggers and how this changes the system's trajectory (outcomes).

As we have already established, causation is context specific; introducing an intervention in different contexts will likely trigger different mechanisms, leading to different outcomes. For instance, people in our socially contrasted neighbourhoods in Montreal and Kingston may react differently to the closures of the Play Streets. In one neighbourhood, adults might see Play Streets as an opportunity to also spend time outdoors. Doing so, their presence might become reassuring for parents fearful of strangers, thus encouraging them to permit more frequent outdoor free-play during street closures. In another neighbourhood, streets closures might give rise to persisting conflicts between Play Street users and drivers, creating uninviting environments for children and other residents. This unanticipated difference in contextual reactions to interventions has important implications for how we consider the design of interventions and their evaluation.

Critical realists do not strive towards the standardisation of interventions (i.e. the same duration, frequency, types of activities, etc.). Instead, they argue that standardisation, in the case of our example, would not significantly change the outcomes in our different types of neighbourhoods, nor would it help with generalisation. On the contrary, tailoring the intervention to the local needs and preferences would help make the intervention more pertinent for those living in that particular context, meaning that tailoring the intervention would help it to couple and embed with each unique context. Indeed, what we can understand from the example is that it is the mechanisms leading to the positive outcomes (the intervention's functions) that need to be replicated from one setting to another, not the intervention package (Hawe et al., 2009).

Critical realism also underscores that the evaluation of an intervention cannot simply be about assessing *if* it is able to generate the desired outcome. Assessing effectiveness does indeed give us clues about *whether* (the intervention per se) might, or might not, work to generate the desired outcome. But the only way to be able to attribute the occurrence, or non-occurrence, of the effects to the intervention is to understand *how* it worked, that is, to open up the black box and uncover how people interpreted and reacted to the street closure (the mechanisms) (Byrne, 2013). Moreover, assessing the conditions under which it did work, as well as the ones under which it did not, helps delineate *why* the intervention is able to work, or not.

This means that every intervention should first be regarded as a case with its mechanisms and outcomes analysed and interpreted within their context (Byrne, 2013). A subsequent cross-case analysis then makes it possible to uncover the key ingredients of the interventions, namely, the mechanisms common to the different environments, as well as the contextual conditions which must (or must not) be present to activate them. Compared to a traditional outcome evaluation, this type of endeavour would allow us to further explain how change has come about, bringing our understanding closer to *what* is really causing the change to occur.

In sum, interventions are not reducible to a pre-determined package, i.e. their visible parts. In the case of *Levelling the Playing Fields*, the intervention is not the mere closure of the Play and School Streets. New ideas about where or how children can play and move about in their neighbourhoods, new opportunities around public space use or new types of interactions between citizens, municipal workers and school staff members, are just a few examples of many possible important, yet less tangible, inputs from the intervention. Moreover, what causes the intended outcome is not an intervention component; it is rather how people interpret and react to the ideas and opportunities offered by the introduction of this component in their lives.

32.3 Conclusions

Some 35 years after the writing of the Ottawa Charter, much of health promotion and its attendant interventions are still seeking to change individual behaviour, despite a rhetoric encouraging us to think about how we can better understand and alter the social context to encourage health-related practices to come about. When it comes to the evaluation of these interventions, the gold standard in public health also remains the randomised control trial. While we would not quibble that, at times, individual behaviour modification interventions and/or RCTs used to evaluate interventions may have their place, we argue that there are important limits to models such as RCTs for answering many of the important questions health promotion seeks to address. We support these arguments by illustrating the importance critical realism places on understanding the complex contextual conditions of interventions that RCTs attempt to "control" away. First, taking account of context in the development of interventions should lead to more appropriate, culturally sensitive, implementable and effective interventions. Understanding how interventions interact with context is a key to understanding how they achieve impact. Second, failure to take account of such interactions is one reason why interventions shown to be effective in one setting fail to achieve similar impacts elsewhere, even if they are replicated faithfully and implemented successfully in the new setting. Third, understanding interactions between intervention and context helps to explain why impacts vary, and in particular, whether the intervention is likely to narrow or widen inequalities in health. Finally, including adequately detailed accounts of context in reports of intervention studies will make them more useful to decision makers interested in implementing, sustaining, transferring and scaling up the interventions, and to researchers developing theoretical models of change underlying improvements in health promotion (Craig et al., 2018).

This brings us to the role that individuals play in our research practice. First, we firmly believe that "It is not programs that make things change, it is people, embedded in their context who, when exposed to programs, do something to activate given mechanisms, and change" (Pawson & Tilley, 1997, cited in Stame, 2004, p. 62). The role that people play in interventions is not just as passive recipients, but as active actors, both in the creation of the intervention and in its unfolding. As we argued throughout, it is therefore necessary to take into account how programs, as complex social interventions, manage to embed themselves in these social contexts by aligning with existing incentive structures and mobilising key members of the community. This process, we would argue, is not just about understanding and changing individuals' health-related behaviours, but involves reflecting on, thinking about, and helping enact change in people's living environment to promote health. Second, a critical realist evaluation epistemology and its attendant demands in terms of citizen participation can itself be salutary through the empowerment process it offers. Health promotion defines itself as "the process of enabling people to increase control over, and to improve, their health" (WHO, 1986). Active engagement in change processes, such as the one we have described with *Levelling the Playing Fields*, may be just as health-producing for the individuals involved as for the children and citizens who will profit from the outcomes of the intervention.

References

Allin, L., West, A., & Curry, S. (2014). Mother and child constructions of risk in outdoor play. [Article]. *Leisure Studies, 33*(6), 644–657. https://doi.org/10.1080/02614367.2013.841746

Bhaskar, R. (2013). *A realist theory of science*. Routledge.

Brockman, R., Jago, R., & Fox, K. R. (2011). Children's active play: Self-reported motivators, barriers and facilitators. *BMC Public Health, 11*, 461. https://doi.org/10.1186/1471-2458-11-461

Byrne, D. (2013). Evaluating complex social interventions in a complex world. *Evaluation, 19*(3), 217–228.

Byrne, D., & Callaghan, G. (2014). *Complexity theory and the social sciences: The state of the art*. Routledge.

Byrne, D., & Uprichard, E. (2012). Useful complex causality. In H. Kincaid (Ed.), *The Oxford handbook of philosophy of social science* (pp. 109–129). Oxford University Press.

Clark, E., & Dumas, A. (2020). Children's active outdoor play:'Good'mothering and the organisation of children's free time. *Sociology of Health and Illness, 42*(6), 1229–1242.

Cortinez-O'Ryan, A., Albagli, A., Sadarangani, K. P., & Aguilar-Farias, N. (2017). Reclaiming streets for outdoor play: A process and impact evaluation of "Juega en tu Barrio" (play in your neighborhood), an intervention to increase physical activity and opportunities for play. *Plos One, 12*(7), e0180172–e0180172. https://doi.org/10.1371/journal.pone.0180172

Craig, P., Di Ruggiero, E., Frolich, K. L., Mykhalovskiy, E., White, M., & on behalf of the Canadian Institutes of Health Research (CIHR)–National Institute for Health Research (NIHR) Context Guidance Authors Group. (2018). *Taking account of context in population health intervention research: guidance for producers, users and funders of research*. NIHR Evaluation, Trials and Studies Coordinating Centre.

Crawford, S. B., Bennetts, S. K., Hackworth, N. J., Green, J., Graesser, H., Cooklin, A. R., et al. (2017). Worries, 'weirdos', neighborhoods and knowing people: A qualitative study with children and parents regarding children's independent mobility. *Health & Place, 45*, 131–139. https://doi.org/10.1016/j.healthplace.2017.03.005

D'Haese, S., Van Dyck, D., De Bourdeaudhuij, I., Deforche, B., & Cardon, G. (2015). Organizing "play streets" during school vacations can increase physical activity and decrease sedentary time in children. *International Journal of Behavioral Nutrition and Physical Activity, 12*(1), 14. https://doi.org/10.1186/s12966-015-0171-y

De Leeuw, E., & Simos, J. (2017). *Healthy cities: The theory, policy, and practice of value-based urban planning*. Springer.

Encarta. (1999). *Encarta world English dictionary*. Microsoft. Bloomsbury.

Francis, J., Martin, K., Wood, L., & Foster, S. (2017). 'I'll be driving you to school for the rest of your life': A qualitative study of parents' fear of stranger danger. *Journal of Environmental Psychology, 53*, 112–120. https://doi.org/10.1016/j.jenvp.2017.07.004

Frohlich, K. L., Corin, E., & Potvin, L. (2001). A theoretical proposal for the relationship between context and disease. *Sociology of Health and Illness, 23*(6), 776–797.

Hawe, P., Shiell, A., & Riley, T. (2009). Theorising interventions as events in systems. *American Journal of Community Psychology, 43*(3–4), 267–276.

Houston, S. (2010). Prising open the black box: Critical realism, action research and social work. *Qualitative Social Work, 9*(1), 73–91.

Lee, Y., Takenaka, K., & Kanosue, K. (2015). An understanding of Japanese children's perceptions of fun, barriers, and facilitators of active free play. *Journal of Child Health Care, 19*(3), 334–344. https://doi.org/10.1177/1367493513519294

Montreal Urban Ecology Center. (2015). *Participatory urban planning : Planning the city with and for its citizen*. Montreal Urban Ecology Center.

ParticipACTION. (2018). *Canadian kids need to move more to boost their brain health*. The ParticipACTION Report Card on Physical Activity for Children and Youth. ParticipACTION.

Pawson, R., & Tilley, N. (1997). *Realistic evaluation*. Sage.

Poland, B., Frohlich, K. L., & Cargo, M. (2008). Context as a fundamental dimension of health promotion program evaluation. In L. Potvin, D. D. McQueen, M. Hall, L. de Salazar, L. M. Anderson, & Z. M. A. Hartz (Eds.), *Health promotion evaluation practices in the Americas* (pp. 299–317). Springer.

Pynn, S. R., Neely, K. C., Ingstrup, M. S., Spence, J. C., Carson, V., Robinson, Z., et al. (2019). An intergenerational qualitative study of the good parenting ideal and active free play during middle childhood. *Children's Geographies, 17*(3), 266–277.

Ridge, T. (2011). The everyday costs of poverty in childhood: A review of qualitative research exploring the lives and experiences of low-income children in the UK. *Children and Society, 25*(1), 73–84.

Rigolon, A. (2016). A complex landscape of inequity in access to urban parks: A literature review. *Landscape and Urban Planning, 153*, 160–169.

Sayer, A. (2000). Key features of critical realism in practice: a brief outline. In A. Sayer (Ed.), *Realism and social science* (pp. 10–28). Sage.

Stame, N. (2004). Theory-based evaluation and types of complexity. *Evaluation, 10*(1), 58–76.

Valentine, G., & McKendrck, J. (1997). Children's outdoor play: Exploring parental concerns about children's safety and the changing nature of childhood. *Geoforum, 28*(2), 219–235.
WHO. (1986). *Ottawa charter for health promotion*. World Health Organization.
Winge, L., & Lamm, B. (2019). Making the red dot on the map-bringing children's perspectives to the city planning agenda through visible co-design actions in public spaces. *Cities & Health, 3*(1-2), 99–110.
Witten, K., Kearns, R., Carroll, P., Asiasiga, L., & Tava'e, N. (2013). New Zealand parents' understandings of the intergenerational decline in children's independent outdoor play and active travel. *Children's Geographies, 11*(2), 215–229.
Zieff, S. G., Chaudhuri, A., & Musselman, E. (2016). Creating neighborhood recreational space for youth and children in the urban environment: Play (ing in the) Streets in San Francisco. *Children and Youth Services Review, 70*, 95–101.

Chapter 33
Using Critical Theory to Research Commercial Determinants of Health: Health Impact Assessment of the Practices and Products of Transnational Corporations

Julia Anaf, Matt Fisher, and Fran Baum

33.1 Introduction

Health promotion, as defined by the WHO Ottawa Charter for Health Promotion (World Health Organization, 1986), is the process of enabling people to increase control over, and to improve, their health. This charter outlined key strategies for health promotion, such as creating supportive environments for health and building healthy public policy, with responsibilities going beyond the purview of the health sector. Therefore, health promotion research is important for devising effective health promotion and disease prevention policies and programmes that can contribute to healthy environments and support individuals to make healthier choices; thereby reducing their risk of disease and disability. Health promotion aims to have population-wide impact and identify ways to eliminate health inequities, improve quality of life and ensure the availability and quality of health care and related services.

Our research approach is informed by a Marxist critical theory interpretation which calls ideologies into question, maintains a focus on unequal power relations in society and seeks to understand and help mediate the social structures through which people are dominated and oppressed (Kincheloe & McLaren, 2000; Thompson, 2017). Researchers within a Marxist frame aim to go beyond describing a phenomenon to interrogate and challenge the powerful social structures that shape population health and generate health inequities (Ng & Muntaner, 2014). This fits well with the health promotion mandate to advocate for change to societal structures that affect health adversely.

J. Anaf (✉) · M. Fisher · F. Baum
Stretton Health Equity, Stretton Institute, University of Adelaide, Adelaide, South Australia
e-mail: Julia.anaf@adelaide.edu.au

L. Potvin, D. Jourdan (eds.), *Global Handbook of Health Promotion Research, Vol. 1*,
https://doi.org/10.1007/978-3-030-97212-7_33

Critical theory directs researchers 'upstream' to examine the social, economic and political structures which lead to health inequities (Bhaskar, 1979). Critical theory requires a focus on the political economy of health, a framework within which questions can be asked about the global economic order and the extent to which it prioritises private profit over public health considerations (Baum, 2005).

TNCs increasingly shape individual and population health by shaping the lived environment; directly through practices and products, and indirectly through policy influence. The impact of TNCs on public health is increasingly being assessed, (Baum & Anaf, 2015) and, as they are now recognised as commercial determinants of health (CDoH) (Kickbusch et al., 2016), regulating their activities is therefore an important task for health promotion and healthy public policy (Baum & Sanders, 2011).

The aim of this chapter is to discuss how we have applied a critical theory perspective as a framework to study the health and environmental harms of the practice and products of TNCs.

33.2 The Purpose of the Research Programme

The main purpose of our research programme has been to research the ways in which TNCs act as CDoH to affect population health and well-being. The main method we have used to achieve this has been to develop, test and apply a corporate health impact assessment (CHIA) framework. The framework was devised during a meeting in Bellagio, Italy, in 2015, funded by the Rockefeller Foundation, and attended by 19 representatives from academia, the corporate sector and civil society (Baum et al., 2016a, b). Recognising that a methodology had been lacking, this joint initiative focused on adapting health impact assessment (HIA) methodologies to better understand and assess corporate health impacts on different communities (Baum, 2011; Baum et al., 2016a, b).

This is an important area of research as, based on their size and influence, TNCs are recognised as the 'primary movers and shapers of the global economy' (Vercic, 2003, p. 177); with TNC revenues now surpassing those of many national governments. By 2018, of the world's top 100 economic revenue collectors, 71 were corporations and 29 were nation states (Oxfam, 2018). Thus, TNCs are able to use their economic position to wield increasing social, economic and political power in both the globalised market economy and within individual countries. Their products and practices have the potential to shape many social and environmental determinants of health such as (inter alia) income, employment conditions, social conditions, food and beverage environments, ecological health and climate change.

TNCs also influence the political and economic conditions that distribute social and economic advantages and disadvantages within and between countries, giving rise to health inequities (Commission on the Social Determinants of Health, 2008). TNCs are drivers of non-communicable diseases (NCDs) by influencing key risk factors such as diet, drug and alcohol use and tobacco smoking and environmental factors such as air pollution (Freudenberg, 2014). It is for these reasons that the corporate entity has been described as 'a distal, macro-level social structure that influences the health of the public' (Wiist, 2006, p. 7).

TNCs can contribute to health inequities if health effects resulting from their practices and products have disproportionate adverse impacts on socially or economically disadvantaged populations, or if they provide greater health benefits to already more advantaged groups (Baum et al., 2016a, b). While there is a large body of research on the health impacts of TNC-related products and practices, such as tobacco, alcohol, ultra-processed foods or pharmaceuticals (Grover et al., 2012), there has been limited research to investigate and assess the health impacts of individual TNCs (Baum et al., 2016a, b).

33.2.1 The Research Framework

We situate our research framework within a broad understanding of the structure of the global capitalist economy and the ways in which it supports the growth, operations and economic and political power of TNCs (Radice, 2014). TNCs act as CDoH, which have been defined as strategies and approaches used by the private sector to promote products and choices that are detrimental to health (Kickbusch et al., 2016; Mialon, 2020). We have extended this definition to include indirect ways by which TNCs can influence policy and government revenues, such as through lobbying, donations to political parties or taxation avoidance (Baum et al., 2016a, b).

Other terms include the 'commercial determinants of ill health'; the 'commercial drivers of ill-health'; the 'commercial determinants of non-communicable diseases' (NCDs); and the 'commercial drivers of NCDs' (Mialon, 2020). Having previously been under-researched, both TNCs and CDoH are now growing areas of research interest in public health (Kickbusch et al., 2016). We adapted HIA and applied a critical theory perspective and a social, economic and ecological view of health to create the CHIA framework.

Our framework adapts well-known HIA methods to the specific task of assessing the health impacts of individual TNCs (Harris et al., 2007). It draws on existing examples of retrospective HIAs to gain the best evidence of likely health impacts, rather than health outcomes (Australian Indigenous Doctors' Association and the Centre for Health Equity Training Research Evaluation University of New South Wales, 2010). HIA involves six stages:

1. Screening, to determine whether an HIA is appropriate or required
2. Scoping, to plan and design the HIA
3. Identifying a profile of a particular community or population likely to be affected by a proposal
4. Assessing, which synthesises and critically analyses the collected information in order to prioritise health impacts

5. Decision-making and recommending action on findings
6. Evaluation and follow-up (Harris et al., 2007).

Our health framing is social, economic and ecological, and we examine each category of impact in term of effects on social determinants of health equity. We also consider the global operating environment within which the TNC operates by examining how international, national or sub-national regulatory practices, or a TNC's corporate social responsibility practices, enable or constrain their health impacts (See Fig. 33.1: The CHIA Framework).

A: How do regulatory structures impact on TNC practices?		
Global/Regional: Regulatory environment; Political & economic environment; International institutions	National: Regulatory environmental; Political & economic environment; Status & capabilities of national government; Social & economic inequalities	Sub-national/Local: Regulatory environment; Regions or population groups especially affected by TNC

B: What are the TNC practices and products that impact on health & equity?		
Structure: Global and national operational structure and size of TNC; supply chain		
Political practices: Actions to influence: Global regulatory or political environment; National regulatory or political environment; Role of industry bodies; Taxation structures; Media	Business practices: Control over supply chain; Labour practices; Taxation payments/profit shifting; Use of litigation; Use of trade/investment treaties to influence national regulations	Products, distribution & marketing: Product types, trends, proportions; Export vs domestic sale; Marketing methods & strategies

C: What is the direct impact of TNC practices on the daily living conditions in countries?				
Workforce & work conditions Workforce; Wages; Health & safety; Living conditions	Social conditions Local goods & services; Local community life	Natural environment Ecological systems; Land, water, pollutants	Health related behaviours Food consumption; Cost of goods	Economic conditions Impacts on national or local economy; Public revenue; Local production systems
Assess potential health impacts from TNCs activities on: area of impact, type of impact (+ve, -ve), populations affected, size of impact, likelihood (if prospective), timing (urgency) is this fair or avoidable?				

D. Recommendations
Recommendations for legislation / policy / practice including who is responsible for taking action, the likelihood that action can be taken, timeframes for taking action

Fig. 33.1 Corporate Health Impact Assessment (CHIA) Framework: conceptual pathways of the health impacts of Transnational Corporations (TNCs) on population health. Reprinted from Anaf et al. (2019), Fig. 1. CC BY 4.0

33.2.2 Applying the CHIA Framework in Our Research

We have tested and applied the CHIA framework in research on: a fast-food TNC, McDonald's in Australia (Anaf et al., 2017); an extractives TNC, Rio Tinto, in Australia, South Africa and Namibia (Anaf et al., 2019); and an alcohol TNC, Carlton and United Breweries in Australia. Based on these studies, we believe that applying the framework across TNCs, industry sectors and/or national jurisdictions has significant potential to generate data for comparative analysis. This could include documenting: the differences in health impacts between TNCs operating in the same or different industry sectors; the different impacts of one TNC in different jurisdictions; and the regulatory structures between countries and resulting differences in TNC practices and health impacts.

33.3 Research Methods and Examples of How They Highlight TNCs' Policies and Practices

Our research methods are designed around the CHIA framework and informed by theory and evidence on social determinants of health and health equity. Our cases focused on both the TNC as a whole and on its operations in specific countries.

We mainly relied on qualitative methods which allow for rich descriptions and explanations of processes in identifiable local contexts (Miles & Huberman, 2009). We used documentary methods such as data from corporate literature; media items relating to the specific TNC and semi-structured interviews. These interviews enabled us to gain views from a wide range of civil society actors including from non-government organisations (NGOs) and trades union, as well as advocates and campaigners who challenged different aspects of the relevant TNC's activities. We have had no success in involving actors from TNCs (more details in the following section). Full details of our methods are available elsewhere (Anaf et al., 2017).

We have also used mixed methods to provide richer analyses. For example, to inform the McDonald's CHIA, we commissioned a spatial and socioeconomic analysis of McDonald's restaurants in Australia using Geographic Information System (GIS) technology which creates, analyses, and displays geographic data on digital maps. To test the findings of the McDonald's CHIA in the public arena, we also conducted research on the broader public's responses to the findings of our CHIA by holding a citizen's jury; one of several deliberative democracy processes that are promoted as ways to engage the public in policy decision-making, to manage community expectations and to increase commitment to public health policy (Street et al., 2014). This jury comprised 15 randomly selected and demographically representative citizens who, through a process of facilitated deliberation, addressed the question of what, if any, regulations should govern the fast-food industry in Australia.

In the Rio Tinto CHIA, we also undertook a comparative demographic analysis between a high-income country (Australia) and two medium-income countries (South Africa and Namibia) to contextualise our findings.

The CHIA on Carlton and United Breweries in Australia includes an epidemiological analysis of population trends in the chronic disease burden attributable to alcohol consumption in Australia. This also allowed us to estimate the disease impact of the particular TNC under assessment and so identify implications for health equity.

33.4 Some Key Findings from Our Research

33.4.1 McDonald's Australia

The spatial and socioeconomic analysis of McDonald's identified that there are approximately 1000 McDonald's outlets in Australia. These were slightly more likely to be located in areas of lower socioeconomic status, and the main consumer groups were children and young people. Therefore, use of this mixed method provided data which highlighted important equity implications that may not have been otherwise identified (Anaf et al., 2017).

Our deliberative democracy process elicited the important finding for policymakers that a majority recommended significantly stronger regulatory controls of major fast-food corporations than that currently practised by Australian governments (Anaf et al., 2018).

The CHIA also identified that McDonald's Australia's workforce conditions are bolstered by Australian employment regulations which include a minimum wage reviewed annually and guarantees a level of worker protection that remains unavailable in some other jurisdictions (Fair Work Commission, 2013). However, despite areas of relatively good performance, our assessments about the adverse health impacts of McDonald's products led us to conclude that the overall health impact of the TNC in Australia was likely to be negative.

33.4.2 Rio Tinto in Australia, South Africa and Namibia

The comparative analysis in this study recognised that, as a global TNC, Rio Tinto works in different socioeconomic contexts ranging from high-income and strongly democratic countries to those with much lower incomes and weaker democratic regimes.

Important regulatory implications were noted, as findings included significant differences between work, health and safety regulations in Australia and Southern Africa. Exact comparisons between jurisdictions are difficult due to factors including the type of mineral produced and the level of mechanisation, but we noted that workplace fatalities in South Africa's mining industry were four times higher than those in Australia. Our analysis also identified that Rio Tinto generally complied with what is needed to meet regulatory requirements in the countries in which it operates, but did not apply its highest corporate standards consistently across the different global jurisdictions.

Rio Tinto's health-related practices were generally of a lower standard in both South Africa and Namibia compared to Australia due to regulatory frameworks being limited, or not as well enforced or resourced, or because union support is weaker. The methodological approach we adopted in the Rio Tinto project therefore helped us to understand and report how differing regulatory frameworks across jurisdictions lead to different impacts on health and equity.

33.5 The Relationship with Industry Actors and Other Participants

We have found that conducting a CHIA may involve engaging with a range of industry, civil society, policy and other actors. While a senior TNC executive from a global food company attended our initial meeting, a key issue for the application of all three CHIAs has been the refusal of any TNC actors to engage in the research and offer corporate perspectives.

Industry representative organisations with TNC members are another potential source of business perspectives, but to date, all those approached have also declined to participate. Arguably, invitations to high-level consultative processes, such as the one held in Bellagio in 2015 (Baum et al., 2016a, b) may be a key to industry engagement.

TNC senior management across industry sectors may perceive public interest research, including CHIAs, as potentially antagonistic to their corporate interests, rather than as an opportunity to promote and defend their existing corporate values and practices such as corporate social responsibility programmes. While we had hoped to engage some industry co-operation, we were also mindful of the possible need to protect the independence of our research, in light of the demonstrated track record of TNCs or peak industry bodies using their power and resources to secure policy positions favourable to their commercial interests, and oppose changes seen to impinge on those interests, including those related to public health (Thorn, 2018). This point is discussed further below.

By contrast, a range of civil society actors have engaged in each of the CHIAs. Our research programme has included examination of the role civil society plays as a watchdog on the practices and products of TNCs that might threaten individual, community or environmental health. We have included civil society players in each of our CHIAs and written on their role in terms of CDoH (Anaf et al., 2020).

Civil society organisations (CSOs) take many forms, including legally constituted organisations, trades union and non-government organisations (NGOs), which operate across or within jurisdictions (Scott, 1981). Each of these types of CSO has been represented in our research, together with more informal groups of concerned citizens, advocates and activists. These actors generally organise around their shared goals to either achieve positive, or resist negative, change (Scott, 1981).

Activists who engaged in the Rio Tinto CHIA also had a range of major concerns. These included challenges to the growing incursion of coal mining into productive agricultural land in eastern Australia with devastating impacts on local communities (Fieldes, 2015). In matters of litigation between civil society activists and TNCs, the CHIA revealed that existing legal structures promote corporate mining interests ahead of the public interest (Anaf et al., 2020). The Rio Tinto CHIA also highlighted the viewpoint of unionists who were advocating for the best interests of workers in the extractives industry in respect of wages and conditions; including work, health and safety in the three countries which were the focus of our research (Industriall Union, 2014a). It revealed the demand by Rio Tinto for 'direct engagement' between management and the work force to limit the influence of third parties including unions (Anaf et al., 2020; Industriall Union, 2014b).

We also mapped data from our case studies on the fast food and the extractives sectors to consider the health impacts on civil society actors and others. We revealed the types of strategies that civil society organisations have adopted to encourage TNCs to act in more health-promoting ways; how effective they have been; and how TNCs have used their power to counteract civil society action. Strategies used by civil society actors included the use of online platforms and social media, and direct action such as street marches, public protests, including at corporate annual general meetings, and taking legal action. The respondents across both studies discussed the rewards and challenges they faced when trying to change TNCs' practices related to health; especially within the context of a neoliberal public policy environment.

By reflecting on the disparity between the willingness of actors from civil society and those from industry to engage in our research, we identified another possible strategy, which was to target current or former TNC employees. However, there is the potential for this approach to be open to criticism by TNCs, with respondents being framed as disgruntled former employees seeking revenge through reputational damage. Such framing is part of a much greater range of strategies engaged by TNCs in different contexts in order to weaken their critics (Freudenberg, 2014).

Regardless of research constraints due to non-engagement by industry, our experience and outputs suggest that assessment of a TNC's health impacts does not depend on participation by TNC or industry-representative staff. The dilemmas of involving TNC actors in research is discussed within a range of other challenges. This is a potential area for future research which is most likely to be effective when considering general regulatory issues rather than focusing on specific TNCs. Public servants engaged in areas of policy relevant to regulating TNCs are another possible group of research participants for a CHIA study. Our studies so far have not sought to engage with public servants extensively due to limited resources.

33.6 Specific Challenges

We identified a range of challenges associated with researching the health impacts of TNCs and for translating the findings. One is complexity due to frequent changes of ownership associated with business mergers, acquisitions and divestments. These are undertaken by TNCs to extend global market reach, to acquire funds or to facilitate strategic sales. For example, mergers are undertaken to potentially increase shareholder value and boost corporate efficiency. Over recent years, the Australian alcohol company, which is the focus of our latest CHIA, has undergone several ownership changes at both the level of the TNC parent body and the Australian company under acquisition (Boyd & Baird, 2019). These and other strategic partnerships among corporations often result in a higher degree of market concentration. This arguably offers corporations undue influence on the market, with commercial power often translating into political influence (Renner, 2000). Given the evidence on the health harms of excessive alcohol use (Collins & Lapsley, 2008; Freyer et al., 2016) a key issue for health equity and for health promotion is the rapid pace of consolidation of beer corporations and therefore their power. This has increased dramatically with the top 10 companies selling more than a quarter of the world's beer in 1980, scaling up to two-thirds of global beer sales by 2017 (Jernigan & Ross, 2020).

In respect of changes of corporate ownership, during the period of our Rio Tinto research within Australia, this TNC sold all its coal mining operations which were an important focus of our study (McPherson, 2017). This included gathering data from respondents who were some of the activists challenging Rio Tinto's coal mining operations. Other activists were representatives of the traditional custodians of the land being mined (ABC News, 2015). The sale reflected a mutually beneficial strategic ownership change of Australian coal assets between two global TNCs (Ong et al., 2017).

Constant corporate ownership changes in any industry sector makes it more difficult to undertake CHIAs; especially when seeking to map the business practices of a particular corporate owner, including their taxation strategies and related liabilities.

33.6.1 The Corporatisation of Universities and Funding Constraints

Another potential challenge for researching TNCs is the increasing corporatisation of universities; a business model which may result in universities not welcoming critical public health research on corporate entities including powerful TNCs. Despite enabling legislation that establishes Australian universities as public institutions with mainly non-commercial functions and goals, these institutions have been transformed over recent decades to largely mirror hierarchical corporate structures within the commercial sector (Pelizzon et al., 2020). Corporations increasingly fund research or research positions within universities and questions have been raised about how this might threaten research independence and integrity and create conflicts of interest (Jureidini & McHenry, 2020; Resnik & Shamoo, 2002). As the wider literature and our own research have revealed, collaborations between industry actors and the university sector create potential conflicts of interest (Bero, 2016; Anaf et al., 2019).

Other research constraints include the possible responses of grant reviewers and funders to university research proposals on CDoH. Our experience suggests that some of these individuals or organisations may criticise or reject such proposals because they perceive them as infeasible (due perhaps to anticipated lack of cooperation from TNCs) or as unlikely to make any difference. Such views may indicate that the actors involved disagree politically with our research aims. Feedback on our applications to national funding bodies have identified TNC's non-participation as a weakness. However, based on our own work, and much earlier wide-ranging research conducted on the world's largest corporation, Walmart, (Brunn, 2006), we query this judgement.

33.6.2 Lack of Engagement by TNC and Industry Actors in Research

As previously noted, another challenge is the refusals by TNC executives and other industry actors to engage in our research. These have been variously expressed by simply ignoring several requests; offering polite refusals; stating that participation cannot be granted 'at the moment'; or making the claim that it is not company 'policy' to engage in research. However, industry refusals have also included a response reflecting veiled hostility and arguable intent to intimidate researchers. For example, one email response refusing an invitation to participate included a statement which suggested a presumption of researcher bias, with this message being conveyed concurrently by email copy to our university's vice-chancellor. While we have not been aware of any pressure to adapt our research to date, and have previously received university funding towards our broader TNC research agenda, arguably this may be a troubling consideration for universities that receive significant corporate funding. Engaging TNC executives is just one example of a much greater challenge of attracting powerful elites as research participants (Harvey, 2015); with their refusal to participate arguably being another expression of corporate power.

33.6.3 *Policy Actors' Reluctance to Impose Comprehensive Regulations*

A further challenge is to research translation concerning the health impact of TNCs. This is due to the potential reluctance of policy actors to confront the full nature and scope of TNCs' health impacts, or to contemplate the kinds of regulatory measures that might be applied to TNC products or practices to reduce those impacts; knowing the kind of political response this is likely to draw from TNCs. In relation to TNC products such as food, tobacco and alcohol, policy actors can, and regularly do, prefer an alternative viewpoint; to view use and health impacts of these products as purely a matter of individual behavioural choices, to be tackled with social marketing campaigns exhorting individuals to adopt a healthier 'lifestyle' (Baum & Fisher, 2014). As Kingdon's Multiple Streams Framework helps us to understand, within the policy-making process the progress of 'problems' and corresponding policy options onto and *up* a government's action agenda will be shaped by decision makers' 'reading' of the political environment and any possible political consequences of such action (Kingdon, 2011).

33.7 The Benefits of CHIA Research

Despite these documented challenges, CHIA research is viable because publicly available corporate documents prove to be a rich source of data on financial value, employment levels, corporate sustainability initiatives and taxation. Civil society documents provide data, including evaluation of corporate social responsibility claims, and union and other campaigns. We also understand that senior corporate and other executives are often expected to speak on behalf of, or be the 'voice' of, the organisation. Researchers may therefore gain nothing more from an interview than could have been garnered from publicly available documents. As has been argued elsewhere, there is a big difference between researchers being offered a personal or candid assessment and 'being quoted the party line' (Welch et al., 2002). The LinkedIn business and employment-oriented online service used for professional networking may identify former employees of TNCs who are not subject to 'gag clauses' and may be prepared to be interviewed.

As researchers, another test is to find an interested audience for our findings. The level of interest is shown by 85 Google Scholar citations of our six TNC-related publications since 2015. We have also used personal, activist and academic networks to disseminate our findings. Fran Baum has had a long involvement with the People's Health Movement (PHM) (and is currently co-chair of the Global Steering Committee) and is able to feed the findings into the PHM's activism. As the UN Binding Treaty on Business and Human Rights is yet to be formally adopted, dissemination of research on the health impacts of TNCs will provide further evidence of the need for such a treaty. Importantly, the Guiding Principles apply to all States and to all business enterprises, both transnational and others, regardless of their size, sector, location, ownership and structure (United Nations Office of the High Commissioner for Human Rights, 2011).

Strategic use of social media platforms is another option we have adopted, including social journalism platforms (Baum et al., 2016a, b), those promoted by our university's own media and communication publicity (Flinders University News Desk, 2019) and radio programmes. The growing focus on CDoH in academia means there is increased interest in our research. Our research group has recently been designated as a WHO Collaborating Centre for the Social, Political and Commercial Determinants of Health (Flinders University, 2020), which signals an interest in the CDoH from the WHO.

The HIA method has therefore allowed us to examine TNCs' global business practices and their local health impacts in particular countries. With or without industry participation in research, TNCs' practices can ultimately be examined through a health and equity lens.

33.8 Conclusions

In the contemporary context of a global capitalist economy, actions by governments or civil society organisations to enable people to increase control over and to improve their health must include attention to the economic and political power, and health impacts of TNCs. The economic power and reach of TNCs means that their products and practices can affect the health of much of the world's population. It also places TNCs in a position where they can influence international agencies, trade agreements and national governments in their own interests. These have a distal effect on health where they prevent or weaken regulation in the public interest to protect public health and reduce health inequities. Furthermore, the adoption of neoliberal principles and practices by many governments can serve to position TNC interests high on their political agenda. However, the impacts of CDoH on population health also affect the rising costs of health care and create incentives for government action on prevention. We have seen governments and international agencies take action on the health impacts of the tobacco industry. To further promote health and prevent disease, this willingness to act needs to be extended into other sectors where TNCs are prominent such as food, alcohol, extractive and pharmaceutical.

It is vital that in the quest for health equity, researching CDoH becomes part of health promotion's research agenda. Our research helps to structure the field of health promotion research by acknowledging that the issue of CDoH is broader than individual TNCs and relates to the global economic and political system that supports their operations and unhealthy behaviours. As health promotion aims to have population-wide impact and identify ways to eliminate health inequities, a CHIA framework can contribute to analysing this environment and highlighting what regulatory measures are likely to be needed. Using this framework, we garnered evidence for socially oriented actors to strengthen their advocacy towards challenging negative health impacts, promoting health and equity and tackling CDoH (Anaf et al., 2020). Such critical analysis will provide information for governments who seek to regulate TNCs' activities in order to further public good.

References

ABC News. (2015). *Bulga Declaration protest in Sydney*. https://www.abc.net.au/news/2015-04-21/bulga-declaration-protest-in-sydney/6407906?nw=0. Accessed 22 Feb 2021.

Anaf, J., Baum, F., Fisher, M., Harris, E., & Friel, S. (2017). Assessing the health impact of transnational corporations: A case study on McDonald's Australia. *Globalization and Health, 13*(1), 7. https://doi.org/10.1186/s12992-016-0230-4

Anaf, J., Baum, F., & Fisher, M. (2018). A citizens' jury on regulation of McDonald's products and operations in Australia in response to a corporate health impact assessment. *Australian and New Zealand Journal of Public Health, 42*(2), 133–139. https://doi.org/10.1111/1753-6405.12769

Anaf, J., Baum, F., Fisher, M., & London, L. (2019). The health impacts of extractive industry transnational corporations: A study of Rio Tinto in Australia and Southern Africa. *Globalization and Health, 15*(1), 13. https://doi.org/10.1186/s12992-019-0453-2

Anaf, J., Baum, F., Fisher, M., & Friel, S. (2020). Civil society action against transnational corporations: Implications for health promotion. *Health Promotion International, 35*(4), 877–887. https://doi.org/10.1093/heapro/daz088

Australian Indigenous Doctors' Association and the Centre for Health Equity Training Research Evaluation University of New South Wales. (2010). *Health impact assessment of the northern territory emergency response*. Australian Indigenous Doctors' Association Canberra.

Baum, F. (2005). Wealth and health: The need for more strategic public health research. *Journal of Epidemiology and Community Health, 59*(7).

Baum, F. (2011). From Norm to Eric: Avoiding lifestyle drift in Australian health policy. *Australian and New Zealand Journal of Public Health, 35*(5), 405–406.

Baum, F., & Anaf, J. (2015). Transnational corporations and health: A research agenda. *International Journal Health Servay, 45*(2). https://doi.org/10.1177/0020731414568513

Baum, F., & Fisher, M. (2014). Why behavioural health promotion endures despite its failure to reduce health inequities. *Sociology of Health and Illness, 36*(2), 213–225.

Baum, F., & Sanders, D. (2011). Ottawa 25 years on: A more radical agenda for health equity is still required. *Health Promotion International, 26*(Suppl 2), ii253–ii257. https://doi.org/10.1093/heapro/dar078

Baum, F., Sanders, D., Fisher, M., & Anaf, J. (2016a). Assessing the health impact of transnational corporations: Its importance and a framework. *Globalization and Health, 12*(27). https://doi.org/10.1186/s12992-016-0164-x

Baum, F., Anaf, J., & Laris, P. (2016b). Big 4 accounting firms a poor prescription for health. *Croakey* (Vol. 2016).

Bero, L. (2016). *Essays on health: How food companies can sneak bias into scientific research*. https://theconversation.com/essays-on-health-how-food-companies-can-sneak-bias-into-scientific-research-65873. Accessed 22 Feb 2021.

Bhaskar, R. (1979). *The possibility of naturalism: A philosophical critique of the contemporary human sciences*. Harvester Press.

Boyd, T., & Baird, L. (2019). Asahi buys Carlton and United Breweries for $16b. In *The financial review*. Nine Entertainment.

Brunn, S. (2006). *Wal-Mart world: The world's biggest corporation in the global economy*. Taylor and Francis.

Collins, D. J., & Lapsley, H. M. (2008). *The costs of tobacco, alcohol and illicit drug abuse to Australian society in 2004/05: Summary version*. Australian Government, Department of Health and Ageing.

Commission on the Social Determinants of Health (2008). *Closing the gap in a generation: Health equity through action on the social determinants of health*. Final Report of the Commission on Social Determinants of Health. World Health Organisation.

Fair Work Commission. (2013). *McDonald's Australia Enterprise Agreement 2013* http://www.sda.org.au/download/enterprise-agreements/MCDONALDS-AUSTRALIA-ENTERPRISE-AGREEMENT-2013.pdf Accessed 23 Sept 2016.

Fieldes, D. (2015). Destroying a village to save... a coal mine. *Red Flag, 2020*.

Flinders University. (2020). *World Health Organization collaborating centre on social, political and commercial determinants of health equity*. https://www.flinders.edu.au/southgate-institute-health-society-equity/who-collaborating-centre. Accessed 11 Sept 2020.

Flinders University News Desk. (2019). *Tips for David vs Goliath protests*. Flinders University of South Australia.

Freudenberg, N. (2014). *Lethal but legal: Corporations, consumption, and protecting public health*. Oxford University Press.

Freyer, C., Morley, C., & Haber, P. (2016). Alcohol use disorders in Australia. *Internal Medicine Journal, 46*(11), 1259–1268. https://doi.org/10.1111/imj.13237

Grover, A., Citro, B., Mankad, M., & Lander, F. (2012). Pharmaceutical companies and global lack of access to medicines: Strengthening accountability under the right to health. *Journal of Law, Medicine and Ethics, 40*(2), 234–250.

Harris, P., Harris-Roxas, B., Harris, E., & Kemp, L. (2007). *Health impact assessment: A practical guide*. Centre for Health Equity Training, Research and Evaluation, UNSW.

Harvey, W. (2015). Strategies for conducting elite interviews. *Qualitative Research*. https://doi.org/10.1177/1468794111404329

Industriall Union. (2014a). *Rio Tinto the ugly truth* (7/10/2014 Ed.). Industriall Union.

Industriall Union. (2014b). *Unsustainable: The ugly truth about Rio Tinto*. Industriall Union.

Jernigan, D., & Ross, C. S. (2020). The alcohol marketing landscape: Alcohol industry size, structure, strategies, and public health responses. *Journal of Studies on Alcohol and Drugs, s19*, 13–25. https://doi.org/10.15288/jsads.2020.s19.13

Jureidini, J., & McHenry, L. (2020). *The illusion of evidence-based medicine*. Wakefield Press.

Kickbusch, I., Allen, L., & Franz, C. (2016). The commercial determinants of health. *The Lancet Global Health, 4*(12), e895–e896. https://doi.org/10.1016/S2214-109X(16)30217-0

Kincheloe, L., & McLaren, P. (2000). Rethinking critical theory and qualitative research. In H. Denzin & Y. Lincoln (Eds.), *Handbook of qualitative research* (2nd ed., pp. 279–313). Sage.

Kingdon, J. W. (2011). *Agendas, alternatives, and public policies*. Pearson Education.

McPherson, S. (2017). China's Yancoal snaps up Rio Tinto's NSW coal mines. *iseekplant.com.au* (Vol. 2020).

Mialon, M. (2020). An overview of the commercial determinants of health. *Globalization and Health, 16*(1), 74. https://doi.org/10.1186/s12992-020-00607-x

Miles, B., & Huberman, A. (2009). *Qualitative data analysis*. Sage.

Ng, E., & Muntaner, C. (2014). A critical approach to macrosocial determinants of population health: Engaging scientific realism and incorporating social conflict. *Current Epidemiology Reports, 1*, 27–37.

Ong, T., Farquar, L., & Connell, C. (2017). Rio Tinto agrees to sell Australian coal unit to China's Yancoal for $3.2b. *ABC News* (25/1/2017).

Oxfam. (2018). Of the world's top 100 economic revenue collectors, 29 are states, 71 are corporates. In *From poverty to power* (3/8/2018 ed.).

Pelizzon, A., Young, M., & Joannes-Boyau, R. (2020). 'Universities are not corporations': 600 Australian academics call for change to uni governance structures. *The Conversation*.

Radice, H. (2014). Transnational corporations and global capitalism: Reflections on the last 40 years. *Critical Perspectives on International Business, 10*(1/2), 21–34. https://doi.org/10.1108/cpoib-02-2013-0004

Renner, M. (2000). Corporate mergers skyrocket. In *Vital signs* (Vol. 2020). Worldwatch Institute.

Resnik, D., & Shamoo, A. (2002). Conflict of Interest and the University. *Accountability in Research, 9*(1), 45–64.

Scott, D. (1981). *Don't mourn for me-organise: The social and political uses of voluntary associations*. Allen & Unwin.

Street, J., Duszynski, K., Krawczyk, S., & Braunack-Mayer, A. (2014). The use of citizens' juries in health policy decision-making: A systematic review. *Social Science & Medicine, 109*, 1–9. https://doi.org/10.1016/j.socscimed.2014.03.005

Thompson, M. (2017). Introduction: What is critical theory? In M. Thompson (Ed.), *The Palgrave handbook of critical theory. Political philosophy and public purpose*. Palgrave Macmillan.

Thorn, M. (2018). Addressing power and politics through action on the commercial determinants of health. *Health Promotion Journal of Australia, 29*(3), 225–227. https://doi.org/10.1002/hpja.216

United Nations Office of the High Commissioner for Human Rights. (2011). *Guiding principles on business and human rights: Implementing the United Nations "protect, respect and remedy" framework*. United Nations.

Vercic, D. (2003). Public relations of movers and shakers: Transnational corporations. In K. Sriramesh & D. Vercic (Eds.), *The global public relations handbook: Theory, research and practice*. Lawrence Erlaum Association.

Welch, C., Marschan-Piekkari, R., Penttinen, H., & Tahvanainen, M. (2002). Corporate elites as informants in qualitative international business research. *International Business Review, 11*(5), 611–628. https://doi.org/10.1016/S0969-5931(02)00039-2

Wiist, W. (2006). Profits, payments, and protections. The anticorporate movement: Rationale and recommendations. *American Journal of Public Health, 96*, 1370–1375.

World Health Organisation. (1986). *The Ottawa charter for health promotion*. https://www.who.int/healthpromotion/conferences/previous/ottawa/en/. Accessed 25 Mar 2019.

Chapter 34
Knowledge Transfer: A Snapshot on Translation Processes from Research to Practices

Valérie Ivassenko, Ioanna Bakogianni, Jan Wollgast, Sandra Caldeira, Vanessa de Almeida, Keli Bahia Felicíssimo Zocratto, Conceição Aparecida Moreira, Daniela Souzalima Campos, Mirela Castro Santos Camargos, Eike Quilling, Maja Kuchler, Janna Leimann, Christina Plantz, Adamandia Xekalaki, Achilleas Attilakos, Alexia Prasouli, and Ioanna Antoniadou-Koumatou

34.1 Introduction

Valérie Ivassenko

As illustrated in the different chapters of this third part, the knowledge produced by research on the practices of decision makers and institutions aims to identify and analyse the political and institutional determinants of individuals' and population's health. This requires a study of how institutions and policymakers at local, regional, national or international levels establish and implement their practices and how these affect people's health. Because health promotion is both ethical and transformative in its aim to contribute to social change for the health of all, health promotion research cannot be limited to the production of knowledge. As the knowledge

Authorship is ordered by appearance of section in the chapter.

V. Ivassenko (✉)
UNESCO Chair and WHO Collaborating Center in Global Health & Education, Clermont-Auvergne University, Clermont-Ferrand, France
e-mail: valerie.ivassenko@uca.fr

I. Bakogianni (✉) · J. Wollgast · S. Caldeira
European Commission, DG Joint Research Centre (JRC), Directorate F – Health, Consumers and Reference Materials, Health in Society Unit, Ispra, VA, Italy
e-mail: Ioanna.BAKOGIANNI@ec.europa.eu

V. de Almeida (✉) · K. B. F. Zocratto · M. C. S. Camargos
Federal University of Minas Gerais, Belo Horizonte, Minas Gerias, Brazil
e-mail: vanessaalmeida@ufmg.br

L. Potvin, D. Jourdan (eds.), *Global Handbook of Health Promotion Research, Vol. 1*,
https://doi.org/10.1007/978-3-030-97212-7_34

produced intends to guide practices and policies, it is therefore crucial to be able to share and transfer this knowledge to the various actors/agents of these practices.

The following four snapshots illustrate different forms and possible responses to this critical issue for health promotion research, namely, knowledge transfer. Make clear, understandable, evidence-based and easily exploitable information available to decision makers working in public health and support policy choices in health promotion: this is the purpose of the "Health Promotion and Disease Prevention Knowledge Gateway" (first snapshot). The accessibility of scientific data is crucial in this field. But beyond making relevant data available, it is also a question of ensuring that actors can translate and use these data to inform and support their practice.

To guide and support political and institutional choices, analysing the design, implementation and evaluation of health policies also constitutes an important resource and a central object of research. Thus, the second snapshot presents the modalities and challenges of the implementation, monitoring and evaluation of health promotion policy in the 853 municipalities of the State of Minas Gerais in Brazil. Here again, it is essential to produce data that is transferable and usable by the main actors. Consequently, the definition of the data and the different indicators must consider both the priorities and purposes of the research itself and, above all, the needs of the various actors involved in implementing these policies. This means assessing the adaptability and relevance of the data produced according to local contexts in a necessarily participatory approach.

The collaborative dimension of health promotion research faces new challenges in projects with an international dimension, such as the European project presented by Eike Quilling. This project aims to support municipalities in the implementation of health promotion policies. Firstly, it seeks to identify the facilitating elements and obstacles to the implementation of measures to create health-promoting environments. Once identified, these elements are then translated and shared through the elaboration of European recommendations to guide and support the development of

C. A. Moreira · D. S. Campos
State Health Department, Belo Horizonte, Minas Gerias, Brazil

E. Quilling (✉) · M. Kuchler · J. Leimann
Department of Applied Health Sciences, Hochschule für Gesundheit, Bochum, Germany
e-mail: eike.quilling@hs-gesundheit.de

C. Plantz
Bundeszentrale für gesundheitliche Aufklärung, Federal Centre for Health Education, Cologne, Germany

A. Xekalaki (✉) · A. Prasouli · I. Antoniadou-Koumatou
Institute of Child Health, Athens, Greece

A. Attilakos
National and Kapodistrian University of Athens, Athens, Greece

Attikon Hospital, Haidari, Greece

these policies and practices at municipal level. The collective and collaborative dynamic is crucial in this generalisation work, which attempts to uncouple the data from their context and extract the universal and transferable aspects.

Finally, knowledge transfer can also take the form of very concrete tools, such as the health booklet distributed to all newborns. The process of producing such a tool in Greece (4th snapshot) illustrates multiple issues involved in such a project. It implies to bring together a large multidisciplinary group of actors to consider the different dimensions of child development, but also of defining and structuring the link between families and the primary care system. Both a guide and a support for monitoring and collecting information, a tool such as the health record thus concentrates political, health and educational functions and issues. It materialises the connection between policies, professionals and families around the child's development.

34.2 Streamlining Knowledge for Better Health Policies: The "Health Promotion and Disease Prevention Knowledge Gateway"

Ioanna Bakogianni, Jan Wollgast, and Sandra Caldeira

The Health Promotion and Disease Prevention Knowledge Gateway is an online resource, created for – and with – decision makers in EU Member States working in the area of public health. Its content reviews and summarises data and knowledge needed to justify investments in health promotion and make public health count in policy prioritisation. It focuses on non-communicable diseases (NCDs), their modifiable risk factors and prevention policies to address them.

Effective health promotion policies are of great importance in the effort to tackle major risk factors for NCDs, such as unhealthy diets, physical inactivity, alcohol and tobacco use. However, controversies on the evidence base, uncertainties, budget constraints and difficulties in balancing disparate interests are common challenges that can hamper public health-minded action by policymakers. To support them in making the case for public health, the European Commission created the Health Promotion and Disease Prevention Knowledge Gateway. The Knowledge Gateway streamlines the wealth of information on public health promotion to provide clear, evidence-based and authoritative information that is understandable and actionable for policymakers (that may well be non-experts in the topics described). While the Knowledge Gateway was created for policymakers, the information and policy recommendations found there (https://knowledge4policy.ec.europa.eu/healthpromotion-knowledge-gateway_en) are also used by academics and the public. We consistently receive positive feedback on its usefulness and the Gateway is among the tools that the European Commission provides its Member States in its efforts to promote public health. Member States use the Knowledge Gateway to inform their decisions in policymaking; as well as a resource of recommendations for the policies to be implemented.

The choice of the research questions included in the Knowledge Gateway is based on input from stakeholders and decision makers in EU Member States regarding their priorities for action in health promotion and non-communicable disease prevention. This is facilitated by the fact that the Gateway is led by two European Commission services, the Joint Research Centre (JRC) and DG Health and Food Safety. So far, the Gateway covers prevention of various non-communicable diseases, including cancer, cardiovascular disease and diabetes and the areas of nutrition, physical activity, alcohol, marketing of foods and beverages, mental health promotion as well as related societal impacts, such as disease burden and health inequalities.

The content is organised in concise, independent, yet inter-linked briefs. Each brief is structured in a similar manner; it includes a definition of each issue and describes its health-related effects, a summary of EU data and recommendations for best practices, actions, as well as examples of recommended and implemented policies that address the topics.

A structured review of authoritative literature selects and identifies reliable and solid sources of information that address specifically the questions in point. The Knowledge Gateway does not provide summaries or analyses of the *latest* peer-reviewed literature; the sources selection follows a tiered approach where pertinent reports and reviews authored or endorsed by authoritative public health-related, international organisations, governmental or supra-governmental bodies, scientific associations and public health professional associations are prioritised. In the absence of such sources, systematic literature reviews from medical and public health peer-reviewed journals are also analysed. This selection ensures that the content is evidence-based and of quality and that the information can be used immediately by policymakers to design and implement well-founded strategies and policies. Each brief is accompanied by a comprehensive bibliography with access to all original sources. The identification of national and EU-based surveys reporting representative data related to the prevalence of the diseases or their risk factors follows a similar approach.

The content created for the Knowledge Gateway is reviewed internally by the JRC, DG Health and Food Safety and/or other relevant European Commission services, and is externally peer-reviewed by renowned experts on the topics. The content is updated periodically and new Briefs are added regularly to reflect developments in the field and respond to the needs of EU policymakers.

The Knowledge Gateway strives for clear and understandable writing for both experts and non-experts and provides policymakers with a unique, trusted "one-stop-shop" where they can find high quality data to support, justify and strengthen the development of policies that underlie health promotion in all its facets.

34.3 A Five-step Process Implementation Evaluation of the State Health Promotion Policy (POEPS) of Minas Gerais, Brazil

Vanessa de Almeida Guerra, Keli Bahia Felicíssimo Zocrato, Conceição Aparecida Moreira, Daniela Souzalima Campos, and Mirela Castro Santos Camargos

This presents the evaluation process of the implementation of the State Health Promotion Policy (SHPP), a recent (2016) and relevant policy in Minas Gerais, the first state in Brazil to institute such policy. The aim was to demonstrate how the policy implementation was developed in the 853 municipalities of Minas Gerais, to subsidize its reorganisation.

Brazil is divided into 26 states and a Federal District, where the capital, Brasília, is located for a total of 27 federal units. Considering the territorial dimensions of the country and the adoption of a universal health system, each federal unit has the responsibility to adapt health policies to their own local reality, supporting the implementation process. Specifically, regarding the SHPP, a routine monitoring and evaluation of health promotion actions is instituted. Federal funding for the implementation of the SHPP is a function of achieving set health indicators

The state of Minas Gerais is divided into 28 Regional Health Units, which allow the principles of regionalisation and decentralisation of the Brazilian National Health System to be implemented. In each Superintendency, there are professionals who accompany and support municipalities in structuring health policies and, among them, health promotion. The study was carried out with the help of the state administration, a health promotion professional resource from each of the state's Regional Health Units and 360 health promotion professionals from the 852 municipalities that joined the State Health Promotion Policy.

This evaluation project was carried out following the cycle of public policy which understands the political process as something dynamic, organised in time and composed of well-defined stages. This allowed aligning knowledge development with the dynamism of the policy implementation process (Dalfior et al., 2015). The implementation, one of the phases of this cycle, is a result of government decision making. It is the phase in which concrete results of public policy are produced (Secchi, 2013). Our implementation evaluation comprised five stages.

The first stage was to collect relevant information through documentary research, based on the documents that instituted the SHPP. The second stage was to develop the policy's logic model and to create an analysis and judgement matrix, two key analytical tools for organising the data and analysing the results while taking into account the context in which the policy was implemented. Meetings were held with the policy state management personnel, to create the logic model, and collect data about the mechanisms involved in the operationalisation of the SHPP at the municipal level. It was possible to visualise the relationships between intervention, implementation and expected results, and it was possible to verify whether there was consistency between the objectives set out in the policy and the design adopted to meet them.

The same strategy was adopted for the preparation of the analysis and judgement matrix, with the participation of representatives from the 28 Regional Health Units in order to value regional diversities and as a way of ensuring that the process happened in a participatory manner, favouring dialogue.

The analysis and judgement matrix mirrored the logic model and comprised criteria and indicators, selected by participants involved. Indicators were selected and defined in three steps: (1) a list of possible indicators was created through face-to-face interviews and translated into a questionnaire; (2) the questionnaire was administered online to 28 participants from the Regional Health Units to filter the relevant indicators, to organise the indicators excluding those considered less relevant, and to list the evaluation criteria for each indicator and (3) the analysis and judgement matrix was formed by dimensions, with their respective sub-dimensions, indicators and criteria, which were valued according to debriefing with participant health promotion professionals. These indicators were used in the collection of primary data.

The third stage was the elaboration of a structured and self-administered questionnaire to collect primary data. The questionnaire was conceived in sections formed by three dimensions of the policy implementation process: (1) structure (human resources, input and administrative management); (2) processes (permanent education, information management, execution of actions and management) and (3) results (resolution by goals). The definition of dimensions originated from the operational strategies provided by the SHPP, to guide implementation in each federal unit. These include: territorialisation, intra- and inter-sectoral articulation, articulation with health care networks, social participation, management, permanent education and communication.

The fourth stage consists in the online data collection with the municipalities, through a representative sample, by population size, proportionally among the 28 Regional Health Units. Secondary data related to the results achieved by the municipalities in the indicators associated with the SHPP were also collected using the State Health Resolutions Management System (SiG-RES). The fifth and final stage comprised the analysis of the data according to the dimensions of structure, processes and results. The assessment of the level of implementation was based on a scoring system accounting for the three dimensions.

The implementation analysis made it possible to describe the path taken in the implementation of the SHPP across Minas Gerais. It allowed the identification of strengths and weaknesses in the implementation process and pointed to areas of supporting interventions. The results obtained contributed to the state management, monitoring and evaluation strategies to enhance the implementation of the SHPP. Results also allowed the academic environment to produce scientific knowledge on health promotion.

The regional health promotion units have been strongly involved in the SHPP since its conception, as well as in assisting in monitoring actions. Professionals in these units were key to the implementation evaluation. They participated in the selection of the relevant indicators for the implementation of the policy based on their experience and observations, in addition to assisting in the mobilisation of key municipal informants to answer the questionnaire.

34.4 Collaborative Health Promotion Research in Europe – Experiences and Relevance for Health Promotion at the Municipal Level

Eike Quilling, Maja Kuchler, Janna Leimann, and Christina Plantz

Within the framework of an EU-wide research project on the objective of promoting healthy living, it was investigated which measures for creating healthy living environments are implemented in the municipal context in the participating European countries.

The creation of healthy living environments is a central approach of health promotion. The research identified facilitating factors and obstacles in the implementation of the health promotion measures and identified which support the local actors may need.

The resulting expertise is incorporated into international recommendations for policy and practice in health promotion, which are published as the result of the EU project with the aim of supporting the creation of healthy living environments. The project accompanies thirteen European countries in the implementation process of self-selected health promotion measures in the municipal setting – and thus offers an increase in knowledge with regard to the generalisability of success factors as well as the use of models and quality criteria. The methodological design of the research is divided into several sequential steps. The participating partners and actors are involved in the process in different ways, in line with the overall collaborative research approach.

Methods

At the beginning of the project, a common conceptual working paper was developed as a basis for the whole process (Quilling et al., 2020). This created a consistent understanding of central topics and terminology of municipal health promotion among all participants. This was developed by a team of experts based on current scientific knowledge and with the participation of all project partners. It formed a joint starting point for the implementation for all parties involved. As one of the first steps of the research process, the research group conducted a rapid review on recommendations for the creation of healthy living environments in the municipal context via a systematic online literature search, which provides an insight into experiences from already implemented international practice projects. In addition, guideline-based expert interviews were conducted with the project partners to gain deeper insight into the methodological and strategic approach of planning and implementing measures. A special focus was placed on goals, obstacles and success factors. The results of the rapid review, together with the aspects generated in the interviews, served as a basis for the formation of initial theses on the topic, which were discussed and concretised in preparation for a Delphi study in an online workshop with the project partners. The two-stage Delphi study aims to build consensus among the participating European actors and their cooperation partners on the generated theses and to produce data on knowledge production process.

Lessons Learned

The collaborative way of working enabled a very productive and promising overall process as well as the generation of practice-relevant results. Even though the comparability of the results seems to be limited at first glance due to the different health systems and structures in the participating thirteen countries, the practical work with the actors showed that the challenges in municipal health promotion are very similar and that they benefit from international exchange of experiences. The common goal as well as the consideration of the wishes and experiences of the participants, which was practiced from the beginning, led to great interest in the project. Networking between the countries was encouraged from the beginning. As a result, the countries were able to learn from each other's experiences already during the process. In some cases, the countries implemented measures that had already been successfully implemented by partner countries. The participatory research of a practice project that was independent in itself brought challenges: contact with the actors involved mainly took place through the management of the accompanied project. Visibility of the research team through participation in meetings and regular, transparent communication of their results and next steps proved beneficial. The flexible design of the research steps promoted international cooperation with various partners and enabled the project to be implemented almost according to plan despite the Covid-19 pandemic. This was mainly due to constant dialogue about current developments and corresponding adjustments, especially in terms of deadlines, as well as a switch to online formats. Another key lesson learned is that the constant identification of opportunities for participation and motivation is essential for such a collaborative project.

Conclusion

This research intends to contribute to making specific challenges and proposed solutions visible for establishing more health equity through health-promoting environments. Each step, both of the project and of the accompanied partner countries, pursues the goal of health promotion and is in turn designed to be participatory. The generated results should serve as recommendations for the creation and implementation of healthy living environments in different countries within Europe, but also beyond the borders of Europe. In addition, they should be understood as a starting point for improving health equity, which can be relevant across projects for all actors with an interface to municipal health promotion.

34.5 Producing and Sharing Knowledge: A Collaborative Work to Produce the New Greek Child Health Booklet

Adamandia Xekalaki, Achilleas Attilakos, Alexia Prasouli, and Ioanna Antoniadou-Koumatou

Introduction

The regular follow-up of children's health and development and support of their parents with their upbringing are an essential element of children's Primary Health

Care (PHC), (Hagan et al., 2008; Hall et al., 2009). Supporting parents and all those involved in the education of children in the development of health capacities is a major public health objective. Among the tools that could be used, the Child Health Booklet (CHB), the health record booklet given to parents of every newborn, is a valuable tool in PHC focusing on regular follow-up of children's health and development, health education and support of parents. In 2016, the task of reforming the CHB was assigned by the Greek Ministry of Health to the Department of Social and Developmental Pediatrics of the Institute of Child Health (ICH), a public research institute.

The aim was to reform the CHB integrating primary care evidence-based guidelines and providing a tool to health professionals and families with an emphasis on prevention, early detection, treatment and promotion of health and well-being of children.

Methods Used

An extended group of specialists, members of the university community, the primary health care sector and the ICH were convened to produce guidelines for PHC practitioners. The group consisted of paediatricians, child's development and mental health experts, an ophthalmologist, an otolaryngologist, a dentist, an endocrinologist and epidemiologists. An extensive review of the literature and practices in selected other countries was carried out. The multidisciplinary approach resulted in producing national guidelines for PHC professionals. The guidelines included health assessment, developmental surveillance and anticipatory guidance. Ages that are appropriate to evaluate the health, development and care needs of the child and family and directions given on the content of the examination at those ages, were specified. Also, recommendations for comprehensive or selective screening in the literature were studied, along with the local health resources and infrastructure to make the necessary adaptations. The American Academy of Pediatrics grading system was used for screening recommendations (American Academy of Pediatrics, 2004). The statement describes three sequential activities in developing evidence-based guidelines: (1) determination of the aggregate evidence quality in support of a proposed recommendation; (2) evaluation of the anticipated balance between benefits and drawbacks when the recommendation is carried out and (3) designation of recommendation strength. The project of developing the guidelines was funded by the European Structural and Investment Funds, in 2014.

The new CHB integrates the primary care evidence-based guidelines, focusing on regular follow-up of children's health and development, health education and support of parents. Since significant changes in the content have been introduced, we are planning to evaluate its implementation.

Fifteen specific ages were recommended and were included in the new CHB for scheduled visits: six ages in infancy (1–2 weeks, 2, 4, 6, 9 and 12–15 months), four ages in toddler and pre-school age (18 months, 2–2.5, 4 and 5–6 years), two in school age (7–8 and 9 years) and three in adolescence (11–12, 14–15 and 17–18 years). In each age, essential elements of physical examination and developmental/behavioural monitoring and anticipatory guidance were proposed. Recommendations for comprehensive or selective screening were made about hearing, vision, congenital heart defects in newborns, developmental dysplasia of the hip, iron deficiency anaemia, dyslipidaemia, chlamydia infections, and risk for sudden death in young athletes. WHO child growth standards and WHO references growth charts were adopted. Written instructions were sent to PHC practitioners by e-mails and seminars were conducted nationwide for optimal use.

The guidelines for PHC practitioners and the new CHB have been approved by the Central Health Council (2017).

Conclusions

The project contributes to advancing health promotion research, because it embraces holistic care and multidisciplinary teamwork and promotes changes in practices and values in the Greek health system. That was a valuable experience since the health system is medical-centred, with medical doctors having minimum experience of collaborating with other primary care workers and vice versa. In addition, it provides specific recommendations regarding the systematic follow-up of children's health and development (ages, screening, growth standards), thus permitting evidence-based paediatric primary care practices and epidemiological comparisons over time.

The new CHB provides an important tool in PHC in terms that an evidence-based practice model is suggested which ensures uniform principles for the systematic follow-up of children's health and development.

References

American Academy of Pediatrics, Steering Committee on Quality Improvement and Management. (2004). Classifying recommendations for clinical practice guidelines. *Pediatrics, 114*, 874–877.

Dalfior, E. T. et al. (2015). *Reflections on implementation analysis of health policies*. Saúde em Debate. Rio de Janeiro (Vol. 39, Issue 104) (pp. 210–225). http://www.scielo.br/pdf/sdeb/v39n104/0103-1104-sdeb-39-104-00210.pdf. Accessed 17 Jan 2018.

Hagan, J. F., et al. (2008). *Bright Futures: Guidelines for health supervision of infants, children, and adolescents* (3rd ed.). American Academy of Pediatrics.

Hall, D., et al. (2009). *The child surveillance handbook*. Radcliffe Publishing.

MINAS GERAIS. (2016). Secretaria de Estado de Saúde de Minas Gerais – SES-MG. Resolução SES/MG n° 5.250, de 19 de abril de 2016. Institui a Política Estadual de Promoção da Saúde no âmbito do Estado de Minas Gerais e as estratégias para sua implementação. https://www.saude.mg.gov.br/images/documentos/Resolu%c3%a7%c3%a3o_5250.pdf. Accessed 19 Sept 2020.

Quilling, E., Babitsch, B., Dadaczynski, K., Kruse, S., Kuchler, M., Köckler, H., Leimann, J., Walter, U., & Plantz, C. (2020). Municipal health promotion as part of urban health: A policy framework for action. *Sustainability, 12*(16), 6685.

Secchi, L. (2013). *Políticas públicas: conceitos, esquemas de análise, casos práticos* (2. ed.).

Part IV
Researching the Practices of Researchers and Innovators

Chapter 35
From the Production to the Use of Scientific Knowledge: A Continuous Dialogue Between Researchers, Knowledge Mobilization Specialists, and Users

Angèle Bilodeau, Marie-Pier St-Louis, Alain Meunier, Catherine Chabot, and Louise Potvin

35.1 Introduction

A significant part of health promotion science is built through systematic observation of practice, informed by relevant theories often drawn from the humanities and social sciences. Conversely, practice strengthens through collective reflexivity and the mobilization and integration of scientific knowledge (Potvin et al., 2008; Potvin & McQueen, 2007). Therefore, the interdependence of expert and practical knowledge, and knowledge sharing between researchers and practitioners, are inherent in, and distinctive of, health promotion. This implies for health promotion research to adopt a continuous and dialogical research–practice posture. Such a dialogical posture becomes essential in other fields of applied research, giving rise to a growing field of practice and expertise, that of knowledge mobilization.

Knowledge mobilization emerged in the 1990s under the term knowledge transfer, mainly using a top-down approach, and has since evolved into an interactive approach. Current definitions characterize this process as knowledge exchange

A. Bilodeau (✉)
School of Public Health, University of Montreal, Montréal, QC, Canada
e-mail: angele.bilodeau@umontreal.ca

M.-P. St-Louis · C. Chabot
Canada Research Chair in Community Approaches and Health Inequalities, School of Public Health, University of Montreal, Montréal, QC, Canada

A. Meunier
Communagir, Montréal, QC, Canada

L. Potvin
School of Public Health, University of Montreal, Montréal, QC, Canada

Centre de recherche en santé publique (CReSP), Université of Montreal and CIUSSS du Centre-Sud-de-l'Île-de-Montréal, Montréal, QC, Canada

L. Potvin, D. Jourdan (eds.), *Global Handbook of Health Promotion Research, Vol. 1*,
https://doi.org/10.1007/978-3-030-97212-7_35

between researchers, decision-makers, practitioners, and other stakeholders as well as its translation into action (Hot et al., 2017; Jones et al., 2015; Mitton et al., 2007; SSHRC, 2019). Since the 2000s, the term knowledge translation has spread beyond Canada, where it emerged and was promoted to represent the knowledge-to-action process (Graham et al., 2006; Miranda et al., 2020; Thirsk, 2018). This dynamic, iterative process includes a wide range of practices such as knowledge synthesis, dissemination, exchange, and application into action, which often involve sustained interactions and reciprocity between knowledge producers and users (CIHR, 2015). The complexity implementing these practices is linked to the diversity of research paradigms and their compatibility with knowledge translation, the need for selecting and adapting knowledge translation to contexts and audiences, and the necessary reciprocity between knowledge producers and users (Armstrong et al., 2007; Dagenais & Mc Sween-Cadieux, 2020; Graham et al., 2006; Mitton et al., 2007). Three main strategies characterize knowledge translation: (1) synthesis, dissemination, and exchange of scientific results in forms suitable to specific audiences (e.g. summaries, stakeholder briefings, educational sessions, and workshops); (2) appropriation and therefore translation of scientific knowledge into practical knowledge and know-how (e.g. practice guides, knowledge brokers, web-based services, tools); and (3) putting knowledge into action (e.g. technical assistance and staff training, auditing and feedback, community of practice) (Armstrong et al., 2007; CIHR, 2015; Hot et al., 2017; SSHRC, 2019). It is generally recognized that these strategies are fostered by a long-term, reciprocal, sustained research–practice relationship reinforced by fair and effective governance (Campbell et al., 2019; Hot et al., 2017; La Rocca et al., 2012; Mitton et al., 2007).

Developing the field of health promotion research which would integrate knowledge mobilization requires research practices that meet the challenges of the dialogical approach of knowledge mobilization and a theory-driven reflection on the know-how to translate knowledge into health promotion (Armstrong et al., 2006; Laurent et al., 2019; Miranda et al., 2020). To this end, this chapter takes a close, reflexive look at the integrated knowledge production and translation processes in our 10-year research program on intersectoral action conducted collaboratively with practice settings. The chapter begins by addressing the research posture and partnership established to conduct the research. The centrepiece of the chapter is a detailed description of the dialogical process between researchers, knowledge mobilization specialists and users in the production of the instruments for knowledge exchange and translation, based on an extensive review of the research program's archives. Then it analyses this process with the lens of the actor–network theory (ANT) which sheds light, inter alia, on the relationship between innovators and designers of technical devices and their users (Akhich et al., 2006; Callon, 1986, 1989; Callon & Latour, 1986, 2012; Latour, 2005).

35.2 Context: A Research and Knowledge Translation Programme on Local Intersectoral Action

Since the 1980s, intersectoral action has emerged as a public-action strategy to deal with the complexity of societal problems. This involves actors from various sectors (education, health, transportation, etc.) and spheres of society (institutions, private enterprises, community organizations, philanthropy) crossing the boundaries of sectors to develop better coordinated or integrated interventions (public policies, programs, initiatives, etc.) (Chircop et al., 2015; Divay et al., 2013; Ferlie et al., 2011). This strategy is widely promoted and used in health promotion. The purpose of our research program was to link the processes implemented by the intersectoral neighbourhood committees in Montreal's boroughs to observable transformations in the living environments. We conducted a series of case studies based on ethnographic methods informed by ANT (Latour, 2005).

The research partnership has been developed according to an approach of "organized reflexivity", whereby participating neighbourhood committees are conceived of as action systems independent of the research system (Potvin & Bisset, 2008). Each system has its own network of actors, processes, instruments, rationality, and objectives (Lefebvre et al., 2016). Research–practice collaboration is shaped in a negotiation space in which the action system is an active, reflexive subject interacting with the research system that observes it. Subjects in this negotiation space include the selection of cases studied, the feasibility of data collection methods, data completion, validation and interpretation of the results, mobilization of the knowledge produced and discussions that contribute to the collective reflexivity. Our research posture adopts the ANT perspective that social actors have, first and foremost, knowledge of themselves, who the other actors are, their social relationships, what they do, and the context in which their actions take place (Callon & Latour, 2012). Social actors construct their representation of reality, what is happening, and the course of events. The researchers' position is to approach practitioners as actors in the research system in that they actively contribute to the construction of the knowledge that the research develops about their practice. The researchers' job is to produce an interpretation of who the practitioners are and what they do in terms of the theory, based on an explicit theoretical referent and the data derived from their observations and provided by informants. The added value of this work is to put forward a theoretically informed perspective of the system of action under study, to draw generic knowledge out of singular realities, to increase generality by generating middle-range theories about local intersectoral action. Then, by submitting this reading of their reality and practice to actors from the field, we can translate theory and experience into an instrumentation that is both contextualized because it is anchored in empirical observations and generalizable through its derivation from a broader theory of action (ANT). This research approach means that testing the validity of research results first requires convincing the actors in the field and, in particular, key informants (Callon & Latour, 2012).

The analysis of local intersectoral action systems using ANT has led to a generic model of the production of the effects of local intersectoral action in living environments (ex. solidarity food market, cycle path). This model shows that local intersectoral networks work by chaining a finite series of typical actions, called transitional outcomes (TOs), which punctuate the progression of the action to its effects. A repertoire of 12 generic TOs was identified and validated. These 12 TOs relate to three key functions of networks: (i) network setup and governance; (ii) self-representing and influencing others; (iii) aligning necessary actors and resources. These TOs are linked in different ways by neighbourhood committees depending on the context and their objectives (Bilodeau et al., 2019).

This knowledge was first shared with research partners and then more broadly with decision makers and practitioners in the field. Since non-researchers do not perform the systematic work of data gathering and analysis from several sites that are performed by researchers, they were first intrigued by this research-generated knowledge about them. They also found that the results made sense for reflecting on their practice and that it could be useful to them. In their view, the research results represent their achievements in a clear way and make it easier to understand and justify the existence and work of the neighbourhood committees. These results also have the potential to support collective reflexivity in order to improve practices. This meets the need for research partners to be equipped with tools for reflexivity and evaluation purposes. However, as they were, these results appear difficult to apply and would require some instrumentation.

35.3 Instruments of Knowledge Exchange and Translation into Action

35.3.1 Knowledge Exchange

With regard to synthesis, dissemination, and knowledge exchange, various products were developed for a range of audiences. Articles have been published in the scientific literature (Bilodeau & Potvin, 2018; Bilodeau et al., 2019; Potvin & Aumaître, 2010; Potvin & Clavier, 2012, 2013). Presentations were given in major scientific and professional conferences where research partners were actively engaged in the preparation and delivery at two of them. In addition, posters have been presented on the research results in each case at these conferences. Subsequently, these posters have been used locally by the neighbourhood committees. These presentations and publications have established the scientific credibility of the knowledge produced which was to be mobilized in practice settings. Concurrently, monographs were published on each case as well as a synthesis aimed at practitioners and decision makers (Bilodeau et al., 2018, 2020). In addition, presentations and training sessions have been organized for specific audiences (decision makers, managers, and practitioners) to reach a wide range of practice settings. All these productions are listed in Appendix.

Although there is a great deal of interest in these results in the practice settings, the actors are not in a position to use them autonomously. The actors expressed interest in having an interactive tool based on research results that would allow them to document their own processes and effects and report on them to third parties, such as in their activity reports. Then research partners embarked with the researchers on the production of an interactive, online tool to make it possible for local authority actors to use the research results.

35.3.2 Practical Knowledge and Know-How

In terms of translating scientific knowledge into practical knowledge, interpersonal skills, and know-how, the online platform *Outil d'appréciation des effets de l'action intersectorielle locale* (https://chairecacis-outilinteractif.org/) and its English version *Tool for Assessing the Effects of Local Intersectoral Action* (https://chairecacis-outilinteractif.org/en) have been produced in close collaboration with practice settings.

35.3.2.1 Production of the Tool

The *Tool* was produced according to a rigorous participatory process and validated with target users. The steering committee created for this project brought together the necessary expertise: two professionals experienced in knowledge mobilization whose role was to plan and coordinate the project, design and carry out the *Tool*'s various production activities, and oversee its deployment; an advisor with Communagir (a Quebec non-profit organization who provides consultant services in community development) whose role was to provide expertise in the various production phases of the *Tool* and support its deployment; and the principal investigator for the research, whose role was to ensure the correspondence between the *Tool* and the knowledge produced by the research.

Translating research results into a user-friendly tool for field practitioners was more complex than expected. Unlike a "black box"-type device that encapsulates knowledge without the user having to understand and master it, practitioners leading intersectoral actions must collectively master several tasks in order to benefit from the research results. They need to: (1) tell the story of their project by highlighting its milestones, i.e. those through which the progression of their action towards the observed effects was achieved, and situate them in time; (2) grasp the meaning of the modelling concepts (in this case, the repertoire of 12 generic transitional outcomes with which to plot the progression of the action towards its effects); (3) interpret singular events on their project timeline in terms of transitional outcomes; and (4) model the chain of key events/transitional outcomes of their project and learn from it. To achieve this goal, the steering committee implemented a three-phase procedure (from October 2016 to October 2019), enlisting at each phase the practical expertise of intersectoral action practitioners.

The first phase consisted of defining the desired characteristics of the *Tool*. To achieve this, four design-workshops were held with a total of 57 participants. These workshops validated the need for a tool and clarified its uses: retrospective (portrait, assessment, accountability process); prospective (action planning); and formative (collective reflection, training; explanation of the consensus-building process). These workshops also established the desired characteristics of the *Tool*: user-friendliness; easy to integrate into practice; a tool that guides the practitioner in its use; and in the form of a dashboard-style action-tracking tool. In addition, an inventory of existing tools and guides that could inspire the steering committee was produced.

The second phase was to design and experiment the prototype of the *Tool*. Based on phase 1, it was determined that the *Tool* would consist of three modules. Module 1—*Taking Ownership of the Foundations of the Tool*— is a self-supporting online training that presents the *ANT concepts mobilized in the Tool and the repertoire of transitional outcomes*. Module 2—*Mapping the Key Events of a Project and Translating them into a Chain of Transitional Outcomes*—contains a facilitator guide for holding a workshop in which participants using the tools included in this module will start modelling their project. Module 3—*Diagramming a Project's Chain of Transitional Outcomes, Culling Out What Has Been Learned, and Integrate Learnings Into Action*—includes a timeline for consolidating the chain of significant events and transitional outcomes, a modelling tool, and a feedback grid. Module 2, the centrepiece of the *Tool*, was produced first. Three laboratory workshops on facilitating the workshop on using the *Tool* were held with three intersectoral bodies that did not participate in the research. The first prototype of the facilitator guide was tested and then improved after each workshop to produce the final version.

The intersectoral bodies that tried out the guide concluded that the session allowed them to take their thinking further, compared to other forms of facilitation already used to produce their project's story. The added value lies in the use of more general concepts (the transitional outcomes) to interpret the events of a project. This led the participants to focus on the actions that made possible significant progress in their project and to deepen their reflection on the meaning and scope of the events by not limiting themselves to the mere sequence of actions in the project's story. The role of the facilitator then appeared to be critical in order to take advantage of the session. The facilitator must be a neutral person from outside the project with experience in intersectoral action and facilitation. The person must be totally dedicated to the facilitation process. Beforehand, the facilitator must familiarize himself or herself with the three modules of the *Tool* and the project's story in order to guide participants. Lastly, participants should be familiar with Module 1, which deals with the basics of the *Tool*.

The third phase was the production of a final version of the *Tool* and its publication online. Based on the previous experience, Module 2 was produced using graphic design to make it user-friendly. Then, Module 1 on theoretical notions was created with PREZI presentation software to make it attractive and efficient. Audio clips in everyday language were produced to explain ANT concepts and to illustrate the 12 transitional outcomes with examples taken from the case studies. Lastly, the instruments of Module 3 were produced, in particular, a series of questions to support collective feedback when modelling a project's chain of transitional outcomes. The *Tool* was launched during a webinar (257 participants) in October 2019 under the responsibility of Communagir, who integrated it into its support activities (https://chairecacis-outilinteractif.org/).

The English version of the *Tool* was produced with the collaboration of Tamarack Institute (a Canadian non-profit organization that supports collaborative action) using a translation committee, including practitioners and a test with target users (October 2019–September 2020). The translation committee was composed of experts in the field familiar with the *Tool* terminology in both languages, i.e. a professional translator; two expert practitioners; the principal investigator for the research project; and the designer of the original *Tool*. The committee's role was to ensure that the wording in the translation conveyed the meaning in its original French version. The pre-testing of the translated *Tool* was intended to ensure that (1) the *Tool* used clear terms and language corresponding to that of the target users; and (2) the users understanding matched with the meaning of the French version. This kind of procedure is necessary because the usability of such tools is highly dependent on their ability to represent professional practice (Bilodeau & Kranias, 2019). The English *Tool* was launched during a webinar (74 participants) held by Tamarack Institute in December 2020. Tamarack hosts the *Tool* on its website and disseminates it in its networks.

35.3.3 Putting Knowledge into Action

In addition to the *Tool*'s intended use, the experience of practitioners with the *Tool* shows a strong tendency to adapt it to their needs. Users can take instruments that are useful to them piecemeal, such as using the feedback grid in Module 3 without first telling their project story. Users have also developed another application of transitional outcomes by using them as indicators on a dashboard to track the action progress as it occurs. Experience also shows that optimal use of the TO repertoire and the *Tool* is often supported by various resources (consultant, trainee, support organization). Professional support and the sharing of experiences between practitioners on a continuous and longer-term basis therefore appear necessary to promote effective implementation of the TOs and the *Tool*. The development and implementation of a community of practice (CP), which is a favourable strategy for this purpose (INSPQ, 2018), is in plan. The aim is to make the *Tool* known, to facilitate its use, and to share user experiences so they could benefit from it. The community of practice is a recognized strategy to support collective learning (Wenger, 2005). It supports the sharing of experiences, resources, and instruments that promote collective problem solving; the belonging to a common practice, and recognition of specific expertise; the development of a common repository of knowledge and tools; and the development and deployment of best practices (Lièvre et al., 2016).

35.4 ANT-Informed Examination of Knowledge Translation Process

Knowledge-translation instruments are cognitive and technical objects that link three categories of entities: the authors of the scientific knowledge and designers of the instruments, the objects that reflect this knowledge, and the practice settings in which they are used (Akrich, 2006a). The translation process thus operates at the confluence of three worlds.

Scientific knowledge is the work of researchers who are historically and socially situated in relation to the phenomena being studied. It results from a translation process through a series of operations that transform original events into scientific writings (e.g. data collection, reduction, analysis, interpretation, validation) and knowledge translation tools (e.g. synthesis, highlighting, popularization, prototyping, testing, modelling) (Callon, 1989). No scientific knowledge is produced without researchers (MacLeod et al., 2019; Rau Steuernagel et al., 2019). In the experience presented, although the researchers followed the action in context and analysed how the actors themselves defined what was happening, the knowledge and knowledge translation tools produced are a representation of the work of the neighbourhood committees by researchers and knowledge mobilization specialists.

Knowledge translation tools belong to the realm of inscriptions. These are translations into physical (e.g. charts, maps, written information, tools) or social (e.g. knowledge brokers) forms that act as intermediaries between knowledge producers and users (Callon, 1991). The characteristic of these intermediaries is to transport knowledge and uses without transforming them (Latour, 2005). In this way, inscriptions stabilize scientific and technical innovations and make them sustainable and portable (Bilodeau & Potvin, 2018; Rau Steuernagel et al., 2019). Inscriptions circulate within a field of action by connecting innovations with networks of actors who are likely to adopt and use them (Callon & Latour, 1986; Callon, 1989).

Lastly, the world of practice refers to human engagement in actions and interactions with others, involving the interpretation of situations, and composing processes within a socio-historical context that gives them structure and meaning (Giddens, 1987; Wenger, 2003). Studying practice and tracing it in the course of social life involve recognizing the disparate elements that are inextricably linked to it (cognitive categories, symbols, techniques, objects, material and social environments, etc.) and that regularly enter into the complex and active processes by which people act and give meaning to the world, their activities, and their lives (Nimmo, 2011).

In our experience, the *Tool* records the knowledge produced by the research in a powerful and meaningful representation: the map of the chains of transitional outcomes up to their effects. This inscription is appreciated in several networks of actors because it clearly and simply communicates what seems messy and confusing at first blush. This inscription is of interest to practitioners who see it as a tool for representing their action and strengthening their argument about its effectiveness. The strength of the inscription is precisely to be able to represent and communicate a complex reality in a readable form in a scope that the interlocutor can easily grasp. It lies in its ability to make the essential visible and to communicate it in a simple way (Allard et al., 2008; Latour, 2006).

35.4.1 Agency of Knowledge Translation Instruments

Because they interconnect researchers and practitioners, knowledge translation instruments exercise a form of agency in that they continually feed and transform the relationship between these two categories of actors. During its development, the *Tool* has been the substrate of a collective learning process between practitioners and researchers, as evidenced by the sequence of iterations between design workshops, laboratory workshops, prototype testing, and successive modifications. The agency of the finalized *Tool* depends, first of all, on its capacity to be an effective vector for users to grasp and adopt the specialized terminology of transitional outcomes included in the *Tool*. The *Tool*'s agency also acts by maintaining interaction between its designers and users through the community of practice. Such instruments exercise their agency within user groups by virtue of the fact that they are equipped with the skills conferred by their designers and that they are capable of producing change. These instruments therefore allow designers to exert influence in user networks without being present. In return, these instruments require user networks to have a set of skills as they introduce new modes of action. These instruments thus bring about change through their circulation in networks of actors (Sayes, 2014).

35.4.2 Usage Scenarios Built in Knowledge Translation Instruments

The more knowledge translation tools encrypt information about their use, the more sophisticated technical objects they become. Consequently, depending on the choices made by their designers, these objects define users' roles to be taken up and the relationships to be established between them, a division of skills, and a suitable framework in which to operate (Callon, 1989). They also establish what is built into the instrument and what is left to the initiative of the users. The malleability of these instruments, which is tested in encounters with users, depends on the choices made by their designers (Akrich, 2006a, b). Through their decisions, the designers also define "*the script from which the future history of the device is to be developed*" (Akrich, 2006a, p. 171). If the conditions under which users are placed do not deviate too much from those established by the designers, the technical object somehow disappears and becomes a "black box" used to produce other knowledge. Otherwise, a gap appears between the expectations of both designers and users and what is actually achieved in action.

The *Tool* defines the roles of facilitator and participant. It was determined that the facilitator should have expertise in intersectoral action and facilitation and, preferably, be from outside the project. They may be practitioners of concerted action (coordinator, community organizer) or consultants with a mandate to do so, i.e. people who are qualified because of their skills and social position. The participants are members of the network hosting a project. It was also determined that the most appropriate setting for the *Tool* workshop was a forum specifically designed for stocktaking and evaluation exercise at the end or during the course of a project. In addition, the designers refined the scenario for using the *Tool* in a carefully developed and tested facilitation guide with target users, rather than leaving it up to the users. They have also provided a grid for interpreting the modelling carried out and making decisions about continuing a project.

35.4.3 The Active Role of Users in Designing Knowledge Translation Tools

Akrich (2006b) argues that an action apprehended and instrumented by the designers of technical objects cannot be reduced to its technical dimension alone. The development of such objects must also take into consideration the users, their environment, and their registers of action, since the action occurs at the meeting of the user, object, and the environment.

The designers of the *Tool* did not, at first glance, have a firm position on the competence of practitioners to use the knowledge produced and on the characteristics of the device that was to instrument them in this task. As a result, target users were called upon to join in the development of the *Tool* and interact with its designers as direct representatives of target users. Various techniques (design workshops, laboratory workshops, prototype testing) were used to gather their experience, views, and feedback. Co-construction of the *Tool* was carried out by knowledge mobilization specialists familiar with the context of use, user practitioners, and the principal investigator for the research. The roles of facilitator and participant, the necessary skills, and the preferred usage scenario were then established with the input of target users. The work to translate the *Tool* into English was carried out in the same spirit by inviting expert practitioners to serve on the translation committee and by pretesting the translation with target users.

When actually using the *Tool,* without modifying it or altering its intended usage scenario, users modify its use somewhat by using the instruments piecemeal for reflexive activities on their project without completing the entire intended scenario. Users are also taking an active role in developing another application, namely, a transitional outcome dashboard that adds a monitoring function to the stocktaking and evaluation functions planned for by the designers. Akrich (2006c) qualifies this form of user intervention as an extension of the instrument insofar as the *Tool* retains its original form and uses, but has added elements that enrich the list of its functions.

35.5 Conclusions

The inefficiency of the linear model of disseminating scientific knowledge from researchers to knowledge mobilization specialists and then to users, has now been established. Alternative models are more sophisticated: they account for the recursiveness between knowledge production and the design and use of translation tools. Moreover, they bring together a diversity of actors with varied skills (Akrich, 2006c).

The experience presented in this chapter shows how complex and demanding such processes are in terms of skills, resources, and innovation. The light shed by ANT shows just how crucial practice settings are to such processes. In this experience, establishing a research partnership with the practice settings and their early involvement in the research was the first step in connecting users with the process of knowledge production, translation, and ultimately, mobilization in practice. Reciprocal and continuous communication between research and practice, instrumented by specialized professionals and techniques, has been the active ingredient in the process of producing knowledge translation instruments, and beyond in the process of putting knowledge into action.

These learnings are of high relevance for health promotion research since it aims to contribute to societal transformation approach engaging citizens and a diversity of social actors. Our experience provides information on the requirement of a reciprocal epistemic posture between research and practice. It also informs about the dialogic space, not only between researchers and practitioners, but also between the diversity of intersectoral actors engaged in health promotion, showing the crucial role of mediation professionals and the specialized methodologies and devices they mobilize to promote and support continuous reciprocal communication.

Acknowledgments

Funding The research program was funded by CIHR 2011–16 ROH115211 and CIHR 2017–20 PJT153093.

The production of the *Tool* benefited financial support from the Fonds des services aux collectivités, Ministère de l'Éducation, de l'Enseignement supérieur et de la Recherche du Québec (Project 2015-010).

The English translation was funded by SSHRC-Connection (Project 611-2019–1023).

Field Partners Three neighbourhood committees participated to the research: the Table de développement social Centre-Sud, the Table de quartier Hochelaga-Maisonneuve and the Table de développement social de Pointe-aux-Trembles.

The four design-workshops on the characteristics of the Tool were performed with 57 participants from Montreal's neighbourhood committees that participated and did not participate in the research.

The three laboratory workshops on facilitating the workshop on using the Tool were performed with three intersectoral bodies: Vivre Saint-Michel en Santé Neighbourhood Committee; the Comité de ressources pour les jeunes familles de la MRC Les Moulins (young families's resource committee); and Action-Gardien, the community joint action table in Pointe-Saint-Charles.

Pretest of the English version of the Tool was performed with five practitioners from the Saskatoon Poverty Reduction Partnership, SK; DC Moves Dufferin County, ON; Human Ecology Manager, Lethbridge, AB; Poverty Reduction Initiatives Community Partnerships, Peel Region, ON; Cities/Team Lead, Cities Deepening Community –Vibrant Communities-Tamarack Institute.

Appendix

List of Productions on the Research Results and the Tool

Presentations of the Research Results in Major Scientific and Professional Conferences

- IUHPE (International Union for Health Promotion and Education) World Conference on Health Promotion, Rotorua, Aotearoa, New-Zealand, 2019
- Canadian Public Health Association Conference, Halifax (NS), Canada, 2017
- Journées d'études internationales du contrat REFLEXISS, Toulouse, France, 2017
- World Congress on Public Health, Melbourne, Australia, 2017
- IUHPE World Conference on Health Promotion, Curitiba, Brazil, 2016
- Journées annuelles de santé publique, Montréal (QC), Canada, 2016
- London School of Hygiene and Tropical Medicine, London, England, 2016
- Communities in Control Workshop, Lancaster, England, 2016
- Sparking Solutions, Ottawa (ON), Canada, 2016
- IFFÉRISS, Université Toulouse 3, Toulouse, France, 2016
- IREPS Auvergne-Rhône-Alpe, Lyon, France, 2019
- Colloque IFRISS, Toulouse, France, 2015.

Posters on the Research Results of the Three Case Studies

Lefebvre, C., Galarneau, M., Bilodeau, A., Potvin, L. (2016). Acting proactively on living conditions through local collaborations: The case of the Initiative montréalaise de soutien au développement social local. Sparkling Solutions Summit on

Population Health Intervention Research, Ottawa, April 25. https://chairecacis.org/fichiers/publications/20160425_im-prim_ang_final.pdf

Galarneau, M., Roy, M., Lefebvre, C., Bilodeau, A., Potvin, L. (2016). La table de quartier Hochelaga-Maisonneuve comme leader d'une action intersectorielle locale porteuse de transformations urbaines. Poster at the 22e World Conference Health Promotion – IUHPE, Curitiba, May 22–26. http://chairecacis.org/fichiers/publications/2-affiche_tab_quartier_hochelaga-maison.pdf

Lefebvre C, Rivest R, Bernard S, Galarneau M, Bilodeau A, Potvin L. (2016). *Éclairage sur le processus de production des effets : l'Initiative montréalaise de développement social local et le cas de la Table de développement social de Pointe-aux-Trembles.* Communication affichée. Poster at the 22e World Conference Health Promotion – IUHPE, Curitiba, May 22–26. http://chairecacis.org/fichiers/publications/affiche_tds_pat_finale_0.pdf

Training Sessions on Research Results and on the *Tool*

A dozen talks on research results have been delivered at the local, regional, and provincial levels, such as the City of Montreal; United Ways Montreal; Dynamo (Quebec nonprofit organization supporting collective action); partners of MI; École ARIMA, ARIMA partnership, University of Montreal; École d'été de Santé publique, McGill University, Montreal.

A workshop on the *Tool* was given at the seminar *Orchestrer l'action intersectorielle: de la mobilisation à l'évaluation*. Journées annuelles de santé publique 2019.

This workshop is integrated into the curriculum of the École ARIMA *Orchestrer l'action intersectorielle*, ongoing since 2021 at the University of Montréal's Faculty of Arts and Science.

The *Tool* is also integrated into the https://espacerezo.ca/ interactive platform on network action.

Webinars on the French and English *Tool*:

- National Collaborating Centre for Methods and Tools /Centre de collaboration nationale des méthodes et des outils, on February 2021.
- February 24 Webinar Audio Recording (French): https://www.youtube.com/watch?v=kekB-pOO8xw
- February 25 Webinar Audio Recording (English): https://www.youtube.com/watch?v=0TfMAXzLmSA
- International Union for Health Promotion and Education/ Union internationale de promotion de la santé et d'éducation pour la santé, on December 2020 and May 2021. https://www.youtube.com/watch?v=tyhPUZVUpFw (French)

References

Akrich, M. (2006a). La description des objets techniques. In M. Akrich, M. Callon, & B. Latour (Eds.), *Sociologie de la traduction Textes fondateurs* (pp. 159–178). Presses des Mines. https://doi.org/10.4000/books.pressesmines.1181

Akrich, M. (2006b). Les objets techniques et leurs utilisateurs. De la conception à l'action. In M. Akrich, M. Callon, & B. Latour (Eds.), *Sociologie de la traduction Textes fondateurs* (pp. 179–199). Presses des Mines. https://doi.org/10.4000/books.pressesmines.1181

Akrich, M. (2006c). Les utilisateurs, acteurs de l'innovation. In M. Akrich, M. Callon, & B. Latour (Eds.), *Sociologie de la traduction Textes fondateurs* (pp. 253–265). Presses des Mines. https://doi.org/10.4000/books.pressesmines.1181

Akrich, M., Callon, M., & Latour, B. (Eds.). (2006). *Sociologie de la traduction. Textes fondateurs*. Presses des Mines. https://doi.org/10.4000/books.pressesmines.1181

Allard, D., Bilodeau, A., & Gendron, S. (2008). Figurative thinking and models: Tools for participatory evaluation. In L. Potvin & D. McQueen (Eds.), *Health promotion evaluation practices in the Americas* (pp. 123–148). Springer.

Armstrong, R., Waters, E., Roberts, H., Oliver, S., & Popay, J. (2006). The role and theoretical evolution of knowledge translation and exchange in public health. *Journal of Public Health, 28*(4), 384–389. https://doi.org/10.1093/pubmed/fdl072

Armstrong, R., Waters, E., Crockett, B., & Keleher, H. (2007). The nature of evidence resources and knowledge translation for health promotion practitioners. *Health Promotion International, 22*(3), 254–260. https://doi.org/10.1093/heapro/dam017

Bilodeau, A., & Kranias, G. (2019). Self-evaluation tool for action in partnership: Translation and cultural adaptation of the original Quebec French tool to Canadian English. *The Canadian Journal of Program Evaluation, 34*(2), 192–206. https://doi.org/10.3138/cjpe.43685

Bilodeau, A., & Potvin, L. (2018). Unpacking complexity in public health interventions with Actor-Network Theory. *Health Promotion International, 33*(1), 173–181. https://doi.org/10.1093/heapro/daw062

Bilodeau, A., Lefebvre, C., Galarneau, M., & Potvin, L. (2018). Quels sont les effets de l'action intersectorielle locale sur les milieux de vie et comment sont-ils produits? In *Le Point sur... l'action intersectorielle* (Vol. 4, pp. 1–8). Centre de recherche Léa-Roback. http://chairecacis.org/fichiers/lea-roback-2018-4.pdf

Bilodeau, A., Galarneau, M., Lefebvre, C., & Potvin, L. (2019). Linking process and effects of intersectoral action on local neighbourhoods: Systemic modelling based on Actor-Network Theory. *Sociology of Health and Illness, 41*(1), 165–179. https://doi.org/10.1111/1467-9566.12813

Bilodeau, A., Lefebvre, C., Galarneau, M., & Potvin, L. (2020). Linking processes and effects of intersectoral action on living environments. In *Focus on... intersectoral action* (Vol. 4, pp. 1–8). Centre de recherche Léa-Roback. http://chairecacis.org/fichiers/publications/focus_on_intersectoral_action_4.pdf. Accessed 25 May 2021.

Callon, M. (1986). Some elements of a sociology of translation: Domestication of the scallops and the fishermen of St. Brieux Bay. In J. Law (Ed.), *Power, action and belief: A new sociology of knowledge?* (pp. 196–223). : Routledge & Kegan Paul.

Callon, M. (1989). Introduction. In M. Dans Callon (Ed.), *La science et ses réseaux. Genèse et circulation des faits scientifiques* (pp. 7–32). La Découverte.

Callon, M. (1991). Techno-economic networks and irreversibility. In J. Law (Ed.), *A sociology of monsters: Essays on power, technology and domination* (pp. 132–161). Routledge.

Callon, M., & Latour, B. (1986). Les paradoxes de la modernité. Comment concevoir les innovations? *Perspective et Santé, 36*, 13–25.

Callon, M., & Latour, B. (2012). Pour une sociologie relativement exacte. In J. Roberge, Y. Sénéchal, & S. Vibert (Eds.), *La Fin de la société. Débats contemporains autour d'un concept classique* (pp. 39–66). Athéna édition. http://www.bruno-latour.fr/sites/default/files/16-SOCIO-RELATIVISTE.pdf.

Campbell, A., Louie-Poon, S., Slater, L., & Scott, S. D. (2019). Knowledge translation strategies used by healthcare professionals in child health settings: An updated systematic review. *Journal of Pediatric Nursing, 47*, 114–120. https://doi.org/10.1016/j.pedn.2019.04.026

Chircop, A., Bassett, R., & Taylor, E. (2015). Evidence on how to practice intersectoral collaboration for health equity: A scoping review. *Critical Public Health, 25*, 178–191. https://doi.org/10.1080/09581596.2014.887831

CIHR. (2015). *Health research roadmap II: Capturing innovation to produce better health and health Care for Canadians. Strategic plan 2014–15 – 2018–19*. Date modified: 2015-04-14. https://cihr-irsc.gc.ca/e/29418.html. Accessed 3rd June 2020.

Dagenais, C., & Mc Sween-Cadieux, E. (2020). La Revue TUC: transfert et utilisation des connaissances dans la francophonie. *Chronique Revues savantes*, February 3. https://www.acfas.ca/publications/magazine/revues-savantes. Accessed 1st June 2020.

Divay, G., Belley, S., & Prémont, M.-C. (2013). Introduction. La collaboration intersectorielle: spécificités, questionnements et perspectives. In *La revue de l'innovation: La revue de l'innovation dans le secteur public, 18*(2), 1–22. https://www.innovation.cc/francais/peer-reviewed/2013_18_2_1_dicay_intro-collaborate-intersect.pdf.

Ferlie, E., Fitzgerald, L., McGivern, G., Dopson, S., & Bennett, C. (2011). Public policy networks and 'wicked problems': A nascent solution? *Public Administration, 89*(2), 307–324. https://doi.org/10.1111/j.1467-9299.2010.01896.x

Giddens, A. (1987). *La construction de la société*. PUF.

Graham, I. D., Logan, J., Harrison, M. B., Straus, S. E., & Tetroe, J. (2006). Lost in knowledge translation: Time for a map? *Journal of Continuing Education in the Health Professions, 26*(1), 13–24. https://doi.org/10.1002/chp.47

Hot, A., Le Govic, R., Deshaies, S., & White, D. (2017). *Traduire les connaissances issues de la recherche pour changer les pratiques de collaboration: un cadre de réflexion tiré de l'expérience ARIMA*. : CRPSI, CIUSSS du Nord-de-l'Île-de-Montréal. https://centreinteractions.ca/publication/traduire-les-connaissances-de-la-recherche-pour-changer-les-pratiques-de-collaboration/. Accessed 1st June 2021.

INSPQ. (2018). *La communauté de pratique un outil pertinent: résumé des connaissances adaptées au contexte de la santé publique*. : Institut national de santé publique du Québec. https://www.inspq.qc.ca/sites/default/files/publications/2351_communaute_pratique_outil_pertinent_resume_connaissance.pdf. Accessed 1st Feb 2021.

Jones, K., Armstrong, R., Pettman, T., & Waters, E. (2015). Knowledge Translation for researchers: Developing training to support public health researchers KTE efforts. Cochrane Update. *Journal of Public Health, 37*(2), 364–366. https://doi.org/10.1093/pubmed/fdv076

La Rocca, R., Yost, J., Dobbins, M., Ciliska, D., & Butt, M. (2012). The effectiveness of knowledge translation strategies used in public health: A systematic review. *BMC Public Health, 12*, 751. https://doi.org/10.1186/1471-2458-12-751

Latour, B. (2005). *Reassembling the social. An introduction to actor–network-theory*. Oxford University Press.

Latour, B. (2006). Les "vues" de l'esprit. Une introduction à l'anthropologie des sciences et des techniques. In M. Akrich, M. Callon, & B. Latour (Eds.), *Sociologie de la traduction Textes fondateurs* (pp. 33–69). Presses des Mines. https://doi.org/10.4000/books.pressesmines.1181

Laurent, A., Ferron, C., Lombrail, P., Berry, P., Frattini, M.O., Berdougo, F. et al. (2019). How to build and share an experiential knowledge in public health? Poster Walks. In 2th European public health conference *Building bridges for solidarity and public health*. Marseille, November 20–23.

Lefebvre, C., Galarneau, M., Bilodeau, A., & Potvin, L. (2016). Au carrefour de la recherche et de la concertation de quartier: un dispositif de recherche adaptatif pour étudier les effets de l'*Initiative montréalaise de soutien au développement social local*. In G. Sénécal (Ed.), *Revitalisation urbaine et concertation de quartier* (pp. 203–225). Presses de l'Université Laval.

Lièvre, P., Bonnet, E., & Laroche, N. (2016). Etienne Wenger – Communauté de pratique et théorie sociale de l'apprentissage. In T. Burger-Helmchen, C. Hussler, & P. Cohendet (Eds.), *Les*

Grands Auteurs en Management de l'innovation et de la créativité (pp. 427–447). Éditions Management & Société.

MacLeod, A., Cameron, P., Ajjawi, R., Kits, O., & Tummons, J. (2019). Actor-network theory and ethnography: Sociomaterial approaches to Researching medical education. *Perspectivies on Medical Education, 8*, 177–186. https://doi.org/10.1007/s40037-019-0513-6

Miranda, É. D. S., Figueiró, A. C., & Potvin, L. (2020). Are public health researchers in Brazil ready and supported to do knowledge translation? *Cad Saúde Pública, 36*(4), 1–5. https://doi.org/10.1590/0102-311X00003120

Mitton, C., Adair, C. E., McKenzie, E., Patten, S. B., & Perry, B. W. (2007). Knowledge transfer and exchange: Review and synthesis of the literature. *The Milbank Quarterly, 85*(4), 729–768. https://doi.org/10.1111/j.1468-0009.2007.00506.x

Nimmo, R. (2011). Actor-network theory and methodology: Social research in a more-than-human world. *Methodological Innovations Online, 6*(3), 108–119. https://doi.org/10.4256/mio.2011.010

Potvin, L., & Aumaître, F. (2010). Les partenariats: espaces négociés de controverses et d'innovations. In L. Potvin, M. J. Moquet, & C. Jones (Eds.), *Réduire les inégalités sociales en santé* (pp. 318–325). Institut National de Prévention et d'Éducation à la Santé.

Potvin, L., & Bisset, S. (2008). There is more to methodology than methods. In L. Potvin & D. V. McQueen (Eds.), *Health promotion evaluation in the Americas. Values and research* (pp. 63–80). Springer.

Potvin, L., & Clavier, C. (2012). La théorie de l'acteur-réseau. In F. Aubry & L. Potvin (Eds.), *Construire l'espace socio-sanitaire. Expériences et pratiques de recherche dans la production locale de la santé* (pp. 75–98). Les Presses de l'Université de Montréal.

Potvin, L., & Clavier, C. (2013). Actor-network theory: The governance of intersectoral initiatives. In C. Clavier & E. de Leeuw (Eds.), *Health promotion and the policy process* (pp. 82–102). Oxford University Press.

Potvin, L. & McQueen, D.V. (2007). Modernity, public health, and health promotion. A reflexive discourse. In: L. Potvin & D. V. McQueen (Eds), *Modernity, public health, and health promotion* (pp 12–20). Springer. http://eknygos.lsmuni.lt/springer/685/12-20.pdf. Accessed 23 Feb 2021.

Potvin, L., Bilodeau, A., & Gendron, S. (2008). Trois défis pour l'évaluation en promotion de la santé. *IUHPE – Promotion & Education, Supp 1*, 17–21. https://doi.org/10.1177/1025382308093991

Rau Steuernagel, C., Engebretsen, E., Kristiansen, H. W., & Moen, K. (2019). Ethnography of texts: A literature review of health and female homosexuality in Brazil. *Medical Humanities, 0*, 1–10. https://doi.org/10.1136/medhum-2018-011544

Sayes, E. (2014). Actor–Network Theory and methodology: Just what does it mean to say that nonhumans have agency? *Social Studies of Science, 44*(1), 134–149. https://doi.org/10.1177/0306312713511867

SSHRC. (2019). *Guidelines for effective knowledge mobilization*. https://www.sshrc-crsh.gc.ca/funding-financement/policies-politiques/knowledge_mobilisation-mobilisation_des_connaissances-eng.aspx. Accessed 1st June 2020.

Thirsk, J. (2018). Knowledge translation. Editorial. *Nutrition & Dietetics, 75*, 341–344. https://doi.org/10.1111/1747-0080.12466

Wenger, E. (2003). *Communities of practice*. Cambridge University Press.

Wenger, E. (2005). *La théorie des communautés de pratique: apprentissage, sens et identité*. Les Presses de l'Université Laval.

Chapter 36
A Critical Health Promotion Research Approach Using the Red Lotus Critical Health Promotion Model

Lily O'Hara and Jane Taylor

36.1 Introduction

This chapter describes and reflects on our program of critical health promotion research. Critical health promotion is focused on social change, challenging oppressive systems, power structures, and dominant discourses (Taylor et al., 2020). It is underpinned by explicit values and principles articulated in seminal health promotion charters and declarations. These values were first recognised in the Ottawa Charter for Health Promotion where social justice and equity were identified as prerequisites for health. Critical health promotion aims to challenge social structures that create and perpetuate health inequities. The objective of our research program is to produce knowledge on the application of critical health promotion processes to address health and well-being priorities. In doing so, we aim to build the critical health promotion research capacity of researchers and researcher-practitioners. The research program is distinctive due to the purposeful application of critical health promotion values and principles in research projects across the four stages of the health promotion practice cycle (community assessment, planning, implementation, and evaluation).

Section two of the chapter describes the epistemological and theoretical foundations of our critical health promotion research program, which is positioned within a constructivist epistemology and underpinned by critical theory, critical systems theory, and critical systems heuristics. The founding project in the research program was the development of the Red Lotus Critical Health Promotion Model (RLCHPM),

L. O'Hara (✉)
QU Health, Qatar University, Doha, Qatar
e-mail: lohara@qu.edu.qa

J. Taylor
University of the Sunshine Coast, Sippy Downs, QLD, Australia

L. Potvin, D. Jourdan (eds.), *Global Handbook of Health Promotion Research, Vol. 1*,
https://doi.org/10.1007/978-3-030-97212-7_36

which is described in section three. Section four presents the application of the RLCHPM in research projects across the health promotion practice cycle.

36.2 Epistemological and Theoretical Foundations of the Research Program

36.2.1 Epistemology

This research program is positioned within constructivist epistemology (Crotty, 1998), which is consistent with our beliefs about the social construction of knowledge and meaning. Although many forms of constructivism have developed over time, the central tenet of constructivist epistemology is that human knowledge and the methods used to develop new knowledge are constructed and not innate (Phillips, 1995). This means that there is no single objective reality, but rather multiple interpretations based on the experiences and existing knowledge of the learner (Crotty, 1998). Constructivism holds that the content of all scientific disciplines, such as the discipline of health promotion, is constructed through the work of scholars and practitioners across the generations, within the context of the social and political environment (Phillips, 1995). Our research program builds on the work of health promotion scholars and practitioners who have been writing about concepts related to critical health promotion for over 30 years.

36.2.2 Critical Theory

Health promotion practice is fundamentally focused on reducing inequity within and between communities (Baum, 2008; World Health Organization, 1986). As such, the theoretical perspective used in this research program is critical theory (Crotty, 1998). Critical theory refers to research, policy, and practice focused on social change to reduce inequities in society through critiquing power relationships and social structures that perpetuate inequity (Porter, 2003). Baum argues that all health promotion research should use critical theory because of its inherent requirement for action that addresses the causes of inequality and thereby contributes to reducing inequity (Baum, 2002).

An influential contemporary critical theorist is German sociologist and philosopher Jurgen Habermas (Morrow & Brown, 1994; Held, 1997), who proposed three knowledge domains that contribute to research processes and outcomes: technical knowledge, practical knowledge, and emancipatory knowledge. The technical knowledge domain, also referred to as instrumental action, denotes the way people use technical knowledge to manage their work environment. The practical knowledge domain, also known as communicative action, denotes knowledge generated through social interaction that enhances interpretation and understanding about social phenomena. Emancipatory knowledge denotes knowledge of the self that is gained through self-reflection. It includes enhanced consciousness and understanding about one's perception of themselves, their role in, and their expectations of social life. This form of knowledge, Habermas contends, results in the liberation of individuals from oppressive social structures (Habermas, 2002, 2004a, b).

Critical theory and other critical approaches are used extensively in health promotion research (see, for example, Alvaro et al., 2011; Simpson & Freeman, 2004; Smyth, 2020). However, this theoretical perspective had not been embedded into existing health promotion models used to guide day-to-day practice (Gregg, 2012). Crosby and Noar (2010) argue that the development of health promotion theory has not kept up with practice because it has been developed in an evidence-based rather than practice-based environment, and is not grounded in practice or easily accessible to practitioners. Whilst health promotion models have included Habermas's technical knowledge domain in terms of knowledge and skills required to conduct community assessments, and plan, implement and evaluate health promotion action (Barry et al., 2012), they have not included the practical and emancipatory knowledge domains (Habermas, 2002, 2004a, b).

36.2.3 Critical Systems Theory

Critical Systems Theory (CST) is a framework that draws together systems thinking and critique. It is increasingly being used in a range of environmental, management and social disciplines to better understand and respond to issues that are complex, large in scale, where there is uncertainty about inherent relationships and types of appropriate actions, and where there is impermanence and imperfection (Bammer, 2003). A historical account of CST by Jackson (1991a) identified five commonly agreed commitments to CST: critical awareness, social awareness, human emancipation, methodological pluralism, and theoretical pluralism (Jackson, 1991b, c; Midgley, 1996).

Critical awareness refers to the need to understand and be able to interrogate the theoretical underpinnings, strengths, and weaknesses of the range of systems theories, methodologies, and their associated techniques and methods. It requires the ability to examine the inherent assumptions and values of existing and proposed systems designs and maps such as strategic plans and social policies and programs. Social awareness requires those that use systems methodologies to consider the social consequences of their use, particularly whose interests are or are not being served. Human emancipation refers to the empowerment of people through the use of participatory methods, for example, participatory action research, action research, and collaborative inquiry, which value active involvement of those who are impacted by particular issues in decision-making processes about those issues. It is focused on the maximum development of the potential of all individuals involved in an initiative (Jackson, 1991c). Methodological pluralism involves the complementary use of systems methodologies that use all the features of CST in their application to problem situations (Jackson, 1991c). CST authors posit that different assumptions underpin different methodologies and that it is appropriate to use a combination of methodologies to respond to different problem situations in different contexts (Midgley, 1996). Theoretical pluralism requires a commitment to the development of systems approaches that reflect an understanding of, and are respectful of differing theoretical positions.

The key mechanism for realising the commitments to CST is critical reflection, which, together with technical expertise, is required for professional competence (Ulrich, 2005; Flood & Romm, 1996). Flood and Romm (1996, 81) define critical reflection as the process of reflecting '... on the relationship between different organisational and societal interests and the dominance of different theories and methodologies'. Ulrich (2005) suggests that critical reflective practice requires engagement in critical reflective discourse for the purposes of emancipation, competent practice, and public benefit.

Ulrich (1987) cautioned that early forms of CST were not necessarily able to realise their emancipatory or critical intent, as they did not offer the practical tools to critically reflect on and deal with the coercive nature of problem situations. He asserts that emancipatory discourse enables citizens to play a role in civil society, but opportunities to participate in civil society are not equitable because there are boundaries around power, knowledge, and decision-making inherent in any discourse driven by those that hold power. This means that the emancipatory intent of CST is often difficult to realise without discursive exploration of the underlying structural inequities (Bammer, 2003; Ulrich, 1987, 2003, 2005). To address this issue, Ulrich proposed a form of CST referred to as critical systems heuristics (Ulrich, 1987, 1988).

36.2.4 Critical Systems Heuristics

Critical Systems Heuristics (CSH) is regarded as the third wave of systems thinking (Stephens et al., 2010). The term heuristic derives from the Greek term *heurisko* which means to assist to discover (Moore, 2001). In this context, the term heuristic refers to the development of practical tools to assist professionals and lay people to engage in critical reflective dialogue about the underlying normative content of systems designs or propositions (Ulrich, 2005). Normative content refers to the accepted and unchallenged value judgements inherent in propositions such as recommendations for action, plans, standards, and evaluative criteria, and the implications of these propositions for those affected by their implementation (Ulrich, 2003, 2005; Ulrich & Reynolds, 2010).

Ulrich's concern is that a proposition to address an issue reflects the value judgements of its creators, and not those of the people with the lived experience of the issue and the consequences of the proposition's application (Ulrich, 1987). Researchers, policymakers, and practitioners who are legitimised through their paid work roles, contribute to decision-making processes about health issues and their solutions, often without input from or consideration of their impact on recipients of such initiatives. Professionals therefore influence the construction of problem situations, their solutions, and consequences for which they are often not accountable. A key aspect of CSH is finding constructive ways to engage with the range of stakeholders and work through the tensions that arise between the various stakeholder perspectives over the course of change processes. Many applied science disciplines, including health promotion, lack the mechanisms required to make explicit the underlying normative content inherent in change processes (Ulrich, 1987; Ulrich & Reynolds, 2010).

CSH aims to improve the quality of scientific study by giving users of a system a voice inside science, rather than having observations about the system constructed solely by experts (Ulrich, 2001). Norman asserts that 'health promotion research and practice recognises that social change is not linear and involves multiple communities of interest working together in a coordinated manner in order to address health problems' (Norman, 2009, 868). Norman advocates for the use of systems methodologies and critical systems heuristics in health promotion practice and research (Norman, 2009). CSH is a practical, applied theoretical framework that is useful in a practical, applied discipline such as health promotion. It is a framework that builds phronesis (Flyvbjerg et al., 2012) or practical wisdom on how to address and act on social problems in a particular context.

There are three ideas central to CSH: 1. the need to develop the critical competence of professionals and lay people to support reflection and discourse; 2. reflective practice, which requires heuristic support for dialogue in the form of critical questioning tools; 3. systems thinking, which, in this context, refers to the need to consider issues from a whole systems perspective by identifying the prior judgements, or values and empirical observations, which are more or less valued in a situation (Bammer, 2003; Ulrich, 2003, 2005). Prior (*a priori*) judgements, referred to as boundary judgements, reflect the multiple assumptions inherent in complex issues. Boundary judgements influence the merit attributed to the different claims within a whole system. Boundary judgements are explored through boundary critique, which is a structured critical dialogue using a heuristic. Boundary critique can occur through self-critical reflection on practice or at an emancipatory level, which challenges the value judgements of those that may not be so open to critical self-reflection (Ulrich, 1987, 2003, 2005). CSH extends the philosophical foundations of CST to incorporate boundary critique as a strategy to ground CST in ethical practice (Bammer, 2003; Ulrich, 2003, 2005) and include heuristic tools to aid genuine dialogue between stakeholders in coercive problem situations (Jackson, 1991a).

36.3 Red Lotus Critical Health Promotion Model

In the beginning were the waters. Matter readied itself. The sun glowed. And a lotus slowly opened, holding the universe on its golden pericarp (Jain & Daljeet, 2006).

36.3.1 Structure of the Red Lotus Critical Health Promotion Model

The red lotus plant (*Nelumbo nucifera*), regarded as 'the most majestic flower abounding in supreme beauty, sublime grace and the aura of transcendence' (Jain & Daljeet, 2006), was selected as the symbol for the Red Lotus Critical Health Promotion Model (RLCHPM), based on the alignment of its biological and cultural qualities with the philosophical, ethical, and technical elements of critical health promotion. In many societies across the world, the lotus plant has culinary, medicinal, and spiritual significance, which are described elsewhere (Gregg & O'Hara, 2007a) (Fig. 36.1).

The RLCHPM has ten interrelated components represented by parts of the red lotus plant: (1) health and well-being status; (2) people's characteristics; (3) environmental determinants of health and well-being; (4) community assessment; (5) planning; (6) implementation; (7) evaluation; (8) sustainability; (9) values and principles system; and (10) critical refection.

The flower pod represents the holistic health and well-being status of people at individual, family, and community levels, including settings such as schools, universities, workplaces, and hospitals. The pod's seeds represent mental, physical, spiritual, social, and any other aspect of health and well-being important to people. The life cycle of the pod symbolises stages in the life course, including the cyclical concept of life and death inherent in many cultures.

The flower stamens represent the characteristics that influence people's level of privilege and life opportunity, including biological (age, sex, genetics, physiological status, skin colour, body size, neurodiversity, physical ability), socio-economic (education, employment, income, housing status, ethnicity, gender, sexuality, citizenship, relationship status), cognitive (knowledge, attitudes, values, beliefs, language), affective (emotions, feelings, moods), and behavioural (physical, mental, social, cultural, spiritual) factors.

These characteristics interact with environmental conditions which are represented by flower petal layer 1 and include social, cultural, economic, commercial,

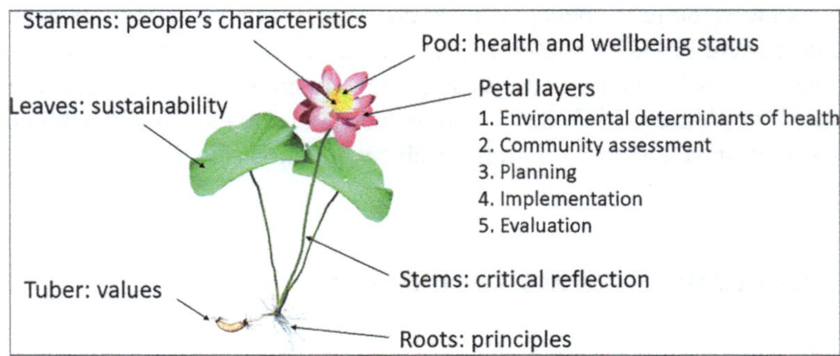

Fig. 36.1 Red Lotus Critical Health Promotion Model

political, built, and natural environments. The next four flower petal layers represent the four stages of the health promotion practice cycle. Community assessment (petal layer 2) involves the identification and prioritisation of health and well-being related felt, expressed, normative, and comparative assets and needs. This involves the collection of a range of evidence via rigorous, credible, and trustworthy research processes.

Petal layer 3 represents planning of critical health promotion action to address the determinants of priority health and well-being issues, in collaboration with primary and secondary co-activists. This includes formative evaluation and the development of process, impact, and outcome evaluation plans. Primary co-activists are those directly affected by the priority health and well-being issue, and secondary co-activists are people and organisations with the resources and capacity to contribute to addressing the priority issue.

Petal layer 4 represents the implementation stage which involves supporting co-activists to implement health promotion action and process evaluation plans, including the establishment of partnerships with other stakeholders, and responding to the need to secure, mobilise, and maintain financial, human, and other resources.

Petal layer 5 represents the evaluation stage which involves actioning the impact and outcome evaluation plans made in the planning stage, and communicating the findings.

The concept of sustainability is represented by the leaves of the plant. Healthy, vibrant leaves are required to ensure the longevity of the plant and its future viability. Likewise, critical health promotion requires health promotion action to result in sustainable improvements in the conditions required for improved health and well-being and reduced health inequities.

The tuber represents the 12 critical health promotion values, and the roots represent their related principles (Table 36.1) (Taylor et al., 2020). The stems represent the critical reflection process, which involves the purposeful reflection on the extent to which the values and principles are evident across the components of the model represented by the flower and leaves. To facilitate the critical reflection process, we have developed a heuristic tool to evaluate the extent of alignment of health promotion practice or research programs with critical health promotion (O'Hara et al., 2015a).

36.3.2 Theoretical Foundations of the Red Lotus Critical Health Promotion Model

The RLCHPM incorporates commitments to critical theory, critical systems theory, and critical systems heuristics, distinguishing it from other health promotion models. The values and principles component of the RLCHPM incorporates an interrelated system of ethical, philosophical, and technical values and principles that characterise critical health promotion, drawn from contemporary health promotion

Table 36.1 Values and principles in the Red Lotus Critical Health Promotion Model

Focus of value and principle	RLCHPM Value	RLCHPM principle – action on the value in practice
Health paradigm	Holistic health paradigm	Seeing health as a complex concept that includes physical, mental, spiritual, social, and cultural aspects of well-being that relate to the whole person.
Program approach	Salutogenic approach	Emphasising salutogenic factors that create and support health, well-being, sense of coherence, happiness, and meaning in life.
Scientific approach	Ecological science	Using the science of ecology, which recognises that: people exist in multiple ecosystems, from the individual, to the family, group, community and population levels; all parts within systems impact on each other; the whole of any system is greater than the sum of the parts.
Who to work with	Focus determined by equity	In recognition that access to health promoting conditions of living is a human right, prioritising work with people and communities that are most marginalised, vulnerable, and disadvantaged based on considerations of equity
Professional role	Working with people as an ally	Working with people as a culturally competent ally and resource who is respectful of all aspects of diversity.
Assumptions about people	Assume people are doing the best for their well-being	Assuming that when left to their own devices, people will do the best for their well-being and that of their families and communities, given their circumstances and available resources.
Basis for practice	Comprehensive use of evidence and theory	Basing health promotion practice on evidence of community assets and needs, sound theoretical foundations, and evidence of effectiveness.
Strategy approach	Portfolio of multiple strategies	Using a portfolio of strategies incorporating all action areas of the Ottawa Charter.
Engagement processes	Empowering engagement processes	Using participatory enabling processes that empower and meaningfully engage people most impacted by an issue in collaborative governance and decision-making to gain increased control over their lives and the determinants of their health and well-being.
Personal autonomy	Respect personal autonomy	Ensuring all relevant parties consent to health promotion change processes and acknowledging and respecting that not all people will choose the same actions.
Beneficence	Maximum beneficence	Actively considering what the benefits of any health promotion change process may be to the full range of beneficiaries.
Non-maleficence	Non-maleficence is a priority consideration	Actively considering what the potential harms of any health promotion change process may be; who may be harmed by the change processes and in what way; taking steps to minimise or avoid this harm; communicating risks involved in a truthful and open manner.

literature (Gregg & O'Hara, 2007b) and international (Barry et al., 2012) and Australian (Australian Health Promotion Association, 2009) health promotion competency frameworks. The inclusion of ethical, philosophical, and technical values and principles responds to criticism in the literature about the lack of attention to ethical and philosophical aspects of health promotion practice (Antonovsky, 1996; Eriksson & Lindström, 2008; Lundy, 2010; Sindall, 2002; St Leger, 2001; Tremblay & Richard, 2011).

Presenting the values and principles as a system highlights their connection to other model components, consistent with the intention of CST (Bammer, 2003; Jackson, 1991c; Midgley, 1996; Ulrich, 1987, 1988) to develop methodologies and frameworks that acknowledge interrelatedness. The inclusion of the values and principles system also responds to the CST requirement to make explicit the underlying normative content inherent in programs (Ulrich, 1987; Ulrich & Reynolds, 2010), including the accepted and unchallenged underlying value judgements of programs (Ulrich, 2003; Ulrich & Reynolds, 2010). The CST commitment to critical awareness calls for researchers and practitioners to increase their consciousness about the normative content of programs, and reflect on the implications for those they are intended to impact (Habermas, 2004a, b; Jackson, 1991c; Midgley, 1996). The RLCHPM includes ethical values related to active engagement of those affected by an issue, and consideration of personal autonomy, beneficence, and non-maleficence (Gregg & O'Hara, 2007a). Failure to enact ethical change processes could result in harmful outcomes and reinforcement of the status quo.

Implicit in the RLCHPM is the CST commitment of methodological pluralism, which refers to the theoretically coherent and carefully considered use of a variety of research methods. The values and related principles of evidence-based practice and system-level evaluation, and community assessment and evaluation stages of the health promotion process all require a variety of approaches and methods for gathering evidence to inform policies and programs and their evaluation.

The critical refection component of the RLCHPM represents the mechanism to reflect on the underlying values and principles across the stages of a health promotion process. Critical reflection is a key CST requirement for professional competence (Ulrich, 2005; Flood & Romm, 1996); however, it is not well-developed among health promotion practitioners (Tretheway et al., 2015). This component aligns with Habermas's emancipatory knowledge domain, which denotes self-knowledge through self-reflection for the purpose of liberating people from oppressive social structures through enhanced understanding about themselves, their role in, and expectations of social life (Habermas, 2004a, b). In the RLCHPM, this is evident in the values and principles related to empowerment, participation, and democratic processes.

Enacting the values and principles and critical reflection components of the model enables researchers and researcher-practitioners to gain greater insight into the nature of their own and others' practice, and advocate for the reorientation of practice to align with the values and principles of critical health promotion. This responds to the three main ideas of Ulrich's CSH: developing critical competence to support reflection; using heuristic tools to support reflective dialogue; and considering issues from a whole system's perspective by making explicit the prior values and empirical observations that are more or less valued in a situation (Bammer, 2003; Ulrich, 2003, 2005).

36.4 Health Promotion Research Projects Using the Red Lotus Critical Health Promotion Model

In the years since publication, we have used the RLCHPM in research projects in three fields of practice (individuals and populations, stakeholders (including practitioners,) and policymakers and institutions) across the health promotion practice cycle. The projects conducted within this research program are presented in Table 36.2. For each project, we present the following: focus of the research; relevant stage of the health promotion practice cycle; examples of critical health promotion values applied in the project and the nature of their application; research design; and new knowledge created and potential translation into critical health promotion practice. Findings from each project are intended to inform the next stage of the health promotion practice cycle, and ultimately be translated into policy and practice. (Table 36.2).

Consistent with the critical health promotion value of working with people rather than on them, we collaborate with people in the community and institutions to plan and conduct health promotion research projects. For example, school-based research projects have involved collaborative planning and implementation with school administrators, teachers, and parents, with shared governance and decision-making. In research projects in primary health care settings, staff were jointly responsible for planning, implementation, governance, and decision-making. Research results are shared with participants in the form of research summaries, presentations, or reports, depending on the nature of the project. This is an ethical obligation consistent with the philosophical value of working with people, which means that people participating in the research also own the results. The specific objectives of each research project are defined by the project researchers in collaboration with the stakeholders in the research setting. Various data collection and analysis methods are used across quantitative, qualitative, and mixed methods projects. Some projects have involved quantitative surveys (online or on paper), with statistical analyses to determine prevalence and relationships. Other projects used semi-structured interviews to collect qualitative accounts of experiences, which were analysed thematically. Quasi experimental pre-test and post-test designs have been used to assess qualitative and quantitative changes in attitudes, values, and practices. We used multimedia critical discourse analysis (Machin & Mayr, 2012) to examine government documents. Three of these projects are described in detail, in order to provide examples of how to use the RLCHP in practice. In each description, the relevant component of the model is included in italics.

Table 36.2 Application of critical health promotion values to research projects

Project title	Focus of research	Health promotion practice cycle stage	Critical health promotion value	Application of critical health promotion value	Research design	New knowledge created and potential translation to practice
Experiences of weight-based oppression	Individuals and populations	Community assessment	Focus determined by equity	Prioritised working with people at higher weights	Narrative inquiry methodology using individual in-depth semi-structured interviews with staff, faculty, and students at Qatar University recruited through purposive sampling; inductive thematic analysis of qualitative data	Evidence of stakeholder perspectives on WBO (O'Hara et al., 2020); evidence base for the design of critical health promotion programs to reduce WBO
			Non-maleficence	Designed questions to use neutral, non-pathologising language about body weight		
			Holistic health paradigm	Explored impact of WBO on physical, mental, spiritual, and social health and well-being		
			Ecological science	Explored exposure to WBO at multiple interacting levels		

(continued)

Table 36.2 (continued)

Project title	Focus of research	Health promotion practice cycle stage	Critical health promotion value	Application of critical health promotion value	Research design	New knowledge created and potential translation to practice
The health and well-being of people in school, university, and town settings	Individuals and populations	Community assessment	Holistic health paradigm and ecological science	Designed instruments to collect data on physical, mental, spiritual, social, and environmental health and well-being at multiple level levels	Two separate studies involving online and in-person cross sectional surveys with university staff, faculty, and students and residents of a small town, respectively, recruited through universal sampling; descriptive and inferential analysis of quantitative data Two separate studies involving fully mixed methods sequential equal status designs using interactive classroom based qualitative data collection activities followed by quantitative surveys with primary school students, parents, and teachers, and secondary school students, respectively, recruited through purposive sampling across whole year groups; deductive thematic analysis of qualitative data and descriptive and inferential analysis of quantitative data	Evidence of the health status, health behaviours, and interactions with health-related environments of people in a university setting (Parker, 2008), town setting (McKinnon, 2008), primary school (Zeven, 2007), and secondary school (Adams, 2008); evidence base for the development of critical health promotion programs in school, university, and town settings

Disordered eating, weight-based oppression and depression in female university students	Individuals and populations	Community assessment	Focus determined by equity	Focused on young women as priority equity group	Online cross-sectional surveys of female students at three universities recruited through universal sampling; descriptive and inferential analysis of quantitative data	Evidence of the extent of disordered eating, weight-based oppression and depression in female university students (O'Hara et al., 2016; Thomas et al., 2016); evidence base for the development of critical health promotion programs to address disordered eating, weight-based oppression and depression in young women
			Ecological science	Explored exposure to WBO at multiple interacting levels		
			Non-maleficence	Designed questionnaires to use neutral, non-pathologising language about body weight		
Everybody in Schools: a Health at Every Size-based program to reduce weight-based oppression, and enhance intuitive eating, joyful movement and self-esteem	Policymakers and institutions	Planning, implementation and evaluation	Working with people as an ally	Co-designed a curriculum unit with teachers (primary co-activists	Co-planning and implementation of a curriculum unit with Grade 3 teachers at one school recruited through purposive sampling, followed by in-depth semi-structured interviews with same teachers; inductive thematic analysis of qualitative data	Everybody in Schools Curriculum Unit (Shelley et al., 2008) and evidence of the positive impact on teachers' knowledge, skills, attitudes, and practice (Shelley et al., 2010); evidence base for the development of future school-based programs
			Salutogenic approach	Designed content to ensure a strength-based orientation		
			Non-maleficence	Designed program to use neutral, non-pathologising language about body weight		

(continued)

Table 36.2 (continued)

Project title	Focus of research	Health promotion practice cycle stage	Critical health promotion value	Application of critical health promotion value	Research design	New knowledge created and potential translation to practice
A professional development (PD) program on critical health promotion for primary health care practitioners	Policymakers and institutions	Planning, implementation and evaluation	Comprehensive use of evidence and theory Empowering engagement processes	Designed, implemented, and evaluated RLCHPM PD strategy Engaged with stakeholders (primary and secondary co-activists) throughout the process	Co-planning and implementation of a PD strategy; evaluation research methodology involving fully mixed methods sequential equal status design using quasi-experimental pre-post program survey using self-administered quantitative questionnaire followed by in-depth semi-structured interviews with a universal sample of employees of a primary health care organisation; descriptive and inferential analysis of quantitative data and deductive thematic analysis of qualitative data	Evidence of the positive impact on practitioners' critical health promotion competencies (Gregg, 2012; Taylor et al., 2015); evidence base for the development of future critical health promotion professional development programs in the primary health care setting
Exploring the use of a critical reflection model with health promotion practitioners	Practitioners	Planning, implementation, evaluation	Working with people as an ally Respect personal autonomy	Worked alongside participants in the critical reflection process Ensured participants determined the extent of their engagement with the critical reflection process	Critical reflection methodology using in-depth semi-structured interviews with health promotion practitioners recruited purposively; deductive thematic analysis of qualitative data	Evidence of the positive impact on critical health promotion practice (Tretheway et al., 2017); evidence base for the development of critical reflection processes for health promotion practitioners

Kids in the Kitchen: a school-based program to enhance food preparation skills and consumption of fruit and vegetables	Policy makers and institutions	Planning, implementation and evaluation	Salutogenic approach	Designed content to ensure a strength-based orientation	Quasi-experimental pre-post program evaluation research involving self-administered in-person questionnaire with universal sample of grade 1 and grade 5 students at one school, and researcher-administered assessment of grade 1 students' food preparation skills; descriptive and inferential analysis of quantitative data	Evidence of the positive impact on children's food preparation skills and consumption of fruit and vegetables (Ritchie et al., 2015); evidence base for the development of future school-based critical health promotion programs
			Comprehensive use of evidence and theory	Used Health Promoting Schools model		
			Portfolio of multiple strategies	Integrated strategies on policy, community action, supportive environments, and personal skills		
			Working with people as an ally	Researcher-practitioner work collaboratively with students, parents, teachers, and school administrators to plan, implement, and evaluate the project		

(continued)

Table 36.2 (continued)

Project title	Focus of research	Health promotion practice cycle stage	Critical health promotion value	Application of critical health promotion value	Research design	New knowledge created and potential translation to practice
Healthy Towns: a community-based program to enhance connections between people, place and green space	Individuals and populations	Planning, implementation and evaluation	Focus on equity	Ensured that projects focused on populations where there was greatest need	Co-planning and implementation of community-based health promotion program with local organisations in four local government areas and process evaluation using analysis of program documentation and survey of project participants using an online questionnaire; content analysis of qualitative data and descriptive analysis of quantitative data	Evidence of positive engagement and satisfaction of local organisations (Taylor et al., 2019); evidence base for the development of community-based critical health promotion programs
			Salutogenic approach	Built on strengths and resources of participating towns		
			Empowering engagement processes	Connected local people (primary co-activists) to contribute to their town's health and happiness		
A yoga program to enhance holistic health and wellbeing of older people in an aged care facility	Individuals and populations	Planning, implementation and evaluation	Focus determined by equity	Focused on older people as priority equity group	Experimental randomised wait-list control pre-post design using researcher-administered physical tests and self-administered questionnaire with older people recruited from a universal study population within a residential aged care facility; descriptive and inferential analysis of quantitative data	Evidence of the positive impact on holistic health and well-being (Vogler et al., 2011); evidence base for the development of critical health promotion programs for older people
			Respect personal autonomy	Ensured that yoga poses were optional and tailored to each participant's choices		
			Maximum beneficence	Provided the yoga program to the control group after the evaluation		

Love your Body: a brief Health at Every Size-informed health promotion activity to enhance mental health and wellbeing of female university students	Individuals and populations	Planning, implementation and evaluation	Focus determined by equity	Focused on young women as priority equity group	Fully mixed methods sequential quantitative dominant design involving quasi-experimental pre-post program evaluation using a self-administered online questionnaire before, immediately after, and 10 weeks after the program, and semi-structured individual interviews at the 10 week follow-up with a convenience sample of female students at one university; descriptive and inferential analysis of quantitative data and content analysis of qualitative data	Evidence of the positive impact on mental health and well-being (O'Hara et al., 2021); evidence base for the development of critical health promotion programs for young women
			Empowering engagement processes	Young women (primary co-activists) designed, implemented, and evaluated the program		
			Comprehensive use of evidence and theory	Strategies based on evidence and theory about brief activities to enhance body positivity		
Narrative review of the weight-centred health paradigm	Policy makers and institutions	Evaluation	Focus determined by equity	Prioritised a topic that inequitably impacts on people at higher weights	Qualitative content analysis of scholarly articles, books, policies, and programs; inductive iterative thematic analysis of qualitative data	3C Framework to build critical competence for a paradigm shift (O'Hara & Taylor, 2018) and evidence of the context, critique and consequences of the weight-centred health paradigm (O'Hara & Taylor, 2018); evidence base for the development of weight-inclusive critical health promotion programs
			Holistic health paradigm, ecological science, beneficence, and non-maleficence	Investigated full range of benefits and harms at multiple levels		

(continued)

Table 36.2 (continued)

Project title	Focus of research	Health promotion practice cycle stage	Critical health promotion value	Application of critical health promotion value	Research design	New knowledge created and potential translation to practice
The extent to which Australian government 'anti-obesity' public health programs are consistent with the values and principles of critical health promotion	Policy makers and institutions	Evaluation	Focus determined by equity	Prioritised a topic that inequitably impacts on people at higher weights	Multimedia critical discourse analysis of weight-related public health initiatives commissioned or produced by the Australian Government or parliament over a 10-year period followed by critical reflection using the health promotion values and principles for heuristic support	Evidence of the discourses present in 'anti-obesity' public health programs; evidence that such programs are not consistent with the values and principles of critical health promotion (O'Hara et al., 2015a, b); evidence base for the development of weight-inclusive critical health promotion programs; and
			All values	Critiqued existing policies and programs		

The RLCHPM as a pedagogical foundation for teaching on the health promotion practice of university graduates	Stakeholders, including practitioners	Evaluation	Empowering engagement processes Maximum beneficence	Gathered graduates' (primary co-activists) perspectives Explored the range of benefits to graduates	Fully mixed methods sequential equal status design using self-administered online questionnaire-based survey with a universal sample of graduates of health promotion degree programs from one university, followed by in-depth semi- structured interviews with a convenience sample of self-selected participants from the same sample; descriptive and inferential analysis of quantitative data and deductive thematic analysis of qualitative data	Evidence of the positive impact on graduates' practice and the relative lack of impact on institutional policies (O'Hara & Taylor, 2020); evidence base for the development of additional support for graduates' critical health promotion practice and integration into institutional policies
The impact of an organisational development strategy to reorient a primary health care service towards comprehensive primary health care	Policymakers and institutions	Evaluation	Empowering engagement processes	Engaged with stakeholders (primary and secondary co-activists) to develop and implement the evaluation plan	Fully mixed methods concurrent equal status design using a self-administered online questionnaire-based survey during and after the implementation of the organisational development strategy, followed by in-depth semi-structured interviews at the same time points, with a purposive sample of employees at a primary health care service; descriptive and inferential analysis of quantitative data and deductive thematic analysis of qualitative data	Evidence of the positive impact on the primary health care service (Costello et al., 2015); evidence base for the development of future critical health promotion organisational development strategies in the primary health care setting

Experiences of Weight-Based Oppression

This health promotion research project was implemented as part of a community assessment (*program stage*) process to gather primary data related to experiences of weight-based oppression (WBO) in a university setting. WBO is a widespread phenomenon that is associated with a range of psychological, physiological, and behavioural harms (O'Hara & Taylor, 2018). Research on WBO is largely absent from the Arab region. The objective of this project was to examine internalised attitudes, values, and beliefs related to body weight, and experiences of external weight-based oppression among a sample of staff, faculty, and students at Qatar University. The study used narrative inquiry methodology involving individual in-depth semi-structured interviews with staff, faculty, and students at Qatar University recruited through purposive sampling. People with larger bodies were approached by the researchers to determine their interest in participating in the study. People with larger bodies or higher weights are subjected to higher levels of intrapersonal, interpersonal, and institutional WBO, which results in inequitable health outcomes. The study prioritised working with people at higher weight (*who to work with determined by equity)*. As researchers, it is an ethical requirement to do no (more) harm (Aphramor 2020, 12 May). We must think carefully about the potential for harm that might arise from our methods for recruitment, data collection, data analysis, and reporting. Of particular consideration in this project was the potential for harm arising from the framing of body weight. Evidence suggests that the use of pathologising language (ob*sity and overw*ight) is problematic and results in poorer health outcomes (Almond et al., 2016; Essayli et al. 2017). As such, we designed interview questions to use neutral, non-pathologising language about body weight (*non-maleficence*). In the interviews, we explored exposure to WBO at multiple interacting levels (*ecological science)* and the impact of WBO on physical, mental, spiritual, and social health and well-being (*holistic health paradigm)*, whilst respecting that people were coping the best they could, given these circumstances (*assuming that people are doing the best for their well-being)*. Inductive thematic analysis was used for the qualitative data generated from the interviews. In weekly meetings, the research team engaged in *critical reflection* with attention to issues related to the adherence to the values and principles as well as quality considerations. This enabled us to reflect on any preconceived ideas and be alert to the potential for imposing our ideas or beliefs over those of the participants. The research project generated evidence of community perspectives on WBO (O'Hara et al., 2020), which provides an evidence base for the design of critical health promotion programs to reduce WBO.

Healthy Towns

The Healthy Towns research project (Primary Health Network, 2021) involved the co-planning, implementation, and process evaluation (*program stage*) of a community-based health promotion project in four local government areas. A working group of stakeholders from primary health care, local government, community and university sectors undertook program planning and implementation. The major strategy was the initiation of an annual awards program that recognised and rewarded the contribution of local community-based organisations to building connections between people, place, and green space. Healthy Towns aimed to build on strengths and resources of participating towns (*empowering engagement processes*). To apply for an award, local community projects had to demonstrate that they were non-discriminatory (*non-maleficence*), aiming to improve the health and happiness of the community (*salutogenic approach*), addressing one or more populations where there was greatest need (*who to work with determined by equity*), sharing learnings and creating connections (*maximum beneficence*), and working towards *sustainability*. We conducted process evaluation using analysis of program documentation and a survey of project participants via an online questionnaire. Content analysis was used for qualitative data and descriptive analysis for quantitative data. At regular meetings, the Healthy Towns working group engaged in *critical reflection* about how critical health promotion values and principles were being applied in the planning, implementation, and evaluation stages of the project. The process evaluation produced evidence of positive engagement and satisfaction of local organisations in the Healthy Towns research project (Taylor et al., 2019), which contributes to the evidence base for the development of community-based critical health promotion programs.

Kids in the Kitchen

Kids in the Kitchen (Ritchie et al., 2015) was a school-based health promotion project that aimed to enhance preparation skills and consumption of fruit and vegetables in students in one primary school. Project planning, implementation, and evaluation (*program stage*) were undertaken by a team of students, teachers, school administrators, parents, and university academics, led by a teacher as the researcher-practitioner (*working with people as an ally*). The 10-week program comprised a *portfolio of multiple strategies* to develop and embed a new food-based unit into the curriculum for grades 1 and 5 that included growing, harvesting, preparing, and communal consumption of fruit and vegetables in the school setting. The program was based on the Health Promoting Schools model (*comprehensive use of evidence and theory*) and was strengths orientated (*salutogenic approach*). Impact evaluation involved quasi-experimental pre-post program evaluation research. Data collection tools were a self-administered in-person questionnaire with a universal sample of grade 1 and grade 5 students, and researcher-practitioner administered assessment of grade 1 students' food preparation skills. Descriptive and inferential analyses of quantitative data were conducted. In regular meetings, the researcher–practitioner and university academics engaged in *critical reflection* about the research elements of the project. The researcher-practitioner also met regularly with school administrators, teachers, and parents to reflect on implementation elements of the project. The research project provided evidence of the positive impact on children's preparation skills and consumption of fruit and vegetables (Ritchie et al., 2015), which contributes to the evidence base for the development of school-based critical health promotion programs.

36.4.1 Enablers and Challenges to Enacting the RLCHPM in Research

Consistent with the value of ecological science, we now reflect on the inter-related multi-dimensional factors that enable and challenge the use of the RLCHPM in health promotion research. Many research opportunities exist within the health promotion practice environment; however, these opportunities are often not taken up because research is seen as being outside the scope of everyday practice. The RLCHPM locates health promotion research within the practice context by positioning community assessment, planning, implementation, and evaluation as research-based practices. The critical health promotion values and principles component of the model ensures consideration of how the values and principles are enacted across all stages of the health promotion process cycle beyond the technical aspects of practice. Explicit consideration of the critical health promotion values and principles ensures they are privileged by researchers and researcher-practitioners in order to inform the research.

At a broader contextual level, the current global health promotion policy environment supports the use of a critical health promotion model in the Anthropocene epoch (Langmaid et al., 2020; Hancock, 2015). The Sustainable Development Goals (United Nations, n.d.), social determinants of health agenda (Lucyk & McLaren, 2017) and the Shanghai Declaration on promoting health in the 2030 agenda for sustainable development (World Health Organization, 2016) all call for more critical responses to health and well-being inequities and ecological priorities through health promotion research and practice, and the RLCHPM provides a mechanism to do so.

Challenges of using the RLCHPM in health promotion research include the need for researchers and researcher-practitioners to understand the critical theoretical foundations of the model. It also requires purposeful consideration and application of relevant critical health promotion values and principles in the design and implementation of health promotion research. There are no current guidelines or checklists for health promotion research that ensure explicit attention to underlying critical health promotion values and principles such as those that exist for other types of research, for example, the PRISMA guidelines for systematic reviews (Page et al., 2021). A further challenge is that researchers who undertake empirical health promotion research do not always explicitly position it within the health promotion practice cycle. For example, empirical research about the prevalence, incidence, determinants, or experiences of health and well-being issues within communities is rarely explicitly positioned within the community assessment stage. The use of the RLCHPH enables the positioning of empirical research within the health promotion practice cycle.

36.5 Conclusions

This chapter described and reflected on our program of critical health promotion research. The objective of our research program is to produce knowledge on the application of critical health promotion processes to address health and well-being priorities. The key elements of our research approach are the use of the RLCHPM as the health promotion framework to design and implement research projects across the four stages of the health promotion practice cycle, and the explicit use of critical health promotion values and principles in this process. Our research program is positioned with a constructivist epistemology and underpinned by critical theory, critical systems theory, and critical systems heuristics. In describing the application of the RLCHPM, we provide guidance to assist other health promotion researchers and researcher-practitioners to apply the model in their own research.

Our critical health promotion research program helps structure the field of health promotion research by contributing to the development of critical competence of researchers and researcher-practitioners. The use of the RLCHPM as the theoretical framework for health promotion research provides the field with a heuristic tool to reflect on the alignment of research practice with critical health promotion values and principles. The ultimate goal of this research program is to reorient health promotion practice towards a more critical approach to address the structural determinants of health and well-being and reduce health inequities.

References

Adams, L. (2008). *Perceptions of Nambour High School students about the factors in their school environment that impact on their health and well-being*. University of the Sunshine Coast.

Almond, D., Lee, A., & Schwartz, A. E. (2016). Impacts of classifying New York City students as overweight. *Proceedings of the National Academy of Sciences of the United States of America, 113*(13), 3488–3491. https://doi.org/10.1073/pnas.1518443113

Alvaro, C., Jackson, L. A., Kirk, S., McHugh, T. L., Hughes, J., Chircop, A., & Lyons, R. F. (2011). Moving Canadian governmental policies beyond a focus on individual lifestyle: some insights from complexity and critical theories. *Health Promotion International, 26*(1), 91–99. https://doi.org/10.1093/heapro/daq052

Antonovsky, A. (1996). The salutogenic model as a theory to guide health promotion. *Health Promotion International, 11*(1), 11–18. https://doi.org/10.1093/heapro/11.1.11

Aphramor, L. (2020). *Reframing health ethics to support liberation*. Accessed 12 May. https://medium.com/@lucy.aphramor/reframing-health-ethics-to-support-liberation-11063da4e46

Australian Health Promotion Association. (2009). *Core competencies for health promotion practitioners*.

Bammer, G. (2003). Embedding critical systems thinking and other integration and implementation sciences in the academy. In *Stream 13: OR/systems thinking for social improvement*. National Centre for Epidemiology and Population Health, The Australian National University.

Barry, M. M., Battel-Kirk, B., & Dempsey, C. (2012). The CompHP core competencies framework for health promotion in Europe. *Health Education & Behavior, 39*(6), 648–662. https://doi.org/10.1177/1090198112465620

Baum, F. (2002). *The new public health* (2nd ed.). Oxford University Press.

Baum, F. (2008). The commission on the social determinants of health: Reinventing health promotion for the twenty-first century? *Critical Public Health, 18*(4), 457–466. https://doi.org/10.1080/09581590802443612

Costello, M., Taylor, J., & O'Hara, L. (2015). Impact evaluation of a health promotion-focused organisational development strategy on a health service's capacity to deliver comprehensive primary health care. *Australian Journal of Primary Health, 21*(4), 444–449. https://doi.org/10.1071/PY14107

Crosby, R., & Noar, S. M. (2010). Theory development in health promotion: Are we there yet? *Journal of Behavioral Medicine, 33*(4), 259–263. https://doi.org/10.1007/s10865-010-9260-1

Crotty, M. (1998). *The foundations of social research: Meaning and perspective in the research process* (1st ed.). Allen and Unwin.

Eriksson, M., & Lindström, B. (2008). A salutogenic interpretation of the Ottawa Charter. *Health Promotion International, 23*(2), 190–199. https://doi.org/10.1093/heapro/dan014

Essayli, J. H., Murakami, J. M., Wilson, R. E., & Latner, J. D. (2017). The impact of weight labels on body image, internalized weight stigma, affect, perceived health, and intended weight loss behaviors in normal-weight and overweight college women. *American Journal of Health Promotion, 31*(6), 484–490. https://doi.org/10.1177/0890117116661982

Flood, R., & Romm, N. (1996). Diversity management: Theory in action. In R. Flood & N. Romm (Eds.), *Critical systems thinking: Current research and practice* (pp. 81–92). Plenum Press.

Flyvbjerg, B., Landman, T., & Schram, S. (2012). Introduction: New directions in social science. In B. Flyvbjerg, T. Landman, & S. Schram (Eds.), *Real social science: applied phronesis* (pp. 1–14). Cambridge University Press.

Gregg, J. (2012). *Development of a health promotion model and the impact evaluation of the model on practitioners' health promotion practice*. University of the Sunshine Coast.

Gregg, J., & O'Hara, L. (2007a). The Red Lotus Health Promotion Model: A new model for holistic, ecological, salutogenic health promotion practice. *Health Promotion Journal of Australia, 18*(1), 12–19. https://doi.org/10.1071/HE07012

Gregg, J., & O'Hara, L. (2007b). Values and principles evident in current health promotion practice. *Health Promotion Journal of Australia, 18*(1), 7–11. https://doi.org/10.1071/HE07007

Habermas, J. (2002). *The structural transformation of the public sphere*. Polity Press.

Habermas, J. (2004a). *The theory of communicative action: Reason and the rationalisation of society* (Vol. 1). Polity Press.

Habermas, J. (2004b). *The theory of communicative action: The critique of functionalist reason* (Vol. 2). Polity Press.

Hancock, T. (2015). Population health promotion 2.0: An eco-social approach to public health in the Anthropocene. *Canadian Journal of Public Health, 106*(4), e252–e2e5. https://doi.org/10.17269/cjph.106.5161

Held, D. (1997). *Introduction to critical theory: Horkheimer to Habermas*. Polity Press.

Jackson, M. (1991a). The origins and nature of critical systems thinking. *Systems Practice, 4*(2), 131–149.

Jackson, M. C. (1991b). Arguments between critical systems thinkers: A critical comment on Flood and Ulrich's "testament". *Systems Practice, 4*(6), 611–614.

Jackson, M. C. (1991c). *Systems methodology for the management sciences*. Plenum Press.

Jain, P. C., & Dr Daljeet. (2006). *Lotus: From a pond to a palace dome*. http://www.exoticindiaart.com/article/lotus

Langmaid, G., Patrick, R., Kingsley, J., & Lawson, J. (2020). Applying the Mandala of health in the anthropocene. *Health Promotion Journal of Australia*. https://doi.org/10.1002/hpja.434

Lucyk, K., & McLaren, L. (2017). Taking stock of the social determinants of health: A scoping review. *PloS One, 12*(5), e0177306. https://doi.org/10.1371/journal.pone.0177306

Lundy, T. (2010). A paradigm to guide health promotion into the 21st century: The integral idea whose time has come. *Global Health Promotion, 17*(3), 44–53.

Machin, D., & Mayr, A. (2012). *How to do critical discourse analysis: A multimodal introduction*. Sage.

McKinnon, J. (2008). *Assessing the holistic health and well being of the Cootharaba Community*. University of the Sunshine Coast.

Midgley, G. (1996). What is this thing called CST? In R. Flood & N. Romm (Eds.), *Critical systems thinking: Current research and practice* (pp. 11–24). Plenum Press.

Moore, B. (2001). *The Australian pocket Oxford dictionary*. Oxford University Press.

Morrow, R., & Brown, D. (1994). *Critical theory and methodology: Contemporary social theory* (Vol. 3). Sage Publications.

Norman, C. D. (2009). Health promotion as a systems science and practice. *Journal of Evaluation in Clinical Practice, 15*(5), 868–872. https://doi.org/10.1111/j.1365-2753.2009.01273.x

O'Hara, L., & Taylor, J. (2018). What's wrong with the 'war on obesity?' A narrative review of the weight-centered health paradigm and development of the 3C framework to build critical competency for a paradigm shift. *SAGE Open, 8*(2), 1–28. https://doi.org/10.1177/2158244018772888

O'Hara, L., & Taylor, J. (2020). *The impact of the Red Lotus Critical Health Promotion model on graduates' health promotion practice*. Paper presented at the Qatar University Annual Research Forum and Exhibition (QUARFE 2020), Doha, Qatar.

O'Hara, L., Taylor, J., & Barnes, M. (2015a). The extent to which the public health 'war on obesity' reflects the ethical values and principles of critical health promotion: A multimedia critical discourse analysis. *Health Promotion Journal of Australia, 26*(3), 246–254. https://doi.org/10.1071/HE15046

O'Hara, L., Taylor, J., & Barnes, M. (2015b). We are all ballooning: multimedia critical discourse analysis of 'measure up' and 'swap it, don't stop it' social marketing campaigns. *M/C Media Culture Journal, 18*(3), 1–11.

O'Hara, L., Tahboub-Schulte, S., & Thomas, J. (2016). Weight-related teasing and internalized weight stigma predict abnormal eating attitudes and behaviours in Emirati female university students. *Appetite, 102*, 44–50. https://doi.org/10.1016/j.appet.2016.01.019

O'Hara, L., Alajaimi, B., & Alshowaikh, B. (2020, October 28). *Experiences of weight-based oppression in Qatar*. Paper presented at the Qatar University Annual Research Forum and Exhibition (QUARFE 2020), Doha, Qatar.

O'Hara, L., Ahmed, H., & Elashieb, S. (2021). Evaluating the impact of a brief health at every size®-informed health promotion activity on body positivity and internalized weight-based oppression. *Body Image, 37*, 225–237. https://doi.org/10.1016/j.bodyim.2021.02.006

Page, M. J., Moher, D., Bossuyt, P. M., Boutron, I., Hoffmann, T. C., Mulrow, C. D., Shamseer, L., et al. (2021). PRISMA 2020 explanation and elaboration: Updated guidance and exemplars for reporting systematic reviews. *BMJ*, n160. https://doi.org/10.1136/bmj.n160

Parker, S. (2008). *Holistic, ecological, salutogenic health and well being of staff and students of the University of the Sunshine Coast*. University of the Sunshine Coast.

Phillips, D. C. (1995). The good, the bad, and the ugly: The many faces of constructivism. *Educational Researcher, 24*(7), 5–12.

Porter, S. (2003). Critical theory. In R. Miller & D. John (Eds.), *The A-Z of social research*. Sage Publications.

Primary Health Network. (2021). *Healthy towns*. https://healthytowns.org.au

Ritchie, B., O'Hara, L., & Taylor, J. (2015). Kids in the kitchen impact evaluation: Engaging primary school students in preparing fruit and vegetables for their own consumption. *Health Promotion Journal of Australia, 26*, 146–149. https://doi.org/10.1071/HE14074

Shelley, K., O'Hara, L., Gregg, J., & Durbridge, T. (2008). *Everybody in schools curriculum unit resource kit*. University of the Sunshine Coast.

Shelley, K., O'Hara, L., & Gregg, J. (2010). The impact on teachers of designing and implementing a health at every size curriculum unit. *Asia-Pacific Journal of Health, Sport & Physical Education, 1*(3/4), 21–28.

Simpson, K., & Freeman, R. (2004). Critical health promotion and education—A new research challenge. *Health Education Research, 19*(3), 340–348. https://doi.org/10.1093/her/cyg049

Sindall, C. (2002). Does health promotion need a code of ethics? *Health Promotion International, 17*(3), 201–203. https://doi.org/10.1093/heapro/17.3.201

Smyth, L. (2020). Social roles and alienation: Breastfeeding promotion and early motherhood. *Current Sociology, 68*(6), 814–831. https://doi.org/10.1177/0011392118807512

St Leger, L. (2001). Building and finding the new leaders in health promotion. *Health Promotion International, 16*, 301–303.

Stephens, A., Jacobson, C., & King, C. (2010). Towards a Feminist-Systems Theory. *Systemic Practice and Action Research, 23*(5), 371–386. https://doi.org/10.1007/s11213-009-9164-6

Taylor, J., O'Hara, L., Barnes, M., & Kassulke, D. (2015). *Evaluating a health promotion training strategy to develop primary health care workers' health promotion capacity*. In *Population Health Congress*. Hobart, TAS, Australia.

Taylor, J., Hudson, P., & Innes, J. (2019). *Healthy towns, happy people process evaluation*. In 23rd World conference on health promotion. Rotorua, New Zealand.

Taylor, J., O'Hara, L., Talbot, L., & Verrinder, G. (2020). *Promoting health: The primary health care approach* (7th ed.). Elsevier Australia.

Thomas, J., Quadflieg, S., & O'Hara, L. (2016). Implicit out-group preference is associated with eating disorders symptoms amongst Emirati females. *Eating Behaviors, 21*, 48–53. https://doi.org/10.1016/j.eatbeh.2015.12.005

Tremblay, M.-C., & Richard, L. (2011). Complexity: A potential paradigm for a health promotion discipline. *Health Promotion International*. https://doi.org/10.1093/heapro/dar054

Tretheway, R., Taylor, J., O'Hara, L., & Percival, N. (2015). A missing ethical competency? A review of critical reflection in health promotion. *Health Promotion Journal of Australia, 26*(3), 216–221. https://doi.org/10.1071/HE15047

Tretheway, R., Taylor, J., & O'Hara, L. (2017). Finding new ways to practise critically: Applying a critical reflection model with Australian health promotion practitioners. *Reflective Practice, 18*(5), 627–640. https://doi.org/10.1080/14623943.2017.1307721

Ulrich, W. (1987). Critical heuristics of social systems design. *European Journal of Operational Research, 31*(3), 276–283. https://doi.org/10.1016/0377-2217(87)90036-1

Ulrich, W. (1988). Systems thinking, systems practice, and practical philosophy: A program of research. *Systemic Practice and Action Research, 1*(2), 137–163. https://doi.org/10.1007/bf01059855

Ulrich, W. (2001). The quest for competence in systemic research and practice. *Systems Research and Behavioral Science, 18*(1), 3–28. https://doi.org/10.1002/sres.366

Ulrich, W. (2003). Beyond methodology choice: Critical systems thinking as critically systemic discourse. *The Journal of the Operational Research Society, 54*(4), 325–342.

Ulrich, W. (2005). *A brief introduction to critical systems heuristics (CSH)*. Milton Keynes: Systems Department and Knowledge Media Institute.

Ulrich, W., & Reynolds, M. (2010). Critical systems heuristics. In M. Reynolds & S. Holwell (Eds.), *Systems approaches to managing change: A practical guide* (pp. 243–292). Springer.

United Nations. (n.d.). *About the sustainable development goals*. United Nations. https://www.un.org/sustainabledevelopment/sustainable-development-goals/.

Vogler, J., O'Hara, L., Gregg, J., & Burnell, F. (2011). The impact of a short-term iyengar yoga program on the health and well-being of physically inactive older adults. *International Journal of Yoga Therapy, 21*(1), 61–72.

World Health Organization. (1986). *The Ottawa Charter for health promotion*. https://www.who.int/healthpromotion/conferences/previous/ottawa/en/

World Health Organization. (2016). *Shanghai Declaration on promoting health in the 2030 agenda for sustainable development*. https://www.who.int/healthpromotion/conferences/9gchp/shanghai-declaration.pdf?ua=1

Zeven, M. (2007). *The perception and relative priority of factors in the school environment that impact on the health and well-being of students attending Glenview State School*. University of the Sunshine Coast.

Chapter 37
Making Reflexivity and Emotions Visible: The Contribution of Logbooks and Polar Semantic Maps in Health Promotion Research

Patrizia Garista and Giancarlo Pocetta

37.1 Introduction

Logbooks and semantic maps are presented here as a means of reflecting and revealing narratives and emotions of members of an interdisciplinary health promotion research team. The paper goes on to consider the impact of making such narratives and emotions visible to the research team on the direction of research projects. During the last 30 years, interdisciplinary health promotion research has moved away from conventional research methods and has shifted to a more innovative approach (Labonte et al., 1999; Koelen et al., 2001; Larouche & Potvin, 2013). Two paradigms which have shaped this transition – the salutogenic model of health development and the constructivist paradigm of knowledge production – guided the design of the present study. According to the salutogenic model, people move towards healthy choices when they are able to recognize and use the available resources (Mittelmark et al., 2017). This capacity is called sense of coherence (SOC). Salutogenic theory may also support "competencies in navigating lifelong learning, such as problem-solving, guidance and reorientation, self-assessment and the communication of emotions, all skills needed for creating a balance between what is learned and what could be shifted into practice" (Garista et al., 2019). Following this perspective, knowledge production incorporates narrative skills, meaning-making, emotional recognition and reflection (Lindström, 1996).

P. Garista (✉)
National Institute of Documentation, Innovation and Educational Research, Rome, Italy

University of Perugia, Perugia, Italy
e-mail: p.garista@indire.it

G. Pocetta
Department of Medicine and Surgery, University of Perugia, Perugia, Italy

L. Potvin, D. Jourdan (eds.), *Global Handbook of Health Promotion Research, Vol. 1*,
https://doi.org/10.1007/978-3-030-97212-7_37

Like any other human practice, scientific research is deeply linked and influenced by participants' reactions. Emotions reveal how knowledge develops. Emotions are closely related to all phases of the research process, particularly when this occurs collaboratively (McLaughlin, 2003; Benozzo & Colombo, 2003). Fundamental to investigating the connection between emotions and knowledge production is the relevance of emotions. "It is not the avoidance of emotions that necessarily provides for high-quality research. Rather, it is an awareness and intelligent use of our emotions that benefits the research process" (Gilbert, 2001, p. 11).

One of the factors that determine the quality of the research itself is the visibility of emotions throughout the research process. The constructivist paradigm invites us to consider all dimensions and connections that are involved in the structuring of knowledge. The systemic perspective, deriving from this paradigm (Bateson, 1972; Kok et al., 2008; Denzin & Lincoln, 2000), calls for innovative methods related to the way researchers represent, experience and live their research activity (Labonte et al., 1999). Moreover, chaos, critical incidents, mistakes, complexity and emotions are all elements which construct experiences, capabilities and new knowledge. Research is a textual practice, a process expressed in language (sometimes a second language) that includes the acts of reading, noting, summarizing, reflecting, rereading and so on. As argued by Labonte et al. (1999), the element of meaning-making is absent from conventional research and narrative approaches appear suitable for filling this gap. Theories on narrative thinking in knowledge building were introduced by Bruner (1993) to explain the human mind and how it works. "We use a *logical thought* when dealing with abstract concepts and formal procedures, and a *narrative thought* to understand and manage social life" (Garista et al., 2015b, p. 747). This is why we naturally create stories to tell to help us make sense of the world around us. This ability to generate stories makes it easier to understand the world and reality, to provide a sense of coherence, to reflect and to recognize resources, assets or critical elements in data collection and interpretation (Bruner, 1993). Knowledge-building and learning occur when we use a narrative thinking style (cognition) but, above all, when we practice reflexivity (individually and within a research community) on what happened and on how they could be managed (meta cognition). Reflection becomes the added value in this methodology. It constructs coherence between the topic to be researched and how research is managed; it promotes a "critical consciousness of preconceptions that influence the way we conduct our business and constrains our understanding of the world and the development of knowledge" (Larouche & Potvin, 2013, p. 64).

The Salutogenic model and the constructivist paradigm suggest the importance to practice reflective research *in-action* and *on-action* (Labonte et al., 1999). A reflective approach to research could lead to deeper analysis of how a community of scholars controls what happens and how they act in a project (Strauss & Corbin, 1990), promoting individual and group empowerment (Fetterman, 2017; Rootman et al., 2001; Freire & Macedo, 1987).

Finally, we should make explicit an ethical issue underpinning the study on the use of reflective writing illustrated in the next paragraphs. *Which aspects in the process management and data sharing should be taken into account when entering in researchers' narratives? What crucial principles of health promotion and constructivism, as participation and sharing, could be guaranteed in a research community without violating privacy and anonymity?*

Data sharing, in a participatory way, is vital for producing new knowledge. At the same time, privacy and anonymity should be ensured. Reflective researchers are invited to agree on data collection and analysis, and design spaces for spontaneous participation in reflective writing.

37.2 Introducing the Use of Logbooks to the Reflective Researcher

37.2.1 The Choice of Logbook Among Narrative Methods

Given these premises, we could consider a variety of approaches and tools through which researchers document and reflect on the research process: interviews, stories, content analysis, cases and various ethnographic methods (Figley, 2001), including writing a logbook to monitor their personal contribution to the project. Among various chronicles' strategies, logbooks are introduced here as a powerful tool for knowledge and capacity-building to facilitate reflection on the research process within a specific program. Biographical storytelling, as a tool for evaluation research, can enhance participation, problem posing, reflection, critical thinking and interpretation. Logbooks, in some publications named *diaries* or *reflective journals*, are usual tools in social and educational work, in higher education and in professional development, as input for reflective practice and empowerment (Scantamburlo et al., 2016). The choice of logbook has its roots in two key trends. Firstly, in historical, cultural and, more specifically, social research and evaluation in which autobiographies, and in particular reticent autobiography, are used (Kenneth Jones, 2000). Secondly, in education, evaluation and action research in health promotion, narrative approaches are common (Labonte et al., 1999; Darlington & Scott, 2002). Kenneth Jones (2000) classifies diaries as either commissioned (solicited) or unsolicited. Our aim is to debate their added value in health promotion research.

Reflective researchers argue about topics (deliverables, outputs, evaluation and data), creating a story of the research, recollecting information and reordering actions and discussions. In other words, investigators structure a plot of the project by using narrative thinking, resulting in a scholar community in which participation and cooperation become practicable. Actions, decisions, discussions, emailing, group working, kick-off meetings, deadlines, writing, presenting reports and results are all activities that make a contribution to determining the life of a researcher in the plot of a project.

In general, the process of research can benefit from the use of the logbook in terms of: assessment of quality and quantity of intervention implementation, clarification of the theoretical pathways through which the intervention will have its intended effect, assessment of contextual factors influencing the delivery and outcomes of the action (Craig et al., 2008). Furthermore, the inclusion of the logbook as a research tool provides an opportunity for self-evaluation, individual and group empowerment. It is also a resource for the collection of latent information and tacit knowledge which would not normally surface through traditional methods.

37.2.2 The Logbook in the Context of an International Project

The context for the present critical reflection on the contribution of logbooks and polar semantic maps in health promotion research is in an international programme involving researchers from several countries, with the objective of defining health promotion competencies and their accreditation (Barry et al., 2012; Garista et al., 2015a, b). Researchers were asked to write a logbook within the evaluation work package. The overall evaluation design of the project included the integration of qualitative and quantitative strategies and tools: Desk research, Monitoring form, Questionnaires, working groups, Delphi, visual methodologies. Among these strategies, a researcher's diary was conceived as an opportunity for self-evaluation oriented towards individual and group empowerment (Fetterman, 2010; Filep et al., 2015; Morrison, 2012; Barry et al., 2012).

The idea of health promotion researchers' logbooks came from our experience of 15 years in training health, social and educational professionals in health promotion, during which we explored the potential of logbooks in higher education. The proposal of using logbooks in a research project will be presented here. It gives us the opportunity of introducing and discussing the strengths and weaknesses of reflective writing and allows us to argue that narratives could be shared and visualized without compromising the privacy of researchers, while providing us the opportunity to reflect on research (Mortari, 2007). Furthermore, polar semantic maps, derived from the data contained within logbooks, offered us the opportunity to use a visual tool which would help us understand the hidden aspects of the research process. In this sense, the logbook is revealed as a tool for disclosing the emotional dimension of the researcher's experience in the process (Filep et al., 2015; Morrison, 2012), which is shaped by a *fluid* health-promoting setting, such as a research community.

37.3 Logbooks and Polar Semantic Maps

37.3.1 Researchers' Engagement: Doing Research with Researchers

Engaging researchers from fields where reflective practice is not a *habitus* can be a challenge, as well as providing an opening for shifting methods from one discipline to another. The more participants get evidence of how information extracted from the logbooks are collected, analysed and shared, the more they feel involved and the more they participate. In our case example, results were communicated to participants and commented on by them, during intermediate meetings. This strategy created a research setting where *reflection on practice is made with researchers*, listening to their needs, expectations and doubts. In one of the project meetings, we noticed that the majority of investigators sent their reflections individually, and only a minority of researchers expressed their preference for sending their logbooks as a team (Box 37.1).

Box 37.1: Introducing a Logbook Within a Research Community
Introducing a logbook within a multidisciplinary research community can be met either with defensive reactions or with enthusiasm. In our case example, the logbook allowed leaders and researchers to feel free to write as much and whatever they wished to share with colleagues. This open task generally works with researchers who are familiar with monitoring their research through reflective tools. During our case example, a more structured format and management of the tool was requested. The reflective activity was contextualized in a multidisciplinary, multi-country and multi-professional group. The logbook proposal addressed two concerns raised by the participants: the content expected in the logbook and hesitations because of time constraints to complete this extra task. Hence, a template with a set of reflective guiding questions was drawn up (Box 37.2). This was accompanied by a covering letter outlining the usefulness of the tool and the procedure to follow when compiling the logbook. This second format could be considered a more structured logbook, guiding the process of reflection with researchers who generally use quantitative or less reflective tools. Guiding questions could be composed in line with the aim of the research, the evaluation design or specific relevant aspects of the research project. According to our experience, for a successful engagement, the task should not be mandatory but proposed as a supplementary tool for achieving a deep comprehension of complex settings.

A total number of 21 individuals were invited to complete the logbook. Every 2 months, a reminder was sent to researchers involved. In the period between the 8th month and the 32nd month of the project, there were 10 calls for sending a new piece of the logbook. All work package leaders, researchers and main collaborating partners were involved. The logbook template was modified during the project development. For instance, for the last entry, questions were slightly modified to guide reflection on other aspects, and therefore a second template was sent with the last call. The return of the logbook was considered as an expression of consent by the participants to include it in the analysis, always safeguarding anonymity. An additional consent for treating data was requested when the research project was already finished (Box 37.2).

Box 37.2: Reflective Questions for Stimulating Writing
Not all researchers felt comfortable with an open task to write something for reflection. Some prefer the following guiding questions. According to our experience, the format for writing should be flexible, negotiated and agreed. In our case example, we proposed the following reflective inputs as a first entry: *What is your role in the project? What are your feelings about the project? How do you think will your contribution to the project be valuable? Do you have any personal objectives to reach by the end of this project? How do you feel about having to complete a logbook?*

Other examples of questions for supporting a narrative thought, in and on the project, were: *How have you contributed to the project lately? What adjective would you use to describe this contribution? Did you come across any particular challenges which made you reconsider your work? Have there been any constraints that limited the development of your work? What do you think about the communication with other partners? Do you feel there is enough collaboration among partners? Is there an event or a situation you would like to share?*

Finally, for the last entry, an overall look at the writing process is investigated by questioning: *looking back at your log in the first entry...have your feelings changed about the project? Do you feel you have achieved/learnt something you weren't expecting to learn? Compiling the log is....*

37.3.2 Becoming "Logbookish" in the "Researcherhood"

The logbook proposal aroused considerable resistance and perplexity, welcomed by some researchers, less enthusiastically by others. The diaries were written in the common language (English) by just less than half of the researchers involved. Someone emphasized the importance of writing experiences in their mother tongue.

The texts were analysed following the Framework Analysis approach and data were presented anonymously in the various group meetings. The Framework Analysis (Ritchie & Spencer, 1994) is considered grounded and inductive because the analytical process moves from pre-set aims, follows structured phases, and finally underlines terms and thoughts collected on the field (Pope et al., 2000). The Framework Analysis involves the following five-step process (Ritchie & Spencer,

1994; Pope et al., 2000; Lacey & Luff, 2007): *familiarization* (immersing yourself in the raw data by reading all the collected materials in order to obtain a first list of key ideas and recurring themes); *identification* of a thematic framework; *indexing* (data coding); *creation of graphs* (abstraction and synthesis of data from different sources of information); *mapping and interpretation* (to define concepts, map the range and nature of phenomena, create typologies, polarities and associations).

Data revealed various experiences regarding participation in an international research group (a sort of "researcherhood" (Barnard, 2019)) that have given space to express thoughts and emotions in relation to the role played in the project (project leader or research contractor) and to participate in what we can define as a research community. First, we consider it to be important to report quotations on feelings of researchers about the task of writing the logbook, describing its weaknesses and strengths.

> We feel that the logbook is not our most important job, but we see the importance of it. (Researcher E)

> The logbook is cathartic but some concerns about anonymity. [...] I am using it to work out my feelings and try to refocus my role. (Researcher B)

> Useful and valuable exercise. Good reflective tool. Will try to complete more often. [...] Compiling this logbook is a good way of reflecting on what has been done and what has been learned. (Researcher A)

> A flimsy mechanism to capture and respect partners' feedback. (Researcher G)

> Fantastic for being aware of where we are. (Researcher D)

> I am convinced for the usefulness of the fieldwork diary as a tool. I make fieldwork diary whenever I'm in a research project. [...] A way to stand still and think, the best we can do in a process this long because if we wouldn't we would lose the connections with reality. (Researcher F)

> Logbookish. (Researcher H)

> I was struck by the creative/innovative way of monitoring and evaluation. (Researcher M)

> I know it is important but also time consuming. And writing about feelings and thoughts is easier in your own language. (Researcher J)

> I think the logbook is also very useful as a 'personal' reflective document and a good integrative mechanism, gives a sense of ownership of the overall project and not just individual work packages. (Researcher I – team logbook)

Secondly, we report also some quotations deriving from questioning about challenges, participation and communication.

> I'm learning to work in a team from a distance, I haven't done this so long before. (Researcher F)

> It might have been useful to get feedback from partners about some decisions points instead of letting the team make these decisions alone. (Researcher E)

> On a personal level I am slightly concerned about the contradictions and complexity of issues this raises particularly in terms of governance of health promotion and where it sits

> as a professional discipline within the wider public health workforce. (Researcher I – team logbook)

> The relationship between this project and national development worry me. (Researcher M)

> I think this teamwork is able to manage and cope with workload. (Researcher O – Team logbook)

> Usually, we discuss about the difficulties and test each other our perplexity in order to share the final decision. (Researcher L).

Some researchers did not express their thoughts on this reflective writing. We can affirm, however, that the tool was appreciated by the partners. Data analysis was very valuable for monitoring the process, and a second reading at the end of the process through the lens of emotional literature in health promotion revealed additional aspects of research life.

37.3.3 Making Reflexivity and Emotions Visible Through Polar Semantic Mapping

Maps based on opposite semantic codes (Wertz et al., 2011; Riley, 2004; Rose, 2001) were an additional tool used for data visualization, protecting privacy and anonymous reflections. The issue of anonymity was discussed extensively within project groups (Box 37.3).

Box 37.3: The Construction of Polar Semantic Maps

In our case example, polar semantic maps were created using opposite concepts coded in the narratives. A map visualizes ideas, thought and data, and could be metaphorical (e.g. an image of a tree with roots, branches, leaves, flowers and fruits to represent knowledge generation) or it could be organized in a geometrical figure. Our example shows several semantic areas created through the intersection of axis. Each axis connects two polarities, creating spatial and mental contexts to place data. A typical axis is Time, which represents a timeline where past and future are opposite sites in the research experience. Another axis example refers to "wellbeing and stressful situations," which are a very common way people feel during their experience in research/learning working group. Likewise, we can add other common opposite dimensions usually described in the narratives regarding the relationship between "the researcher and participants," or "the researcher and colleagues." Other examples of categories for creating a polar semantic axis are "communication/lack of communication" or "theoretical/methodological aspects of the research." The choice is not fixed or predetermined. On the contrary, using the Framework Analysis approach, we were able to identify routine codes, and in the end, we selected the polarities and the axis that could be intersected to place different thoughts and experiences in a meaningful way.

The first map was drawn up after the first 4 entries (month 8) (Fig. 37.1). The second map summarizes the last 6 entries and was constructed in the 34th month of the Project (Fig. 37.2). Contents centred on the Project, rather than on emotional dynamics and work relationships, may indicate a more task-oriented approach by researchers and whether researchers chose a more narrative style or shorter fragmented answers,

The positions of the key topics within these areas are not unintentional. On the contrary, the closer an element is to a polarity the more relevant it is to it. Data placed within a figure created a meta-narrative of the research community, making latent dimensions visible, as emotions, creating connections, supporting empathy and empowerment. The maps encouraged logbook writing. Following the first uncertainties and resistances, during the return of data anonymously, the interest and appreciation for the research logbook has grown, defined by someone as "cathartic," capable of raising relational and emotional aspects that can impact the involvement and personal commitment both in the research project in question and with respect to one's career in general. Emotions explicated by investigators were various. For example, the *Fear* of possible failure (the transfer of professional competencies accreditation system into the professional European health promotion reality); the *Distrust* in the acceptance of the program recommendations by the health systems of the various countries; the *Frustration* linked to the misunderstanding of one's commitment by other colleagues and the organizational environment. On the other hand, positive emotions empowered the team, as the sense of *Satisfaction* and *Gratification* in feeling a leading part of a research community committed to a project deemed capable of bringing forward one's own discipline. Emotions also

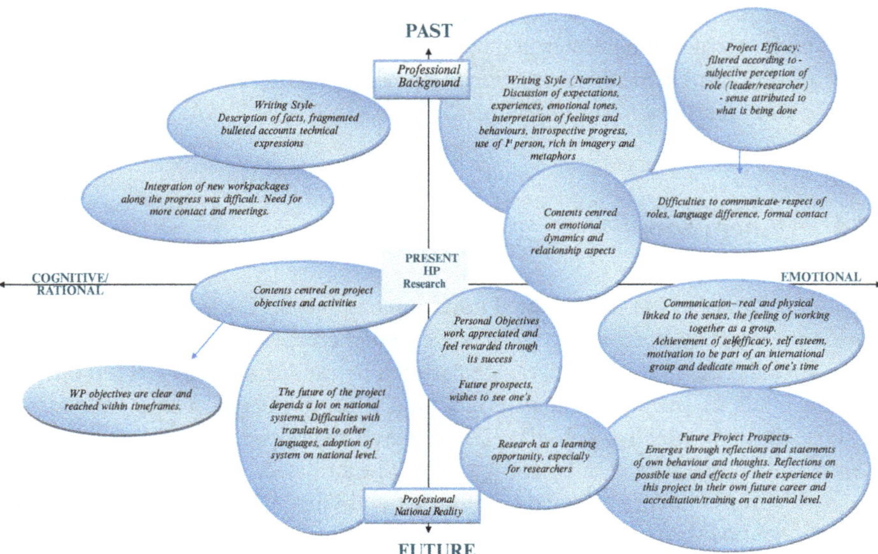

Fig. 37.1 Map 1: reflections on the research process

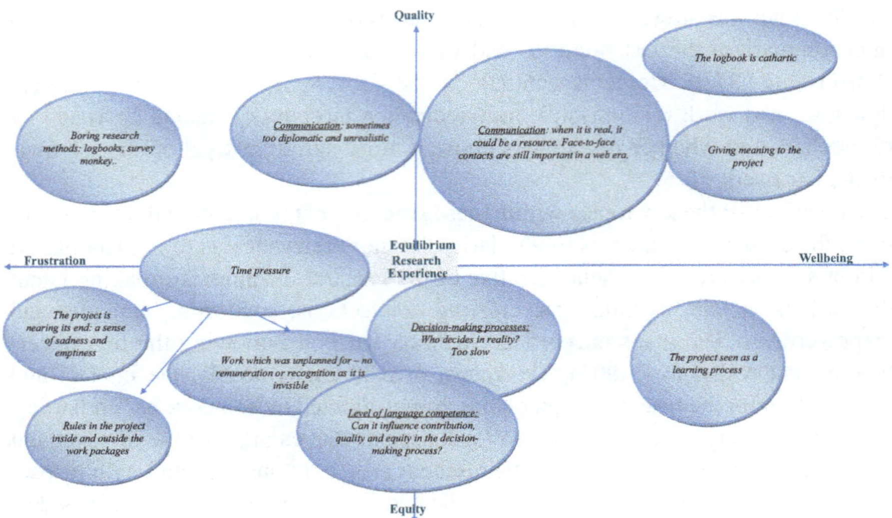

Fig. 37.2 Map 2: the research experience

describe the need to connect one's own research experience within the project to the rest of one's own professional life.

In sum, Logbooks and Polar Semantic Maps were experienced by the researchers in a positive way and proved to be effective as a research process, which include all of the most important principles of health promotion. Furthermore, it could be defined as: *participatory* (by way of researchers' contribution in defining the logbook format); *holistic* (the evaluation proposal connects the rational dimension with the emotional dimension, and the influence of the community environment to the individual); *empowering* because it generated a sense of satisfaction and of belonging to project aims and process; *critical* (showing natural tensions in knowledge building from frustration to well-being).

37.4 Conclusions

Engaging researchers in professional development, through reflective writing, provides an interesting context for a discourse on coherence between the topic to be researched and the research experience narrated by multidisciplinary and multicultural members of an international programme. The salutogenic paradigm became the lens through which to observe the research experience as a context where resources and assets need to be recognized and mobilized. Our starting point was that health promotion practice and research are embodied in practitioners' and communities' stories whose elements are often "emotionally laden" (Ferrer & Mendes, 2018, p. 1). Among narrative approaches, the use of logbooks and polar semantic maps reveal emotions and represent tacit knowledge, introducing an analytical function in research which generates reflections and ideas to guide the direction of the project. We have demonstrated that awareness of their presence and their role by means of reflective research strategies, is of crucial importance because of the potential for making a positive impact on the research process.

The contribution of logbooks and polar semantic maps make to structuring health promotion research is due to the way that reflective writing encourages and supports reflective *skills* among researchers. Researchers need to reflect and discuss the strengths and weaknesses of their research routines, by adopting tools capable of documenting and evaluating their work and which are also able to reveal latent aspects of their well-being promotion inside this fluid community. Establishing connections between the values and aims of health promotion and the contents and methods of research processes in this field must be a fundamental and distinctive objective for those who are called upon to design, manage and evaluate health promotion research. Health Promotion Research needs to innovate continuously, coping with complex and changing health issues. Reflexivity should be seen as a key competence in the management of complex and evolving situations. From this perspective, logbooks have shown to work well in this study. They are suitable tools at all levels of health promotion research for "mobilizing professional knowledge [...] promoting participation and empowerment [...] reorienting the practices [...] questioning one's own assumptions [...] innovating research perspectives" (Larouche & Potvin, 2013).

Acknowledgements We would like to express our sincere gratitude to all the researchers of the CompHP Project. We would also like to acknowledge Professor Margaret M. Barry, Dr. Barbara Battel-Kirk and Dr. Erika M. Pace for their encouragement and invaluable suggestions.

References

Barnard, A. (2019). Developing researcherhood: Identity tensions and identity work of women academics reflecting on their researcher identity. *Forum Qualitative Sozialforschung/Forum: Qualitative Social Research, 20*(3, Art. 9). https://doi.org/10.17169/fqs-20.3.3238

Barry, M., Battel-Kirk, B., Davison, H., Dempsey, C., Parish, R., Schipperen, M., & on behalf of the COMPHP Partners. (2012). *The CompHP project handbook*. International Union for Health Promotion and Education (IUHPE).

Bateson, G. (1972). *Steps to an ecology of mind*. Jason Aronson.

Benozzo, A., & Colombo, M. (2003). Le emozioni nella ricerc-azione. *Ricerche di Psicologia, 3-4*, 93–109.

Bruner, J. (1993). *Acts of meaning*. Harvard University Press.

Craig, P., Dieppe, P., McIntyre, S., Nazareth, I., & Petticrew, M. (2008). Developing and evaluating complex interventions: Medical Research Council guidance. *British Medical Journal, 337*, a1665.

Darlington, Y., & Scott, D. (2002). *Qualitative research in practice. Stories from the field*. Open University Press.

Denzin, N., & Lincoln, Y. (2000). *Handbook of qualitative research* (3rd ed.). SAGE Publications.

Ferrer, R., & Mendes, W. (2018). Emotion, health decision making, and health behaviour (Editorial). *Psychology & Health, 33*(1), 1–16. https://doi.org/10.1080/08870446.2017.1385787

Fetterman, D. M. (2010). *Etnography step-by-step* (3rd ed.). SAGE.

Fetterman, D. M. (2017). Transformative empowerment evaluation and Freirean pedagogy: Alignment with an emancipatory tradition. *Pedagogy of Evaluation, 155*, 111–126. https://doi.org/10.1002/ev.20257

Figley, C. (2001). From the series editor. In K. Gilbert (Ed.), *The emotional nature of qualitative research*. CRC Press LLC.

Filep, C., Thompson-Fawcett, M., Fitzsimons, S., & Turner, S. (2015). Reaching revelatory places: The role of solicited diaries in extending research on emotional. *Area, 47*(4), 459–465. https://doi.org/10.1111/area.12217

Freire, P., & Macedo, D. (1987). *Literacy: Reading the word and the world*. Bergin and Harvey.

Garista, P., Pace, E., Barry, M., Contu, P., Battle-Kirk, B., & Pocetta, G. (2015a). The impact of an international online accreditation system on pedagogical models and strategies in higher education. *REM – Research on Education and Media, 7*(1). https://doi.org/10.1515/rem-2015-0006

Garista, P., Sardu, C., Mereu, A., Campagna, M., & Contu, P. (2015b). The mouse gave life to the mountain: Gramsci and health promotion. *Health Promotion International*, 746–755. https://doi.org/10.1093/heapro/dau002

Garista, P., Pocetta, G., & Lindström, B. (2019). Picturing academic learning: Salutogenic and health promoting perspectives on drawings. *Health Promotion International, 34*(4), 859–868. https://doi.org/10.1093/heapro/day027

Gilbert, K. (2001). Introduction: Why are we interested in emotions? In K. R. Gilbert (Ed.), *The emotional nature of qualitative research*. CRC Press LLC.

Kenneth Jones, R. (2000). The unsolicited diary as a qualitative research tool for advanced research capacity in the field of health and illness. *Qualitative Health Research, 10*(4), 555–567.

Koelen, M., Vaandrager, L., & Colomer, C. (2001). Health promotion research: Dilemmas and challenges. *Journal of Epidemiology and Community Health, 55*(4), 257–262.

Kok, G., Gottlieb, N., Commers, M., & Smerecnik, C. (2008). The ecological approach in health promotion programs: A decade later. *American Journal of Health Promotion*, 437/441. https://doi.org/10.4278/ajhp.22.6.437

Labonte, R., Feather, J., & Hills, M. (1999). A story/dialogue method for health promotion. Knowledge development and evaluation. *Health Education Research Theory and Practice, 14*, 39–50.

Lacey, A., & Luff, L. (2007). *Qualitative research analysis*. The NIHR RDS for the East Midlands.

Larouche, A., & Potvin, L. (2013). Stimulating innovative research in health promotion. *Global Health Promotion, 20*(2), 64–69. https://doi.org/10.1177/1757975913490428

Lindström, B. (1996). *Forming a salutogenic learning model*. Nordic Health Promotion Research Conference, Bergen.

McLaughlin, C. (2003). The feeling of finding out: The role of emotions in research. *Educational Action Research, 11*(1). https://doi.org/10.1080/09650790300200205

Mittelmark, M. B., Sagy, S., Eriksson, M., Bauer, G. F., Pelikan, J. M., Lindström, B., & Espnes, G. A. (Eds.). (2017). *The handbook of salutogenesis*. Springer.

Morrison, C. A. (2012). Solicited diaries and the everyday geographies of heterosexual love and home: Reflections on methodological process and practice. *Area, 44*(1), 68–75. https://doi.org/10.1111/j.1475-4762.2011.01044.x

Mortari, L. (2007). Il Diario di Ricerca. In L. Mortari (Ed.), *Cultura della Ricerca e Pedagogia* (pp. 227–238). Carocci.

Pope, C., Ziebland, S., & Mays, N. (2000). Analysing qualitative data. *British Medical Journal, 320*, 114. https://doi.org/10.1136/bmj.320.7227.114

Riley, H. (2004). Perceptual modes, semiotic codes, social mores: A contribution towards a social semiotic of drawing. *Visual Communication, 3*(3), 294–315.

Ritchie, J., & Spencer, E. (1994). Qualitative data analysis for applied policy research. In A. Bryman & R. Burgess (Eds.), *Analyzing qualitative data*. Routledge.

Rootman, I., Goodstadt, M., Potvin, L., & Springett, J. (2001). A framework for health promotion evaluation. In I. Rootman (Ed.), *Evaluation in health promotion. Principles and perspectives* (European series; n. 92) (Vol. 92, pp. 7–40). WHO Regional Publications.

Rose, G. (2001). *Visual methodologies*. SAGE Publications Ltd.

Scantamburlo, G., Vierset, V., Bonnet, P., Verpoorten, D., Delfosse, C., & Ansseau, M. (2016). Electronic logbook: Learning tool and teaching aid for the evaluation of learning activities. *Revue Médicale de Liège, Apr, 71*(4), 210–215.

Strauss, A., & Corbin, J. (1990). *Basics of qualitative research: Grounded theory procedures and techniques*. SAGE.

Wertz, F., Charmaz, K., McMullen, L., Josselson, R., Anderson, R., & McSpadden, E. (2011). *Five ways of doing qualitative analysis*. The Guilford Press.

Chapter 38
Steering Committee: A Participatory Device to Support Knowledge Flow and Use in Health Promotion

Marianne Beaulieu, Alix Adrien, Clément Dassa, Louise Potvin, and The Comité consultatif sur les attitudes envers les PVVIH

38.1 Introduction

Despite large-scale investments in research and development and the generation of a high number of scientific results, these results are rarely utilized or adopted in practice (Green et al., 2009). As a result, there is a persistent gap between research and action. This research-action gap is particularly problematic for health promotion stakeholders who seek to strengthen community actions to ensure "full and continuous access to information, learning opportunities for health, as well as funding support." (WHO, 1986) It is essential to find solutions to bridge the gap between "what we know and what we do" (Graham & Tetroe, 2009, p. 46).

The Comité consultatif sur les attitudes envers les PVVIH

M. Beaulieu (✉)
Faculty of Nursing, Université Laval, Québec, QC, Canada

VITAM – Centre de recherche en santé durable, Québec, QC, Canada
e-mail: marianne.beaulieu@fsi.ulaval.ca

A. Adrien
Direction régionale de santé publique, Centre intégré universitaire de santé et de services sociaux du Centre-Sud-de-l'Île-de-Montréal, Montréal, QC, Canada

Department of Epidemiology, Biostatistics and Occupational Health, McGill University, Montréal, QC, Canada

C. Dassa
School of Public Health, Département de médecine sociale et préventive, University of Montreal, Montréal, QC, Canada

L. Potvin
School of Public Health, University of Montreal, Montréal, QC, Canada

Centre de recherche en santé publique (CReSP) Université de Montréal and CIUSSS du Centre-Sud-de-l'Île-de-Montréal, Montréal, QC, Canada

L. Potvin, D. Jourdan (eds.), *Global Handbook of Health Promotion Research, Vol. 1*,
https://doi.org/10.1007/978-3-030-97212-7_38

Usually, this research-action gap is attributed to a knowledge transfer problem or to the fact that, while scientific knowledge and practical knowledge are complementary, they are fundamentally different. Van de Ven and Johnson (2006) suggested another way to understand this situation, "namely, that the gap between theory and practice is a knowledge production problem" (p. 803). From this perspective, a steering committee, which is a participatory research device, is a promising way to close this gap because of the co-creation processes that arise from the participation of all stakeholders at every step of the research (Brownson et al., 2006; Campbell, 2010; Cargo & Mercer, 2008; Colditz et al., 2008; Israel et al., 1998; Scharff & Mathews, 2008; Vingilis et al., 2003). This ensures the formulation of research questions that are relevant for action and have real-world applicability, the creation of realistic research designs and data collection procedures, the generation of results that are more useful and meet real needs, and a deeper interpretation of the context.

Participatory research approaches aim to bring the two worlds of knowledge production and knowledge "use" together to allow information to be shared among different stakeholders who wish to solve a problem or advance a cause. This in turn facilitates integrated knowledge translation (IKT), which requires "the development of a relationship between academic researchers and practitioners and/or policymakers for the purposes of collaboratively engaging in a mutually beneficial research project or programme of research" (Kothari & Wathen, 2013, p. 188).

In this collaboration, knowledge translation is thought of, not as a relatively linear or cyclical process (Ward et al., 2009), but as a complex dynamic process involving various stakeholders that builds and evolves as the research project unfolds (Green et al., 2009; Lavis et al., 2003). Iterative communication processes also allow for continuous consultation with an audience that is interested in the proposed strategies and ready to use them. This leads to multidirectional exchanges involving two aspects: knowledge flow and knowledge utilization (KFU). As Zhuge (2002) explains:

> A knowledge flow is a process of knowledge passing between people or knowledge processing mechanism. It has three crucial attributes: direction, content and carrier, which respectively, determine the sender and the receiver, the sharable content and the media that can pass the content.

According to Stetler (2001), "research [knowledge] utilization is the process of transforming research knowledge into practice." (p. 272) Research results are used in three distinct forms. *Instrumental use* refers to direct and concrete applications designed to carry out interventions and support specific decisions (Beyer, 1997; Estabrooks, 1999). *Conceptual or cognitive use* involves the use of research for general enlightenment and potentially to change ways of thinking (Beyer, 1997; Estabrooks, 1999). Here, the influence is more indirect and less precise than with instrumental use (Beyer, 1997). *Symbolic or strategic use* is the use of research as a political or persuasive tool to legitimize a position or influence the practice of others (Beyer, 1997; Estabrooks, 1999). The scope of the KFU depends not only on the relationships and interactions between the stakeholders (Greenhalgh et al., 2004) but also on the relevance of the knowledge produced and the extent and diversity of the professional networks involved (Barreteau et al., 2010; Bowen et al., 2005; Cowan & Jonard, 2004; Fritsch & Kauffeld-Monz, 2010; Granovetter, 1983; Innvaer et al., 2002; Jansson et al., 2010; Liu, 2011; Loew et al., 2004; Lomas, 2007; Mitton et al., 2007; Reagans & McEvily, 2003; Singh, 2005; Sorenson et al., 2006; Vingilis et al., 2003).

This chapter presents a case study of a specific participatory device, namely a steering committee, and examines its contribution to KFU. This research addresses HIV stigmatization, which is a priority for both government and community organizations (Coalition des organismes communautaires québécois de lutte contre le sida, 2011; Ministère de la Santé et des Services sociaux du Québec, 2003). Hence, a steering committee bringing together different interest groups was created to consider the issue. More specifically, the patterns of knowledge flow within the professional networks are analysed below, as is the way in which the research results were used.

38.1.1 Role of a Steering Committee in KFU

Previous studies have emphasized partnerships between two specific groups of stakeholders, namely researchers and policymakers (Brownson & Jones, 2009; Lavis et al., 2003). However, community organizations and healthcare professionals are also key stakeholders in ensuring the sustainability of interventions (Kothari & Armstrong, 2011; Mallonee et al., 2006). Although these stakeholders may have different perspectives, expectations, and values, they are motivated by the common ultimate goal of participating in a knowledge co-creation approach (Jull et al. 2017; Kothari & Wathen, 2017; Nguyen et al., 2020). Their participation is facilitated by social interactions through frequent meetings or regular exchanges over a period of time. This is often formalized in a specific device, such as a steering committee that is involved on an ongoing basis as the research progresses (Koné et al., 2000; Newman et al., 2011).

38.1.2 Knowledge Access Method

While some consider IKT to be epistemologically neutral (a research approach rather than the object of research), others associate it more with a social constructivist epistemology (research concerning relationships and partnerships between knowledge producers and knowledge users) (Nguyen et al., 2020). This chapter reflects the second perspective. In addition to explaining "how individuals integrate and apply new knowledge," it also seeks to reveal "the ways in which individuals and groups participate in the creation of their perceived social reality" (Thomas et al., 2014). Indeed, it highlights the role of social relationships not only in the flow of knowledge but also in its transformation. From the perspective of a knowledge producer (or researcher), "knowledge" arises directly from research results, i.e. a research result IS knowledge. In contrast, once research results are produced, they may be transformed by users into useful and relevant knowledge. This means that knowledge users engaged in a steering committee do more than simply "use knowledge" in a passive manner; they participate actively in its transformation and play a role more akin to "knowledge mobilisers (people who move knowledge into action)" (Ward, 2017). These transformations, which were observed particularly in instrumental and strategic uses, show that "knowledge" is a social construct. This is consistent with several knowledge mobilization models that present "a collaborative or co-productive view of knowledge mobilization involving the continual shaping and re-shaping of knowledge between parties." Thus, partnerships between knowledge producers and knowledge users aimed at co-constructing "knowledge" in IKT call into question the notion of "expertise," revealing it to be shared among the stakeholders (Kothari & Wathen, 2013).

38.2 Documenting KFU

A PhD student in health promotion (M. Beaulieu) was interested in the contribution of participatory approaches in improving KFU. Therefore, she included in her doctoral work a population survey on the stigmatization of people living with HIV in 2010, and a steering committee (participatory device) of 11 members from various backgrounds who had six mandates (see Table 38.1). Several members had been recommended by the research coordinator of the provincial coalition of HIV community organizations. Others were identified by the research team as leaders whose expertise may be relevant to the committee's work. Committee members were also recruited on the basis of their interest in HIV stigma. The committee met over a period of 3 years. In addition to their formal meetings, there were frequent emails and telephone conversations (at least once per month) before, during and after the survey.

Two scientific productions were analysed. The first was a short outreach article on trends in HIV knowledge between 1996 and 2010. This article was written a few weeks after the survey ended (July 2010), at a committee member's suggestion. It was published in the Quebec AIDS Foundation bulletin. This article included a bar graph and short narrative which concluded that HIV knowledge decreased significantly from 1996 to 2010. The second was a preliminary research report shared with the steering committee nearly 6 months after the survey ended (November 2010). This draft was discussed at a committee meeting, where members asked questions regarding the statistical analyses and results tables to be sure they understood and interpreted them correctly. The report (approximately 50 pages) presented the complete survey results along with tables and bar charts. It identified new forms of stigmatizing attitudes towards PLHIV and target groups for awareness interventions.

Table 38.1 Committee members' profiles and committee mandates

<table>
<tr><th>Committee members</th><th>Group affiliation</th><th>Mandates</th></tr>
<tr><td>A</td><td>Government agency</td><td rowspan="11">1. Identify new concerns about attitudes towards PLHIV in the general population of Quebec and define the research questions.
2. Ensure the social relevance of the research questions.
3. Participate in the development of the measurement scale.
4. Contribute to the interpretation of the research results and formulate recommendations.
5. Disseminate the results in their networks.
6. Review publications.</td></tr>
<tr><td>B</td><td>PhD Student</td></tr>
<tr><td>C</td><td>Person living with HIV</td></tr>
<tr><td>D</td><td>Person living with HIV</td></tr>
<tr><td>E</td><td>Community organization</td></tr>
<tr><td>F</td><td>Community organization</td></tr>
<tr><td>G</td><td>Government agency</td></tr>
<tr><td>H</td><td>Community organization</td></tr>
<tr><td>I</td><td>Community organization</td></tr>
<tr><td>J</td><td>Healthcare professional</td></tr>
<tr><td>K</td><td>Healthcare professional</td></tr>
</table>

To document KFU in the steering committee, three sources of data were used to triangulate the findings. First, semi-structured interviews were conducted with the steering committee members (n = 11) to explore the dissemination and use of the research results. Second, the proceedings of the five formal committee meetings were analysed. Third, Google and media (newspapers, television) searches were conducted using specific keywords ([attitudes towards PLHIV], [knowledge of HIV transmission], and "A" & "B"). The results present KFU in terms of knowledge flow between senders and receivers and its scope as well as KT facilitators and barriers.

38.3 Examining KFU Through Two Scientific Productions

38.3.1 Outreach Article

The paths for the outreach article (Fig. 38.1) reveal that B was the first sender and that two committee members disseminated the article: F and G. As expected, F published the article in the Quebec AIDS Foundation bulletin for donors.

> I suggested publishing the survey results in a [Foundation] bulletin (...) This is interesting because it is a different format, which is addressed to the general population of 7,000 donors. There is an English and a French version. (...) [In the article], there is a small table

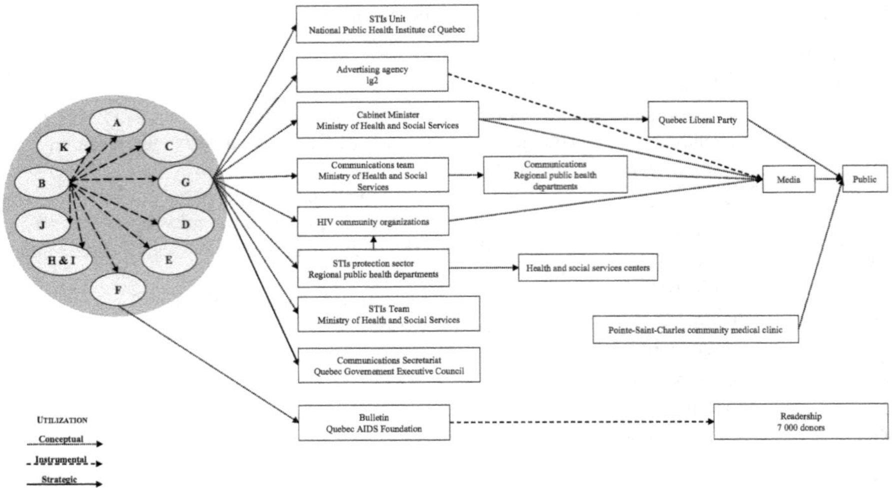

Fig. 38.1 Paths of outreach article results. (Adapted from Beaulieu, 2014)

> in which we presented the results of the survey. (...) It is a place where one really has to make sure that the writing is generic and accessible. B was asked to write it to ensure that there was no bias, it's always better when a researcher does the writing.
>
> (F, community organization)

Meanwhile, G had emailed the article in its original form (conceptual use) to three types of partners: (1) public and parapublic agencies involved in the fight against sexually transmitted infections (STIs), (2) decision makers in the provincial government's Executive Council and an advertising agency and (3) community organizations. It is noteworthy that several receivers in G's network became secondary-senders and even tertiary-senders.

The outreach article was used by G for different reasons depending on the receiver targeted. He used it with decision makers to obtain funding (strategic use) to plan a provincial awareness campaign with the advertising agency (conceptual use). Most of the secondary-senders used the article results to announce the World AIDS Day awareness campaign (press release) or published articles on what it is like to live with HIV in 2010 (conceptual use). Only the advertising agency used the results directly to design the provincial awareness campaign (poster and radio messages) (instrumental use).

> We used the research data to convince the Communications team to argue with the government Communications Secretariat. (…) For the advertising agency it was: 'Here are the data we have.' This was the starting point to produce the message. (...) [The] message [was] general and resulted in a poster showing a man working in his office full of people hiding: behind plants, behind the water fountain.
>
> (G, government agency)

Most of the paths converged towards the media and ultimately targeted the general public. The outreach article's paths (Fig. 38.1) show that several transactions between senders and receivers are often necessary before reaching the general public. In addition, publication of the article enabled organizations/individuals outside the committee to use the research results in multiple ways without being in direct contact with a committee member (mainly through conceptual use).

38.3.2 *Preliminary Research Report*

The paths for the preliminary research report (Fig. 38.2) reveal that B was the first sender and that the majority of committee members transferred part of the information. There were three different profiles of receivers for the results presented in the preliminary version of the research report: (1) community organizations (youth centre, HIV prevention), some PLHIV and Gay Pride participants, (2) public and parapublic organizations and (3) an advertising agency. In only a few cases, receivers became secondary-senders to eventually reach the general public. Very few examples of KU by organizations or individuals outside the committee were identified.

Compared to the outreach article, the results of the preliminary research report led to a wider range of uses in the committee. Engagement in the conceptual use of the results took place on a more individual basis, especially for the committee members from community organizations, as they reflected on their professional practice and compared their lay experience with the scientific data. For others, engagement in the conceptual use involved sharing the results with colleagues in more or less formal contexts or adapting their intervention messages. For example, one committee member from a public agency sent the preliminary research report to a decision maker (Deputy Minister of Health) so that he could prepare for media interviews (conceptual use). Another member said:

> We relied on the results of the survey to convey information better. For example, in the case of our workshops, we tell people: 'You know that for people of a certain age, they say such a thing. This can have such a result, you need to know such a thing.' So we adapt the

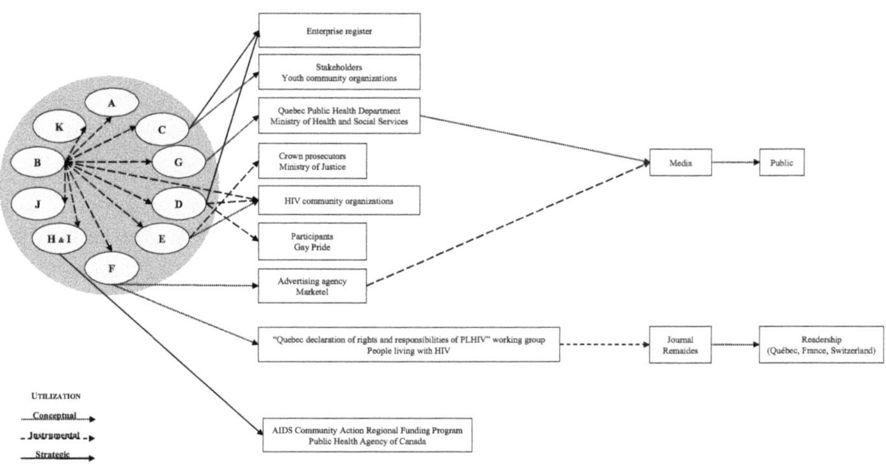

Fig. 38.2 Paths of preliminary research report results. (Adapted from Beaulieu, 2014)

> information. (...) It's not that I systematically disseminate the survey results but it will help me to understand certain behaviors better and (...) improve how I intervene in some situations.
>
> (H, community organization)

Instrumental uses took different forms, such as Gay Pride awareness posters as well as scientific conferences and publications. They also led to a shift in community interventions and the development of a training session for HIV community groups. The knowledge generated throughout the survey was used by a committee member (community organization) to target and design awareness campaigns.

> In January, I organized [a training day], (…) that we called 'Acting together against stigma and discrimination.' (...) B and D joined forces to present the preliminary survey results to community stakeholders, to inform them about the public's attitudes and to introduce them in a format they could use later. It thus directly helped to build capacity. There were about sixty participants in this training, it was a large audience. There was a time for sharing and questions, discussions with B at the end.
>
> (E, community organization)

As for strategic use of the preliminary report results, only a minority of the committee members, particularly PLHIV and community groups, tried this. Some created written material to advocate against HIV criminalization with Crown prosecutors, while others used the results to support their efforts to sustain existing program funding and to create a new community group.

> I used [the results] to create a group with D and someone else. (...) We founded an organization and we relied in part on the research results to justify our raison d'être, to draft the project (...) and to get funding. Somewhere in the results of the study it says there is still education to do.
>
> (C, PLHIV)

Unlike with the outreach article, committee members worked together to plan actions (B & D organized a provincial training session for HIV community organizations while C & D registered a new community group). In terms of scope, Fig. 38.2 suggests more limited scope and more direct, simple and personalized sender-receiver transactions. Rather than observing paths converge on some receivers (media, public), there is a plurality of KF directly initiated by committee members.

38.3.3 Experience of Participation and KFU

Most of the committee members explained that since they were involved in formulating questions and the research design, the results obtained were especially important for them. Moreover, the relevance of the analyses, the presentation of the results, and access to an official published document (research report) contributed to the conceptual use of the results. They also noted that they were more likely to use the results just by being part of the committee since they were more familiar with the investigation.

> We actively participated [in the process], we assisted in formulating questions, and we also helped to select themes. It made it easier for us to adopt this tool because we were in there right from the start.
> (H, community organization)

Others spoke of the close relationship with the researcher, which gave them an opportunity to question the researchers about the results and to receive immediate and clear explanations regarding their interpretations. They also believed that this relationship allowed for unusual access to precise and timely data, which seemed to favour an instrumental use of the research results.

> There were representatives from different levels. (...) And [B] had the patience to explain, to get everyone on the same level to deliver these results. I remember an anecdote where E (...) said: 'I'm not good with numbers, it's Chinese to me.' It was difficult to understand the statistics clearly and precisely. [B] could still get everyone on the same level and we realized it was possible to interpret the graphs and tables of statistical data.
> (I, community organization)

> According to the research, HIV transmission knowledge regressed on some aspects. I had a relationship with [B] so I could say, 'Is there a way to get more details about these data?' B has always shown great generosity in regard to needs I might have, which were not necessarily the needs of the committee. (...) So the fact that we had very accurate data at some point, it was very useful to guide the campaign.
> (G, government agency)

38.4 Discussion

This chapter describes a knowledge-sharing approach focusing on the flow and utilization (instrumental, cognitive and strategic) of research results. More specifically, it examines the partnership and functioning of a participatory device involving stakeholders with different profiles engaged in a long-term dialogue. It highlights some challenges, but also provides some important lessons for health promotion research.

First, it is important for health promotion researchers to adopt an engaged posture (Beaulieu et al., 2018) rather than the traditional posture of 'knowledge producer' in order to foster the utilization and dissemination of knowledge in collaboration with a steering committee. This suggests that, in addition to participating in the production of knowledge, researchers are in an unusual position at the interface between science and practice. Meaningful (Bowen & Graham, 2013) and reciprocal (Petras & Porpora, 1993) interactions over a long period of time transform the researcher into a resource person, whom other members can turn to with formal or informal questions and requests (Innvaer et al., 2002), which in turn fosters understanding, and utilization of the results. Thus the researcher is not only engaged in the research process but also becomes a true change agent (Checkoway, 2013), who collaborates in different actions taken by the committee members to produce and explain high-quality scientific results in lay terms in a timely manner

(Brownson et al., 2013). This is essential to support evidence-informed policy and practice in health promotion. However, some may view this proximity as problematic and even dubious due to the researchers' apparent lack of intellectual independence (Grey, 2001). Researchers who use participatory components in their projects do not necessarily share this view, which entails maintaining a distance from their research subject. To combat such criticisms, however, their methodological rigour must be flawless.

The composition of advisory committees benefits from including different profiles of stakeholders in order to expand the uses and impact of the knowledge. With a variety of profiles, diverse views can be reflected; for example, members may be university researchers, stakeholders from agencies/public organizations, representatives of community organizations and individuals who could be positively or negatively affected by the research results (Dukma et al., 2007; Greenwood et al., 1993; Guba & Lincoln, 1989; Israel et al., 1998, 2005; Payne, 1999; Schulz et al., 2000). Far from being perceived as having a passive role, the committee members are active participants from the public health system (Kohatsu et al., 2004). It does not take long for their mobilization and active involvement in the research process to affect their thoughts and professional practices, which in turn expands the influence of the scientific results in their respective networks. In addition, how the knowledge was used differed according to the committee members' profiles. For example, there were more instrumental and strategic uses of the research results among community partners, which suggests that they could play an active part in closing the gap between research and practice (Kothari & Armstrong 2011; Mallonee et al., 2006). Although this diversity has considerable advantages, it can also be a major challenge. For example, members may have opposing interests in participating in the research, which requires coordination of and skilful negotiations between the differing points of view in order to reach compromises between the partners at different steps in the research project: developing the objectives, interpreting the results, disseminating the results and deciding which actions to take. In this context, it is not enough for researchers to be effective in producing 'science'; from time to time, they must also act as 'mediators' in interpersonal relationships to maintain mobilization and a healthy work environment.

38.5 Conclusions

In this chapter, we have presented a case study illustrating the contribution of a specific participatory device, namely a steering committee composed of stakeholders from different environments, to KFU. This committee was involved at every step in developing the project: formulating the research questions, developing the measurement scale, planning the data collection, analysing the data and disseminating the results. We discovered that the interactions on the steering committee fostered a variety of uses and transformations of the research results into knowledge that was useful and relevant to the practices of the stakeholders involved.

These findings suggest that mobilizing a steering committee to lead and design research projects is a real benefit for health promotion research. In fact, this type of participatory device is the incarnation of a founding principle in health promotion, namely the participation of different stakeholders to study and solve complex problems.

References

Barreteau, O., Bots, P. W. G., & Daniell, K. A. (2010). A framework for clarifying "participation" in participatory research to prevent its rejection for the wrong reasons. *Ecology and Society, 15*, 1.

Beaulieu, M. (2014). *Attitudes stigmatisantes envers les personnes vivant avec le VIH : développement et validation d'un instrument de mesure intégrant un dispositif participatif* (Thesis/Dissertation). Université de Montréal.

Beaulieu, M., Breton, M., & Brousselle, A. (2018). Conceptualizing 20 years of engaged scholarship: A scoping review. *PLoS ONE, 13*(2), e0193201.

Beyer, J. M. (1997). Research utilization: Bridging the gap between communities. *Journal of Management Inquiry, 6*, 17–22.

Bowen, S. J., & Graham, I. D. (2013). From knowledge translation to engaged scholarship: Promoting research relevance and utilization. *Archives of Physical Medicine and Rehabilitation., 94*(1 Suppl), S3–S8.

Bowen, S., Martens, P., & The Need to Know Team. (2005). Demystifying knowledge translation: Learning from the community. *Journal of Health Services Research & Policy, 10*, 203–211.

Brownson, R. C., & Jones, E. (2009). Bridging the gap: Translating research into policy and practice. *Preventive Medicine, 49*, 313–315.

Brownson, R. C., Kreuter, M. W., Arrington, B. A., & True, W. R. (2006). Translating scientific discoveries into public health action: How can schools of public health move us forward? *Public Health Reports, 121*, 97–103.

Brownson, R. C., Fielding, J. E., & Maylahn, C. M. (2013). Evidence-based decision making to improve public health practice. *Frontiers in Public Health Services and Systems Research, 2*(2), Article 2.

Campbell, B. (2010). Applying knowledge to generate action: A community-based knowledge translation framework. *Journal of Continuing Education in the Health Professions, 30*, 65–71.

Cargo, M., & Mercer, S. L. (2008). The value and challenges of participatory research: Strengthening its practice. *Annual Review of Public Health, 29*, 325–350.

Checkoway, B. (2013). Strengthening the scholarship of engagement. *Journal of Higher Education Outreach and Engagement., 17*(4), 7–22.

Coalition des organismes communautaires québécois de lutte contre le sida. (2011). *Réglements généraux*. Coalition des organismes communautaires québécois de lutte contre le sida.

Colditz, G. A., Emmons, K. M., Vishwanath, K., & Kerner, J. F. (2008). Translating science to practice: Community and academic perspectives. *Journal of Public Health Management and Practice, 14*, 144–149.

Cowan, R., & Jonard, N. (2004). Network structure and the diffusion of knowledge. *Journal of Economic Dynamics and Control, 28*, 1557–1575.

Dumka, L. E., Mauricio, A. M., & Gonzales, N. A. (2007). Research partnerships with schools to implement prevention programs for Mexican origin families. *Journal of Primary Prevention, 28*(5), 403–420.

Estabrooks, C. A. (1999). The conceptual structure of research utilization. *Research in Nursing & Health, 22*, 203–216.

Fritsch, M., & Kauffeld-Monz, M. (2010). The impact of network structure on knowledge transfer: An application of social network analysis in the context of regional innovation networks. *Annals of Regional Science, 44*, 21–38.
Graham, I. D., & Tetroe, J. M. (2009). Getting evidence into policy and practice: Perspective of a health research funder. *Journal of the Canadian Academy of Child and Adolescent Psychiatry, 18*(1), 46–50.
Granovetter, M. (1983). The strength of weak ties: A network theory revisited. *Sociological Theory, 1*, 201–233.
Green, L. W., Ottoson, J. M., García, C., & Hiatt, R. A. (2009). Diffusion theory and knowledge dissemination, utilization, and integration in public health. *Annual Review of Public Health, 30*, 151–174.
Greenhalgh, T., Robert, G., Macfarlane, F., Bate, P., & Kyriakidou, O. (2004). Diffusion of innovations in service organizations: Systematic review and recommendations. *Milbank Quarterly, 82*, 581–629.
Greenwood, D. J., Whyte, W. F., & Harkavy, I. (1993). Participatory action research as a process and as a goal. *Human Relations, 46*(2), 175–192.
Grey, C. (2001). Re-imagining relevance: A response to Starkey and Madan. *British Journal of Management, 12*(Special Issue), S27–S32.
Guba, E., & Lincoln, Y. (1989). *Fourth generation evaluation*. Sage.
Innvaer, S., Vist, G., Trommald, M., & Oxman, A. (2002). Health policy-makers' perceptions of their use of evidence: A systematic review. *Journal of Health Services Research and Policy, 7*, 239–244.
Israel, B. A., Schulz, A. J., Parker, E. A., & Becker, A. B. (1998). Review of community-based research: Assessing partnership approaches to improve public health. *Annual Review of Public Health, 19*, 173–202.
Israel, B. A., Parker, E. A., Rowe, Z., Salvatore, A., Minkler, M., López, J., … Halstead, S. (2005). Community-based participatory research: Lessons learned from the centers for children's environmental health and disease prevention research. *Environmental Health Perspective., 113*(10), 1463–1471.
Jansson, S. M., Benoit, C., Casey, L., Phillips, R., & Burns, D. (2010). In for the long haul: Knowledge translation between academic and nonprofit organizations. *Qualitative Health Research, 20*, 131–143.
Jull, J., Giles, A., & Graham, I. D. (2017). Community-based participatory research and integrated knowledge translation: Advancing the co-creation of knowledge. *Implementation Science, 12*(1), 150.
Kohatsu, N. D., Robinson, J. G., & Torner, J. C. (2004). Evidence-based public health: An evolving concept. *American Journal of Preventive Medicine, 27*(5), 417–421.
Koné, A., Sullivan, M., Senturia, K. D., Chrisman, N. J., Ciske, S. J., & Krieger, J. W. (2000). Improving collaboration between researchers and communities. *Public Health Reports, 115*, 243–248.
Kothari, A., & Armstrong, R. (2011). Community-based knowledge translation: Unexplored opportunities. *Implementation Science, 6*, 59.
Kothari, A., & Wathen, C. N. (2013). A critical second look at integrated knowledge translation. *Health Policy, 109*(2), 187–191.
Kothari, A., & Wathen, C. N. (2017). Integrated knowledge translation: Digging deeper, moving forward. *Journal of Epidemiology and Community Health, 71*(6), 619–623.
Lavis, J., Ross, S., McLeod, C., & Gildiner, A. (2003). Measuring the impact of health research. *Journal of Health Services Research and Policy, 8*, 165–170.
Liu, C.-H. (2011). The effects of innovation alliance on network structure and density of cluster. *Expert Systems with Applications: An International Journal Archive, 38*, 299–305.
Loew, R., Bleimann, U., & Walsh, P. (2004). Knowledge broker network based on communication between humans. *Campus-Wide Information Systems, 21*, 185–190.

Lomas, J. (2007). The in-between world of knowledge brokering. *British Medical Journal, 334*, 129–132.

Mallonee, S., Fowler, C., & Istre, G. R. (2006). Bridging the gap between research and practice: A continuing challenge. *Injury Prevention, 12*, 357–359.

Ministère de la Santé et des Services sociaux du Québec. (2003). *Stratégie québécoise de lutte contre l'infection par le VIH et le sida, l'infection par le VHC et les ITSS*. Ministère de la Santé et des Services sociaux du Québec.

Mitton, C., Adair, C. E., McKenzie, E., Patten, S. B., & Perry, B. W. (2007). Knowledge transfer and exchange: Review and synthesis of the literature. *The Milbank Quarterly, 85*, 729–768.

Newman, S. D., Andrews, J. O., Magwood, G. S., Jenkins, C., Cox, M. J., & Williamson, D. C. (2011). Community advisory boards in community-based participatory research: A synthesis of best processes. *Preventing Chronic Disease, 8*, A70.

Nguyen, T., Graham, I. D., Mrklas, K. J., Bowen, S., Cargo, M., Estabrooks, C. A., Kothari, A., Lavis, J., Macaulay, A. C., MacLeod, M., Phipps, D., Ramsden, V. R., Renfrew, M. J., Salsberg, J., & Wallerstein, N. (2020). How does integrated knowledge translation (IKT) compare to other collaborative research approaches to generating and translating knowledge? Learning from experts in the field. *Health Research Policy and Systems, 18*, 35.

Payne, J. (1999). *Researching health needs: A community-based approach*. Sage.

Petras, E. M., & Porpora, D. V. (1993). Participatory research: Three models and an analysis. *The American Sociologist, 24*(1), 107–126.

Reagans, R., & McEvily, B. (2003). Network structure and knowledge transfer: The effects of cohesion and range. *Administrative Science Quarterly, 48*, 240–267.

Scharff, D. P., & Mathews, K. (2008). Working with communities to translate research into practice. *Journal of Public Health Management and Practice, 14*, 94–98.

Schulz, A. J., Israel, B. A., Selig, S. M., Bayer, I. S., & Griffin, C. B. (2000). The research perspective: Development and implementation of principles for community-based research in public health. In T. A. Bruce & S. U. McKane (Eds.), *Community-based public health: A partnership model* (pp. 53–69). American Public Health Association.

Singh, J. (2005). Collaborative networks as determinants of knowledge diffusion patterns. *Management Science, 51*, 756–770.

Sorenson, O., Rivkin, J., & Fleming, L. (2006). Complexity, networks and knowledge flow. *Research Policy, 35*, 994–1017.

Stetler, C. B. (2001). Updating the Stetler Model of research utilization to facilitate evidence-based practice. *Nursing Outlook, 49*, 272–279.

Thomas, A., Menon, A., Boruff, J., Rodriguez, A. M., & Ahmed, S. (2014). Applications of social constructivist learning theories in knowledge translation for healthcare professionals: A scoping review. *Implementation Science, 9*, 54.

Van De Ven, A. H., & Johnson, P. E. (2006). Knowledge for theory and practice. *The Academy of Management Review, 31*(4), 802–821.

Vingilis, E., Hartford, K., Schrecker, T., Mitchell, B., Lent, B., Bishop, J., & Consortium for Applied Research and Evaluation in Mental Health. (2003). Integrating knowledge generation with knowledge diffusion and utilization: A case study analysis of the Consortium for Applied Research and Evaluation in Mental Health. *Canadian Journal of Public Health, 94*, 468–471.

Ward, V. (2017). Why, whose, what and how? A framework for knowledge mobilisers. *Evidence & Policy, 13*(3), 477–497.

Ward, V., House, A., & Hamer, S. (2009). Developing a framework for transferring knowledge into action: A thematic analysis of the literature. *Journal of Health Services Research & Policy, 14*, 156–164.

World Health Organisation. (1986, November 21). *Ottawa charter for health promotion: First international conference on health promotion Ottawa*.

Zhuge, H. (2002). A knowledge flow model for peer-to-peer team knowledge sharing and management. *Expert Systems with Applications, 23*, 23–30.

Chapter 39
Reflections on Health Promotion Research in the Field of Health-Promoting Health Care: The What, Why, and How of the Viennese Tradition

Daniela Rojatz and Birgit Metzler

39.1 Introduction

The Viennese tradition of research and scientific support for health care organizations as relevant settings for health promotion has its roots in the Ottawa Charter and started with a model project in a Viennese hospital more than 30 years ago (Nowak et al., 1999). Since then, a group of researchers around principal investigator Jürgen M. Pelikan has been contributing to realizing the vision of reorienting health services towards health promotion, as called for in the Ottawa Charter (WHO, 1986), through research, scientific support, and consulting of health care organizations and networks.

Although research group members and the research context (due to changing institutes) have significantly changed over time[1], the mission has remained the same: to contribute to the reorientation of health services towards health promotion through research and scientific support of practice and policy in Austria and internationally. In this chapter, the current project leaders for health-promoting hospitals and health services and health-promoting primary care units (PCUs) reflect on developments to date and their current research practices addressing the following issues:

- Health care organizations as distinctive research objects

[1] From the Ludwig Boltzmann Institute for Sociology of Health and Medicine (1979–2008) to the Ludwig Boltzmann Institute Health Promotion Research (2008–2016), to the Austrian National Public Health Institute (2016–onwards)

D. Rojatz (✉) · B. Metzler
Austrian National Public Health Institute, Vienna, Austria
e-mail: Daniela.Rojatz@goeg.at

L. Potvin, D. Jourdan (eds.), *Global Handbook of Health Promotion Research, Vol. 1*,
https://doi.org/10.1007/978-3-030-97212-7_39

- Health promotion in health care organizations
- The sociological paradigm underlying the research program
- Researching health care organizations
- The research program contributions.

39.2 Health Care Organizations as Research Objects

The Viennese research tradition focuses on the impact of organizations on the health of individuals and the conditions and possibilities of health promotion interventions in and by these organizations. In line with the Ottawa Charter (WHO, 1986), health care organizations are chosen as the research object to support the reorientation of health services towards health promotion.

What reorientation means and aspires can be interpreted differently. It can be understood as the implementation of health promotion measures in health care organizations in addition to other services ('add-on') (i.e. health promotion in the health care organization). But it can also be understood as the implementation of health as a decision criterion in core processes of the organization ('add-in') (i.e. health-promoting health care organization). For applying the add-on approach, it is sufficient to select health promotion measures and implement them in form of a project. The add-in approach is about a fundamental cultural change, which requires capacity development within and outside the organization (Pelikan & Dietscher, 2015a). The Viennese research tradition pursues the second objective.

For the reorientation of health services towards health promotion, it is important to understand the specifics of the respective health care organization (Pelikan, 2007b). Organizations represent a relevant environment for people. Moreover, organizations create essential conditions for health (Pelikan & Dietscher, 2015b). Like any other organization, health care organizations are founded for a specific purpose. Hospitals and primary care units (PCU) can be regarded as health care organizations, founded to treat diseases to regain health. Health care organizations are usually frequented by human beings when there is a health problem that they cannot manage themselves or within their households (Bhuyan, 2004; Pandey, 2018).

Health promotion research in the field of health-promoting health care has started with hospitals and has recently been expanded to primary care.

Hospitals are conceptualized as 'professional organizations, which are typically expert-driven, skills-oriented, and based on professional-client interactions that are very hard to monitor and supervise by organizational management' (Wieczorek et al., 2015). To fulfil their main function of curing and caring, hospitals are offering diagnostic, therapeutic, and care services for patients, provided by professional staff members in interactive situations. Moreover, hospitals are differentiated multi-stakeholder organizations in which the stakeholders differ in their interests and possibilities to influence relevant structures and processes of a hospital, follow different logics and specific concepts of evidence (Pelikan, 2007b). This is supported by the ideas of Glouberman and Mintzberg (2001), according to whom hospitals are characterized by four competing 'worlds' of nursing care, medical cure, management, and trustees. The potential of hospitals for health promotion can be actualized by orienting 'their governance models, structures, processes, and culture to optimize health gains of patients, staff and populations served and to support sustainable societies' by using a comprehensive settings approach (Nutbeam & Muscat, 2021).

Primary care units (PCU) are a new development in Austria and go back to the new primary care concept of 2014 (Bundesministerium für Gesundheit, 2014). These multi-professionally staffed units are intended to complement the dominating individual medical practices. The core team consists of general practitioners, nurses, and other professional groups (including office assistants, social workers, physiotherapists, occupational therapists, logopedic therapists) according to regional needs. The primary care act (*PrimVG,* 2017) defines health promotion, prevention, and health literacy are tasks of these new PCUs. As a result, PCUs can provide more comprehensive care for patients and focus more on social and mental health determinants than individual medical practices (BMASGK, 2019; Bundesministerium für Gesundheit, 2014).

Although hospitals and PCUs share a similar basic purpose (treatment of diseases to gain health) and challenges in terms of health promotion (disease orientation, evidence understanding), they possess some structural differences. This is partly due to the respective organizational characteristics and, as can be seen from the example of Austria, also to divided legislative and administrative competencies: While responsibility for hospitals is held by the federal government and the provinces, for PCU, it lies with the social insurance system and partially the provinces. Therefore, approaches of reorientation towards health promotion can only be transferred from one setting to the other to a limited extent. This in turn has implications for research-practice collaborations and the research approach to be taken.

39.3 Health Promotion in Health Care Organizations

The Ottawa Charter emphasizes a reorientation of health services to support a change of attitudes and organizations in such a way that an orientation towards the needs of the human being as a holistic personality becomes possible (WHO, 1986). This requires a change in health care organizations.

The potential of health care organizations for health promotion lies especially in the following areas:

- With the increase in chronic diseases, it is no longer enough to treat diseases, but also to address the non-medical health needs and health resources of patients.
- Health problems lead people to health services. This opens a window of opportunity for health promotion for patients and their caring relatives.
- A large number of people are employed in the health sector, which offers big opportunities for workplace health promotion.

- The orientation of central health care organizations towards health promotion can have a role model effect and thus contribute to a cultural change in society.

As settings in which a large number of people work and which are visited for cure and care, health care organizations can reach large segments of the population (Pelikan and Dietscher 2015a):

- The patient role often comes along with a focus on health, which provides an opportunity to empower patients and involve them in treatment processes as co-producers of their health. This way, the autonomy of the patients, the quality of treatment, and thus the clinical outcome can be improved, but also disease–and health-related changes in behaviour and situation can be initiated.
- Hospitals and, to a lesser extent, PCUs also employ considerable numbers of staff and are particularly stressful places for them physically, mentally, and socially, which leads to a variety of health risks (e.g. accidents, occupational diseases, stress). Health promotion and disease prevention are therefore especially indicated for staff.
- As purchasers and consumers of substantial quantities of goods and services, hospitals affect the health of the population in the region. By choosing products and services with a more favourable health and ecological balance, hospitals can improve their health impact and contribute to environmental sustainability. Primary care units are in close contact with the local community and provide services aligned to their needs.

Health-promoting health care organizations contribute to (BMGFJ, 2008):

- Short-, medium-, and long-term health gain for patients, staff, and the population.
- The integration of health promotion as a guiding and decision-making criterion in health care organizations.
- Further development of existing processes and structures in a health-promoting manner or health-promoting (quality) management of service provision.
- Strategic repositioning by introducing additional health-promoting services.
- Sustainable environments.

Individuals, community groups, health professionals, health services, and governments share the responsibility for health-promoting health services and have to work together towards a health care system contributing to the pursuit of health (WHO, 1986). Thus, reorienting health services needs a cooperative or participatory approach.

However, there are a few tensions that arise when linking health promotion and health care organizations:

- The purpose of health care organizations is primarily the treatment of diseases, i.e. they are rather disease- or risk-oriented than health-oriented. However, especially in the case of chronic diseases (particularly those related to lifestyle), a mainly curative, disease-oriented treatment is no longer sufficient. A health orientation also addresses people's non-medical health needs and resources to improve their health.

- Concerning evidence, medicine and health promotion have different ideas and possibilities to demonstrate effects. Thus, it is difficult for health promotion research to relate to the concept of medical evidence (Pelikan & Dietscher, 2015a).

The research contributes to overcoming these tensions and realizing the potential of health-promoting health care.

39.4 Applying a Sociological Perspective on the Reorientation of Health Services: The Viennese Model of Health-Promoting Health Care Organizations

The Viennese research tradition is rooted in sociology, especially in the sociology of health and organizations. Theories and concepts are influenced by Luhmann's systems theory (Luhmann, 1984), Antonovsky's salutogenesis approach (Antonovsky, 1996), and Donabedian's quality development framework (Donabedian, 1988). Strategies for influencing health can be based on health or illness, on maintaining or improving health (c.f. Table 39.1). These strategies can be well combined. Depending on the setting, a different strategy mix may be appropriate.

Regarding health care organizations as settings allows to apply the settings approach of health promotion (Nutbeam, 1986). Settings are 'the social context in which people engage in daily activities, in which environmental organizational and personal factors interact to affect health and well-being' (Nutbeam, 1986). People can use and shape this social context and thus not only create but also solve problems related to health (Nutbeam, 1986).

Usually, an organization is assigned to a setting. The setting itself can only be addressed for health promotion via its assigned organization (i.e. hospital or PCUs), as these have the agency to shape the setting and the capacity to interact with the environment of the setting. Accordingly, setting development is always also organizational development (Pelikan & Dietscher, 2015b). Health promotion action can relate to means of organizational development and to promote health by reaching people as well as through interaction of different settings with the wider community (Nutbeam, 1986). The overall aim is to reorient these settings towards health.

To achieve sustainable and comprehensive development of settings such as hospitals and PCUs, health promotion must be integrated into the organizational decision-making premises. The organizational core of these settings is used to

Table 39.1 Strategies to influence health

Strategies oriented on	Disease	Health
Maintaining health	Prevention of disease	Health protection
Gaining health	Treatment of disease	Health promotion

Adapted and translated from Pelikan (2007a)

address and improve health determinants. Changes can therefore be achieved by decisions regarding the physical and social environment of the setting as well as by decisions that affect the behaviour of persons, e.g. through information, education, training, and motivation. People are generally easier to influence than social systems.

A simple action model, referencing the work of Kurt Lewin and James Coleman, was developed to show how settings can improve people's health (Pelikan, 2007a) (c.f. Table 39.2). It distinguishes between system (e.g. hospital, PCU) and environment on the one side, and between opportunity structure (of a behaviour, of an action) and selection culture (aims, goals, preferences) on the other. Crossing these dimensions leads to four different determinants of action or behaviour: At the system level, ability (e.g. education, training) and willingness (e.g. aims, goals, preferences), and at the environmental level, opportunities (e.g. resources, infrastructure) and values/norms (e.g. legislation). All four determinants are essential for the successful execution of an action. Therefore, interventions should ideally address ability, willingness, opportunities, and values/norms alike or use an assessment to determine which determinants should be given priority.

The settings approach makes it possible to address all four determinants with a bundle of coherent strategies (by structural, cultural, system/organizational, and environmental development), thus enabling sustainable effects. Different interventions are suitable for each dimension. Health-promoting setting development is then a combination of health-promoting structural and cultural, systems, and environmental development (Pelikan, 2007a). Providing definitions, strategies, standards, and tools contribute the structural development. Regulations and statutes facilitate cultural development.

One key thesis in reorienting health services is that health care systems can be understood as a complex of strongly interrelated professional practice, research, and supporting policy (Pelikan, 2017). Research and scientific support are therefore related to supporting and informing policy and practice (c.f. Fig. 39.1). Since implementing systematic change requires multiple domains, multiple levels are addressed (local, national, international) (Harnett, 2018).

Table 39.2 Model of action

Prerequisite for action	Opportunity structure	Selection culture	Possibility of intervention
System	Ability	Willingness	System development
Environment	Opportunities	Values and norms	Environmental development
Possibility of intervention	Structural development	Cultural development	Setting development

Adapted and translated from Pelikan (2007a)

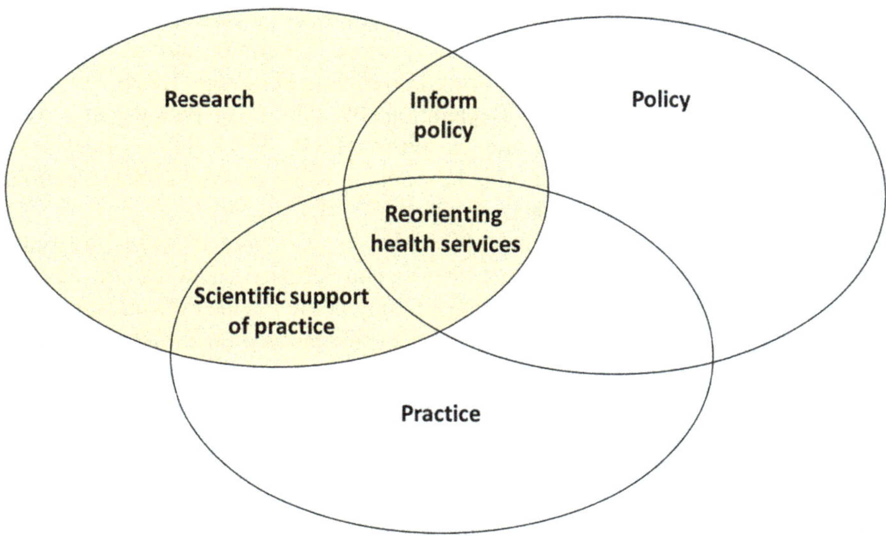

Fig. 39.1 Research to support policy and practice

39.5 Researching Health Care Organizations: Producing and Sharing Knowledge of Health-Promoting Health Services

Our research program on the reorientation of health services has started with a WHO model project in a hospital setting in the late 1980s. Using methods of organizational development and quality management, strategies, standards, and indicators were developed to support the re-orientation of hospitals towards health promotion. Support was also given to the establishment of health promotion networks at regional, national, and international levels. Currently, the team at the Austrian National Public Health Institute provides scientific support at the regional level to the Vienna Alliance for Health Promotion in Health Care Institutions and at the national level to the Austrian Network of Health Promoting Hospitals and Health Services (HPH). At the international level, the team scientifically prepares and coordinates the international conferences of the International HPH Network.

The initial work had a rather visionary character and became increasingly systematic and application-oriented (Pelikan, 2007b). Tools from organizational development and quality management were used to integrate health promotion in professional – medical-led – health care organizations. From the outset, the health promotion of the organization- as-a-whole with its most relevant stakeholder groups, i.e. patients (and their relatives), staff, and the local community, were the focus.

For hospitals, a concept for the practical implementation of health promotion was developed at the initiative of WHO/Europe. With the WHO model project (1989–1996), a research group based at the Ludwig Boltzmann Institute for the

Sociology of Health and Medicine in Vienna scientifically planned, consulted, and evaluated the first model hospital to pilot the concept of health-promoting hospitals. In 1990, the International Network of Health Promoting Hospitals (HPH) was initiated. In 1991, with the Budapest Declaration, the first HPH policy paper was adopted (Network of Health Promoting Hospitals [HPH], 1991). Next to the definition and objectives of health-promoting hospitals, it listed criteria for participation in a European Pilot Hospital Project.

In this project (1993–1997), the HPH approach was piloted in 11 European countries. As a result of the project, the Vienna Recommendations on Health Promoting Hospitals were adopted, which strongly promoted the network approach (LBIMGS, 1997). Networks at regional, national, and international levels have been established as a central strategy to support setting-oriented health promotion.

In 1996, a national network was established in Austria with the support of the Federal Ministry of Health. Since 2006, the Austrian HPH Network has been a registered association (ONGKG) and has a section 'Tobacco-free Hospitals', followed by a section 'Baby-friendly Hospitals' in 2010 with internationally developed certification programs. Including its section members, the ONGKG currently (2020) comprises more than 60 member institutions. Since its foundation, the Viennese research group provides scientific support for the network and organized knowledge exchange and transfer (e.g. via annual national conferences, workshops, newsletters, website).

From 2000 onwards, the quality development approach was pursued more intensively within the framework of the International HPH Network. For example, 18 core strategies that provide a conceptual overview of all possible contents of HPH and seven implementation strategies were developed (Pelikan et al., 2006). In line with the improvement of quality aspects, standards and indicators for self-assessment of health-promoting hospitals were developed to support the existing networks and member hospitals in their reorientation (Pelikan & Dietscher, 2015a). An important milestone for knowledge production and exchange was also the constitution of HPH as an association under Swiss law in 2008 with good relations to the WHO and the expansion of the membership to other health services. Since then, research has been increasingly called upon to provide the basis for cooperation between different health care services.

The definition of standards, strategies, and indicators formed the basis for an international evaluation study on the implementation of health promotion in health services (Pelikan et al., 2011). In a dissertation based on this study, a framework for the effectiveness of health promotion networks was elaborated (Dietscher, 2012).

Since 2016, when the research team was integrated in the Austrian National Public Health Institute, research work has become more policy- and practice-oriented, and scientific work has declined. At the regional and national levels, the focus is on scientific and strategic support of the respective networks (Vienna Alliance for Health Promotion in Health Care Institutions, Austrian HPH Network). This includes the scientific conception and coordination of workshops and conferences to promote the exchange among network members, the publication of newsletters to strengthen knowledge transfer, and addressing priority topics. In 2019, for example, the development of a recognition procedure for age-friendly health care services in accordance with international standards has started. Together with HPH members and external experts, the International HPH Network developed a new set of standards in the sense of a broader range of umbrella standards, which were published by the end of 2020.[2] The research group was also actively involved in this process.

In contrast to work in hospital settings, research in the field of primary care is more fragmented and still in the fledgling stages. From 1998 to 2001, the European research project 'Health Promotion in General Practice and Community Pharmacy', commissioned by the European Commission and funded by the Austrian Health Promotion Fund, was conducted under Austrian lead by the Ludwig Boltzmann Institute. Methods applied were conceptional work towards definitions of health promotion in general practice and community pharmacy and a literature review. To support the capacity building for the reorientation, a European database on health promotion projects was established. Moreover, a European conference was organized to support the commitment and cultural development for the reorientation.

However, it took until 2016 before the reorientation of primary care towards health promotion gained renewed attention in Austria. The Austrian Health Promotion Fund commissioned a pilot study. Based on a literature review evidence on health promotion measures in general practices was compiled and the health promotion practice of general practitioners in Austria was explored using qualitative methods. Recommendations were derived, including the development of a framework for a health-promoting PCU (Rojatz et al., 2018a, b). An attempt was made to start the public discourse on the topic by publishing a fact sheet and presenting the results at relevant national congresses.

Another milestone is an action research project (2018–2021), financed by the Austrian Health Promotion Fund together with the umbrella organization of the Austrian Social Insurance. In the sense of a comprehensive salutogenic public health approach in primary care, health promotion, disease prevention, and health literacy are defined as services of primary care and should be systematically implemented. The objective of the project is to make these services comprehensible, meaningful, and manageable for the PCU's funders and for the PCU team by applying Antonovsky's concept of sense of coherence (1996) adapted to the Austrian context. Continuous exchanges with primary care practitioners and funders allow identifying opportunities to support the implementation of the three services. This support includes reviewing scientific literature and models of good practice to develop tools to inform and support policy and practice decisions (Rojatz et al., 2018a).

As part of the project, exchange forums were established at the federal level (Austrian Health Promotion Fund, Austrian Social Insurance, Federal Ministry of Health) and with funders (regional social insurance and health funds) in the federal provinces. These exchange forums were important to identify and address the

[2] https://www.hphnet.org/standards/

current support needs of financiers and decision-makers. Preliminary project results are presented at workshops and conferences to promote the discourse on health promotion and to receive feedback and attune the products to the needs.

In the first step, the framework for an ideal model of health-oriented PCU was developed (Rojatz et al., 2018b). It recognizes three target groups (patients, PCU team, community) and three action areas (organizational development of PCU towards a health-promoting workplace; integrating health promotion, disease prevention, and health literacy measures into PCU; and cooperation with local services and initiatives to initiate and implement measures in the region of the PCU).

After the elaboration of an ideal model of health-promoting PCU, PCUs need support in the start-up phase to ensure that health promotion, disease prevention, and health literacy are integrated from the outset. Therefore, a blueprint for the health care concept was developed, which shows where health promotion, disease prevention, and health literacy could be considered (Sprenger et al., 2018).

Finally, PCUs are supported by a starter toolkit (Rojatz et al., 2021). Evidence-based and easy-to-implement health promotion, disease prevention, and health literacy services were identified, selected, and compiled to a starter toolkit for PCU teams. The aim is to make health promotion, disease prevention, and health literacy comprehensible, meaningful, and manageable for them.

In 2020, the Austrian Social Health Insurance Fund launched a health promotion and prevention strategy for the systematic guidance of PCUs. Currently, the project results are integrated into this guidance process. Furthermore, it is scientifically supported to contribute to a systematic implementation of the services of health promotion, disease prevention, and health literacy.

Moreover, the Austrian National Public Health Institute is commissioned to support the integration of public health services into primary care by WHO. One deliverable refers to a guidance document for the definition of health promotion and prevention services in primary care. Health promotion and prevention services, along with the essential public health operations (EPHO) (WHO Europe, 2012), were compiled as a basis for national and regional service-level agreements (WHO Region Office for Europe, in press).

39.6 The Research Program Contributions

Since health services are regarded as a complex of strongly interrelated professional practice, research, and supporting policy, the contribution so far is described along with these three areas (c.f. Fig. 39.1). This research program is linked to contributions in three areas of health promotion.

39.6.1 Contributing to Health Promotion Research Through Theory Development

The need for further theory development was identified and has been so far, at least partially addressed. This includes definitions of key concepts like health and health promotion.

The question of what 'health' is, is crucial since the approach of health care services is usually limited to the treatment of disease. Work is underway in developing a conceptual understanding based on a system-theoretically oriented concept of health and the relationship between health and illness. Accordingly, health is more fundamental than disease and can be promoted even if illness exists (Pelikan, 2007a).

Another research need concerns the relationship between 'health promotion and salutogenesis' and 'salutogenesis and participation'. Antonovsky's salutogenesis approach (Antonovsky, 1996; Eriksson and Lindström 2008) is often considered as a theoretical background for health promotion. Efforts have been made to apply salutogenesis to hospitals (Dietscher et al., 2017; Pelikan, 2017) and primary care (Rojatz et al., 2022). The application can refer to salutogenic health orientation (the main interpretation for health promotion), the salutogenic model, or the concept of the sense of coherence (SOC) (Pelikan, 2017).

With the emergence of the health literacy concept, the question of the relationship between health promotion and health literacy (and subsequently between health literacy and salutogenesis) is increasingly being raised (Gugglberger, 2019). Health literacy is understood to be an essential determinant of health. Not all health promotion measures increase health literacy (e.g. offer healthy and eco-friendly food in hospitals). At the same time, not all measures to increase health literacy are health promotion. Health literacy can be interpreted against the background of the concept of SOC (Nowak & Rojatz, 2020).

39.6.2 Contribution to Health-Promoting Practice Through Structural Development

Over the past 30 years, especially in the hospital sector, contributions have been made to the development of definitions, strategies, standards, and indicators that are intended to make it easier for hospitals and networks of hospitals and health services to orient themselves towards health.

The use of the network approach and the scientific support of regional and national networks as well as the collaboration with international networks enable a continuous exchange with practice, the identification of new topics, and the processing of these. Due to limitations in space, just a few are highlighted – especially focusing on patient participation, an issue not fully realized yet.

Based on the self-help-friendly hospital approach developed in Germany, a model and stepwise approach to strengthening the cooperation between health-promoting hospitals and self-help groups was developed (Forster et al., 2013). The model was taken up by the New Haven recommendations on partnering with patients, families, and citizens to enhance performance and quality in health-promoting hospitals (International Network of Health Promoting Hospitals and Health Services et al. 2016; Christina Wieczorek et al., 2018).

In cooperation with Austrian hospitals, a concept for health-literate health care organizations and an assessment tool were developed and piloted (Dietscher & Pelikan, 2016). The concept and assessment tool were later adapted for PCU (ÖPGK, 2019) and might provide the basis for a concept and certificate of a health-promoting PCU.

The Viennese research group has contributed to the development of the global HPH approach both conceptually (by defining core strategies and strategies for implementation) and practically (by supporting implementation through developing and promoting topics and tools).

This holds true for PCUs at the national and regional levels. However, unlike hospitals, in the newer field of PCU, support is not provided at the network level (as such does not exist), but at the level of PCU financiers. Tools are developed, piloted, and enhanced in a participatory approach (Rojatz & Atzler, 2020).

39.6.3 Contributing to Policy Development

The contribution of the Viennese research group to the development of supportive political frameworks for reorientation refers, on the one hand, to the creation of own products and, on the other, to the contribution of expertise in strategic processes and documents of other actors. The actual research focuses on the integration of public health services in primary care. A guidance document for the integration of health promotion and prevention services was developed (WHO Regional Office for Europe, in press), which can provide the basis for national service level agreements in primary care.

To initiate processes and policy dialogues towards health-promoting health care in health care settings, a knowledge base on incentives for doing health-promoting health care will be elaborated.

At the national level, the Vienna research group's expertise in the fields of health promotion, prevention, and health literacy is also in demand to support strategic processes and policy developments. For example, it contributed to the Health Quality Act of 2005 (Gesundheitsqualitätsgesetz, 2004), which stipulates that health care must be provided in a health-promoting environment. More recently, the research group contributed to the revision of the National Action Plan on Physical Activity, where it was asked to comment on and supplement the chapter on health services.

39.6.4 Major Learnings for the Reorientation of Health Services

Major learnings for our 30-year research program can be summarized as follows:

Reorienting health services towards health promotion needs continuous support, even if definitions, strategies, standards, and tools are developed and provided.

At the level of organizational settings, but also at the policy level, the realization of health-promoting health care organizations requires the development of sustainable structures, such as supporting policy frameworks and concepts for financing health promotion activities – otherwise, it remains dependent on the idealism of individual actors.

A key aspect of health promotion that is still underexposed is the cooperation with or participation of users of health services and their local communities. As stated above, attempts have been made, but effective implementation is not yet in sight.

Participation and involvement of health service users contribute to a comprehensible, meaningful, and manageable health service. This also leads to the question of how salutogenesis can be better linked with organizational development and quality management approaches.

In general, it is necessary to observe trends and future developments (e.g. digitalization, aging society, pandemics) to prepare topics and respond in due time.

39.7 Conclusions

This chapter highlighted the research practices in the field of health-promoting health care as they have been developed and established in Vienna for more than 30 years. Based on the Ottawa Charter's call to reorient health services towards health promotion (WHO, 1986), practice-oriented research strived to contribute to health-promoting health care. Within the framework of health and organizational sociology, systems theory, setting approach, salutogenesis concept, and quality development approaches were combined and applied to develop models, concepts, and tools for the practical implementation of the aspired reorientation of health services. Besides, a multi-level network on regional, national, and international levels – mainly with health care organizations (practice) and policy has been established, which enables to recognize current developments, trends, and challenges quite quickly and to get involved in their processing.

The research approach helped structure the field of health promotion research and practice in several ways. Through the multi-level approach (regional, national, international), it is possible to learn about different practical approaches and challenges in the implementation of health promotion, e.g. on the international level. This in turn provides stimulus and support for regional developments and vice versa. The cooperation with institutions from the field enables access to the current needs of health care organizations, which are addressed using scientific methods. The developed tools can be piloted due to the good cooperation in the health care organizations and further developed based on the results. In this way, research retains its independent function and contributes to advancements in health promotion practice in health care settings.

Acknowledgement We would like to thank Peter Nowak and Jürgen Pelikan for their insight into their long-standing expertise in the field of health-promoting health care and Benjamin Marent and Charlotte Klein for reviewing the manuscript.

References

Antonovsky, A. (1996). The salutogenic model as a theory to guide health promotion. *Health Promotion International, 11*(1), 11–18.

Bhuyan, K. (2004). Health promotion through self-care and community participation: Elements of a proposed programme in the developing countries. *BMC Public Health, 4*, 11. https://doi.org/10.1186/1471-2458-4-11

BMASGK. (2019). ÖSG 2017 – Österreichischer Strukturplan Gesundheit 2017 inklusive Großgeräteplan gemäß Beschluss der Bundes-Zielsteuerungskommission vom 30. Juni 2017 inklusive der bis 27. September 2019 beschlossenen Anpassungen. Verfasst von der Gesundheit Österreich GmbH (GÖG) im Auftrag der Bundesgesundheitsagentur, Wien.

BMGFJ. (2008). *Gesundheitsfördernde Krankenhäuser und Gesundheitseinrichtungen: Konzept und Praxis in Österreich*. Bundesministerium für Gesundheit, Familie und Jugend.

Bundesgesetz über die Primärversorgung in Primärversorgungseinheiten (Primärversorgungsgesetz PrimVG). (2017).

Bundesgesetz zur Qualität von Gesundheitsleistungen (Gesundheitsqualitätsgesetz – GQG). (2004).

Bundesministerium für Gesundheit. (2014). "Das Team rund um den Hausarzt". Konzept zur multiprofessionellen und interdisziplinären Primärversorgung in Österreich. 2014, Beschlossen in der Bundes-Zielsteuerungskommission am 30. Juni. Bundesgesundheitsagentur und Bundesministerium für Gesundheit, Wien http://bmg.gv.at/cms/home/attachments/1/2/6/CH1443/CMS1404305722379/primaerversorgung.pdf

Dietscher, C. (2012). *Interorganisational networks in the settings approach of health promotion. The case of the International Network of Health Promoting Hospitals and Health Services (HPH)*. University of Vienna.

Dietscher, C., & Pelikan, J. (2016). Gesundheitskompetente Krankenbehandlungsorganisationen. *Prävention Und Gesundheitsförderung, 11*(1), 53–62. https://doi.org/10.1007/s11553-015-0523-0

Dietscher, C., Winter, U., & Pelikan, J. M. (2017). The application of salutogenesis in hospitals. In M. B. Mittelmark, S. Sagy, M. Eriksson, G. F. Bauer, J. M. Pelikan, B. Lindström, & G. A. Espnes (Eds.), *The handbook of salutogenesis* (pp. 277–298). Springer. https://doi.org/10.1007/978-3-319-04600-6

Donabedian, A. (1988). The quality of care: How can it be assessed? *JAMA, 260*(12), 1743–1748.

Eriksson, M., & Lindström, B. (2008). A salutogenic interpretation of the Ottawa Charter. *Health Promotion International, 23*(2), 190–199. https://doi.org/10.1093/heapro/dan014

Forster, R., Rojatz, D., Schmied, H., & Pelikan, J. M. (2013). Selbsthilfegruppen und Gesundheitsförderung im Krankenhaus - eine entwicklungsfähige Allianz für Gesundheit. *Prävention Und Gesundheitsförderung, 8*(1), 9–14.

Glouberman, S., & Mintzberg, H. (2001). Managing the care of health and the cure of disease – Part I: Differentiation. *Health Care Management Review, 26*, 56–69.

Gugglberger, L. (2019). The multifaceted relationship between health promotion and health literacy. *Health Promotion International, 34*(5), 887–891. https://doi.org/10.1093/heapro/daz093

Harnett, P. J. (2018). Improvement attributes in healthcare: Implications for integrated care. *International Journal of Health Care Quality Assurance, 31*(3), 214–227. https://doi.org/10.1108/IJHCQA-07-2016-0097

International Network of Health Promoting Hospitals and Health Services, Plentree, & GmbH, G. Ö. (2016). *The New Haven Recommendations on partnering with patients, families and citizens to enhance performance and quality in health promoting hospitals and health services*. https://www.hphnet.org/wp-content/uploads/2020/03/The-New-Haven-Recommendations.pdf

LBIMGS. (1997). *Wiener Empfehlungen zu Gesundheitsfördernden Krankenhäusern*. https://dngfk.de/wp-content/uploads/2018/02/1997-wiener-empfehlungen.pdf

Luhmann, N. (Ed.). (1984). *Soziale Systeme. Grundriss einer allgemeinen Theorie*. Suhrkamp.

Network of Health Promoting Hospitals (HPH). (1991). *Budapester Deklaration Gesundheitsfördernder Krankenhäuser*. http://www.ongkg.at/downloads-links/downloads.html

Nowak, P., & Rojatz, D. (2020). *Konzept und Umsetzungsmaßnahmen der Gesundheitskompetenz: Kommunikation in der Krankenversorgung*.

Nowak, P., Lobnig, H., Krajic, K., & Pelikan, J. (1999). Case study Rudolfstiftung Hospital, Vienna, Austria – WHO-Model Project "health and hospital". In J. Pelikan, M. Garcia-Barbero, H. Lobnig, & K. Krajic (Eds.), *Pathways to a health promoting hospital. Experiences from the European Pilot Hospital Project 1993-1997* (pp. 47–66). Conrad Health Promotion Publications.

Nutbeam, D. (1986). Health promotion glossary. *Health Promotion International, 1*(1), 113–127. https://doi.org/10.1093/heapro/1.1.113

Nutbeam, D., & Muscat, D. M. (2021). Health promotion glossary 2021. *Health Promotion International*. https://doi.org/10.1093/heapro/daaa157

ÖPGK. (2019). *Selbsteinschätzungsinstrument für Gesundheitskompetenz in Primärversorgungseinheiten*. https://oepgk.at/wp-content/uploads/2019/09/selbsteinschaetzungsinstrument-pve.pdf

Pandey, K. (2018). From health for all to universal health coverage: Alma Ata is still relevant. *Globalization and Health, 11*, 62. https://doi.org/10.1186/s12992-018-0381-6

Pelikan, J. M. (2007a). Gesundheitsförderung durch Organisationsentwicklung. Ein systemtheoretischer Lösungszugang. *Prävention Gesundheitsförderung, 2*, 74–81.

Pelikan, J. M. (2007b). Health promoting hospitals – Assessing developments in the network. *Italian Journal of Public Health, 4*(4), 261–270. https://doi.org/10.2427/5864

Pelikan, J. M. (2017). The application of Salutogenesis in healthcare settings. In M. B. Mittelmark, S. Sagy, M. Eriksson, G. F. Bauer, J. M. Pelikan, B. Lindström, & G. A. Espnes (Eds.), *The handbook of Salutogenesis* (pp. 261–266). Springer. https://doi.org/10.1007/978-3-319-04600-6

Pelikan, J.M., & Dietscher, C. (2015a). *Gesundheitsförderung und Krankenhaus*. Leitbegriffe Der Gesundheitsförderung Und Prävention.BzgA. https://doi.org/10.17623/BZGA:224-i046-1.0

Pelikan, J.M., & Dietscher, C. (2015b). *Organisationsentwicklung als Methode der Gesundheitsförderung*. Leitbegriffe Der Gesundheitsförderung Und Prävention. BzgA. https://doi.org/10.17623/BZGA:224-i083-1.0

Pelikan, J.M., Krajic, K., Dietscher, C., & Nowak, P. (2006). *Putting HPH policy into action*. Working paper of the WHO Collaborating Centre on health promotion in hospitals and health care. http://www.ongkg.at/downloads-links/downloads.html

Pelikan, J. M., Dietscher, C., Schmied, H., & Röthlin, F. (2011). A model and selected results from an evaluation study on the International HPH Network (PRICES-HPH). *Clinical Health Promotion – Research and Best Practice for Patients, Staff and Community, 1*(1), 9–15. https://doi.org/10.29102/clinhp.11003

Rojatz, D., & Atzler, B. (2020). Wie neue Versorgungsformen zu mehr Gesundheit beitragen können – Primärversorgung gesundheitsorientiert gedacht. *Soziale Sicherheit, 3*, 108–112.

Rojatz, D., Nowak, P., & Christ, R. (2018a). The Austrian health care reform: An opportunity to implement health promotion into primary health care units. *Public Health Panorama, 04*(04), 627–631.

Rojatz, D., Nowak, P., Rath, S., & Atzler, B. (2018b). *Primärversorgung neu: Krankheitsprävention, Gesundheitsförderung und Gesundheitskompetenz. Grundlagen und Eckpunkte eines Idealmodells für PVE-Team und Finanzierungspartner.* Gesundheit Österreich. https://goeg.at/sites/goeg.at/files/inline-files/EckpunkteIdealmodell_0.pdf

Rojatz, D., Rath, S., Holzweber, L., Atzler, B., & Nowak, P. (2021). *Krankheitsprävention, Gesundheitsförderung und Gesundheitskompetenz in der Primärversorgungseinheit. Info-Mappe*. Dachverband der österreichischen Sozialversicherungen und Fonds Gesundes Österreich. https://www.sozialversicherung.at/cdscontent/load?contentid=10008.746765&version=1619434739

Rojatz, D., Nowak, P., Bahrs, O., & Pelikan, J. M. (2022). The application of salutogenesis in primary care. In M. B. Mittelmark et al. (Eds.), *The handbook of Salutogenesis*. Springer, Cham.

Sprenger, M., Stigler, F., Rojatz, D., & Nowak, P. (2018). *Krankheitsprävention, Gesundheitsförderung, Gesundheitskompetenz in der Primärversorgung. Ausfüllhilfe für PVE-Gründer/innen zum Musterversorgungskonzept*. Gesundheit Österreich.

WHO. (1986). *Ottawa charter for health promotion*. https://doi.org/10.1038/scientificamerican0604-48

WHO Europe. (2012). European action plan for strengthening public health capacities and services. *European Journal of Public Health*. https://doi.org/10.1093/eurpub/ckw169.061

WHO Regional Office for Europe (in press): Primary care and public health services: specification of health promotion and disease prevention services in primary care – guidance document. WHO Regional Office for Europe

Wieczorek, C. C., Osrecki, F., Dorner, T., & Dür, W. (2015). Hospitals as professional organizations: Challenges for reorientation towards health promotion. *Health Sociology Review, 24*(2), 123–136.

Wieczorek, C. C., Nowak, P., Frampton, S., & Pelikan, J. M. (2018). Strengthening patient and family engagement in healthcare – The New Haven recommendations. *Patient Education and Counseling, 101*(8), 1508–1513.

Chapter 40
Addressing the Complexity of School Health Promotion Through Interdisciplinary Approaches: An Invitation to Think Wildly About Research

Deana Leahy

40.1 Introduction

As I sat down to decide on a focus for my chapter proposal, I was in the midst of finalizing an edited book entitled *Social theory in health education: Forging new insights in research* (Leahy et al., 2020a). In our chapter *Why do we need social theory in health education*? (Leahy et al., 2020b) I, with my co-editors, argued that it was time that we, as researchers, embraced the idea of thinking wildly about health education research. In choosing to 'think wildly' about research, we borrowed from a number of critical scholars and embraced their calls to move outside of our usual disciplinary orbits and habits that tend to trap us in a repetitious cycle of interesting, but ultimately limited, thought. We were inspired by Lauren Berlant (2011) and her book *Cruel Optimism* where she stated that "long term problems of embodiment within capitalism, in the zoning of the everyday, the work of getting through it, and the obstacles to mental and physical flourishing are less successfully addressed in the temporalities of crisis and require other frames for elaborating context of doing, being and thriving" (p. 105). Berlant's words here and indeed her book have much to offer those of us invested in researching and understanding health and how best to support it. Wendy Brown (2005) in her book *Edgework: Critical essays on the politics of knowledge* provocatively asks us to pay attention to our various theoretical alliances, critical or otherwise, and question how they serve to prevent us from embracing the wildness of thinking beyond the immediate order. Similarly, Jack Halberstam (2014), in his lecture *'Notes on wildness'*, asks us to develop a different relationship to thought that is so often driven by the formulaic so

D. Leahy (✉)
School of Education, Culture and Society, Faculty of Education, Monash University, Melbourne, Victoria, Australia
e-mail: deana.leahy@monash.edu

L. Potvin, D. Jourdan (eds.), *Global Handbook of Health Promotion Research, Vol. 1*,
https://doi.org/10.1007/978-3-030-97212-7_40

as new meanings might arise. Taken together, the aforementioned authors compel us to explore what Rasmussen (2020) quite simply refers to as the 'boundaries of our own thinking'. The invitation to think wildly will mean different things to different people depending on the starting point. For some, it might simply mean questioning the theories and methods we rely on and hold dear to our hearts and, rather than returning to them time and time and time again, we might look elsewhere. For others, it might mean stepping outside of our disciplinary echo chambers to engage with other disciplinary perspectives – in this case about school food. The different calls taken together have been significant in shaping my research over time. They are by no means the only critical voices. There is of course a long line of critical health scholars who have drawn on different disciplines and different social theories to examine health promotion politics, practices and pedagogies. Unfortunately, many of those voices though fail to gain traction in the field for various reasons that I will return to in the conclusion to the chapter.

The purpose of this chapter is to provide a case study of how one research team heeded the call to think wildly about research at different times in a project that investigated the everyday experiences of school food programmes. Across Australia and indeed many other countries, schools are considered to be key settings to intervene in children and parent's food practices. Our research sought to examine how children and families experienced the various interventions directed at them by schools. The research starting point is perhaps for some, in and of itself, indicative of a different approach given we weren't trying to measure the behavioural effects of an intervention study, rather we were interested in the experiences of everyday school food programmes. In presenting the case study, I have divided the chapter into three main sections. In the first section, I provide an overview of the background to the research project and our methodology. In the second section, I provide an overview of our research findings and highlight the different and necessary theoretical resources we drew from to help us make sense of what was a very complex and multifaceted data. Finally, I conclude with some reflections about the research project and the promise of interdisciplinarity and thinking wildly for research in health promotion. Whilst thinking wildly is necessary – it isn't always easy. Thinking wildly and outside of our disciplinary areas in research is difficult and it can create a range of issues for researchers related to accessing funding through to publishing. There are also other difficulties to contend with when you find yourself working in fields that are resistant to uncertainty, ambiguity and that hold very tightly to ideas about what counts as knowledge (Warin & Zivkovic, 2019).

40.2 Children as Health Advocates: Introducing Our Research Project

The backdrop to our research is provided by the obesity epidemic and the role that schools are expected to play in obesity prevention. In the field of health promotion, schools unquestionably considered to provide an important platform for dealing with the various health crises of the day (Gard & Pluim, 2014). So, when the World Health Organization announced, nearly 25 years ago now, that we had an obesity epidemic on our hands, schools were called upon to act as key sites for prevention and intervention. As health promotion researchers began to grapple with the best ways for schools to fulfil their roles, critical health scholars from Australia, New Zealand, the United Kingdom, Canada and the United States began to draw attention to the problematic effects of school responses. Specifically, they were finding that programmes fuelled by obesity prevention imperatives adopted highly individualized approaches that ignored the social determinants of health. This meant that programmes tended to be characterized by instrumental approaches that adopted a narrow focus on physical activity and eating, including weighing children and insisting students kept food diet diaries (Burrows et al., 2002; Gard & Wright, 2001; Leahy & Harrison, 2004). In hindsight, critical scholars (me included) were simply reporting back that the various efforts made by health promotion were having an impact on schools. Whether we liked it or not, the lifestyle approach was the model that was dominating what schools were doing. Research that has continued to examine the effects of the obesity epidemic on schools has revealed an ever-increasing myriad of programmes and practices directed at curbing obesity. For example, research from Australia, New Zealand, the US (Pluim et al., 2018) and the UK (Harman & Cappelini, 2015) has discussed the practice of lunchbox policing, where teachers inspect children's lunchboxes, surveilling their contents. Implicitly, and sometimes quite explicitly, lunchbox inspections provide teachers and health promoters with an opportunity to 'reach into' the family in an attempt to change both children's and family food practices. As part of the practice, teachers have sent notes home to parents about the poor state of their child's lunchbox. They have also publicly shamed 'bad' lunchboxes during lunchtimes and in parent assemblies and school newsletters (see Burrows & Wright, 2020; Harman & Cappelini, 2015; Pike & Leahy, 2012).

The obesity epidemic has produced a myriad of what Wright and Harwood (2009) have termed new biopedagogies that attempt in some way to curb the obesity epidemic. However, it is important to note that existing health biopedagogies were also being called on – slightly remodelled and redeployed for different purposes. Leahy and Pike's (2015) ethnographic research in health education classrooms, for example, revealed how teachers had adapted a pedagogical strategy used in Nancy Reagan's inspired drug education classrooms 'Just say no to drugs' and transformed it into an obesity prevention strategy 'Just say no to pies'. Kids in classrooms were practising assertiveness skills and their non-verbal hand gestures in role plays where they were being asked to practice pie refusal skills. Other strategies were also being re-deployed as prevention tactics. Health advocacy was one such strategy. Whilst health advocacy had been an approach of the new public health since the early 1980s (Peterson & Lupton, 1996), in 2003, it was identified as a key approach that could be harnessed in the fight against obesity. Specifically, the *Healthy Weight 2008: Australia's Future* report argued for children and teenagers to become advocates of healthy eating within families as an intervention method directed towards curbing obesity (Commonwealth of Australia, 2003). In order to realize this ambition, schools were going to be required to develop the requisite knowledge and skills required for child health advocacy work.

It is within this context that the research project *Children as Health Advocates: Assessing the Consequences* study was conceived. As governments and health promoters suggested that child health advocacy could provide a strategy to help solve obesity, we had noted that there was very little literature that had explored how this call was being taken up by schools and by children. Significantly, there was a gap in understanding about whether or not the intended messages were being transported home. As the title of the project suggests we were interested to find out about the consequences of the strategy. Importantly, we wanted to understand the impact school food programmes and child health advocacy imperatives were having on families, particularly mothers who are largely responsible for everyday family food practices (Maher et al., 2010; Warin et al., 2014).

40.3 The Research Team and Methodology

40.3.1 The Team

The research project was conceptualized, developed and led by Professor JaneMaree Maher, who is a sociologist in the Faculty of Arts at Monash University. Her research expertise includes gender, families and consumption. The team could be categorized as largely hailing from the social sciences, though we had diverse methodological and theoretical expertise. We had a number of sociologists from the Faculty of Arts at Monash University with expertise in health, gender, consumption and families as well as researchers from Faculties of Education with expertise in school health education, health curriculum and pedagogy. Given the nature of the research problem, the diverse expertise of the team was essential if it wanted to make sense of a health promotion strategy that effectively extends across schools to families and back again.

40.3.2 Our Methods

Our methodology drew inspiration from childhood studies, sociology and geography and focused explicitly on children and family experiences of school food programmes. Our decision to concentrate on children and their family was related to the gap we had identified in the literature. We already knew a lot about schools. What we did not know much about were the effects of everyday school programmes on children and their families. In designing and doing our research, we were committed to the idea of 'peopling policy' – something that seems to be gaining more momentum in the field health promotion. In order to develop insights into people's everyday experiences, we employed a qualitative methodology that utilized semi-structured interviews and collecting visual data (following Lomax, 2015; Nyberg, 2019; O'Connell, 2013). We gave children an iPad for a week and asked them to take photos of food in their home. In asking children to do this, we were effectively inviting them to be co-researchers. We were committed to an approach that was child centred as we wanted children to decide what was important to take photos of and to use their photos to lead the discussion in our interviews (Nyberg, 2019; O'Connell, 2013).

The research was conducted in 2018. The study involved interviewing 67 children from 50 families across a range of demographics and family types in rural and urban areas in Victoria, Australia. One child in each family was provided with an iPad at the initial interview and invited to photograph or film food events in the family context. A second follow-up interview involved interviewing the child using the iPad videos and photographs as prompts and asking general questions about food in the family home and at school. Both interviews also involved talking with the parents and asking questions about their experiences of school food policies and practices and how and when these were communicated to the family. At times, the interviewer found themselves in a three-way or four-way conversation with children and parents at dining tables or in lounge rooms. Overall, we completed 100 interviews and collected over 500 photos and movies. Data were analysed in a number of ways. An excel spreadsheet was used to organize the photographs and video material into themes – for example, lunchboxes, celebrations, fridges. QSR NVivo was used to manage the large data set and to code across the interviews and visual data.

40.4 Our Findings: School Food Programs

Given our interest in school–family–food nexus the conversations and photos and movies kids took all related to their experiences of school food programmes and food in everyday family life. Whilst it is impossible to capture all of our findings in this chapter, I will highlight our major findings with a focus on data related to school food programmes.

Before doing that though, one important contextual 'piece of the puzzle' that will be helpful to international readers trying to understand school food practices in Australia is that Australian schools on the whole do not provide food for children unlike in many other countries. This means that children more often than not take a packed lunch to school as well as their snacks. Children can also purchase food at a canteen or kiosk if they don't bring food with them. This is dependent though on whether the school has a canteen and how many days it is open. The combination of bringing food from home or possibly purchasing it provides a rather unique opportunity for Australian policymakers via different policy actors (teachers) to reach into daily food practices.

Our research revealed that food is entangled in the everyday schooling in a myriad of ways. The infographic in Fig. 40.1 visualizes the different families' accounts of the various school programmes they were exposed to via their primary schools. Each numbered segment represents a single family and the different school food programmes and events they talked about in their interviews. The pattern of shading indicates that for some children and their families there are multiple food initiatives operating in the school. Whereas for others, there were very few programmes. Whilst it is clear from the diagram that there is variation across schools, what is not obvious in Fig. 40.1 is the variation in offerings within individual schools. We discovered this variation by talking to families who had multiple children at the same school. Families with more than one child at the school talked about the different experiences and offerings based on their child's year level and teacher and time at the school. For example, some parents pointed out how different food programmes and initiatives had started and then stopped over the time that their children attended the school.

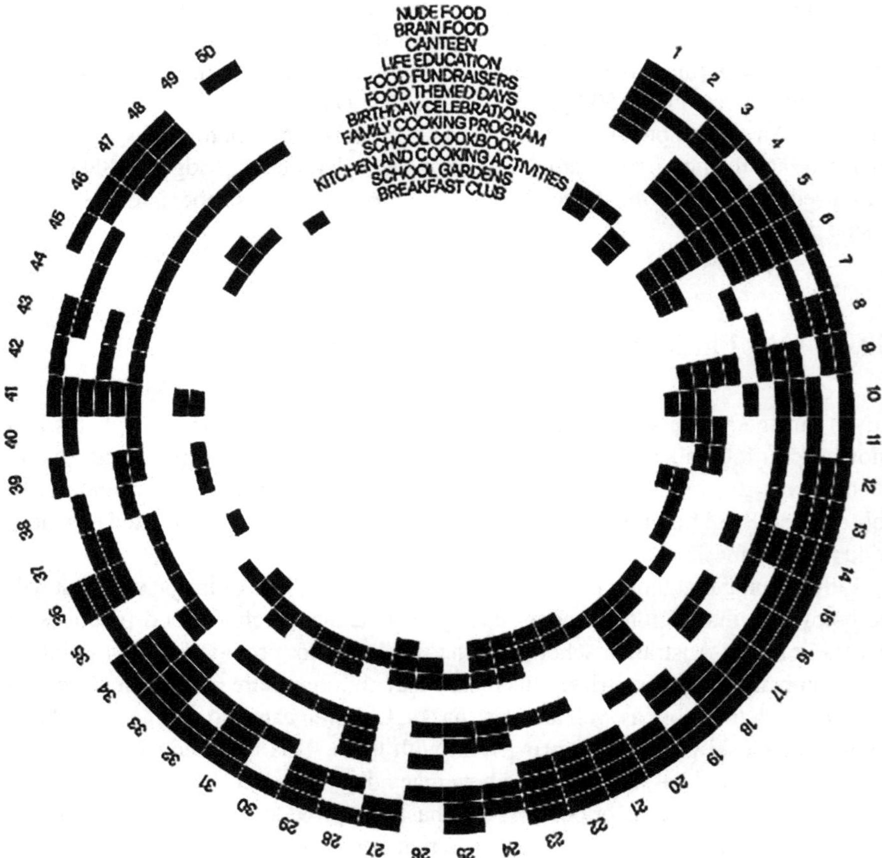

Fig. 40.1 Taking stock of school food initiatives. (Schooling Food, 2019)

A common theme throughout our conversations was how haphazard schools were in their attempts to regulate, and educate about, food choice and consumption. Participants discussed different examples to highlight the inconsistencies they experienced. For example, some talked about how the attention that was paid to lunchboxes and healthy eating seemed to have little bearing on the fact that they were often asked to sell chocolate or soft drinks as fundraisers for the school. Others talked about how their children at the same school experienced very different rules about lunch boxes depending on what grade they were in, and what teacher they had. Different teachers across grade levels meant that children were exposed to different regulations around places of eating and monitoring of food brought to school.

Throughout our many discussions about the multitude of school food programmes and activities, families reported that there was very little formal nutrition or food education (see Maher et al., 2020). Children and families ($n = 20$) did, however, talk about the Life Education Program, an external health education provider that arrives in a van and visits primary schools for short periods of time. Life Education has been a key feature of health education in Australia and New Zealand for over 40 years. Exposure to this programme seemed to be something that was more present for children in the early years of schooling. Despite being involved in the programme, children's knowledge about health and food rarely extended beyond simple understandings of what are considered to be healthy and unhealthy foods. In contrast to formal curriculum, children and their families talked a lot about other food programmes, including nude food, brain food, garden and cooking programmes. Despite the programmes operating largely as extra curricula offerings, the programmes impacted on children's understanding of food. For example, children could recite what their school considered to be brain food or nude food, though again their understandings were limited. Overall, in lieu of any formal ongoing quality health, food or nutrition education, schools tended to rely on a variety of extra curricula programmes.

Across the various fragmented programmatic arrangements in schools, we found no evidence of any programme that utilized child health advocacy as a tactic for obesity prevention. We asked about it, but the overwhelming response was that it 'wasn't a thing' anyone had been a part of. There were examples of where kids were given newsletters to take home or parents were sent information about what the school considered to be healthy snacks and lunches or rules about what kinds of food their children could bring to school. Some schools invited parents to attend assemblies or be part of cookbook or gardening initiatives. But our participants made no mention of any attempt made by teachers to recruit children as health advocates. From all accounts, the everyday attempts at food education and regulation did not provide the conditions required for an initiative like child health advocacy to flourish.

40.5 Using Social Theory to Make Sense of the Messiness of Everyday School Food Programmes

How to make sense of the diverse range of programmes that existed in our family's schools? We turned to two main bodies of literature to help us think about the state of school food. First, we drew inspiration from the emerging interdisciplinary field of food pedagogies (see Flowers & Swan, 2016). Drawing on this scholarly field, each programme or food activity could be understood as either a formal or informal site of learning which form part of a constellation of school food pedagogies that have emerged and/or transformed over time because of the 'obesity epidemic' (see Flowers & Swan, 2016). Each food pedagogy has its own set of ambitions which effectively provides its pedagogical force, which in turn informs the programmatic strategies that get utilized. Adopting this approach meant that we were able to look beyond the usual site of the classroom where pedagogy normally resides to think about how school assemblies, school fundraising efforts, brain food snack programmes, canteens and even children's lunchboxes operate as diverse food pedagogies. This was important for our study given that formal curriculum did not feature in family conversations and we needed to be able to think about how the other school food programmes functioned in lieu of formal curriculum time. It allowed us to contemplate the different knowledges and affects that were produced by each programme which helped us make sense of the different messages and the contradictions our participants talked about.

However, food pedagogies on their own as a conceptual device was not enough to help us make sense of the messiness of school food and its many different configurations across and within schools. We needed some other theoretical resources to help us unpack what the data was telling us about the fragmented and contradictory tales being told by families about their experiences of school food programmes. To help us think about the school programme data, we turned to the Foucauldian inspired field of governmentality studies given its focus on questions related to how the population is governed. This in turn enabled us to think about the various food pedagogies as sites of regulation as they all functioned to purposefully shape particular kinds of behaviours or dispositions of students, but also families. More significantly, governmentality studies enabled us to make sense of the messiness of school food programmes. In previous research, governmentality studies had been drawn on to make sense of the messiness of classroom health education pedagogies (see Leahy, 2014; Leahy & Pike, 2015) and the role of corporations in school health (see Powell, 2014). We wanted to consider what governmentality studies, and particularly the conceptual device of governmental assemblages offered us as we try to forge an explanation for the multiple but varied school food programmes and experiences that featured throughout our participant interviews.

The concept of governmental assemblages emerged out of Foucault's theorizing about contemporary modes of governance or, in his words, the 'conduct of conduct' (see Foucault, 1991). Governmentality scholars, in particular Nikolas Rose and Mitchell Dean have elaborated on Foucault's work to develop his ideas on governmentality. In their various writings, Rose (2000, 2001) and Dean (2010) further developed the conceptual idea that contemporary government is made up of an ensemble of institutions and procedures, working in various lash ups or independently. What this means for our analysis is that we actually should expect to see a range of programmes, from diverse organizations, operating in schools. Whilst on the surface some might imagine this to reflect a 'rational ordering' as the different programmes all appeared in their various singular forms to have a logical order and many adhered to what might be considered the basic tenets we associate with health promotion. However, in the everyday of schooling, when the constellation of food pedagogies are in motion, students and their families find themselves grappling with a diverse and often competing understandings that emerge from different places and organizations because each programme has different ambitions and strategies.

The other issue to consider is that in the everyday of schooling, and in particular in classrooms, is that food pedagogies can hybridize as they are enacted. The drug education strategy of 'Just saying no to pies' I referred to earlier in the chapter provides a good example of what is meant here by hybridization. Whilst we weren't in schools observing food pedagogies in motion in this particular study, it was clear from our data that food pedagogies were indeed hybridizing. The Nude Food Program provides a good case in point. In our study, 38 families out of the 50 reported that they were subjected to the Nude Food programme. Nude Food programmes are connected to Nude Food Movers, a product range produced by Smash Enterprises, an Australian lunch box manufacturer (https://www.nudefoodmovers.com.au). In 2010, Smash Enterprises partnered with *Nutrition Australia* to launch Nude Food Day, as a way to encourage healthy lunches and minimize waste. The initiative reflects a trend of corporate interests merging with health promotion agencies to engage in the everyday work of health promotion and thus governing health via lunchboxes[1] Whilst lunchboxes have been a favourite site of intervention for health promotion for some time (see Harman & Cappelini, 2015; Pike & Leahy, 2012; Pluim et al., 2018), the fact that Nude Food's co-creators manufacture lunchboxes designed specifically for the Nude Food programme is significant. The Nude Food programme was implemented in different ways across schools, and even within schools. Some schools in our study, for example, were Nude Food schools, that is, all food brought to school needed to be 'nude', that is unpackaged every day. Some ran the programme once a week (Nude Food Tuesday), some once a term and others once a year. Some even held 'surprise' Nude Food Days, where children and parents were only told the day before that 'tomorrow is Nude Food Day'.

Parents said they found the Nude Food lunch boxes useful, with their tiny compartments and containers convenient for 'brain food' and snacks. However, parents also described the tireless 'hunt' for many lost small containers and lids. When components went missing, parents had to replace whole lunch boxes. Nude Food Day also sparked anxiety in some parents, spurring trips to school lost property and

---

[1] See Powell (2014) for a more extensive critique of the lash up of multinational corporations and health education.

last-minute runs to the grocery store, tearing packaging off at home before packing food into containers in order to meet the Nude Food standards. Some children and parents described the fear of turning up to school with food in wrappers when it was Nude Food Day. During our interviews, we met 6-year-old Emily who attended a Nude Food school. When Emily was in prep, her mother packed a wrapped muesli bar in her lunch box. Emily realized her mother's mistake as soon as she opened her lunch. Terrified that she would be told off, she ran outside and buried the offending muesli bar in the school garden. We heard several stories like Emily's from other children and families.

While some of the talk around appropriate food to be included in lunchboxes engaged with food knowledge about healthy and unhealthy foods, the school information around nude food seemed to draw primarily on an environmental discourse of sustainability (that is the avoidance of single use plastic). In contrast, the children's talk about nude food programmes was more likely to be characterized by references to regulatory practices – the desire to reduce the amount of rubbish at school and also punishments and rewards for individuals and school classes for their compliance. In some children's minds, Nude Food was about rubbish. The initial intention of the programme had hybridized, in that further locally based ideals for the programme became entangled in the programme. We might even be tempted to say in some cases that the original intentions for the Nude Food Program were 'lost in translation' as they made their way from the creators of the programme to the intended audiences as the focus on healthy eating and sustainability had been displaced in the everyday enactment of the programme by a focus on managing rubbish in schools.

In some ways the messiness of Nude Food, and School Food in general, was to be expected as governmentality scholars have for some time told us that contemporary approaches to governing the population that are made up of ad hoc arrangements of agencies, actors, knowledges and practices ultimately result in a broad range of heterogeneous and fragmented approaches (Dean, 2010; Moore & Valverde, 2000; Rose, 2000). Research that has utlized governmentality studies to examine school-based health education has flagged this as well (Leahy, 2014; Powell, 2014). Our research though provided new insights from children and families about their experiences of effects and affects of programmatic efforts to govern children and family food practices.

40.5.1 The Promises and Pitfalls of Thinking Wildly and Interdisciplinary Research

Our research findings provide significant food for thought for both policymakers and policy actors, including principals, teachers, health promotion and organizations that contribute to the (re) transformation of school foodscapes in response to the ongoing obesity epidemic. The data presents us with the problem of complexity. However, rather than trying to eschew complexity, we embrace it following Warin and Zivkovic (2019), recognizing that it is an inevitable part of what it is to intervene in any health problem. Part of that complexity can be attributed to the prevailing neoliberal policy conditions that have reduced the role of the state in health promotion and enabled corporations, agencies and a myriad of other actors to get involved in, and benefit from, health promotion. Additionally, schools and teachers are required to respond to a crisis, but have little if any funding to support their response. Schools find themselves in a position where they have to fundraise, so their canteens and other fundraising efforts have to make a profit for them. They find themselves having to balance profits with health. All this whilst they are surveilling what children bring from home in their lunchboxes and trying to intervene in family food practices. The school–family–food nexus simply adds to the complexity of this work. Our research points to the need for us to develop more sophisticated and nuanced insights into the everyday policies and practices of school health promotion from multiple viewpoints, including teachers, canteen workers, principals, children, parents and community partners and stakeholders.

To be able to engage with the complex work of health promotion in any setting, our research invites us to rethink the business-as-usual approach to health promotion and research. John Law (2014, p. 2) in a commentary about mess in social science research, tells us that traditional research methods are inadequate to describe things that are 'complex, diffuse and messy'. Even the recent Lancet Commission on the Global Syndemic of Obesity acknowledges that the current approach to obesity prevention is failing and that obesity needs to be looked at in a much wider social and political context. The report urges for a radical rethink of business models, food systems, civil society involvement, and national and international governance to address the syndemic. To achieve this, we are going to need to think wildly and rethink our research methods and our theoretical alliances. We are going to need some new research tactics.

The reality is that we will need more than new tactics, interdisciplinary thinking and innovative methods that can help us grasp the interplay of health, people, policies and programmes. We are going to need more enabling structures. Bromham et al. (2016), for example, highlight how interdisciplinary research, whilst a hothouse for innovation is perceived to have poorer funding success. Warin and Zivkovic (2019) too, highlight the difficulties experienced by social scientists in having their research taken seriously in the field of public health. This can mean that articles that engage with different theoretical and methodological tools are not read by researchers in public health or health promotion. There are examples of where some journal editors balk at the idea of a sociologically informed article even going so far as to reject it because it is either too complicated or not what they are looking for. Additionally, University internal structures aren't always conducive to interdisciplinary research. Barriers exist across university departments that can prohibit researchers forging teams outside of their department drive financial codes and processes. There are without doubt significant barriers to embracing thinking wildly in health promotion research. But if we are interested in dealing with complexity and failure that are mainstays in our field we are going to need to think wildly and commit to working out ways how we might "assemble all knowledge practices and compare them, without privileging one over the other [and this could mean], a very useful way may emerge for us to reimagine obesity, and to find new ways to address it" (Warin & Zivkovic, 2019, p. 215).

Acknowledgements I would like to thank the Child Health Advocates research team; Professor Jane Maree Maher, Professor Jo Lindsay, Professor Jan Wright, Dr Claire Tanner and Dr Sian Supski. The very inception of the project was an act of thinking wildly in school food research and health promotion. The interdisciplinary team provided a lot of food for thought that will undoubtedly continue to seed many other projects and papers over time.

References

Berlant, L. (2011). *Cruel optimism*. Duke University Press.

Bromham, L., Dinnage, R., & Hua, X. (2016). Interdisciplinary research has consistently lower funding success. *Nature (London), 534*, 684–687.

Brown, W. (2005). *Edgework*. Princeton University Press.

Burrows, L., & Wright, J. (2020). Biopedagogies and family life: A social class perspective. In D. Leahy, K. Fitzpatrick, & J. Wright (Eds.), *Thinking with theory in health education* (pp. 19–32). Routledge.

Burrows, L., Wright, J., & Jurgensen, J. (2002). 'Measure your belly' New Zealand children's constructions of health and fitness. *Journal of Teaching in Physical Education, 78*, 39–48.

Commonwealth of Australia. (2003). *Healthy weight 2008: Australia's future*. Department of Health and Ageing.

Commonwealth of Australia. (2018). *Obesity epidemic in Australia: Final Report,* https://www.aph.gov.au/Parliamentary_Business/Committees/Senate/Obesity_epidemic_in_Australia/Obesity/Final_ReportAccessed 10 Dec 2020.

Dean, M. (2010). *Governmentality*. Sage.

Flowers, R., & Swan, E. (2016). *Food Pedagogies*. Taylor and Francis. https://doi.org/10.4324/9781315582689.

Foucault, M. (1991). Governmentality. In G. Burchell, C. Gordon, & P. Miller (Eds.), *The Foucault effect: Studies in governmentality* (pp. 87–104). Harvester Wheatsheaf.

Gard, M., & Pluim, C. (2014). *Schools and public health: Past, present, future*. Lexington Books.

Gard, M., & Wright, J. (2001). Managing uncertainty: Obesity discourses and physical education in a risk society. *Studies in Philosophy and Education, 20*, 535–549.

Halberstam, J. (2014). *Notes on wildness (This is not a manifesto)* https://hemisphericinstitute.org/en/enc14-5-minute-manifestos/item/2608-enc14-5min-halberstam.html Accessed 10 Dec 2020.

Harman, V., & Cappelini, B. (2015). Mothers on display: Lunchboxes, social class and moral accountability. *Sociology, 49*, 764–781.

Law, J. (2014). Working well with wickedness. CSESC (Centre for Research on Socio-Cultural Change) working paper. http://www.cresc.ac.uk/publications/working-well-with-wickendess. Accessed 1 Nov 2020.

Leahy, D. (2014). Assembling a health[y] subject: Risky and shameful pedagogies in health education. *Critical Public Health, 24*, 171–181.

Leahy, D., & Harrison, L. (2004). Health and physical Education and the production of the 'at risk self'. In J. Evans, B. Davies, & J. Wright (Eds.), *Body knowledge and control: Studies in the sociology of physical education and health* (pp. 130–139). Routledge.

Leahy, D., & Pike, J. (2015). 'Just say no to pies': Food pedagogies, health education and governmentality. In R. Flowers & E. Swan (Eds.), *Food pedagogies* (1st ed., pp. 169–182). (Critical Food Studies)). Routledge.

Leahy, D., McCuaig, L., Burrows, L., Wright, J., & Penney, D. (2016). *School health education in changing times: Policies, pedagogies and partnerships*. Routledge.

Leahy, D., Fitzpatrick, K., & Wright, J. (2020a). *Social theory and health education: Forging new insights in research.* (Critical studies in health and education). Routledge.

Leahy, D., Fitzpatrick, K., & Wright, J. (2020b). Why do *we need social theory in Health education?* In D. Leahy, K. Fitzpatrick, & J. Wright (Eds.), *Social theory and health education: Forging new insights in research (Critical studies in health and education).* Routledge.

Lomax, H. (2015). Seen and heard? Ethics and agency in participatory visual research with children, young people and families. *Families, Relationships and Societies, 4*, 493–502.

Maher, J. M., Fraser, S., & Wright, J. (2010). Framing the mother: Childhood obesity, maternal responsibility and care. *Journal of Gender Studies, 19*, 233–247.

Maher, J., Supski, S., Wright, J., Leahy, D., Lindsay, J., & Tanner, C. (2020). Children, 'healthy' food, school and family: The '[n]ot really' outcome of school food messages. *Children's Geographies, 18*(1), 81–95. https://doi.org/10.1080/14733285.2019.1598546

Moore, D., & Valverde, M. (2000). Maidens at risk: 'date rape drugs' and the formation of hybrid risk knowledges. *Economy and Society, 29*(4), 514–531. https://doi.org/10.1080/03085140050174769

Nyberg, M. (2019). Children's pictures of a good and desirable meal in Kindergarten – a participatory visual approach. *Children & Society, 33*, 471–487.

O'Connell, R. (2013). The use of visual methods with children in a mixed methods study of family food practices. *International Journal of Social Research Methodology, 16*, 31–46.

Peterson, A., & Lupton, D. (1996). *The new public health: Health and self in the age of risk.* Allen & Unwin.

Pike, J., & Leahy, D. (2012). School food and the pedagogies of parents. *Australian Journal of Adult Learning, 52*, 434–459.

Pluim, C., Powell, D., & Leahy, D. (2018). Schooling lunch: Health, food, and the pedagogicalization of the lunch box. In S. Rice & A. G. Rud (Eds.), *Educational dimensions of school lunch: Critical perspectives* (pp. 59–74). Palgrave Macmillan.

Powell, D. (2014). Childhood obesity, corporate philanthropy and the creeping privatisation of health education. *Critical Public Health, 24*, 226–238.

Rasmussen, M. L. (2020). Working with social theory in health education? In D. Leahy, K. Fitzpatrick, & J. Wright (Eds.), *Social theory and health education: Forging new insights in research (Critical studies in health and education).* Routledge.

Rose, N. (2000). Government and control. *British Journal of Criminology, 40*, 321–339.

Rose, N. (2001). The politics of life itself. *Theory, Culture and Society, 8*, 1–29.

Schooling Food: An exhibition. (2019). www.schoolingfood.com Accessed 12 Dec 2020

The Lancet Commission. (2019). The global syndemic of obesity, undernutrition, climate change: The Lancet Commission report. https://www.thelancet.com/commissions/global-syndemic. Accessed Nov 3 2020.

Warin, M., & Moore, V. (2020). Epistemic conflicts and Achilles' heels: Constraints of a university and public sector partnership to research obesity in Australia. *Critical Public Health, 31*(5), 617–628. https://doi.org/10.1080/09581596.2020.1761944

Warin, M., & Zivkovic, T. (2019). *Fatness, obesity and disadvantage in the Australia suburbs: Unpalatable politics.* Palgrave Macmillan.

Warin, M., Zivkovic, T., Moore, V., & Davies, M. (2014). Mothers as smoking guns: Fetal overnutrition and the reproduction of obesity 1. In *Obesity, eating disorders and the media* (1st ed., pp. 73–89). Routledge.

Wright, J., & Harwood, V. (2009). *Biopolitics and the 'Obesity Epidemic'.* (Routledge Studies in Health and Social Welfare). Taylor and Francis.

Chapter 41
Fitting Health Promotion Research with Real-Life Conditions: Viability Evaluation

Charlotte Decroix, Charlotte Kervran, Linda Cambon, and François Alla

41.1 Introduction

Health promotion interventions (actions, programmes, organizations, policies) are generally complex, presenting researchers with a real methodological challenge (Alla, 2018). They require research designs that facilitate understanding of the mechanisms and processes and allow the implementation and conditions of routinization, transfer and scaling up of the intervention to be analysed (Cambon et al., 2013; Chen, 2010). Consideration of principles inherent to health promotion must be added to this challenge, such as participation (which implies the production of knowledge not only "about" but also "with" the users) and incorporating the needs of a variety of stakeholders in a "health for all" perspective (World Health Organization (WHO), 1986).

These challenges require research methodologies adapted to health promotion interventions for which "classical" research designs derived from clinical research show their limitations (Tarquinio et al., 2015). In this perspective, Chen developed a model of integrative validity which recognizes three types of validity: internal

C. Decroix · C. Kervran
Bordeaux University, Inserm, Bordeaux Population Health Research Center, Bordeaux, France

L. Cambon
Bordeaux University, Inserm, Bordeaux Population Health Research Center, Bordeaux, France

Prevention Chair, ISPED, University of Bordeaux, Bordeaux, France

F. Alla (✉)
Bordeaux University, Inserm, Bordeaux Population Health Research Center, Bordeaux, France

CHU de Bordeaux, Bordeaux, France
e-mail: francois.alla@u-bordeaux.fr

L. Potvin, D. Jourdan (eds.), *Global Handbook of Health Promotion Research, Vol. 1*,
https://doi.org/10.1007/978-3-030-97212-7_41

validity, external validity and viable validity. Viable validity is defined as "*the extent to which an evaluation provides evidence that an intervention is successful in the real world*" (Chen, 2010). Questioning the viability of an intervention may be considered a prerequisite for any effectiveness study to avoid the risk of initiating interventions that are not transferable or generalizable in the real world at the end of the research process (Chen, 2010).

After reviewing the value of the integrative validity model, this chapter discusses the need for evaluative research questions related to viable validity as early as possible in the process of developing complex health promotion interventions through pilot studies. We then examine the different viability criteria. Through different examples, we attempt to propose a conceptual, methodological and operational perspective to evaluate and allow for the viability of an intervention in a pilot study.

41.2 The Notion of Viable Validity

41.2.1 The Campbellian Validity Model (Campbell and Stanley): Approach and Limitations

Health research is imbued with Campbell and Stanley's (1963) post-positivist model of validity. This model distinguishes between two types of validity: internal and external (Campbell & Stanley, 1963). The first "*asks whether, in this specific experimental instance, the intervention made a difference*"(Chen, 2010), while the second "*asks whether an experimental effect is capable of generalization, and if so, to what populations, settings, or treatment and measurement variables*" (Chen, 2010). The decision to study interventions in a highly controlled setting or as close as possible to real-life conditions increases internal validity in the former and external validity in the latter. In this context, Campbell and Stanley recommended a stepwise approach to evaluative research, beginning with an internal validity analysis to examine the intervention's potential efficacy under experimental conditions, followed by an external validity study to investigate how it maintains effectiveness in "everyday" conditions (Campbell & Stanley, 1963) in parallel with or in anticipation of dissemination. Drug development is based on this model, for instance. A randomized controlled trial demonstrates the efficacy of a drug (phase III trial) before it can be marketed, possibly followed by phase IV studies that evaluate its safety and efficacy in real life.

There is a tendency to opt for clinical research paradigms and methods to evaluate health promotion interventions. However, this approach has major limitations, some of which were identified by Chen, e.g. this type of internal validity-focused approach does not produce information that can be extrapolated or that is sufficiently relevant to stakeholders to influence their decisions (Cronbach, 1982), and stakeholders' views and needs are insufficiently taken into consideration (Chen, 2010).

This is inconsistent with the principles of responsiveness to people's needs and preferences and the participation inherent in health promotion (WHO, 1986). It is in this context that Chen proposed an alternative model to that of Campbell and Stanley (Campbell & Stanley, 1963), namely, the integrative validity model (Chen, 2010).

41.2.2 *The Integrative Validity Model*

The integrative validity model is based on a combination of the principles set out in the Campbellian model and the need to incorporate elements that guarantee useful and relevant results for stakeholders, thus reducing the "*gap between the academic and practical communities on interventions*" (Chen, 2010). As noted in Table 41.1, this model adopts the concepts of internal and external validity and adds the notion of viable validity.

Referring to the views and interests of stakeholders, viability is defined as "*the extent to which an evaluation provides evidence that an intervention is successful in the real world.*" It thus aims to

- Question whether an intervention is deployable beyond a research context by organizations and stakeholders involved in current practice
- Analyse whether, in the experience of stakeholders, an intervention is "*practical, affordable, suitable, evaluable, and helpful in the real world*" (Chen, 2010)

Table 41.1 From the Campbellian model to the model of integrative validity, according to Chen (2010)

	Campbellian validity model	Main changes between models	Integrative validity model (Chen, 2010)
Internal validity	*"asks whether, in this specific experimental instance, the intervention made a difference"*	> Emphasis on objectivity of results	*"the extent to which an evaluation provides objective evidence that an intervention causally affects specified outcomes"*
External validity	*"asks whether an experimental effect is capable of generalization, and if so, to what populations, settings or treatment and measurement variables"*	> Clarification of the limits of the concept, with a focus on (a) the stakeholders' point of view and interest; (b) the notion of the real world > Concerns viability in addition to effectiveness	*"the extent to which evaluation findings of effectiveness can be generalized from a research setting to a real-world setting or from one real-world setting to another targeted setting"*
Viable validity		> Addition: (a) from the perspective and interest of stakeholders; (b) from the notion of the real world > Prerequisite for the study of other validities	*"the extent to which an evaluation provides evidence that an intervention is successful in the real world"*

Chen anchors this model in an approach that he defines as bottom-up (as opposed to the Campbellian model, which he defines as top-down), considering that the study of viable validity is a prerequisite for the internal and external validity evaluation. Indeed, what is the point of mobilizing actors and employing resources to assess efficacy and effectiveness if the intervention cannot be transferred or generalized to everyday practices? (Chen, 2010).

41.2.3 Relevance of the Integrative Validity Model to Health Promotion Research

In the field of Population Health Intervention Research (PHIR), the bottom-up model predicated on the real world is all the more relevant since population health interventions (actions, programmes, organizations, policies) are generally considered to be complex (Moore et al., 2015). This complexity is characterized in particular by the multiple components that interact both with one another and with the context to produce effects (Hawe & Potvin, 2009; Moore et al., 2015). The intervention and the implementation context continually interact, leading to the consideration of an interventional system rather than a delineated intervention (Cambon et al., 2019). This raises the question of what makes an intervention effective in a specific context that will also make it effective in a variety of other conditions (Cambon et al., 2019; Minary et al., 2018). The question is related to issues of intervention transferability and scaling up. For instance, if context is a determinant of outcome, are outcomes obtained in one experimental setting transferable to another setting? In other words, what is the use of an "effective" intervention under experimental conditions that cannot be encountered in real life (Treweek & Zwarenstein, 2009)?

41.3 The Viability Study: A Key Element in Pilot Studies

The Medical Research Council (MRC) identified several non-linear phases in the development and evaluation of complex interventions (Craig, Dieppe et al., 2008):

- The development phase: identifying the evidence base, identifying or developing theory, the modelling process and outcomes
- The feasibility and pilot phase: testing procedures, estimating recruitment and retention, determining sample size
- The evaluation phase: assessing effectiveness and cost-effectiveness, understanding the change processes
- The implementation phase: dissemination, surveillance and monitoring, long-term follow-up

Consistent with a bottom-up health promotion approach and considering intervention viability as a prerequisite to any evaluation of efficacy/effectiveness means that viable validity must be studied as early as possible in the innovation process, generally right from the pilot stage.

41.3.1 What Do We Mean by 'Pilot Study'?

Pilot studies aim to gather information in order to do something on a larger scale (Thabane et al., 2019). The term pilot study is well established in biomedical research, and so-called phase III pilot studies are routinely conducted (Thabane et al., 2010).

The situation is more ambiguous in PHIR, where a pilot study refers to different objects (Thabane et al., 2019). While clinical research pilot studies are designed to prepare for a trial, in PHIR, pilot studies may involve the preparation of an intervention and/or a trial (or an evaluation) (Thabane et al., 2019). For trial and/or evaluation preparation, pilot studies are clearly standardized (e.g. CONSORT extension specifically for pilot trials (Eldridge, Chan et al., 2016). Consensus and methods seem to be less precise about intervention preparation, which is a key issue for PHIR (Thabane et al., 2019).

41.3.2 What Knowledge Do We Need to Support the Scaling-up Process and How to Produce It?

Unlike some commonly deployed interventions where the evaluator adopts observational methods, we focus on pilot studies of new interventions, whether developed by researchers and/or stakeholders. In 2016, a consortium of twenty-five international experts in PHIR and complex interventions met at a workshop organized by the Coordinated Action for Public Health Intervention Research (ACRISP) to "*promote exchanges between researchers from different disciplines due to the complexity of the field, which requires an interdisciplinary approach*" (Moore et al., 2019; Thabane et al., 2019). It covered issues related to pilot studies, with the experts identifying several objectives for pilot studies of "new" complex interventions, in addition to piloting a trial/evaluation (Thabane et al., 2019). These included:

- Studying the viability of the intervention in the given context
- Explaining the intervention theory. Intervention theory can be defined as "*the set of beliefs and assumptions that undergird program activities […]. They are the hypotheses on which people, consciously or unconsciously, build their program plans and actions*" (Weiss, 1997). According to the intervention-based paradigm, all interventions are based on theories which need to be made explicit to ensure the relevance of the intervention and to achieve the desired outcomes.

These goals align closely with the challenges of transferability and scaling up, since the development of intervention theory (Cambon & Alla, 2019; Moore et al., 2019) and the study of viability help to define the conditions in which an intervention is likely to work, including the influence of its implementation environment (context).

Some dimensions of viability (e.g. programme acceptability from the beneficiaries' perspective) form an integral part of the intervention system, involving context – intervention interactions that trigger (or not) (a) mechanism(s) producing (or not) certain effects. Considering the viability of an intervention as a key factor in its transfer, it seems crucial to analyse viability as early as possible in the innovation process. Moreover, when studying the transferability of complex interventions, a core concern is to distinguish between the adaptable form of the intervention according to the context and the "key function" essential to producing effects (Hawe et al., 2004). Thus, studying transferability highlights intervention components that can be adapted to various contexts and can strengthen its viability while maintaining effects.

Inset 1 illustrates how some aspects of viability are absolute conditions for implementing an intervention in the real world, and the importance of investigating it as early as possible in the intervention development process, in other words, right from the pilot phase.

Inset 1 – PERL project (Early Childhood Research-Action in Lorraine)
In a peri-urban area of north-eastern France marked by unfavourable socio-economic indicators, a primary prevention intervention in perinatal care based on tailored support for families showed positive results on child development (Fidry et al., 2014). To address the transfer or scaling up of this intervention, adaptations were required to facilitate its embedding in common practice, notably by incorporating the support available within the current health system resources (support initially provided by a psychiatric psychologist, then by a team of nurses from the Maternal and Child Protection Department).

These adaptations gave rise to the PERL project (Early Childhood Research-Action in Lorraine), designed to mesh the results of the study into a universal family health policy (Buchheit et al., 2019). In this context, nurses at the Maternal and Child Protection Department support families through home visits until a child is 4 years old. The visits are split into three stages and supervised by a psychologist.

In parallel to the effectiveness evaluation of PERL, in the first year of the intervention's rollout, an assessment was made to examine the processes and mechanisms at play. Contextual difficulties were encountered regarding the feasibility and acceptability of PERL by stakeholders adopting the intervention, temporarily jeopardizing its rollout. Taking the example of one of the issues encountered, namely, the place of recommendations made by nurses in the PERL project, the results show that unlike the trend towards standardization or an instructions-grounded process, the PERL approach considers parents as experts with respect to their own child, offering them support to develop awareness of their own capacity and skills in raising their child. This health promotion practice, designed to empower parents, challenges individual and cultural representations in terms of child-rearing, the legitimacy of professionals considered to know what is best for a child and the standards to which these professionals refer. When such practices are part of a health promotion approach, it is essential that they are shared with professionals offering support to families within a legal framework that allows them to apply such principles.

The investigations highlight the fact that while for some professionals this approach (aimed at limiting recommendations) represents a continuity of practice, for others it is unacceptable for several reasons, e.g. professionals' belief in the importance of giving advice and their responsibility to provide it, reflecting as much their professional conscience as their legal responsibility; professionals' identification of an expertise expectation by families with respect to support; guilt with regard to the feeling of being useful in a context where care resources are limited.

This example highlights the importance of a shared vision of the relevance of the intervention, both in terms of its nature and methods if the intervention is to be adopted and deployed. Without this, even if effective, its dissemination will fail. It is therefore essential to investigate the intervention's acceptability by the actors in the field, their appropriation of the intervention, and the feasibility of its deployment and viable validity criteria, even before evaluating its effectiveness, thereby helping to avoid interventions that are not transferable or generalizable in the real world (i.e. in contexts other than the study context).

While pilot studies offer golden opportunities for studying viability, the latter can be questioned at all stages of the innovation's development. From the beginning of the intervention development, when the intervention levers are being developed, the viability analysis can be incorporated using elements from the literature and/or interviews with stakeholders in the field. This involves considering known conditions of the levers' effectiveness. For example, financial incentives have proven to be an effective lever for smoking cessation among pregnant women (Higgins & Solomon, 2016; Lumley et al., 2009). However, in some countries, many women are opposed to this intervention strategy (Lynagh et al., 2011), indicating a lack of viability in these contexts. In such instances, this lever should be removed from the intervention theory. Viability studies also have their place in the evaluation (whatever the design: realistic evaluation, randomized trials, process evaluation…) or the dissemination of the intervention by re-examining viability as it is deployed in the various contexts.

41.3.3 What Criteria for Viability?

For Chen, "*viable validity refers to stakeholders' views and experience regarding whether an intervention program is practical, affordable, suitable, evaluable and helpful in the real-world*" (Chen, 2010). One of the aims of this chapter is to define these criteria by illustrating their operationalization in the pilot studies of two projects: the "Tobacco-Free Health Support Center" (L.A.S.T) and "Accompagne-moi."

The aim of L.A.S.T is to enhance support for smokers against their addiction to tobacco by implementing incremental pathways between the Tobacco-Free Health Support Centres (L.A.S.T, first-line care offer: https://www.last-na.fr/) and other resource centres (second line of care for so-called complex patients). The "Accompagne-moi" programme is designed to improve the quality of childcare centres and to promote children's social skills from an early age. We will return to each criterion on the basis of the viability studies carried out during the pilot studies of these two programmes, with a breakdown presented in Table 41.2.

Helpful "Can the intervention program (1) recruit ordinary clients without paying them to participate, (2) does it have a clear rationale for its structure and linkages connecting an intervention to expected outcomes, and (3) do ordinary clients and other stakeholders regard the intervention as helpful in alleviating clients' problems or in enhancing their well-being as defined by the program's real-life situations? In this context, 'helpful' refers to whether stakeholders notice or experience progress in alleviating or resolving a problem." In the context of the "Accompagne-moi" health promotion programme, 'helpful' includes its capacity to respond to a need and demand from the population, where an adapted response is lacking. This is addressed by studying the programme's effects as perceived by early childhood professionals and parents. In L.A.S.T, this issue concerns whether the proposed organization can help carers to manage their patients' smoking cessation and whether it meets the expectations and needs of smokers.

Affordable "An additional question is whether decision-makers view the intervention program as affordable?" and whether the intervention "can recruit and/or retain ordinary clients." In "Accompagne-moi," the issue is defined around two aspects: an impossibility to access the intervention or a refusal to participate. The aim was to study the facilitating conditions and the barriers to the participation in the programme, together with the participants' adherence through to completion. It also involved understanding the reasons why some professionals refused to participate or dropped out of the programme. Finally, there was a focus on children's access to the programme. While access appears universal for pre-school children, the differential involvement of professionals as a function of the children or the parents' investment may have an impact on children's access. In the context of L.A.S.T., this issue concerns: (a) the means implemented between 1st and 2nd referral health professionals, and (b) evaluation of the barriers and levers (financial, geographical, socio-cultural, environmental) that could influence the accessibility of health professionals and beneficiaries to the proposed organization and thus their involvement in the programme.

Practical and Suitable The first criteria asks "whether ordinary practitioners – rather than research staff – can implement an intervention program adequately," and the second, "whether the intervention is suitable for ordinary implementing organizations to coordinate intervention-related activities." These criteria can be perceived as an intervention's potential to be integrated into current practice in relation to the

Table 41.2 Questions relating to each viability criterion in the framework of the "Accompagne-moi" and L.A.S.T. programme pilot studies

Criteria	Chen (2010)	Questions – viability study	
		"*Accompagne-moi*"	"L.A.S.T"
Helpful	"Can the intervention program (1) recruit ordinary clients without paying them to participate, (2) does it have a clear rationale for its structure and linkages connecting an intervention to expected outcomes, and (3) do ordinary clients and other stakeholders regard the intervention as helpful in alleviating clients' problems or in enhancing their well-being as defined by the program's real-world situations?"	What is the stakeholders' perception of the effects of the "*Accompagne-moi*" programme? How does this programme respond (or not) to a need and a demand?	Does the proposed intervention help caregivers to manage their patients' smoking cessation? Does the proposed intervention provide the support expected by patients who smoke?
Affordable	"An additional question is whether decision-makers view the intervention program as affordable" and if the intervention "can recruit and/or retain ordinary clients"	Is the programme accessible and affordable (or not) for the different stakeholders (crèches, early childhood professionals and children)?	Can first-line care professionals exchange and be sustained by a secondary care professional? How are they organized between the 1st and 2nd line of care? Does the organization setup have financial consequences on the professionals' activity or structures? Can patients have access to 2nd line structures? Do patients encounter geographical and financial barriers in their progress within the organization?

(continued)

Table 41.2 (continued)

Criteria	Chen (2010)	Questions – viability study	
		"Accompagne-moi"	"L.A.S.T"
Practical	"Whether ordinary practitioners – rather than research staff – can implement an intervention program adequately"	How are early childhood professionals and programme providers able to implement *"Accompagne-moi"* on a day-to-day basis? How does the programme fit in with the everyday practices of early childhood professionals, childcare centres and the wider education system?	Is the proposed intervention method integrable into the common practice of carers? Are the tools made available to caregivers applicable in the practices of each job sector?
Suitable	"Whether the intervention is suitable for ordinary implementing organizations to coordinate intervention-related activities"		Are the patient care modalities suitable for them? Are the tools made available to them adapted to the everyday practices of caregivers? Do they feel that the support provided for this proposed organization is sufficient?
Evaluable		What is the feasibility of a future large-scale randomized cluster trial? What are the conditions for conducting such a trial, if applicable?	To what extent is the organization able to produce objective results in terms of health and its determinants?

deployment context. They can be examined from various perspectives, such as the potential to deploy the intervention at organizational level, the perception of the intervention as a continuity or a change of paradigm (as in the PERL example above), the partnership dynamic, or the acceptability of the intervention and its appropriation (stakes, contents…) by the stakeholders. In "Accompagne-moi," the aim is to understand how, for early childhood professionals, the programme fits into common practice, and to study the factors that facilitate and hamper its implementation. Attention is paid to the place of research in the professionals' perception of "Accompagne-moi" deployment, and their interest in taking part in it as a routine. The purpose of the study with regard to the practical criterion of L.A.S.T. is to assess whether the intervention proposed to carers (including the tools) can be integrated into their everyday practice. It examines whether the organization is adapted to the criteria considered suitable by the health system and L.A.S.T. professionals and determines whether the given organization is institutionalized and scalable between the different stakeholders beyond the pilot stage.

Evaluable In LA.S.T., this involves analysing available data to see if outcome indicators exist in current practices. For "Accompagne moi," evaluability is considered as the capacity of the intervention to produce objectively measurable results, looking at the feasibility of a future large-scale randomized cluster trial and the conditions for carrying out such a trial, if applicable.

41.4 How to Conduct a Viable Validity Analysis?

There is no defined standard for understanding viability since the integrative viability model, underpinned by a contingency perspective, is not described as a universal method. Rather, it emphasizes the combination of methods, in particular the use of mixed methods (Chen, 2010). On this basis, we have undertaken half a dozen viability studies that provide concrete operational experience, enabling us to illustrate this aspect.

41.4.1 The Problematization Process

A viability study has the advantage of being both an object of research and a pragmatic object that corresponds to the challenges common to researchers, field actors and decision-makers alike. While many terms exist (evaluation, evaluation-research, action-research, population health intervention research (PHIR), etc.), with more or less consensual boundaries and development according to the field, it is essential to understand the framework within which the viability study is conducted. The framework and the perspective guide the issues, the problematization, and the choice of methods to be adopted, consistent with the purpose of the knowledge sought. For PHIR and evaluative research, the following distinctions are explicitly made (Ferron, 2017; Potvin, 2014):

- In the first, the knowledge produced by the research is general in nature and the intervention's transferability is explicitly studied (in our example, the pilot study of the "Accompagne-moi" programme),
- In the second, the knowledge produced is the basis for a judgement regarding the intervention (with respect to predefined criteria) on which decisions concerning the latter will be made (Ferron, 2017). In our example, this is the L.A.S.T. pilot study.

As in all research projects, the first phase of the study of viability in PHIR is that of problematization, which allows the angle from which the phenomena are studied and the way in which they are questioned to be clarified (Van Campenhoudt et al., 2017).

Likewise, the prospects for deploying the intervention beyond the viability study should be considered right from the problematization phase, notably: What are the issues (scientific, political…) for the actors, decision-makers and researchers involved in the viability study? How can the results of the viability study be integrated into the transfer and/or scaling up options (potential to adapt the intervention to the context, willingness/capacity of actors to question the innovation according to the results…)? In the context of a pilot study, is it a pilot of the intervention, a trial, or both?

In the "*Accompagne-moi*" example, the programme concerns the adaptation of two interventions developed and routinely adopted in Quebec. Its deployment in France is the result of a partnership between an association that recognized a need in French childcare centres, and researchers and actors in Quebec. The two initial interventions were designed on the basis of evidence and have been the focus of several studies (e.g. a cluster-randomized trial (Larose et al., 2019)). The data found in the literature clearly show how this programme responds to a problem (e.g. the quality of the environment in which a child evolves during the first 1000 days of life is decisive for his/her future development (Heckman, 2008)). Nevertheless, many questions arise before the large-scale rollout of the programme can be considered in a new cultural and organizational context in France. Thus, a pilot study is being conducted in order to clearly examine the programme's viability and transferability.

From another perspective, the L.A.S.T. pilot study is the focus of an evaluation of the organization's deployment within a given catchment area, with an assessment of its organizational effectiveness (analysis of changes in target health professionals' practices) and its viability. The study aims to identify the elements required to make improvements that will be useful to the intervention and to adapt its implementation procedures with a view to a planned rollout on a regional scale on completion of the evaluation.

41.4.2 Interest in Studying Viability in Different Research Approaches

Depending on the evaluation framework, the prospects for deploying an intervention after the pilot study (the prospect of scaling up, if applicable, in terms of routine or research, the possibility to adapt the intervention or a protocolized intervention that is not very adaptable), the researchers' epistemological positioning, and the resulting research/evaluation question(s) will give rise to different designs and methods.

With regards to L.A.S.T., for example, viability is investigated in the light of predefined criteria within an evaluation context, including the indicators, sources and reference system for each viability criterion. The accessibility study, for instance, detailed three conditions to describe the intervention as accessible for patients (e.g. the second recourse structures are open to all, regardless of economic and social factors). The resulting data sources apply mixed methods. Qualitative data come from semi-directive interviews with professionals registered in the L.A.S.T. system and beneficiaries, and seek to explore the five viability criteria according to partially predefined themes. Quantitative data are mainly collected from the patient files of the 2nd line structures and from a patients' progress monitoring tool. The evaluation thus allows us to cover the issues raised with respect to predefined criteria.

In "*Accompagne-moi*," the viability and transferability study is split into two stages:

1. An exploratory stage, based on various sources: literature review, exploratory interviews with the stakeholders who helped to initiate the rollout of "*Accompagne-moi*" in the French context, a documentary study.
2. A more in-depth stage through: (1) semi-directive interviews aimed at understanding how the programme is experienced by the implementers and early childhood professionals from the various childcare centres that benefit from the programme; (2) focus groups with parents to examine their perceptions of the relevance of such a programme.

41.4.3 Study of Viability: An Objective for Stakeholder-Researcher Co-Construction

The PHIR has a cognitive goal of knowledge production, but also an operational one in terms of decision-making support. Thus, from our perspective, PHIR only makes sense if the results are conveyed in decision-making and in practice (Alla & Kivits, 2015; Cambon & Alla, 2014). To this end, alternative methods to traditional research models, such as the integrative validity model rooted in a bottom-up approach, are needed to produce usable evidence. This is the very purpose of knowledge transfer. The partnership must be the glue that holds the knowledge transfer together (Cambon & Alla, 2014). All too often seen as a downstream device or an "after-sales service" for research, knowledge transfer requires the involvement of users of the research results as soon as the research idea is formalized. This implies developing a decision-maker/researcher partnership through an interactive approach, with communication between actors and researchers that enables the removal of organizational barriers via ongoing interaction and an iterative understanding of one another's needs. Without wishing to turn field actors into researchers or vice versa, it requires the joint development of conditions to generate evidence that is not only valid but also useful and adapted to action and decision-making (Alla & Kivits, 2015, Cambon & Alla, 2014).

By integrating the stakeholders' viewpoint and constraints regarding whether the intervention is "practical, affordable, suitable, evaluable and helpful in the real world" (Chen, 2010), the viability study is fully anchored (a) in the social utility perspective of the research, (b) from the perspective of taking stakeholders' needs into account in the "health for all" objective of health promotion. In our viability study examples of the L.A.S.T. and "*Accompagne-moi*" programmes, different levels of collaboration are present, from consulting with stakeholders through interviews to stronger anchoring in co-construction, such as the organization of seminars that draw stakeholders together around various issues. These approaches accompany the challenge of participation, aiming to produce knowledge not only "on" but "with" people. While the role of partnership co-construction is central to PHIR, its operationalization is manifold and raises crucial questions as to the nature and balance of the "actor/researcher/decision-maker" partnership. The latter thus becomes a major factor in the success of a PHIR project (Alla & Kivits, 2015).

41.5 Conclusions

PHIR has been described as the "science of solutions," which is complementary to the "science of problems" (Potvin et al., 2014). The expression "science of solutions" underscores the operational nature of research, since one of the goals of the latter is for field practitioners and policymakers to apply its results. Viable validity is perfectly anchored in this perspective since it is "*the extent to which an evaluation provides evidence that an intervention is successful under real-world conditions*" (Chen, 2010). The study of viability should be considered at the earliest possible stage in research issues linked to the development of health promotion interventions. Indeed, as stated earlier, what is the point of developing or demonstrating the effectiveness or generalizing interventions "off the field" if they are not transferable to the "real world?"

Thus, viability is a core issue in health promotion research. This evaluation helps to structure and strengthen the innovation process, adding an essential step in the process, from the development of the intervention to its scaling up. Given its purpose, viability is also a useful communication tool between researchers and stakeholders, helping to operationalize the partnership ambition of health promotion research.

Inset 2: Chapter's contribution to structuring the field of health promotion research

- Health promotion interventions are generally considered as complex, requiring adapted research approaches.
- The integrative validity model recognizes internal and external validities as well as viable validity.
- Viable validity aims to produce evidence that "an intervention is successful in the real world."
- The study of viability should be considered as early as possible in the research process aimed at developing new interventions.
- This approach anchors the PHIR in a bottom-up, partnership-based approach.

Acknowledgments The authors would like to thank the research team implementers and stakeholders in the "L.A.S. T" programme: Rébecca Ratel, Margaux Fontan, Nolwenn Stevens, Estelle Clet, the MERISP team and the Coordination Régionale Addictions Nouvelle-Aquitaine; in the "Accompagne-moi" programme: Sylvana Côté and the Association Ensemble pour l'Education de la Petite Enfance; in "PERL": Sophie Buchheit, Bernard Kabuth, Fabienne Ligier, Joëlle Kivits, and the conseil départemental de Meurthe-et-Moselle.

References

Alla, F. (2018). Challenges for prevention research. *European Journal of Public Health, **28***(1), 1.

Alla, F., & Kivits, J. (2015). Public health international research: Research scientist-field worker partnership, interdisciplinarity and social role. *Santé Publique, **27***(3), 303–304.

Buchheit, S., Colombo, M.-C., Fidry, E., Ligier, F., & Decroix, C. (2019). Lunévillois : Développement de l'enfant et accompagnement à domicile. *La santé en action, **447***.

Cambon, L. & F. Alla (2014). Recherche interventionnelle en santé publique, transfert de connaissances et collaboration entre acteurs, décideurs et chercheurs. Questions de santé Publique. EDK. Montrouge, France, Rercherche en Santé Publique.

Cambon, L., & Alla, F. (2019). Current challenges in population health intervention research. *Journal of Epidemiology and Community Health, **73***(11), 990–992.

Cambon, L., Minary, L., Ridde, V., & Alla, F. (2013). A tool to analyze the transferability of health promotion interventions. *BMC Public Health, **13***, 1184.

Cambon, L., Terral, P., & Alla, F. (2019). From intervention to interventional system: Towards greater theorization in population health intervention research. *BMC Public Health, **19***(1), 339.

Campbell, M. J., & Stanley, J. (1963). *Experimental and quasi-experimental designs for research*. Rand McNally & Company.

Chen, H. T. (2010). The bottom-up approach to integrative validity: A new perspective for program evaluation. *Evaluation and Program Planning, **33***(3), 205–214.

Craig, P., Dieppe, P., Macintyre, S., Michie, S., Nazareth, I., Petticrew, M., & G. Medical Research Council. (2008). Developing and evaluating complex interventions: The new Medical Research Council guidance. *BMJ, **337***, a1655.

Cronbach, L. J. (1982). *Designing evaluations of educational and socila programs*. Jossey-Bass.

Eldridge, S. M., Chan, C. L., Campbell, M. J., Bond, C. M., Hopewell, S., Thabane, L., Lancaster, G. A., & P. c. group. (2016). CONSORT 2010 statement: Extension to randomised pilot and feasibility trials. *Pilot and Feasibility Studies, **2***, 64.

Ferron, C. (2017). *Recherche interventionnelle en promotion de la santé. La promotion de la santé, comprendre pour agir dans le monde francophone* (P. d. l'EHESP. ed., pp. 443–455).

Fidry, E., Claudon, P., Saint-Gilles, S. S., & Sibertin-Blanc, D. (2014). Prendre soin du bébé et de sa famille : Une expérience de recherche–action en périnatalité. *Neuropsychiatrie de l'Enfance et de l'Adolescence, **62***, 154–162.

Hawe, P., & Potvin, L. (2009). What is population health intervention research? *Canadian Journal of Public Health, **100***(1), Suppl I8–Suppl 14.

Hawe, P., Shiell, A., & Riley, T. (2004). Complex interventions: How "out of control" can a randomised controlled trial be? *BMJ, **328***(7455), 1561–1563.

Heckman, J. J. (2008). Role of income and family influence on child outcomes. *Annals of the New York Academy of Sciences, **1136***, 307–323.

Higgins, S. T., & Solomon, L. J. (2016). Some recent developments on financial incentives for smoking cessation among pregnant and newly postpartum women. *Current Addiction Reports, **3***(1), 9–18.

Larose, M. P., Ouellet-Morin, I., Vitaro, F., Geoffroy, M. C., Ahun, M., Tremblay, R. E., & Cote, S. M. (2019). Impact of a social skills program on children's stress: A cluster randomized trial. *Psychoneuroendocrinology, **104***, 115–121.

Lumley, J., Chamberlain, C., Dowswell, T., Oliver, S., Oakley, L., & Watson, L. (2009). Interventions for promoting smoking cessation during pregnancy. *Cochrane Database of Systematic Reviews*, (3), CD001055.

Lynagh, M., Bonevski, B., Symonds, I., & Sanson-Fisher, R. W. (2011). Paying women to quit smoking during pregnancy? Acceptability among pregnant women. *Nicotine & Tobacco Research, **13***(11), 1029–1036.

Minary, L., Alla, F., Cambon, L., Kivits, J., & Potvin, L. (2018). Addressing complexity in population health intervention research: The context/intervention interface. *Journal of Epidemiology and Community Health, **72***(4), 319–323.

Moore, G. F., Audrey, S., Barker, M., Bond, L., Bonell, C., Hardeman, W., Moore, L., O'Cathain, A., Tinati, T., Wight, D., & Baird, J. (2015). Process evaluation of complex interventions: Medical Research Council guidance. *BMJ, **350***, h1258.

Moore, G. F., Cambon, L., Michie, S., Arwidson, P., Ninot, G., Ferron, C., Potvin, L., Kellou, N., Charlesworth, J., Alla, F., & Discussion, P. (2019). Population health intervention research: The place of theories. *Trials, **20***(1), 285.

MRC. (2012). *Developing and evaluating complex interventions: New guidance*. Medical Research Council.

Potvin, L. (2014). Définir la recherche interventionnelle en santé des populations Recherche interventionnelle contre le cancer Paris.

Potvin, L., Petticrew, M., & Cohen, E. R. (2014). Population health intervention research: Developing a much needed science of solutions. *Preventive Medicine, **61***, 114–115.

Tarquinio, C., Kivits, J., Minary, L., Coste, J., & Alla, F. (2015). Evaluating complex interventions: Perspectives and issues for health behaviour change interventions. *Psychology & Health, **30***(1), 35–51.

Thabane, L., Ma, J., Chu, R., Cheng, J., Ismaila, A., Rios, L. P., Robson, R., Thabane, M., Giangregorio, L., & Goldsmith, C. H. (2010). A tutorial on pilot studies: The what, why and how. *BMC Medical Research Methodology, **10***, 1.

Thabane, L., Cambon, L., Potvin, L., Pommier, J., Kivits, J., Minary, L., Nour, K., Blaise, P., Charlesworth, J., Alla, F., & Discussion, P. (2019). Population health intervention research: What is the place for pilot studies? *Trials, **20***(1), 309.

Treweek, S., & Zwarenstein, M. (2009). Making trials matter: Pragmatic and explanatory trials and the problem of applicability. *Trials, **10***, 37.

Van Campenhoudt, L., Marquet, J., & Quivy, R. (2017). *Manuel de recherche en sciences sociales*. Malakoff.

Weiss, C. H. (1997). How can theory-based evaluation make greater headway? *Evaluation Review, **21***(4), 501–524.

World Health Organization (WHO). (1986). *The Ottawa charter for health promotion*. WHO.

Chapter 42
A Systems Approach to the Coproduction of Evidence for Health Promotion

Therese Riley, Kim Jose, Kate Garvey, and Michelle Morgan

42.1 Background

Health promotion evidence is often created in the contexts of multisectoral partnerships. Partnerships have been a mainstay of health promotion practice since the Ottawa Charter. The process of empowering communities and individuals to *set priorities, make decisions, plan strategies and implement them to achieve better health* (World Health Organization, 1986) requires health promotion practitioners to

T. Riley (✉)
Therese Riley Consulting, Melbourne, Victoria, Australia

The Australian Prevention Partnership Centre, The Sax Institute, Sydney, New South Wales, Australia

Mitchell Institute, Victoria University, Footscray Park, Victoria, Australia
e-mail: therese.riley@vu.edu.au

K. Jose
Menzies Institute for Medical Research, University of Tasmania, Hobart, Tasmania, Australia

K. Garvey
The Australian Prevention Partnership Centre, The Sax Institute, Sydney, New South Wales, Australia

Department of Health, Tasmanian Government, Hobart, Tasmania, Australia

Department of Public Health, LaTrobe University, Bundoora, Victoria, Australia

M. Morgan
The Australian Prevention Partnership Centre, The Sax Institute, Sydney, New South Wales, Australia

Department of Health, Tasmanian Government, Hobart, Tasmania, Australia

School of Geography, Planning, and Spatial Sciences, University of Tasmania, Hobart, Tasmania, Australia

L. Potvin, D. Jourdan (eds.), *Global Handbook of Health Promotion Research, Vol. 1*,
https://doi.org/10.1007/978-3-030-97212-7_42

work collaboratively with communities to enact change.[1] Traditionally, partnerships have been formed to facilitate research into the design or evaluation of specific health promotion programmes or services. Here partnerships are often created from existing networks with like-minded organisations or individuals. Increasingly, research funding bodies also expect researchers to partner with knowledge users (Smits & Denis, 2014) (i.e. policymakers/managers, practitioners, or community members/patients) as a way to facilitate research that is more socially and contextually appropriate with immediate relevance (see Canadian Institutes of Health Research, 2020; National Health and Medical Research Council, 2016).

Navigating the health promotion research landscape has become increasingly complex. Factors that have contributed to this complexity include: inclusion of more stakeholders in the research process (multisectoral partnerships), an increasing focus on the contexts in which evidence is created and the roles and practices of research that often reinforce institutional boundaries. This means that we need to understand the practice of health promotion research as a complex system.

Complexity-based evidence recognises the research process as a complex system, whereby the social conditions in every part of the research process is characterised by many and varied interrelationships between people, organisations and perspectives, along with feedback loops, non-linearity and the adaptive capacity to evolve and change over time (see Patton, 2011). There are three systems thinking ideas that scholars agree are integral to understanding complexity: boundaries, interrelationships and perspectives (Reynolds et al., 2018; Williams & Hummelbrunner, 2010). Integrating these ideas into our research processes and designs will draw our attention to the boundaries that are created when research is designed and implemented, the perspectives that we privilege or ignore and the interrelationships between all facets of research (Reynolds et al., 2018; Williams & Hummelbrunner, 2010).

42.1.1 Boundaries of Research Evidence

Researchers, policymakers, practitioners and community members come to the research process with expectations of roles, skills and practices based on previous experiences and cultural understandings. In the dominant biomedical model of research to practice trajectory, researchers are to be independent and objective.

[1] While there is an abundance of research on intersectoral collaboration, along with tools to measure the nature and quality of our partnerships, this is not the focus of this chapter. See:

- Joss and Keleher (2011). Partnership tools for health promotion: are they worth the effort? *Global Health Promotion, 18*(3), 8–14. https://doi.org/10.1177/1757975911412402
- VicHealth. (2016). *The partnerships analysis tool: A resource for establishing, developing and maintaining partnerships for health promotion.* Victorian Health Promotion Foundation. Retrieved October 20, 2020 from https://www.vichealth.vic.gov.au/media-and-resources/publications/the-partnerships-analysis-tool

Policymakers are best placed to integrate evidence into decision-making. Practitioners translate research in the contexts of their practice and community members are the ultimate beneficiaries of new knowledge. These boundaries appear straightforward but must be challenged if we are to embrace a new way of creating evidence: coproduction. The *coproduction* and/or codesign of health promotion initiatives or research, denotes an "equal and reciprocal relationship" (Boyle & Harris, 2009) between various people and sectors (Blomkamp, 2018; Boyle & Harris, 2009). A more 'coequal' relationship suggests that researchers must rethink their role in the research process. It requires that researchers, policymakers and practitioners must share responsibility for sense-making, priority setting and resource allocation.

Hilger et al. (2018) studied a typology of research roles in laboratories. These are reflective scientist, facilitator, change agent and (self) reflexive scientist. Such a typology expands the roles of researchers/scientists away from scientific technique and more to the 'social dynamics' at play when partnering with others in research. These dynamics are critically important when negotiating issues such as data sharing, conflicts of interest, data analysis and interpretation. In the absence of a genuine attempt to open the black box of research practices, we are destined to continue to reproduce evidence and ideologies that are "expert-driven, authoritarian and disempowering" (Davies & Macdonald, 1998, p. 209). This tension and opportunity is exemplified by the current preoccupation with 'big data' and data linkage, whereby administrative or other data from different sources are linked to create a new, richer dataset. Linking datasets, such as health with socioeconomic, geospatial or environmental datasets, has generated new insights into health outcomes (Wellcome Trust, 2015), but it may need to be supplemented by other forms of data to fully understand different outcomes for specific population groups (Blok et al., 2017; Bornakke & Due, 2018). Large-scale data linkage research may seem at odds with more participatory and collaborative research approaches, but the considerations and structures required to support the process have facilitated cross-sectoral and cross-institutional engagement. The deployment of methods that identify high-level patterns along with those that create context-specific explanations are providing new insights, and also reveal the complex nature of health promotion efforts. Time will tell as to whether these new forms of engagement facilitate a more "equal and reciprocal relationship" (Boyle & Harris, 2009, p. 11) between stakeholders or reinforce old boundaries. What it does demonstrate is that regardless of method, more dynamic research roles and practices such as 'facilitator' and 'change agent' are important (Hilger et al., 2018).

While many agree that the role of researchers is changing, others point to the challenges associated with more 'coequal' relationships with research partners (Oliver et al., 2019). According to Oliver et al. (2019), these challenges emerge within the practice of coproduced research. Research practices such as defining research questions and collecting and analysing data can raise issues such as conflicting priorities and agendas amongst stakeholders and the allocation of resources in support of research. They point out the professional risks to researchers and policymakers from being co-opted by political interests to feeling used by the research process (Oliver et al., 2019). Others have embraced the opportunities of coproduced research to interrogate and expose the processes by which data is interpreted and analysed (Gillard et al., 2012). In doing so, they challenge academic conventions and force a deep reflection on what we know and how we know it. Gillard et al. (2012), in a study of their own coproduction processes, identify six characteristics of knowledge building such as a transdisciplinary approach, revealing and reflecting on the social processes of knowledge production and the dynamic (re) negotiations that take place during all phases of the research process. However, there is no doubt the risks outlined by Oliver et al. (2019) are real, and the need to surface such tensions is important. These 'costs' are the product of work at the boundaries between sectors (e.g. researchers and policymakers) where parties can retreat to their own institutional cultures to make sense of such challenges. The trap is a self-referencing loop that reinforces boundaries rather than opening new spaces for coproduction. At play here is perhaps the most impenetrable boundary of all: the concept of evidence itself.

42.1.2 Interrelationships – The Dynamics of Evidence

We agree that health promotion with a focus on individual and communal behaviours, requires different forms of evidence. Yet the scientific hierarchy of evidence (that underpins evidence-based medicine) emphasises experimental methods, and quantitative data collection and analysis. It is reductionist in nature, involving the identification of linear cause and effect relationships. Much has been written about the inappropriateness of traditional quantitative data analysis approaches for understanding human experience and the determinants of health (Raphael, 2000; Raphael & Bryant, 2000). Reductionist approaches fail to grapple with the complexity of health promotion practice. Health promotion efforts do not unfold in predetermined predicted ways due to the many factors at play during implementation. The nature of evidence derived from such efforts needs to draw on the contexts in which it exists and could be acted upon. This is consistent with arguments regarding the research–practice gap, which highlights that 'evidence' created outside a practice context struggles to be implemented within one (see Westerlund et al., 2019).

Green (2008, p. 120) argues that one of the reasons for this 'disconnect' is the "fallacy of the empty vessel." That is, 'evidence' is poured into the empty vessel that is the practitioner. Such an assumption ignores all the forms of knowledge and evidence that come to bear on the actions and decisions of practitioners. Evidence that is instrumental (traditional scientific), interactive (derived from lived experience – ethnographic), critical (reflective – reflection and action [see Raphael (2000) building on the work of Park (1993]) and derived from a range of perspectives. Addressing complex issues requires flexibility in the type of evidence that is drawn upon and created. In a study of the nature of evidence in an obesity prevention programme in the UK, Goodwin et al. (2013, p. 110) found that in the absence of an evidence base, stakeholders "…largely drew on anecdotal evidence, consultation, local knowledge and practitioner expertise and routine local and national indicators." It is reasonable to believe that in dynamic and complex settings, it would be almost impossible to have an established evidence base behind every practice decision. Indeed, Goodwin et al. (2013) point out that evidence is shaped by local contexts, but this can be misaligned to broader population-level outcomes or evaluations. Aligning different forms of evidence for different purposes requires a more 'coequal' participatory process. Green (2008) called for ongoing engagement with practitioners and communities in a 'participatory process' of generating evidence. We agree that participatory approaches are needed in the generation of new evidence.

42.1.3 Perspectives in Research Evidence

In the context of complexity-based evidence, we need to embrace methodological and theoretical pluralism and draw others into our inquiry processes (Midgley, 2011; Raphael, 2000). This involves extending our evidence boundary even further than the contexts of health promotion practice. We must work with the range of knowledge forms and evidence that come to bear on health promotion decisions and apply methods and processes that genuinely draw in a range of stakeholders and perspectives. New insights frequently arise when we include non-traditional research partners whose experience and/or expertise challenges the underlying assumptions that underpin research practice. Conducting research that embraces methodological pluralism, involves multisectoral partnerships and encourages a range of perspectives, is not easy. Research-funding bodies frequently fail to recognise the additional time, resources and skills such approaches require, but our experience highlights the invaluable learnings gained from employing these approaches for health promotion research. They help us to situate our work within a broader context that is subject to multiple influences, incorporates the expertise of many into our health promotion evidence base, and better attends to the unpredictable, messy, and disorderly nature of the world.

In the following section, we present four case-study projects and share our reflections on how these projects grappled with complexity (implicitly or explicitly). We invite you into our messy world of research decisions and reflections.

42.2 Case Illustrations and Reflection

The four cases below illustrate a range of health promotion research practices from more traditional evaluations of health promotion programmes (case illustration 1, School Breakfast Programs) and research partnerships generating evidence to support policy and practice (case illustration 2, Tassie Kids) to more participatory approaches where stakeholders engage with and question the evidence (case illustration 3, Alcohol Harms) to the development and implementation of a range of systems thinking tools and methods (case illustration 4, Prevention Tracker) that challenge many of the central tenets of what constitutes good science. Each of the cases was conducted in Australia and the health challenges addressed by these cases are described elsewhere.

42.2.1 School Breakfast Program

Australian schools have no history of subsidised meal provision, but in the past decade, there has been a growing trend towards schools offering breakfast programmes on site. Funding for these programmes varies for each Australian state and generally, breakfast programmes have no eligibility criteria. This study was conducted in the Australian state of Tasmania where the funding available to assist schools establish School Breakfast programmes between 2011 and 2014 was no longer available. Researchers were interested in understanding why and how schools established these programmes and their perceived benefits. Adopting a multiple case study design in five primary schools, the perspectives of students, parents, teachers and support services staff were captured. This research project was instigated by researchers with an advisory group consisting of representatives from the Departments of Health and Education, and a parent representative body.

Reflections on the School Breakfast Program This research programme reflects a traditional approach to evaluation of a health promotion programme in a key health-promoting setting for children. Initiated and funded by researchers, the research was supported by health and education representatives, but it was not driven by them and coproduction or codesign elements were not strongly embedded in the research process. While the perspectives of key stakeholders (i.e. children, parents, teachers, principals, funders) were captured as part of the research process, the lack of relational or systemic infrastructure to support knowledge utilisation by policymakers and key decision-makers has limited how the knowledge generated by this study has been used, despite it having clear relevance to a range of end users. If we had engaged these groups in the research from the beginning, it may have resulted in more immediately relevant findings to those who have most at stake.

In addition, the research raised questions about the changing expectations and responsibilities of schools in Australia, highlighting the role school breakfast programmes play in the broader family and/or child social support system (Jose, Vandenberg, et al., 2020b). This critical social support role of schools has been revealed internationally as a consequence of school closures arising in response to the COVID-19 pandemic. Concerns have been raised about the lack of access to school meals for children in countries such as the UK and India, and the potential impact on the well-being of children and their families (see http://www.oecd.org/coronavirus/policy-responses/combatting-covid-19-s-effect-on-children-2e1f3b2f/). How an individual programme, delivered within a localised setting, fits within the broader system are important considerations that are frequently beyond the scope of health promotion evaluations guided by linear programme logic models and focused on more immediate programme impacts (Prevention and Population Health Branch, 2010). The 'scope' of research and evaluation is often considered a hard boundary, rather than an opportunity to reflect on and critique the boundary itself (see Ulrich & Reynolds, 2010) – what questions or perspectives are not asked or listened to because of the scope?

While it remains important to evaluate the local impact and effectiveness of health promotion programmes, situating and monitoring a programme within the broader context and identifying how it aligns (or not), and interacts, with other parts of the system can offer important insights about why a programme behaves the way it does. This offers an opportunity to readjust the programme to ensure it gets better traction within the system, and it can also help anticipate unintended consequences which can then be accounted for.

42.2.2 *Tassie Kids*

The Tassie Kids study investigated pathways through universal early childhood services from the health and education sectors and the impact of service use on child development. The partnership between researchers from the Telethon Kids Institute, the University of Tasmania and managers/policymakers from the Tasmanian Departments of Education, Health, and Premier and Cabinet used population-wide linkage of Tasmanian administrative datasets from health and education to capture service patterns and ethnographic methods that captured how practitioners were engaging with families and each other.

Reflections on the Tassie Kids Study The Tassie Kids study was a partnership between researchers and policymakers and managers in the early childhood service system who were interested in improving the well-being and development of all Tasmanian children. Linking administrative data from universal early childhood services from health and education for the first time revealed the developmental circumstances that influenced children's outcomes (Taylor et al., 2020) and the complex service pathways taken by pre-school-age children through universal services. Ethnographic methods embedded in practice and community captured engagement strategies (Jose, Taylor, et al., 2020a) and approaches to collaborative practice from the perspectives of practitioners and parents. Research designs that are flexible and responsive are critical if researchers are to respond to new and emerging policy and practice questions (Patton, 2015). The Tassie Kids study demonstrates the power of linking administrative data for research purposes, but the process takes time and is inherently inflexible, requiring identification of datasets and variables of interest at the outset. While these challenges were offset by the inclusion of ethnographic methods that were more flexible and responsive, the lack of synchronicity between the two approaches, existing data hierarchies and different understandings of what constitutes evidence has hampered the integration of findings to date.

The insights generated by Tassie Kids are of interest and relevance to families, practitioners, and communities as well as policymakers and researchers. Findings have been shared with researchers via conferences and academic publications and with policymakers and key decision makers via annual partner meetings and departmental presentations. These opportunities were built into the research process. In contrast, sharing findings with local service managers, service providers and families was less systematic and generally occurred informally, as part of the ethnographic research process. Oliver et al. (2019) note that communicating with disparate end users is challenging as their needs and interests differ. However, structuring this into the research process from the beginning may have avoided the misalignment of variables and impacts of interest to the range of stakeholders. Bringing diverse stakeholders together to determine variables or outcomes relevant across systems may bring us closer to understanding the complex impact of health promotion.

42.2.3 Dynamic Simulation Modelling of Alcohol-Related Harms

Dynamic simulation modelling can support decision-making when tackling complex health problems. Integrating various data sources, dynamic simulation modelling can be used by policymakers and others to test possible impacts of different interventions or policy scenarios prior to implementation (Atkinson et al., 2015). Between 2017 and 2018, the Australian Prevention Partnership Centre, in partnership with the Tasmanian Department of Health, developed a dynamic simulation model to test the likely impacts of a range of policies and programmes to reduce alcohol-related harms in Tasmania. A participatory approach was used to develop the model, which involved integrating various data sources and engaging a diverse range of stakeholders who were central to decision-making about alcohol policy in Tasmania.[2]

Reflections on Dynamic Simulation Modelling of Alcohol-Related Harms Building on work done in New South Wales (Atkinson et al., 2015), a participatory approach was taken to build the dynamic simulation model of alcohol-related harms in Tasmania. Facilitated by the Tasmanian Department of Health, this approach involved bringing together diverse stakeholders, including researchers, policymakers from a range of government agencies (including health, economic development, education, justice, sport and recreation, transport and treasury), non-government organisations and service providers. While these stakeholders all have

[2] For more information regarding the project, see The Australian Prevention Partnership Centre, preventioncentre.org.au

roles related to reducing alcohol-related harms, they previously had limited interaction, and brought different perspectives, insights, and data sources, to the table.

Bringing together such diverse stakeholders and maintaining their engagement in the project required a significant investment of time to establish and build relationships. In addition to the various meetings and workshops which occurred frequently over the 18-months to build the model and ground it within the Tasmanian context, one of the members of the core project team made additional contact with key stakeholders to foster those relationships. This contact provided an opportunity to build trust and to have more open conversations about competing priorities, which in turn enabled the establishment of shared priorities and agreement on the boundaries and limitations of the project. Overall, stakeholders reported that the participatory process was valuable, and resulted in deeper engagement with the evidence base and strengthened relationships.

While involvement in the participatory process increased stakeholders' understanding of the complexity of reducing alcohol-related harms and it enabled them to see the bigger picture, the most significant revelation for some was how important their role in addressing this problem was.

Building the model involved integrating various evidence sources provided by stakeholders involved in the project. These sources included practice experience, research, expert knowledge and population-based behavioural and demographic datasets. Bringing together data sources highlighted data gaps and coding issues and that the use of traditional data sources privileged the issues and interventions this data pertained to. For example, in the absence of consistent alcohol-related community injury data, community-based interventions were not able to be included in the model. The participatory process enabled these limitations to be surfaced, and stakeholders were able to engage with and contest the evidence, make their assumptions explicit, and hear from other perspectives in the room.

The resultant dynamic simulation model enabled stakeholders to test a range and combination of possible interventions to reduce alcohol-related harms before implementing them, taking into account the dynamic interaction between risk factors, interventions and the local context. Due to the perceived technical nature of the model interface, few stakeholders have used it independently despite having access to it, perhaps limiting the value of the insights gained. This perception highlights yet another challenge of traditional research practices – the endpoint. If we want new evidence to emerge from participatory processes investigating complex problems, we may need to be more flexible in how we transition from one stage to the next. This project highlighted the importance of facilitation skills by the core team leading the research project, as well as the need to build more capacity locally in the use of technical methods such as dynamic simulation modelling.

42.2.4 Prevention Tracker

An initiative of the Australian Prevention Partnership Centre, Prevention Tracker aimed to describe, guide and monitor system change efforts in the chronic disease prevention systems of four communities across Australia. Researchers partnered with 1–2 lead agencies in each of the communities and formed advisory groups to assist in adapting the methods to the various community contexts. Prevention Tracker tackled the vexed question of what a prevention system looks like at a community level and what it might take to bring about change to strengthen that system. The project applied a range of systems thinking methods and inquiry processes from social network analysis to causal loop diagrams and system action learning. It was designed to build a picture of local prevention systems through the use of various methods and data synthesis techniques. The methodology is described in detail elsewhere (Riley et al., 2020).[3]

Reflections on Prevention Tracker The Prevention Tracker case highlights many of the challenges faced by health promotion practitioners every day. They grapple with complex situations by drawing on multiple forms of knowledge to devise actions while being flexible and responsive to new opportunities that emerge during their work. Prevention Tracker was designed to reflect this responsive practice by adopting methodological flexibility, thus ensuring emergent situations and diverse community contexts to be accommodated as recommended in systems approaches (See Burns, 2007). Methods were adapted to meet community timelines and sought the assistance of local experts in the design and implementation of the study (Riley et al., 2020). Methods such as group model building and community workshops privileged the views and experiences of those in the room. Such views sat alongside evidence gathered and derived from outside the community via traditional research techniques. These (potentially) competing forms of evidence were reconciled through data synthesis processes and a commitment to ongoing problem solving – what do we know now and what do we do next? (Riley et al., 2020)

Prevention Tracker embraced methodological and theoretical pluralism (Midgley, 2011) as a way of working that provided the flexibility to draw on multiple methods and perspectives in the pursuit of a deeper understanding of the nature of prevention systems and how to intervene in dynamic practice contexts (Riley et al., 2020). Applying such a range of systems-inspired methods required access to a variety of researchers and skill sets. This was enabled through the large network of researchers connected to The Australian Prevention Partnership Centre (Wutzke et al., 2017), but may not be available in the same way for others. In other words, being flexible with the range and type of methods applied to address complex problems requires researchers to be trained differently (multi-methods) or for networks of researches

---

[3] For more information regarding the project, see The Australian Prevention Partnership Centre, preventioncentre.org.au and Riley et al. (2020)

to work together (see Riley et al., 2020). In addition, research governance structures such as ethical review boards are not so well equipped for research that is responsive to changing circumstances (Riley et al., 2020).

42.3 Discussion

While health promotion practice has had to embrace complexity and uncertainty in response to our growing understanding of the interrelationships between the systems influencing the health of populations, the process of managing the resulting uncertainty, flexibility and non-linear relationships are yet to be reflected in research practice.

The case illustrations presented here and their approaches highlight the need for researchers to engage with uncertainty and complexity in the same way that health-promoting practitioners have had to in order to respond to the complex social and health problems faced by communities and the broader population. Systems scholars argue that confronting complexity head on requires acceptance of methodological and theoretical pluralism and drawing others into our inquiry processes (Midgley, 2011). The rich insights generated when apparently disparate methods such as data linkage and ethnography are combined, as in the Tassie Kids study, are testament to the benefits of this approach. The case illustrations outlined here demonstrate the limitations that arise when we fail to do so, as well as the approaches needed to capture the uncertainty and complexity inherent in the systems under investigation.

The coproduction and codesign processes previously outlined demand that researchers engage with multiple perspectives throughout the research process, requiring researchers with the skills and capacity to engage with, manage and reconcile multiple perspectives (Facer & Enright, 2016). Research roles such as 'facilitation' (Hilger et al., 2018) are critically important along with a willingness to accept and work with the range of evidences within the system (Goodwin et al., 2013). The resulting outcomes can be the generation of new insights from research and practice (Midgley, 2011), as well as the correction of power imbalances between researcher and researched (Facer & Enright, 2016; Sibbald et al., 2014; Wallerstein et al., 2017). All the case illustrations described here incorporated multiple perspectives, either as research participants (Tassie Kids, School Breakfast Program), as part of the design and implementation process (Tassie Kids, Alcohol Harms, Prevention Tracker) or as a part of the decision-making processes around methods and data use (Alcohol Harms and Prevention Tracker). However, the systems approach and methodologies adopted by the Alcohol Harms and Prevention Tracker studies enabled knowledge to be generated together and shared with multiple stakeholders during the research process. This required not only researchers but policy-makers, practitioners and community to be engaged (to varying degrees) in the process of knowledge generation and interpretation. While not all stakeholders were involved in each phase of the research to the degree described by Gillard et al.

(2012), both projects worked with the social dynamics of research roles as described by Hilger et al. (2018). Engaging with multiple perspectives as well as multiple methodologies and approaches is critical if the evidence base is going to inform policy and practice, address the needs of those whom services are designed to serve and enable the cross-sectoral action required to promote the health and well-being of individuals, communities and populations. Importantly, insights gained or knowledge created through coproduction processes, are more likely to be actionable as they prompt self-reflection on the nature of evidence in a range of practice contexts.

Long-term relationships of trust embedded in community are the foundation for effective health promotion practice. Yet little attention is paid to the relational infrastructure required to engage in health promotion research. This infrastructure of relationships, skills and knowledge are central to collaborative research practice and knowledge mobilisation (Cheruvelil et al., 2014; Facer & Enright, 2016; McIsaac & Riley, 2020), but the mechanisms to support this for research practice are less developed than they are for health promotion practitioners. Short-term funding cycles, ethics processes, the turnover among key policymakers and managers along with changing priorities and expectations can make it difficult to develop long-term research relationships. Researchers and policymakers/managers commonly find themselves having to 'create' new relationships and partnerships in response to targeted funding rounds. Of the four case illustrations described here, the Tassie Kids study had the strongest pre-existing researcher/end user relationships. This existing relational infrastructure assisted with conducting the research and has facilitated some elements of knowledge mobilisation, but it is too early to say if it will result in changes in policy or practice. In contrast, the Alcohol Harms and Prevention Tracker studies involved a range of stakeholders some of whom had not previously worked together, but the methods supported the building of key relationships demonstrating a willingness to consider diverse forms of evidence and adapt methods to changing circumstances. Funding processes need to better reflect the resources (including time), capacity and skills to build trusting research relationships and recognise these relationships as critical research 'outputs'.

The need for a 'flexible' approach to research design is rooted in the understanding that complex systems adapt and evolve. If, as we are suggesting, health promotion practice is adaptive as efforts coevolve within their contexts, then research too must take on this approach. In theory, it looks logical. We collect data, adapt methods, consider what we have learned and what to do next. In practice, most of our research systems, from employment arrangements to ethical review boards, are inflexible. Our case illustrations show these challenges. The School Breakfast Program applied a more traditional (and familiar) approach to programme evaluation, only realising towards the end of the project that some key stakeholders were not engaged to better enable knowledge mobilisation. The impact of the findings could not be fully realised as contracts expired, and people move on to other projects. In Prevention Tracker, a flexible approach was embraced, where methods were adapted overtime to align with the needs of community partners and the ebbs and flows of community life. However, this flexibility came at a cost. It required continuous problem solving (see Riley et al., 2020) and ongoing engagement with ethical review boards. Time was also a factor in Prevention Tracker, with not all facets of Prevention Tracker implemented in all communities. Flexibility of study design and methods is possible, but difficult, when in the context of rigid research governance environments. This has been recognised by others advocating for co-designed research (Goodyear-Smith et al., 2015).

If we accept the importance of a relational infrastructure in which to implement flexible research designs where complexity and uncertainty can prevail, then ongoing reflection and adaption is the glue that keeps it together and on track. We understand that in most research projects, reflective practice will be the norm. It is how we problem-solve when things go wrong. However, if evidence generation is a dynamic social process (Hilger et al., 2018), we need to be aware of when and how to (re) negotiate all aspects of the research. Our case illustrations highlight the importance of 'moments in time' when reflection can lead to new data, new methods, stronger relationships and immediately actionable insights. The opportunity to challenge the data in the Alcohol Harms project could have been a flashpoint resolved by authority (those in power have the final say). Instead, it created a space in which to reflect and reconsider the nature of the data leading to new insight and further investigations.

While challenging in practice, the coproduction of research supports researchers and knowledge end users to generate and build evidence that is more relevant, actionable and useable for all. When done through the lens of *complexity,* coproduced research is enhanced. *Complexity-based evidence* attends to the emergent and non-linear dynamics of the research context, embraces methodological and knowledge pluralism, and gives attention to:

- The *boundaries* that are created when research is designed and implemented
- The *perspectives* that we privilege or ignore
- The *interrelationships* between all facets of the research

While these ideas are innate in systems and complexity methodologies (see Midgley, 2011; Reynolds et al., 2018; Williams & Hummelbrunner, 2010), there is no reason why they cannot be integrated into more traditional research methods. We believe they can assist in ensuring researchers are asking the right sort of questions and generating evidence applicable to a range of possible users.

42.4 What Have We Learned?

To build complexity-based evidence, we encourage others to:

- Extend your evidence boundary to include **various forms of evidence** and **diverse perspectives**. No one method or approach will capture everything, but the process of working together and negotiating boundaries, can be as important as the 'data' itself;

- Engage with **flexible study designs** that can adapt to changing circumstances and new knowledge during the research process;
- **Work with research governance bodies**, such as ethical review boards, to support and encourage more flexible study designs;
- Give attention to the **relational component** of all research. It is the interrelationships between all stakeholders, knowledges and perspectives that will lead to new and perhaps more relevant evidence. Building actionable knowledge and insight with those that have the power to act is likely to enable change across the system in new and unpredictable ways;
- **Build relationship and systems thinking capacities** in research roles and practices to work towards the shared goals of partnerships and embrace complexity. This capacity includes facilitation and negotiation skills, as well as capacities to use specific systems tools, methods and practices; and,
- Embrace a **learning mindset** and continually **reflect, learn and adapt** throughout the research process.

The multitude of existing frameworks addressing different elements of the research process (research design, codesign and coproduction, analysis, reporting of findings) imply that these considerations can be embedded by following checklists and employing specific strategies (advisory bodies, stakeholder consultations). Our experience highlights the unpredictable and iterative nature of applying these approaches in practice and their dependency upon the interrelationship between researchers and their partners. It is the commitment to and employment of the principles that underpin these aspects of health promotion research that appear critical rather than strict adherence to a particular approach that creates the possibility of generating new knowledge and unique insights of value to all involved.

Acknowledgements We gratefully acknowledge The Australian Prevention Partnership Centre for the use of the Tasmanian Dynamic Simulation Model and Prevention Tracker projects as case illustrations. The Australian Prevention Partnership Centre is funded by the NHMRC, Australian Government Department of Health, ACT Health, Cancer Council Australia, NSW Ministry of Health, South Australian Department for Health and Wellbeing, Tasmanian Department of Health and VicHealth. The Prevention Centre is hosted by the Sax Institute. We acknowledge the Telethon Kids Institute and the University of Tasmania along with the Tasmanian Department of Education, Department of Health, and Department of Premier and Cabinet for the use of the Tassie Kids study as a case illustration. This work does not necessarily reflect the view of the government departments involved in the research. We acknowledge the Menzies Institute for Medical Research, University of Tasmania for the use of the School Breakfast Program project.

The Tassie Kids study was supported by the Australian National Health and Medical Research Council Partnership Project Grant (APP1115891). The School Breakfast Program study was supported by the University of Tasmania Research Enhancement Grants Scheme (S0023829).

We also want to acknowledge the Muwinina people in Tasmania and the Boon Wurrung people in Victoria who are the traditional Aboriginal owners and custodians of the lands upon which this chapter was written.

References

Atkinson, J.-A., Page, A., Wells, R., Milat, A., & Wilson, A. (2015). A modelling tool for policy analysis to support the design of efficient and effective policy responses for complex public health problems. *Implementation Science, 10*(26). https://doi.org/10.1186/s13012-015-0221-5

Blok, A., Carlsen, H. B., Jørgensen, T. B., Madsen, M. M., Ralund, S., & Pedersen, M. A. (2017). Stitching together the heterogeneous party: A complementary social data science experiment. *Big Data & Society, 4*(2), 2053951717736337. https://doi.org/10.1177/2053951717736337

Blomkamp, E. (2018). The promise of co-design for public policy. *Australian Journal of Public Administration, 77*(4), 729–743. https://doi.org/10.1111/1467-8500.12310

Bornakke, T., & Due, B. L. (2018). Big–thick blending: A method for mixing analytical insights from big and thick data sources. *Big Data & Society, 5*(1), 2053951718765026. https://doi.org/10.1177/2053951718765026

Boyle, D., & Harris, M. (2009). *The Challenge of Co-Production: How equal partnerships between professionals and the public are crucial to improving public services*. Retrieved October 20, 2020 from https://neweconomics.org/uploads/files/312ac8ce93a00d5973_3im6i6t0e.pdf

Burns, D. (2007). *Systemic action research: A strategy for whole systems change*. The Policy Press.

Canadian Institutes of Health Research. (2020). *Patient engagement in research resources*. Retrieved October 20, 2020 from https://cihr-irsc.gc.ca/e/51916.html

Cheruvelil, K. S., Soranno, P. A., Weathers, K. C., Hanson, P. C., Goring, S. J., Filstrup, C. T., & Read, E. K. (2014). Creating and maintaining high-performing collaborative research teams: the importance of diversity and interpersonal skills. *Frontiers in Ecology and the Environment, 12*(1), 31—38. https://doi.org/10.1890/130001

Davies, J., & Macdonald, G. (1998). Beyond uncertainty: Leading health promotion into the 21st century. In J. Davies & G. MacDonald (Eds.), *Quality, evidence, and effectiveness in health promotion: Striving for certainties*. Routledge.

Facer, K., & Enright, B. (2016). *Creating living knowledge: The connected communities programme, community university relationships and the participatory turn in the production of knowledge*. University of Bristol/AHRC Connected Communities. Retrieved October 20, 2020 from https://connected-communities.org/wp-content/uploads/2016/04/Creating-Living-Knowledge.Final_.pdf

Gillard, S., Simons, L., Turner, K., Lucock, M., & Edwards, C. (2012). Patient and public involvement in the coproduction of knowledge: Reflection on the analysis of qualitative data in a mental health study. *Qualitative Health Research, 22*(8), 1126–1137.

Goodwin, D. M., Cummins, S., Sautkina, E., Ogilvie, D., Petticrew, M., Jones, A., Wheeler, K., & White, M. (2013). The role and status of evidence and innovation in the healthy towns programme in England: A qualitative stakeholder interview study. *Journal of Epidemiology and Community Health, 67*(1), 106–112. https://doi.org/10.1136/jech-2012-201481

Goodyear-Smith, F., Jackson, C., & Greenhalgh, T. (2015). Co-design and implementation research: Challenges and solutions for ethics committees. *BMC Medical Ethics, 16*, 78. https://doi.org/10.1186/s12910-015-0072-2

Green, L. W. (2008). Making research relevant: If it is an evidence-based practice, where's the practice-based evidence? *Family Practice, 25*(Suppl 1), i20–i24. https://doi.org/10.1093/fampra/cmn055. Epub 2008 Sep 15.

Hilger, A., Rose, M., & Wanner, M. (2018). Changing faces – factors influencing the roles of researchers in real world laboratories. *Gaia, 27*(1), 138–145.

Jose, K., Taylor, C. L., Venn, A., Jones, R., Preen, D., Wyndow, P., Stubbs, M. L., & Hansen, E. (2020a). How outreach facilitates family engagement with universal early childhood health and education services in Tasmania, Australia: An ethnographic study. *Early Childhood Research Quarterly, 53*, 391–402. https://doi.org/10.1016/j.ecresq.2020.05.006

Jose, K., Vandenberg, M., Williams, J., Abbott-Chapman, J., Venn, A., & Smith, K. J. (2020b). The changing role of Australian primary schools in providing breakfast to students: A qualitative study. *Health Promotion Journal of Australia, 31*(1), 58–67. https://doi.org/10.1002/hpja.259

Joss, N., & Keleher, H. (2011). Partnership tools for health promotion: Are they worth the effort? *Global Health Promotion, 18*(3), 8–14. https://doi.org/10.1177/1757975911412402

McIsaac, J.-L. D., & Riley, B. L. (2020). Engaged scholarship and public policy decision-making: A scoping review. *Health Research Policy and Systems, 18*(1), 96. https://doi.org/10.1186/s12961-020-00613-w

Midgley, G. (2011). Theoretical pluralism in systemic action research. *Systemic Practice and Action Research, 24*, 1–15. https://doi.org/10.1007/s11213-010-9176-2

National Health and Medical Research Council. (2016). *Statement on consumer and community involvement in health and medical research, consumers health forum of Australia*. National Health and Medical Research Council. Retrieved October 20, 2020 from https://www.nhmrc.gov.au/about-us/publications/statement-consumer-and-community-involvement-health-and-medical-research

Oliver, K., Kothari, A., & Mays, N. (2019). The dark side of coproduction: Do the costs outweigh the benefits for health research? *Health Research Policy and Systems, 17*(1), 33. https://doi.org/10.1186/s12961-019-0432-3

Patton, M. Q. (2011). *Developmental evaluation: Applying complexity concepts to enhance innovation and use*. The Guilford Press.

Patton, M. Q. (2015). *Qualitative research & evaluation methods: Integrating theory and practice* (4th ed.). SAGE.

Prevention and Population Health Branch. (2010). *Evaluation framework for health promotion and disease prevention programs*. Victorian Government Department of Health. Retrieved October 20, 2020 from https://www2.health.vic.gov.au/about/publications/policiesandguidelines/Evaluation-framework-for-health-promotion-and-disease-prevention-programs

Raphael, D. (2000). The question of evidence in health promotion. *Health Promotion International, 15*(4), 355–367. https://doi.org/10.1093/heapro/15.4.355

Raphael, D., & Bryant, T. (2000). Putting the population into population health. *Canadian Journal of Public Health, 91*, 9–12.

Reynolds, M., Sarriot, E., Swanson, R. C., & Rusoja, E. (2018). Navigating systems ideas for health practice: Towards a common learning device. *Journal of Evaluation in Clinical Practice, 24*(3), 619–628.

Riley, T., Hopkins, L., Gomez, M., et al. (2020). A systems thinking methodology for studying prevention efforts in communities. *Systemic Practice and Action Research*. https://doi.org/10.1007/s11213-020-09544-7

Sibbald, S. L., Tetroe, J., & Graham, I. D. (2014). Research funder required research partnerships: A qualitative inquiry. *Implementation Science, 9*(1), 176. https://doi.org/10.1186/s13012-014-0176-y

Smits, P. A., & Denis, J.-L. (2014). How research funding agencies support science integration into policy and practice: An international overview. *Implementation Science, 9*(1), 28. https://doi.org/10.1186/1748-5908-9-28

Taylor, C. L., Christensen, D., Stafford, J., Venn, A., Preen, D., & Zubrick, S. R. (2020). Associations between clusters of early life risk factors and developmental vulnerability at age 5: A retrospective cohort study using population-wide linkage of administrative data in Tasmania, Australia. *BMJ Open, 10*(4), e033795. https://doi.org/10.1136/bmjopen-2019-033795

Ulrich, W., & Reynolds, M. (2010). Critical systems heuristics. In M. Reynolds & S. Holwell (Eds.), *Systems approaches to managing change: A practical guide* (pp. 243–292). Springer.

VicHealth. (2016). *The partnerships analysis tool: A resources for establishing, developing and maintaining partnerships for health promotion*. Victorian Health Promotion Foundation. Retrieved October 20, 2020 from https://www.vichealth.vic.gov.au/media-and-resources/publications/the-partnerships-analysis-tool

Wallerstein, N., Duran, B., Oetzel, J. G., & Minkler, M. (2017). On community-based participatory research. In N. Wallerstein, B. Duran, J. G. Oetzel, & M. Minkler (Eds.), *Community-based participatory research for health: Advancing social and health equity* (3rd ed., pp. 3–16). Jossey-Bass.

Wellcome Trust. (2015). *Enabling data linkage to maximise the value of public health research data: Full report*. Wellcome Trust. Retrieved October 20, 2020 from https://wellcome.org/sites/default/files/enabling-data-linkage-to-maximise-value-of-public-health-research-data-phrdf-mar15.pdf

Westerlund, A., Nilsen, P., & Sundberg, L. (2019). Implementation of Implementation science knowledge: The research-practice gap paradox. *Worldviews on Evidence-Based Nursing, 16*(5), 332–334. https://doi.org/10.1111/wvn.12403

Williams, B., & Hummelbrunner, R. (2010). *Systems concepts in action: A practitioner's toolkit.* Stanford University Press.

World Health Organisation. (1986, November 21). *Ottawa Charter for Health Promotion First International Conference on Health Promotion Ottawa.* Retrieved October 20, 2020 from https://www.healthpromotion.org.au/images/ottawa_charter_hp.pdf

Wutzke, S., Redman, S., Bauman, A., Hawe, P., Shiell, A., Thackway, S., & Wilson, A. (2017). A new model of collaborative research: Experiences from one of Australia's NHMRC partnership centres for better health. *Public Health Research and Practice, 27*(1), e2711706.

Chapter 43
Researching the Aesthetics of Health Promotion Interventions: Reflections on Fit to Drive, a Long-Running Road Safety Education Program

Kerry Montero and Peter Kelly

43.1 Introduction

The scene: a suburban secondary school in Melbourne, Australia. In a large auditorium a group of senior students, 15–16 years old, are participating in a road safety health promotion workshop. At the front of the auditorium are eight of their peers, six girls and two boys, who have been enlisted as volunteers to recreate the circumstances that led to a fatal crash involving young people after a late-night party. Four chairs represent the overcrowded car, containing too many passengers, with two boys squashed in the rear 'boot'. The crash, based on an actual event that had taken place in recent times, had involved classic health risk behaviours and decisions, complex motivations, and peer influence – factors that would be all-too-familiar to the young audience.

Later the students will participate in small group sessions, facilitated by young ('near-peer') university graduate students, where these choices and behaviours are discussed and debated. The students are moved by the story and the far-reaching consequences for all involved, are engaged in the moral questions, and will passionately argue the respective responsibilities and choices in the scenario.

This scenario describes part of a workshop in a long-running school-based road safety program, *Fit to Drive* ('F2D'), targeting senior secondary students in schools in Victoria (Australia). The scenario illustrates and brings together some of the key concerns of this chapter: how do we as health promotion practitioners and researchers understand, account, and plan for the impact of the – unacknowledged, but significant – aesthetic dimensions of any health promotion activity? How do we do

K. Montero (✉)
Freelance Academic, Brunswick East, VI, Australia
e-mail: kamontauk@gmail.com

P. Kelly
School of Education, Deakin University, Melbourne, VI, Australia

L. Potvin, D. Jourdan (eds.), *Global Handbook of Health Promotion Research, Vol. 1*,
https://doi.org/10.1007/978-3-030-97212-7_43

research that captures these, and other dimensions of health promotion, that are often elusive, or rendered absent?

The aesthetic dimensions of the activity described in the scenario are present in the ways it stimulates the senses, engages the imagination, and arouses empathy. There is visual appeal in watching the scene-setting: humour in the antics of the young people; the comedy of many bodies squashing into a car; the drama, indeed tragedy, of the unfolding story. The scenario forms a foundation for students to critically reflect on the actions and decisions of the young people leading up to the crash. And for the role-play participants, a heightened quality to this awareness, and profound feelings experienced after participating in the re-creation of the overcrowded car, and learning of the young people's fate.

Health promotion and education that aims to change individual behaviours is firmly grounded in the complementary disciplines that constitute the research and practice relevant to the targeted issue (in road safety, for example, engineering, epidemiology, medicine, sociology, education, behavioural psychology). There is scant acknowledgement, however, of the importance of understanding the aesthetic considerations in any given health intervention. As we have discussed in much greater detail elsewhere, the problem of young people and road safety, and the engagement of young people in road safety education, is grounded in, and is understood through, the lens of traditional models of health education and health promotion that draw principally on psychological theories of behaviour change and road safety science (Montero & Kelly, 2016). Less attention has been paid to the aesthetics, modes and process, of meaning-making in relation to road safety, and, by extension, to other targeted health behaviours.

In previous work (Montero & Kelly, 2016) we have reflected on the elements that 'make up' the totality of the F2D experience as a health promotion program, and how they come together to create meaning. There, we explored distinct features of the health promotion event as 'theatre', the (use) of stories, the place of emotions and rationality, the shared group space, and road safety as tragedy. A key focus for our research was to understand and analyse the ways in which meaning in relation to road safety, risk and decision-making is constructed, by means of health promotion activities and methods, within the F2d program. Understanding the ways that meaning is constructed within a learning environment is essential to the understanding of the efficacy – or otherwise – of health promotion and health education. In our research, we engaged with particular phenomenological traditions to explore the relationship between our thought, and language, and the experience of bodies and movement in the F2D small group workshop – the embodied meaning-making that occurs in this learning space.

Elsewhere (2016) we have discussed how our work in the field of school-based health promotion has been influenced, in various ways, by the field of studies in Science, Technology and Society (STS), particularly the work of John Law (2004). This analytical approach has opened up productive avenues for thinking about what are often overlooked dimensions of health promotion and education. The work of John Law (2004) and colleagues, and particularly Law's suggestions for 'capturing complexity' in social research, has provided a productive framework for our research and analysis, and has informed our interpretation of the complex ways that knowledges about risk and road safety are constructed within the F2D. In our research, we captured and analysed the participants' encounters with the workshop as it unfolded across the half-day. We paid attention to, not only the content of the messages, but also the embodied experience of the workshop for participants, and to the institutional time and space of the school in which the program is situated.

In this chapter, we draw on this detailed research and analysis of the Fit to Drive program over several years. We begin with a brief description of F2D and the research context, and then explore some of the insights arising from our focus on the deeper dimensions of engagement and meaning-making within health promotion programs.

Extending this discussion of aesthetics, we open up questions about what is made 'present', what is made 'absent', and what is made 'absent-as-other' (Law, 2004) in road safety education, and more broadly, in health promotion. We draw on this analysis, and previous work (Montero & Kelly, 2020), to explore the place of speed, cars, and the human relationship to the machine – the 'human-car-machine assemblage'. Referencing the work of philosopher Rosi Braidotti on technology and the body (Braidotti, 2000, 2006) as well as John Law's (2004) work on the relevance of the Baroque, we describe an innovative road safety project that allows us to imagine an alternative vision of this configuration.

43.1.1 The Research Context: Fit to Drive Program

Fit to Drive (F2D), is a schools-based health promotion program addressing road trauma prevention targeted at young adult drivers and passengers who are significantly overrepresented in road crashes in the state of Victoria, Australia (Montero & Spencer, 2009, 2016). A distinctive feature of Fit to Drive is that it uses trained university undergraduates as 'near-peer' road safety education facilitators and ambassadors to enable and motivate young people to be safer road users. The main focus of the program is a half-day (4-h) road safety education event where Year 11 (senior school) students participate in large group presentations by police, emergency service workers, and community representatives, interspersed with small group discussion workshops that are peer-led and facilitated by trained university students (Spencer & Montero, 2011). The workshops incorporate varied activities and modes of engagement, aiming to equip the young people with largely rational, cognitive, 'risk-based', knowledge, attitudes, and skills to make safe decisions related to motor vehicle use (Spencer & Montero, 2013).

Our aim, in researching F2D, was to understand how the program 'worked'. How did the health promotion and education practices and methods – the philosophy, strategies, and techniques – combine to produce (new) knowledges about road safety and risk in the program participants?

Specifically, our research aimed to understand how knowledges about young people, risk, and road safety are collectively constructed in the workshops. Such knowledges will necessarily be shaped by, or formed within, received understandings of road safety – influenced by current dominant expert discourses, as well as media and other populist representations. Our analysis of Fit to Drive therefore entailed an examination of the different ways the problem of young people and road safety has been named, and how these are given expression in the workshop.

In our analysis, we drew on data we collected over more than 4 years, which included workshop observations, detailed field notes and reflections, video and audio recorded data (interviews, filmed facilitated workshops, filmed presentations), interviews with students, facilitators and program coordinators, and analysis of student evaluation and feedback following each workshop. We also consulted diverse sources of F2D program documentation, for example, records of meetings, and the processes involved in planning, delivery, evaluation, and revision of this program. This was combined with personal reflections on the authors' experiences during a long engagement with the program. From the perspective of practitioner – researcher with a long history in the design and development of the program – this engagement needed to be accounted for in the research through the adoption of reflexive, practitioner research methods (Richardson, 1998). This included a full account of their role within the program, and the ways the information, experience, and reflective practice made available by their intimate involvement with the program over its history influenced and shaped their perspectives and interpretations (for a much fuller account of these activities, see Montero, 2013; Montero & Kelly, 2016).

43.1.2 Reflections on the Aesthetics of Health Promotion and the Embodied Nature of Meaning-Making

Undertaking an extensive and detailed engagement with the embodied, the aesthetic dimensions of the young people's experience of the program, in our research, we sought to understand the ways in which young people make some sense of – give meaning to – the stories, the logics, the practices, and activities that give form to Fit to Drive.

We drew upon theorists in the fields of phenomenology (Gadamer, 2006; Gendlin, 1962, 1995; Merleau-Ponty, 2008; Todres, 2007), pragmatist philosophy (James, 1899, 2010; Johnson, 1987, 2007), as well as educational theory (James, 1899; Jarvis, 2006), cultural studies (Lupton, 1998, 1999a, b, 2004), social psychology (Jessor, 1987, 1991), and sociology (Kelly, 2011, 2012) to consider certain dimensions of the embodied meaning-making that occurs in the workshops: language, the place and uses of emotion, the 'aesthetic' dimension of the health promotion practices, and the production of knowledge/s in relation to road safety.

A critical engagement with processes and practices of meaning-making in this specific health education context opened up new ways of understanding the students' embodied experience(ing) of the workshop. Meaning, we are reminded by

Mark Johnson, comes into being within the textured experiencing of the 'physical, biological, social, embodied, world' (Johnson, 2007, p. 94). As the philosopher Eugene Gendlin (1962) notes, the process of meaning-making is interactional, and part of the process of experiencing. The interaction occurs not just at the level of the embodied self, but also with, and within, the social world. Embodied meaning-making is inter-relational and inter-subjective, and, in this sense, is always present in health promotion interventions. However, this dimension tends to be little recognised, and rarely emphasised within the limits of reasoned, rational decision-making paradigms.

These ideas challenge certain understandings of reason and rationality as being somehow disembodied, as being located predominantly in an individual's cognitive capacities. The assumption of the existence of a disembodied mind is a persistent idea that is rooted within a western, specifically Cartesian, mind/body dualism and associated models of knowing and meaning-making (see Damasio, 1999, 2005; Midgley, 2003, 2006). What was revealed in the workshops was the embodied, emotional, aesthetic, dimensions of the ways in which we apprehend and make sense of the world and transform our understandings. The transformative impact of the workshop, we argued, is located in the bodily experience of the shared group space. Meaning is 'assembled' in the group 'encounter' (Gubrium & Holstein, 2009), and occurs within a dynamic flow of meaning-making that is deeply rooted in the aesthetic, bodily experience of being part of this grouping in this space.

We explored the ways that language is embedded within this embodied, dynamic flow. The character of our embodiment, argues Mark Johnson (2007, p. 94), shapes both what and how we think: there is a 'felt quality' to logical relations prior, and necessary to thinking: '... every thought implicates a certain bodily awareness'. Language is an embodied, physical act, interpreted through the embodied experiencing of the words (James, 1890/1950, 1:245–246, cited in Johnson, 2007, p.96). There is a 'felt sense' conveyed by words, syntax and expression, and concepts themselves have a *felt meaning* (Gendlin, 1995). Much of this felt meaning, the embodied experience, that is present in the interactions, responses, language, and movement of the young people in the workshops will be troubling, unsettling. And this unsettling is a necessary prelude to learning.

We stay with this unsettling to reflect on questions of the body in road safety and the character of its entanglement in the contemporary cultural relationship with the motor vehicle.

43.1.3 'It's Fun to Speed': The Human-Car-Machine-Assemblage

In the previous section, we explored the aesthetic, embodied nature of knowing, of meaning-making. The body, and all it encompasses – desires, fragilities, capacities, limits, possibilities, consequences, implications – is intricately and intimately entangled with the diversity of human relationships with the motor vehicle. In the discussion that follows we consider some of the ways in which the diverse entanglements of the body in the social, material, and cultural space are reflected in road safety education. Law's (2004) work offers a way to explore the *gatherings and bundlings* that constitute our experience and understandings of speed and the human-car-machine-assemblage: our embodied, aesthetic, erotic entanglements with this assemblage (see Montero & Kelly, 2016, 2020).

We have noted the marked absence in road safety education of any direct reference to the powerful meanings and symbolic status of the motor car in contemporary culture. The culturally symbolic significance of the car, with the associated imagery of machine, technology, power, and speed, is afforded no sanctioned place in the cultural iconography of the F2D road safety program. The potent and pervasive presence of the motor vehicle in our cultural imagination is never made present in the workshop, though it forms a distinct part of the 'hinterland' (Law, 2004) of road safety programs (VicRoads, 2006; Spencer et al., 2006). And yet the dominant 'idea' of the car, and its aesthetic and erotic dimensions, play a significant role in shaping the context in which people approach the act of driving, of being in a motor vehicle, of entangling with the human-car-machine assemblage: 'the car is partly constitutive of who it is to be "us". The centrality of the motor car in our culture is both taken-for-granted and idealised' (Paterson, 2007, p. 123).

We undertook a detailed examination of the group discussion-based activities in the F2D workshops to explore and reflect on questions regarding what is made 'present', 'absent' and 'absent as Other' (Law, 2004) in health promotion and road safety education. One example involved the description and analysis of a facilitated group activity in which students explored their values and beliefs in relation to road use and motor vehicles. This activity, in which students passionately debated the statement 'It's fun to speed', highlights some of the key ways in which certain features of driving, such as pleasure, fun, excitement, identity, are 'made absent; in road safety education and promotion (see Montero & Kelly, 2016, 2020).

In our work (Montero & Kelly, 2016, 2020), we have reflected on the complex social, cultural, and 'moral' dimensions of the car and driving in modern culture. Road safety education – public campaigns and targeted education – reveal and reflect different, sometimes fundamentally divergent, imaginaries with respect to the human relationship to the car/machine. The students, for instance, describe, recall, re-experience powerfully embodied memories of 'speeding' – mostly in the context of the motor car, but also other experiences of 'speeding' such as fun park rides, 'extreme' sports, and other forms of 'edge-work' (Lyng, 2008). The responses to the simple statement in the workshop activity reveal the powerful and complex relationship of people to motor vehicles, and to speed, a relationship historically embedded in rich cultural meanings and associations.

In this work, we have drawn on Klaus Theweleit's (1996) discussions of the erotic and aesthetic dimensions of the Fascist psyche that imagine the machine as a 'means to resolve the problems of the body' and of desire. We argued that the aesthetic-erotic dimensions of this imaginary, powerfully manifested in the early twentieth-century Futurist and Fascist sense of 'speed' as a positive force, aesthetic ideal, and object of desire, continue to play a significant role in shaping the context in which people (young and old) approach the act of driving and being in the motor vehicle. And consequently, there arise a series of tensions related to the absences, in schools-based health education with young people, of desire, aesthetics, and erotics, that characterise much of these historical and contemporary human entanglements with what we have referred to as the 'the human-car-machine-assemblage'.

The F2D program – like all educational endeavours – gathers, assembles, and bundles particular objects, relations, knowledges, to produce a 'reality' about cars, speed, and young people. F2D makes certain objects and relations present, and in so doing, renders others absent – manifestly and as Other. 'Speed' is made present in the program – and in road safety education more generally – as risk, as danger – with the associated negative connotations of irresponsibility, immaturity, and lack of care and regard for others. Speed as fun, as desire, as aesthetic and erotic experiencing is manifestly absent. The posing of the discussion starter 'It's fun to speed' is never truly about 'speed as fun' being made present. In the context of the program it is a fleeting way-stop to the representation of speed as risk and danger. Its presence, its purpose, is to throw into relief, to illuminate, these realities.

What is absent-as-Other in this bundling are ideas of speed that are representative of cultural values that are embedded in the expressions of personal and collective identities, particularly (though not exclusively) among many young males: testing the power of cars and engines; using the car as a technology of dominance; and as an extension of personal (masculine) power. In the Australian, hard male culture, it could be argued, speed, and driving, is Thanatos (the death drive) in action (see Smith, 2014). Young people who may not necessarily share these values will likely find themselves entangled with these cultural and social lines of force as they shape the performance, embodiment, and affectivity of their identities. They may, in short, get caught up, against their inclination and judgment, in dangerous driving situations. Being entangled – wittingly or not – with the human-car-machine-assemblage is part of modern(ist) subjectivities.

43.1.4 Health Promotion, the Baroque, and Possibilities for Re-thinking the Body in the Human-Car-Machine Assemblage

Taking the significance of the machine and speed in contemporary culture as a point of departure, we drew on key concepts from Gilles Deleuze and Rosi Braidotti to further explore cultural imaginaries and discourses of the body, their relationship to the motor vehicle, and how these imaginaries play out in schools-based road safety education, where the aesthetics and erotics of the human-car-machine-assemblage are made absent – 'manifestly' and as 'Other'.

In her essay 'Teratologies', post-humanist philosopher Rosi Braidotti (2000) extends the interrogation of the human-machine assemblages to examine the rapidly evolving developments in mechanical, biological, and digital technologies, and links this to what she refers to as a 'teratological imaginary'. Braidotti (2000, p. 156) alerts us to the diverse manifestations of the late postmodern fascination with the 'monstrous', the 'mutant', the hybrid. This contemporary preoccupation continues the historical obsession with the 'freak' and the 'monster', while responding to, and incorporating into these imaginaries, new manifestations of the hybrid possibilities (and realities) produced by developments in technologies (Braidotti, 2000, p. 157 and Braidotti, 2006, 2011).

Braidotti (2000, p.158), while recognising the liberating, therapeutic, and creative possibilities of 'hybrid' bodies, identities, and ways of being, and the technologies that make them possible, provides a trenchant critique of the political and cultural complexities inherent in such a project. In post-modernity, we are witnessing the 'simultaneous overexposure and disappearance of the body', accompanied by a 'deep anxiety about the bodily roots of subjectivity'. Braidotti (2000, pp.160–161) argues that in post-modernist discourse about the body, there is a 'techno-hype' that reveals a tendency towards 'the denial of the materiality of the bodily self'. The 'techno-hype', she argues, 'needs to be kept in check by a sustainable understanding of the self: we need to assess more lucidly the prices we are prepared to pay for our technological environments'. Braidotti argues that we need to develop a more nuanced understanding of the body that recognises boundaries and limitations' (Braidotti, 2000, p. 160).

Braidotti (2000, p.163) suggests that contemporary expressions of the 'monstrous imaginary' occur in the context of a conservative 'anti-maternalist' backlash and crisis of masculinity, associated with hard male cultural symbols and affiliations with misogynist imagery and language. The rejection of, and hostility to, the maternal-feminine is an expression of a 'technological culture [that] expresses a colder and more depersonalised kind of sensibility.' 'Whether we like it or not, and most of us do not, we are made to desire the interface human/machine' (Braidotti, 2000, pp.168–169).

These perspectives lead us to ask: if this *hard-culture,* nihilistic aesthetic is a dominant cultural reference point for the understanding and thinking about the human-car-machine-assemblage, then what are the alternatives for understanding and interpreting these entanglements? Is the 'hard-male' death-drive aesthetic in the human-car-machine-assemblage the inevitable expression of the human relationship to the machine? Are there other orientations, other ways of thinking, of imagining our relationship to technology? How do we 'break through' (Law, 2011) established ways of knowing to open up other ways, other modes, of understanding, experiencing? These questions are potentially productive in the context of school-based health education with young people, and can reveal the shifting relations between what is made present, what is manifestly absent, and what is absent as Other in these health education interventions.

Taking up some of these questions we introduced John Law's (2011) exploration of techniques of the baroque, and the possibilities this offers for opening up different ways of exploring the human-car-machine-assemblage and its place in health education with young people. In his *Assembling the Baroque*, Law (2011, p. 5) is interested in exploring distinctive features of the baroque in order to illuminate possibilities for opening up different kinds of thinking about contemporary questions. Here the baroque refers to the style, alongside the techniques that are predominantly, though not solely, associated with a particular historical period in western cultural history. For Law (2011, p. 4), a study of the 'techniques of the baroque' may give rise to 'questions that resonate with urgent intellectual and political agendas'; the baroque may provide a 'possible resource for thinking about [these] questions'.

Two of the techniques of the baroque that Law describes have been particularly useful in our research, in thinking through questions of the human-car-machine assemblage and the ways it manifests in road safety education. The first pertains to 'knowing', and the partial nature of any practice of knowing and understanding. The baroque, Law (2011, pp. 9–10) argues, recognises, and accepts that each 'practice of understanding', any given form of experience, is necessarily partial, because: 'what we recognise is partial' This means there are multiple avenues or possible entry points for understanding. The quest for understanding is located in different places. Takes different forms. Is agile, and requires readiness to move between different modes of understanding. For Law (2011, p. 7), heterogeneity – which involves 'mobilising all the media available to it' – becomes a necessary technique of the baroque. The baroque assembles – renders visible – many forms and media at once. For example, opera mobilises ballet and art; music performance mobilises dance and architecture. All the senses are engaged in the quest for understanding and experiencing.

Second, Law (2011) identifies, along with other theorists – most notably Deleuze (2006), in his study of Leibniz and the baroque – that a central feature, technique, and symbol of the baroque is the fold. In place of the hard, contained edges and boundaries prevalent in some elements of the human-car-machine-assemblage, the baroque 'works by undoing boundaries'. And creating overflows. The baroque revels in the existence, the proliferation of overflows – 'in multiple and material forms' (Law 2011, p. 6), and thus provides a counterpoint to the hardness, edges, and rigidity of various forms of human-car-machine-assemblage.

For many writers/theorists, the baroque offers a window into a different sensibility, a different way of seeing, understanding, and experiencing. For Law, it is also a resource, one that may be useful in re-thinking contemporary problems and questions. One that may suggest interesting possibilities when trying to make sense of the cultural and political conditions that create different orientations to, and manifestations of, the human-car-machine-assemblage.

43.1.5 *Viewing Road Trauma from 'Inside and Outside': Introducing 'Graham'*

With these questions in mind, we have been interested in the implications of an innovative collaborative road safety education project targeting the general population, but with a particular focus on road trauma prevention in young people. The initiative sponsored the Transport Accident Commission (TAC) in Victoria, Australia, involved collaborations between road crash investigation experts, road trauma surgeons, and the celebrated Australian artist Patricia Piccinini. Working with these experts, Piccinini created a slightly larger-than-life-size sculpture of 'Graham' – a figure who represents an imagined, human, embodied form – external and internal – that has 'evolved' to withstand the force of a car or motorcycle crash.

The 'Graham' exhibition, featuring the imposing sculpture accompanied by interactive displays (TAC, 2016), has travelled around art galleries in Victoria, to be viewed by members of the public and school children. 'Graham', 'monster'-like, posed in a casual seated position, is suggestive of a passenger in a car, arm draped over the back of the seat. 'Graham' is designed to represent what humans would need to become if evolutionary possibilities were given time to fashion the body into a form that could survive a crash. Monstrous, distorted, he is still recognisably human. His chest is bulky, to shield the ribs and organs; his head, neck, and face oversized – to protect brain and facial bones. Graham's skull is a more exaggerated form of normal human skull – 'a lot bigger, almost helmet-like' with 'inbuilt crumple zones that would absorb the energy on impact' (Piccinini, 2016). His facial features, flattened, obscured, recede into the almost concave shape of the head.

The ribs are prominent – the ribcage has additional airbags which on impact would expel a liquid to take the force of a collision. The body, to protect itself, to maintain its integrity, needs to be able to crumple, fold, contract, absorb. Additional concertina-ed layers of spongy flesh offer extra protection for Graham. There are various internal anatomical adaptations that would be required to protect the organs, bones and other tissues in the event of a vehicle crash. These anatomical details are revealed through portals in the interactive display, and appear simultaneously familiar and grotesque. They are distortions of the familiar shapes, textures, arrangements below the surface of our human body. They serve to remind the viewer of the wondrously intricate configurations of the human internal anatomy. To remind us that the internal human form consists of infinite folds, pleats, caverns. A boundlessness within the ostensibly finite mass of the body.

In these ways, we suggested that Graham embodies the baroque. The character of the baroque is deeply enmeshed in the dense and textured materiality of his bodily form. The bulky mass of his figure is grounded, anchored in his setting. However, Graham's exposed body simultaneously suggests the infinite pleats and spongy matter within.

The 'Graham' exhibit entails an encounter for the viewer that represents a 'baroque' approach to understanding, and, as such, an alternative aesthetic encounter. As viewers, we 'move between modes of sensing and experience' (Law, 2011, p.10), and so engage different forms of understanding. We observe from a perspective that is both 'inside and outside'. We gaze, and reflect on, the monstrous form. At the same time, we are invited to view 'inside'. To encounter the hidden folds and configurations that are designed to protect the body, and contemplate the implications for road crash victims.

The proposition posed by the Graham project is that too many of us behave as if we do not know what our body is *not* capable of. That the body is not capable of withstanding a force of a car crash at high speed, or even moderate speed. Graham represents a new way of understanding ('knowing') road safety and road trauma. The creature appears invincible. He has, after all, 'evolved' to withstand injuries in a crash. Yet, his invincibility reminds us of our vulnerability. Graham, with his seemingly endless folds and pleats, his obelisk-like aura of timelessness, also, paradoxically, invites contemplation of the entanglements, mysteries, and possibilities of our 'techno-teratological universe'.

In this sense, he functions as a counter-point to those elements of the human-car-machine assemblage which deny the materialities of the body. Graham represents a disconnection from, and then re-connection with, what it means to be an embodied, en-fleshed human.

43.1.6 Road Safety, Health Promotion, and the Human-Car-Machine-Assemblage: Re-imagining Health Promotion Research

In revisiting the work that we have done over a number of years, we have, in this chapter, presented an approach to health promotion research that provides for the development of new conceptual and theoretical insights and understandings in the design and 'doing' of health promotion and education and research. Our hope is that this research may contribute to the creation of opportunities for the development of deepened, and richer, understandings of youth health promotion, with particular reference to the aesthetic dimensions of health promotion practice: embodied meaning-making, the place of emotion, story, theatre. With reference, also – critically – to what is made 'present, absent and absent as other' (Law, 2004) in health promotion.

Alert to what is made present, absent, absent-as-other in health education and promotion, we have explored speed, the aesthetics, and the erotics of the human-car-machine assemblage. We have asked, for instance, how might our questioning and critique of the cultural significance of speed, and the human-car-machine assemblage connect to more prosaic concerns about what we do in school-based health education with young people?

The F2D program – like all educational endeavours – gathers, assembles, and bundles particular objects, relations, knowledges, to produce a 'reality' about cars, speed, and young people. F2D makes certain objects and relations present, and in so doing, renders others absent – manifestly and as Other. 'Speed' is made present in the program – and in road safety education more generally – as risk, as danger – with the associated negative connotations of irresponsibility, immaturity, and lack of care and regard for others. Speed as fun, as desire, as aesthetic and erotic experiencing is manifestly absent. The posing of the discussion starter 'It's fun to speed' is never truly about speed as fun being made present. In the context of the program it is a fleeting way-stop to the representation of speed as risk and danger. Its presence, its purpose, is to throw into relief, to illuminate, these realities.

What is absent-as-Other in this bundling are ideas of speed that are representative of cultural values that are embedded in the expressions of personal and collective identities, particularly (though not exclusively) among many young males: testing the power of cars and engines; using the car as a technology of dominance; and as an extension of personal (masculine) power. Young people who may not necessarily share these values will likely find themselves entangled with these cultural and social lines of force as they shape the performance, embodiment, and affectivity of young people's identities. They may, in short, get caught up, against their inclination and judgment, in dangerous driving situations. Being entangled – wittingly or not – with the human-car-machine-assemblage is part of modern(ist) subjectivities.

In this context, the figure of 'Graham' provides an opportunity to reconsider the assumptions at work in school-based road safety education. 'Graham' is overburdened with tensions, and paradoxes, and implied questions about 'the prices we are prepared to pay for our technological environments' Braidotti (2000). Failing the biotechnological developments that would permit the Graham-like mutations that would make humans 'crash-proof', we come up against the limits of the human body, and collide 'head-on' with many of the contradictions of our diverse entanglements with the human-car-machine-assemblage. We are compelled to recognise and accept the embodied nature of the human, our limits and vulnerabilities. Approached from this perspective, elements of the human-car-machine-assemblage are revealed as manifestations of the potential for 'nihilism and self-destruction'. They imply a rejection of, a flight from, the limits and boundaries, the 'enfleshed complexities', of what we know as the human (Braidotti, 2000, pp. 158–161).

Graham, with his seemingly endless folds and pleats, his obelisk-like aura of timelessness, also, paradoxically, invites contemplation of the entanglements, mysteries, and possibilities of our 'techno-teratological universe'. Invites us to consider anew how bodies, desires, pleasures, uncertainties, fears, mysteries, contradictions, and tensions populate and complexify the things that we make present, manifestly absent, and absent as Other when we do school-based health education with young people.

43.2 Conclusions

As a morning's health promotion program based in a senior secondary school setting, Fit to Drive may be functionally written up as a series of activities, presentations, and small group sessions. In many respects, such an account would mirror or represent any number of similar schools-based health promotion activities, workshops, interventions. Health promotion research taking such a program as its subject will characteristically focus on processes of implementation, evidence of effectiveness, and on elements such as program logic, content, targeted messages, behavioural intentions. However, this sort of description and analysis, while integral to the task of understanding and evaluating health promotion interventions, would not capture the ways in which the whole workshop, in becoming an assemblage of fragments of story, theatre, facts, voices, images, movement, and personal interactions, becomes in this process an entity that transforms into something that gains its purpose and identity in the particular meshing and correspondences of its constituent elements. A combination of elements that come together to become an assemblage that has its own distinctive aesthetic quality. Such research is unlikely to capture and reveal the aesthetic dimensions that are, as we have argued here, integral to the process of meaning-making, where meaning-making, in turn, is intrinsic to the production of (new) knowledges in health education, and deeply rooted in the aesthetic, bodily experience of the intervention.

We may find the 'aesthetic' in the stories, theatre, other forms of meaning-making. In the embodiment, feelings, the 'felt sense' of the experience where such meaning-making occurs; in the embodied process that is language. We find it in the 'aesthetics' of the influential cultural models and images that form the hinterland of interventions, such as the human-car-machine-assemblage; in assembling alternative aesthetics – opposing the 'hard culture', nihilistic, hard-edged aesthetic, with an aesthetic that embraces the human, the material, and the vulnerable dimensions of relationships with the machine. We may find the 'aesthetic', also, in the ways of knowing that are to be found, for instance, in the techniques of the baroque.

In this chapter, we have drawn on our deep engagement with these aesthetic dimensions of the F2D program to consider what an extensive and detailed engagement with the embodied, the aesthetic, means for trying to understand the ways in which young people engage with and make sense of the array of information, activities, interactions, and other encounters that constitute a health promotion intervention. In doing so, we have endeavoured to open up ways of approaching health promotion research that may complement and extend traditional concerns of such research.

References

Braidotti, R. (2000). Teratologies. In C. Colebrook & I. Buchanan (Eds.), *Deleuze and feminist theory* (pp. 156–172). Edinburgh University Press.
Braidotti, R. (2006). *Transpositions: On nomadic ethics*. Polity Press.
Braidotti, R. (2011). *Nomadic Theory. Embodiment and sexual difference in contemporary feminist theory*. Columbia University Press.
Damasio, A. (1999). *The feeling of what happens. Body and emotion in the making of consciousness*. Harvest.
Damasio, A. (2005). *Descartes' error: Emotion, reason and the human brain*. Penguin.
Deleuze, G. (2006). *The Fold. Leibniz and the Baroque*. London; New York: Continuum.
Gadamer, H.-G. (2006). *Truth and method*, Second, revised edition, Continuum, London New York.
Gendlin, E. (1962). *Experiencing and the creation of meaning: A philosophical and psychological approach to the subjective*. Free Press of Glencoe.
Gendlin, E. (1995). Crossing and dipping: Some terms for approaching the interface between natural understanding and logical formulation. *Mind and Machines, 5*, 547–560.
Gubrium, J. A. & Holstein, J. F. (2009). *Analysing narrative reality*. Sage: Thousand Oaks.
James, W. (1890/1950). *The Principles of Psychology*. 2 vols. New York: Dover.
James, W. (1899). *Talks to teachers on psychology: And to students on some of life's ideals*. Longmans, Green.
James, W. (2010). *The heart of William James, edited and with an introduction by Robert Richardsn*. Harvard University Press.
Jarvis, P. (2006). *Towards a comprehensive theory of human learning. Lifelong learning and the learning society Vol. 1*. Routledge.
Jessor, R. (1987). Risky driving and adolescent problem behaviour: an extension of problem-behaviour theory. *Alcohol Drugs & Driving, 2*, 1–12.
Jessor, R. (1991). Risk behavior in adolescence: A psychosocial framework for understanding and action. *Journal of Adolescent Health, 12*, 597–605.
Johnson, M. (1987). *Body in the mind: The bodily basis of meaning, imagination and reason*. The University of Chicago Press.
Johnson, M. (2007). *The meaning of the body*. The University of Chicago Press.
Kelly, P. (2011). Breath and the truths of youth at-risk: Allegory and the social scientific imagination. *Journal of Youth Studies, 14*(4), 431–447.
Kelly, P. (2012). The brain in the jar: A critique of discourses of adolescent brain development. *Journal of Youth Studies, 15*(7), 944–959.
Law, J., (2011). *Assembling the Baroque*. CRESC Working Paper Series Working Paper No. 109 http://www.cresc.ac.uk/publications/assembling-the-baroque.
Law, J. (2004). *After method: Mess in social science research*. Routledge.
Lupton, D. (1998). *The emotional self. A sociocultural exploration*. Sage Publications.
Lupton, D. (1999a). *Risk*. Routledge.
Lupton, D. (1999b). Monsters in metal cocoons. 'Road rage' and cyborg bodies. *Body & Society, 5*(1), 57–72.
Lupton, D. (2004). Pleasure, aggression and fear: the driving experiences of young Sydneysiders. In W. Mitchell, R. Bunton, & E. Green (Eds.), *Young people, risk and leisure: Constructing identities in everyday life* (pp. 27–42). Palgrave Macmillan.
Lyng, S. (2008). Edgework, risk and uncertainty. In J. O. Zinn (Ed.), *Social theories of risk and uncertainty: An introduction* (pp. 106–137). Blackwell.
Merleau-Ponty, M. (2008). *Phenomenology of perception*. Routledge Classics.
Midgley, M. (2003). *Heart and mind. The varieties of moral experience*. Routledge.
Midgley, M. (2006). *Science and poetry*. Routledge Press.
Montero, K. (2013). *An examination of young people's understandings of risk and risk-taking in relation to road safety*. Unpublished thesis.

Montero, K., & Kelly, P. (2016). *Young people and the aesthetics of health promotion: Beyond reason, rationality and risk*. Routledge.

Montero, K., & Kelly, P. (2020). Young people and the human-car-machine-assemblage: Aesthetics, erotics and other lessons for school-based health education. *Discourse: Studies in the Cultural Politics of Education*. https://doi.org/10.1080/01596306.2020.1740916

Montero, K. & Spencer, G. (2009). Fit to drive: an innovative peer education approach to road safety in schools. *The first Asia-pacific conference on health promotion and education*.

Montero, K. & Spencer, G. (2016, May 17–19). Key elements in the development and delivery of a community based multi stakeholder approach to road safety education for young adult road users. *Proceedings of the 2016 international conference road safety on five continents*.

Paterson, M. (2007). *Automobile politics, ecology and cultural political economy*. Cambridge University Press: Cambridge.

Piccinini, P. (2016). An exclusive interview with Patricia Piccinini…. and 'Graham', Art Almanac, http://www.art-almanac.com.au/an-exclusive-interview-with-patricia-piccinini-and-graham/ (interview) accessed 08-12-2016

Richardson, L. (1998). Writing: a method of inquiry. In N. K. Denzin & K. Lincoln (Eds.), *Collecting and interpreting qualitative materials* (pp. 959–978). California Sage Publications.

Smith, Z. (2014). *Sex and wheels: Zadie Smith on JG Ballard's Crash* https://www.theguardian.com/books/2014/jul/04/zadie-smith-jg-ballard-crash. Accessed 18 Oct 2020.

Spencer, G., & Montero, K. (2011, September). *Empowering youth in schools to be safer road users; peer-led by undergraduates*. Australian Council of Road Safety Conference.

Spencer, G. & Montero, K. (2013, May 15–17). Creating sustainable community partnerships to promote road safety in schools: Case study: Fit to drive (F2D). *Proceeding of the 16th international conference road safety on four continents*.

Spencer, G., Montero, K. & Rowland, B. (2006). *Fit To Drive: a program to enhance the safety of young drivers*. Unpublished report, Melbourne.

Theweleit, K. (1996). *Male fantasies Volume 2. Male bodies: psychoanalysing the white terror*. University of Minnesota Press: Minneapolis.

Todres, L. (2007). *Embodied enquiry: Phenomenological touchstones for research, psychotherapy and spirituality*. Macmillan Palgrave.

Transport Accident Commission. (2016). *Introducing Graham*. https://www.tac.vic.gov.au/about-the-tac/media-room/news-and-events/2016/introducing-graham. Accessed 24 Nov 2016.

VicRoads (2006). *Kids on the move. Traffic safety education for primary schools*. VicRoads Kew.

Chapter 44
Researchers as Policy Entrepreneurs for Structural Change: Interactive Research for Promoting Processes Towards Health Equity

Alfred Rütten, Jana Semrau, Natalie Helsper, Lea Dippon, Simone Kohler, and Klaus Pfeifer

44.1 Introduction

Health promotion is understood as a "strategy" for social change towards better health for all and as a "field of practices" with research as one fundamental type of practice (Brownson et al., 2018; Nutbeam, 2003). As certain structures of social practices persistently preserve health inequalities, a strategy as well as a social practice for structural change is essential for health promotion (Wilkinson, 1996; Frohlich & Potvin, 2008; Abel & Frohlich, 2012; Brown et al., 2019). The approach presented in our chapter builds on an interaction-knowledge-to-action methodology (Rütten et al., 2017; Holmes et al., 2017; Rütten & Gelius, 2013) systematically linking research practice with the practices of policymakers, professionals, and population groups. Following this approach, researchers, in cooperation with other stakeholders, act as "policy entrepreneurs" in order to orient and support structural changes that promote health for all and, by doing so, co-produce new knowledge on these fundamental processes.

There are different reasons for researchers to function as policy entrepreneurs. For example, researchers interested in applying the knowledge they produce and the evidence they provide (e.g. supporting evidence-based policymaking, Mintrom, 2019; Béland & Katapally, 2018) may have to interact with other fields of practices in order to get their knowledge transferred. Moreover, such interactive approaches may also be an appropriate strategy for knowledge production.

In health promotion, researchers have to deal with complex systems and therefore responsive research strategies are important (Hawe, 2015; Baum et al., 2006;

A. Rütten (✉) · J. Semrau · N. Helsper · L. Dippon · S. Kohler · K. Pfeifer
Department of Sport Science and Sport, Friedrich-Alexander-University Erlangen-Nuremberg, Erlangen, Bavaria, Germany
e-mail: alfred.ruetten@fau.de

L. Potvin, D. Jourdan (eds.), *Global Handbook of Health Promotion Research, Vol. 1*,
https://doi.org/10.1007/978-3-030-97212-7_44

Hawe et al., 2004). In general, the role of policy entrepreneurs has been investigated intensively (Frisch-Aviram et al., 2020; Faling et al., 2018) and studies on this topic already exist in health promotion research (Söderberg & Wikström, 2015; Guldbrandsson & Fossum, 2009). However, in previous studies policy entrepreneurs were predominantly political and administrative actors. Research-based policy entrepreneurship has been found in only a few cases (Faling et al., 2018, p. 401). In addition, the vast majority of studies focus on the early stages of the policy process (e.g. problem definition, issue framing) (Faling et al., 2018; Unwin et al., 2017), whereas studies on the role of policy entrepreneurship in the stage of health promotion implementation are lacking (Moloughney, 2012). This chapter contributes to the ongoing debate by specifying the role of researchers regarding policy entrepreneurship and focuses especially on policy implementation processes.

The knowledge generated by our approach relates to the assessment of necessary conditions that enable researchers to act as policy entrepreneurs for innovative health promotion practice. Further, it relates to an outline and a test of selected policy implementation strategies as well as to a preliminary analysis of potential implications and outcomes.

Using a health promotion case study in Germany that focuses on physical inactivity and health inequalities, we illustrate how research practice can bridge national policies and recommendations with the practices of local communities and populations. We show how health promotion research can be designed to connect research practices with practices of local stakeholders and policymakers. Furthermore, we will report on processes of interactive-knowledge-to-action which are part of the co-production of new evidence-based guidelines and the co-production of structural changes for better health for all.

44.2 Definition of the Policy Problem

"Problem definition" is a distinctive component of policy entrepreneurship with various relevant aspects (Rochefort & Cobb, 1993, 1995): Some of the prominent strategies of policy entrepreneurs (e.g. issue promotion, issue framing, agenda-setting; Faling et al., 2018; Mintrom & Norman, 2009) are related to this important phase of policymaking processes.

In Germany, physical activity (PA) promotion was not considered as a relevant policy issue at the national level until the early 2000s, but some milestones were reached in the last decade. Particularly relevant are the development of National Recommendations for PA and PA promotion (Rütten & Pfeifer, 2016) and the enactment of a "prevention law" in 2016 (Bundesgesetzblatt Teil I Nr. 31, 2015).

Both documents share a focus on health equity. The National Recommendations evaluated the impact of PA interventions on health equity and concluded that equity can be "promoted by means of interventions geared directly to socially disadvantaged groups as well as interventions that facilitate active involvement of the target groups in decisions regarding the design and implementation of the intervention"

(Rütten & Pfeifer, 2016, p. 114). The prevention law refers to the problem of health inequality and the need for structural change. Moreover, it obliged health insurances to spend a considerable amount of money per year on setting-based health promotion focusing on structural issues and reducing health inequalities.

However, PA interventions at the local level usually do not systematically consider scientific knowledge on potential effects on health equity. This crucial point of the National Recommendations for PA and PA promotion is not implemented yet. In 2017–2018, national and regional implementation structures were established through the prevention law, but implementation of corresponding approaches at the local level is still lacking. There are structural boundaries between practices of policymaking at different levels (e.g. national, local) and domains (e.g. sport, health) in Germany that may have blocked the local implementation of both National Recommendations and the law so far. Thus, we will investigate the respective contexts and conditions and subsequently indicate potential windows of opportunity for cross-boundary policy entrepreneurship.

44.3 Relevant Contexts and Conditions

While PA policies and recommendations along with the relevant legislation were developed at the international and national levels, the local context remains the arena for the implementation of PA promotion approaches (at least in Germany). PA infrastructures are built and maintained by local communities, PA programs are offered by local sports clubs, local councils decide on local PA policies, and stakeholders, policymakers, and population groups implementing PA promotion are mostly located at the local level.

Besides the vertical diversity of political competencies, the implementation of PA promotion is influenced by different policy domains. Of course, both the sports sector and the health sector are important. Moreover, city planning is a relevant domain regarding PA infrastructures, and if socially disadvantaged populations are considered as a target group, sectors responsible for social policy, youth policy, and policies focusing on older people may be important as well. Thus, a horizontal diversity of political competencies across a variety of domains exists.

Consequently, key functions of policy entrepreneurship may be related to overcoming vertical and horizontal boundaries and developing bridges between policies, resources, key actors, and social practices of different contexts. For example, a function could be to facilitate an expansion of policies and resources from the national health sector to the local arena (different level) in order to support the development and implementation of innovative PA promotion structures by local communities. State sport policy (different domain) may promote this process by lobbying for such support at the national level and by providing additional resources to the local implementation process.

44.4 Aligning Research and Policy Agendas from National to Local Level

Policy entrepreneurs use different strategies to overcome vertical and horizontal boundaries and to support intended policy changes. Besides "issue promotion" and "issue framing," a frequently used approach is coalition building (Faling et al., 2018; Meijerink & Huitema, 2010). In health promotion, transdisciplinary methods are relevant, and such coalition building may lead to new partnerships for health promotion innovation (Rütten et al., 2017; Stokols, 2006; Haire-Joshu & McBride, 2013; Bergmann et al., 2012). In addition, "leading by example" (e.g. a pilot project on successful policy implementation) and "manipulating or transforming institutions" (e.g. initiating new intra- and/or inter-organizational routines) are important for successful policy entrepreneurship (Faling et al., 2018, pp. 404–407; Meijerink & Huitema, 2010, p. 21; Mintrom & Norman, 2009, p. 653).

Although all strategies were relevant in our case study, issue promotion and networking (as a first step to coalition building) were predominant in the early stage. In the attempt to disseminate and implement the German PA recommendations researchers applied a systematic activation approach to engage relevant stakeholders (Rütten et al., 2018). In 2017, the researchers organized two workshops with 60–80 participants plus subsequent working group meetings to develop links to policymakers, professionals, and NGOs from different levels (local, state, national) and domains.

The workshops served three purposes: (1) to introduce the PA recommendations to the stakeholders; (2) to engage stakeholders in drafting materials, which allowed the recommendations a broader reach among multipliers; and (3) to develop initial strategies for dissemination and implementation of the recommendations (Rütten et al., 2018, p. 5).

With the policy outcomes of these early processes, important federal policies acknowledged the recommendations and proposed ways to their implementation. For example, the Conference of the Health Ministers of the German states passed a resolution endorsing the dissemination and implementation of the PA recommendations and proposed their inclusion within the Federal Prevention Act measures (Rütten et al., 2018, p. 6). Moreover, reference to the recommendations was also included in the guideline document of the statutory health insurances.

44.5 Windows of Opportunity

Theories of the policymaking process describe the crucial role of "windows of opportunities" for "policy entrepreneurs" and their attempts to connect diverse streams of research, policy and politics (Bakir & Jarvis, 2017; Kingdon, 1997). In our case study, a key momentum related to a situation created by the German prevention law (launched in 2016). Among other things, the law obliged health insurances to spend about 150 million euros per year on setting-based health promotion focusing on structural issues and aiming to reduce health inequalities. However, the implementation of corresponding approaches at the local level proved to be extremely difficult. On the one hand, the health insurances did not want to leave the money to communities and the approaches available to them. On the other hand, the local routines of health insurances were aligned with individual approaches and were inadequate for structural health promotion as prescribed by the law.

In 2018, this situation opened a window of opportunity for researchers who developed National Recommendations for PA and PA promotion, and to start the activation and implementation process. Four major conditions encouraged the researchers to serve as entrepreneurs for health promotion innovation in Germany. (1) The research stream underlying the PA recommendations showed strong evidence for community-based approaches focusing on structural changes towards health equity. (2) The health insurances needed support to approach the local level in order to fulfil the prevention law. (3) Both insufficient knowledge and conflicting politics between governmental institutions and health insurances let the latter search for support of independent, credible, and evidence-based research. (4) Key actors from both governmental sectors and health insurances considered PA promotion as a timely and exemplary health promotion issue.

Against this background, two key players in the German healthcare system, i.e. the National Association of Statutory Health Insurance Funds (GKV-Spitzenverband), (as umbrella organization of health insurances), and the Federal Center of Health Education (a specialist authority within the portfolio of the German Ministry of Health) offered to fund for a pilot project on implementing the PA recommendations. Moreover, the nationwide project KOMBINE (see below), which included German communities from rural to metropolitan areas and focuses on structural change and health equity, was also considered as a pilot for the implementation of the new prevention law.

44.6 Co-production of a Conceptual Framework

The broader strategies applied in the early stages of our case study (raising awareness and support for the PA recommendations and starting a network with potential stakeholders/partners) prepared the ground for more intensive strategies such as "coalition building," "leading by example" and "transforming institutions" applied in the later process. Such strategies were used in the pilot project KOMBINE (German acronym for "Community-Based PA Promotion to Implement National Recommendations"). From 2018 to 2020, researchers cooperated in KOMBINE with local stakeholders and policymakers as well as with representatives from socially disadvantaged population groups.

In the first phase of KOMBINE, a common conceptual framework for implementing the PA recommendations was developed (Kohler et al., 2021). Knowledge from both public health and policy sciences was applied to design this phase. Theory and research from interactive knowledge-to-action approaches in public health have underlined the need for integrating scientific evidence derived from research practice and "practice-based evidence," i.e. practices that populations, stakeholders, and policymakers consider as relevant for health promotion (Chambers et al., 2013; Glasgow et al., 2012; Green, 2006). Moreover, strategies of policy entrepreneurship such as "issue linking" (Brouwer & Biermann, 2011, p. 5) and "issue framing" (Faling et al., 2018, p. 406) build on an integration of knowledge, ideas, and concepts from different stakeholders, levels, and domains as well.

In a series of workshops and working group meetings, local stakeholders and policymakers from 11 out of 16 states in Germany discussed their specific experiences on facilitators, barriers, and needs in community health promotion, focusing on PA and health equity. Based on an interactive knowledge-to-action approach, the process started with an introduction of the National PA recommendations as well as a presentation of local PA promotion projects as good practice examples (one from a rural area, a medium-sized city, a metropolis). Afterwards, three working groups were formed with participants divided into groups according to the type and size of their community.

Participants in each working group discussed three questions regarding community-based PA promotion with a focus on people with social disadvantages. (1) "What works in practice?", (2) "What are the barriers?" and (3) "What needs for action do you see in the promotion of PA?". This dialogue's first important outcome was a catalogue of nine key components for successful and sustainable community health promotion (see Fig. 44.1). An inductive approach, which clustered all

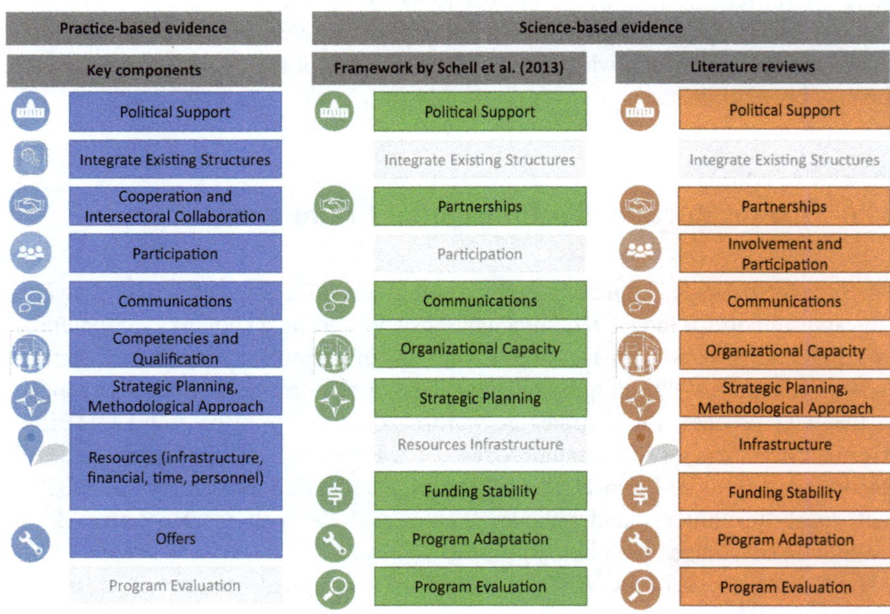

Fig. 44.1 Consensus between practice-based evidence and science-based evidence (Kohler et al. 2021)

findings by content/meaning regarding "facilitators," "barriers," and "needs" led to the identification of these components. Next, we compared the nine key components (representing "practice-based evidence") with updated literature reviews (representing "science-based evidence") on effective and sustainable community-based PA promotion among socially disadvantaged groups (developed in a working group during previous projects) (Abu-Omar et al., 2017; Messing & Rütten, 2017; Rütten et al., 2016). Additionally, we compared the nine key components with the core domains of the sustainability framework for public health programs by Schell et al. (2013).

As Fig. 44.1 indicates, the level of agreement between the practice-based catalogue of key components with the science-based evidence turned out to be very high. For example, the key components political support (e.g. awareness and integration of political decision-makers), cooperation and intersectoral collaboration (e.g. connections between stakeholders of different sectors) or strategic planning and methodological approaches (e.g. a structured approach for planning and implementation), were supported by research and were also identified by stakeholders as important for all types of communities.

Subsequently, the consensus on the key components was embedded in the development of an action-oriented framework for community-based PA promotion. This framework was also developed "bottom up" in successive working group meetings. For each working group (rural, urban, metropolis) the meetings were structured in four stages: (1) the working groups discussed the nine key components; (2) the introduction of a 3-phase action-oriented framework based on common steps in health promotion was presented; (3) the participants assigned the key components to an appropriate phase in the framework; (4) and finally generated a consensus statement. Based on the results of discussions about the role and relevance of each key component in different phases, the original 3-phase framework needed to be extended into a 6-phase action-oriented framework. The process was completed during a second workshop, where the 6-phase action-oriented framework was discussed again, finalized, and agreed upon by all participants (shown in Fig. 44.2). Measures of participatory evaluation are embedded in the overall process.

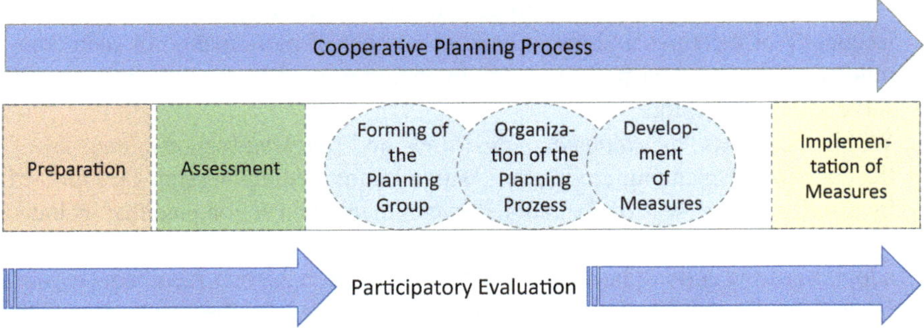

Fig. 44.2 6-phase action-oriented framework for community-based PA promotion (Kohler et al. 2021)

44.7 Co-production and Evaluation of Structural Changes Towards Health Equity

To set the framework into innovative practice, the six phases were implemented in six pilot communities in the second phase of KOMBINE. These were selected using a systematic sampling procedure. The sample is composed of three rural communities, two middle-sized cities, and one metropolis from different regions in Germany. Stakeholders from these communities already participated in the first phase of KOMBINE and contributed to the development of the framework.

44.7.1 Implementation of the 6-Phase Action-Oriented Framework

The following section describes the content and the implementation of each phase in the six pilot communities.

- The "*preparation phase*" comprises the identification of relevant stakeholders, first talks in the community, and the definition of the Kickoff format (e.g. the timeframe and location of the first meeting with all stakeholders) for the local project. Further, it includes the formation of a steering committee and prepares the conduction of the assessment.
- The "*assessment phase*" considers available data from four dimensions of PA: PA behaviour (e.g. prevalence, organization), infrastructure (e.g. offers, facilities), citizen participation (e.g. citizens' initiatives), and PA policy (e.g. political resolutions). Data are collected and analyzed collectively by stakeholders and the research team.
- "*Forming a planning group*" addresses the identification and selection of participants for a cooperative planning group with different stakeholders (administration, politics, citizens) from various domains. Among other things, the process includes getting to know each other and developing a shared understanding of KOMBINE.
- "O*rganization of the planning process*" includes decisions about the scope and frequency of meetings and the maximum number of participants. In each community, a local contact person is appointed and trained by the research team to serve as co-moderator.
- Within the phases "*development of measures*" and "*implementation of measures,*" the cooperative planning group starts with a brainstorming (session 1), followed by priority setting (session 2), and the development of an action plan that includes implementation steps, time frames, responsibilities, indicators (session 3 to 5), the adoption of the action plan by all cooperative planning group members (session 6), and finally the implementation of measures based on the action plan. The cooperative planning group is accompanied by the steering committee of key stakeholders, which oversees the whole cooperative planning process.

44.7.2 Evaluation Approach in the Six Pilot Communities

Evaluation consists of five components: input, process, output, outcome, and impact.

- *Input evaluation* considers the local context, starting conditions, and resources in each community. The assessment thereby collects information about the four dimensions of PA promotion with local partners. In addition, the input evaluation assesses available data about health status and health inequalities. Qualitative interviews are conducted with systematically chosen key informants from the community for a deeper understanding of the local context.
- *Process evaluation* assesses the development of measures and PA promoting structures during the implementation process. The researchers collect meeting minutes and lists of attendance, document phone calls, and take field notes about the cooperative planning process. It further contains regular reflective dialogue within the KOMBINE research team, the steering committee, and the cooperative planning group. Based on these dialogues, decisions about the ongoing process and necessary adaptations are made.
- *Output evaluation* assesses the developed PA promoting measures based on the actions plans. Furthermore, it uses participatory approaches to assess the implementation of these measures by means of the predefined indicators for successful implementation.
- *Outcome evaluation* assesses the effects of both the cooperative planning process and the implemented PA promoting measures on individual and population-based indicators. For example, "pragmatic evaluation measures" (Glasgow & Riley, 2013) are used by the local partners to evaluate participants of new PA offers. Additional outcome evaluation by the research team focuses on determinants of PA (e.g. new networks and infrastructures).
- *Impact evaluation* assesses the effect of the overall process on structural level indicators (i.e. politics, organizational routines in administration) and health inequality. Data are collected i.e. via qualitative interviews and local reports and are compared with input evaluation data.

Due to the COVID-19 pandemic, the final implementation processes (phase 5/6) were interrupted in all communities. Accordingly, the outcome and impact evaluation had to be postponed to 2021. Nevertheless, initial results of other evaluation components can be reported.

As an output of the cooperative planning process, PA promoting measures were developed in all dimensions of PA promotion within all six communities. For example, in the *dimension of PA behaviour* one rural community is planning the establishment of swimming classes in a public school in a socially disadvantaged neighbourhood. For improving the *infrastructure*, one of the pilot cities plans a multi-generational play–/physical-activity-ground developed in cooperation with socially disadvantaged people. This concept can be implemented in different neighbourhoods and allow the transfer to different locations. To foster *citizen participation,* another rural pilot community is organizing a local participatory process with people with social disadvantages to jointly develop approaches for PA promotion. The metropolis is working in the *PA policy dimension* on an overall strategy for PA promotion to establish new structures for PA promotion.

Effects of the cooperative planning process were assessed by an online questionnaire with standardized questions and options for open comments. While this survey is still ongoing, the first results from four out of six communities showed that all communities formed planning groups with about 25–30 participants, consisting of representatives of the administration, political stakeholders, multipliers, experts, and citizens. In the urban communities, representatives of the administration accounted for the largest percentage in the planning group, followed by multipliers and experts. Compared to the urban communities, rural areas had a higher number of elected representatives. Involving people from disadvantaged groups presented a challenge in all communities.

A majority of participants in the four communities agreed that the cooperative planning meetings enabled a useful exchange and a successful intersectoral approach. Further, half of the participants indicated improved political support for PA promotion through the planning process and the measures developed. Open comments supported the need and usefulness of the cooperative planning process for promoting PA, but also showed that some participants lacked more support and viewed the required time for meetings critically.

Furthermore, the COVID-19 pandemic stopped the implementation process of the developed PA measures in all communities. Some participants viewed this as detrimental for the further implementation of KOMBINE.

44.8 Discussion and Conclusions

In our case study, we explored the potential role of research-driven policy entrepreneurship as a strategy and practice of social change towards health equity (Faling et al., 2018; Mintrom & Norman, 2009; Brouwer & Biermann, 2011). In the specific context of health promotion in Germany, we found several conditions relevant for policy entrepreneurship (Faling et al., 2018).

At first, our approach had to deal with a condition of *"institutional overlap,"* which refers to the authority involved within different levels and/or domains over the issue (Faling et al., 2018, p. 409). As indicated above, different levels of government (local, state, national) as well as different domains (e.g. sport, health) are involved in the development and implementation of health promotion strategies focusing on physical inactivity and health inequality in Germany. The opportunities for policy entrepreneurship in a situation of institutional overlap are mainly related to various starting points. For example, if the sports sector at the local level is politically reluctant, less competent, or lacks the resources to address PA and health equity issues, policy entrepreneurs may find better entry points (e.g. policies, actors) in the health sector at the national or state level.

Another condition of policy entrepreneurship discussed in the literature is related to the interpretation of an issue "as requiring a multisector or level approach" (Faling et al., 2018, p. 409). In our case study, the two key policy documents (national PA recommendations, prevention law) recognize the need for intersectoral approaches to address physical inactivity and health inequalities (Rütten & Pfeifer, 2016, pp. 111–112; Bundesgesetzblatt Teil I Nr. 31, 2015, p. 1368). The opportunities related to this condition refer to the readiness of actors from relevant levels and domains to perceive cross-boundary strategies and integrative approaches of policy entrepreneurs as "salient, legitimate and credible" (Faling et al., 2018, p. 410). Accordingly, our approaches of aligning policy agendas from different levels and domains could count on a generally high degree of acceptance by relevant policymakers and stakeholders.

The "existence of a *power vacuum* or *knowledge gap* around an issue" (Faling et al., 2018, p. 410) is a potentially enabling condition as well. In Germany, a "power vacuum" regarding PA promotion exists at the national level, as governmental organizations have no authority over "sport for all activities" (authority of states and communities). Only one large NGO (German Olympic Sport Federation) claims national authority but has no authority regarding PA beyond sports activities (e.g. "physically active transportation"). In addition, a "knowledge gap" regarding PA exists at the national level but even more at the local level. Policymakers are looking for scientific expertise, which may lead to an increasing authority of researchers as consultants and support the role of researchers as policy entrepreneurs.

Further conducive conditions found by Faling et al. (2018, p. 410) refer to "focusing events" at a level or a domain different from the actual issue arena. Such events may provide opportunities to involve relevant actors and/or to "exert pressure on the issue arena." In our case study, certain events organized by sports ministries at the state level (e.g. different meetings with relevant political statements and a conference on PA recommendations and PA promotion issues) put some pressure on agencies from the national level. For instance, those events were helpful to mobilize key actors from the national health sector. In particular, the development of the National PA recommendations was indirectly supported by those events. Other focusing events were located at the national level but were helpful to mobilize agencies at the local level. For example, a decision made by a national board for the implementation of the prevention law to exclusively focus on implementation strategies in the community setting and subsequent conferences on this topic led to a more active involvement of communities.

Against the background of the German context and the conditions discussed so far, our case study results indicate that research-based policy entrepreneurs may be in a position to initiate and direct networks of stakeholders from different levels and domains in order to bridge vertical and horizontal boundaries, and to support the development of new health-promoting structures.

Though potentially successful as a health promotion strategy, the discussion of the case study should also reflect the adequacy of research-based policy entrepreneurship as a distinctive research strategy. There are two main reasons justifying the researcher's role as a policy entrepreneur from a scientific perspective. First of all, policy entrepreneurship opens up specific options in knowledge production. Following Kurt Lewin's famous methodological advice: "if you want truly to understand something, try to change it," policy entrepreneurship from researchers is a kind of scientific field study that contributes to our empirical knowledge on policy processes. Researcher's own experience of real-world policymaking is full of peculiarities that invite a scientific reflection. For example, researchers as policy entrepreneurs apply strategies of policymaking such as "partial mutual adjustment" (Lindblom & Woodhouse, 1993) and by doing so may gain new insight into how the use of scientific evidence could be improved in the real policy world. Secondly, policy entrepreneurship of researchers may be distinctive for the implementation of scientific evidence from health promotion research. For example, after many years of intensive approaches in communicating scientific recommendations of PA with only very limited impact on the PA behaviour of the population, Canadian researchers developed stakeholder-based activation strategies and more interactive and cooperative approaches similar to those applied in our case study in order to get their messages across (Tremblay et al., 2020; Gainforth et al., 2013). Moreover, such research-based policy entrepreneurship was also a key element in the process of developing "integrative evidence" as outlined above in the section on "co-production of a conceptual framework."

Key challenges for researchers as policy entrepreneurs should also be mentioned. Specific capacities are already needed to be a policy entrepreneur (e.g. Mintrom, 2019) but to be a researcher at the same time is even more demanding. As have been outlined above, research-based policy entrepreneurs must be able to build coalitions which includes building trust with different actors, and they must value and enable the true participation of stakeholders in knowledge production. Such prominent roles of researchers in policymaking may be especially challenging in situations where conflicting interests arise. On the one hand, these might put them in the role of a mediator. On the other hand, researchers' own interest in implementing scientific evidence implies that they act as "broker" as well. In addition, their research interest in the production of new knowledge on health promotion implementation gives them another role of a participant observer. In order to fulfil these different roles appropriately and to manage potential role conflicts both training and experience in participatory action research, cooperative planning, and transdisciplinary methods may be necessary. Research-based policy entrepreneurship should also be accompanied by multi-facet evaluation that provides opportunities for self-reflexivity. In addition, more scientific publications on concepts and methods applied in research-based policy entrepreneurship would be helpful to increase the feedback of new insights into the scientific system and to open up a scientific discussion of such approaches by the health promotion research community. To conclude, future research (Mintrom, 2020) should explore the role of research-based policy entrepreneurs in the field of health promotion in more depth, in terms of their characteristics, their used strategies, their impact on producing new scientific knowledge as well as on promoting structural change in different contexts towards health for all.

44.9 Challenges and Achievements

In the final section, we will first outline the challenges that we faced throughout the whole process. We will then conclude with some of the achievements that can be reported so far.

44.9.1 Challenges

Some key challenges of our case study are related to timeline issues. We mainly focused on activities from 2016 to 2020, but it was indicated that these build on earlier phases of policy entrepreneurship, which helped to define the policy problem of physical inactivity and health inequality at the national level in the last decade (Rochefort & Cobb, 1993; Rütten et al., 2013). Moreover, activities related to the implementation and evaluation of sustainable structural changes in the pilot communities, the expansion and further establishment of a supportive national policy coalition, and the scaling-up of successfully piloted approaches are already planned for the next four years (see below). An overall time frame of research-driven policy entrepreneurship from 10 to 15 plus years does not usually fit with single funding streams that may limit research activities to 1–3 years only. Accordingly, in our case study, several successful funding proposals and funding from different institutions were needed to allow researchers to act more or less continuously as policy entrepreneurs over the whole period (Rütten et al., 2018).

Conflicting timelines of research and policy agendas turned out to be challenging as well. For example, the foreseen one-year timeframe of the KOMBINE research plan to implement the 6-phase action-oriented framework in pilot communities, in some cases collided with the timelines of the local decision-making processes within the communities and hindered the start of pilot projects.

Moreover, with the COVID-19 pandemic, a new issue suddenly interrupted the local policy agenda in most local project activities for several months. Conflicting timelines were also a challenge in cooperation with key national institutions that supported the project.

In particular, the considerably long timeframe that researchers (based on scientific evidence) had foreseen pertaining to changes in structures and reaching sustainability of new routines, collided with expectations on a limited time investment and resources by funders and key national actors. Three years for KOMBINE was a compromise, but given the first evaluation results, this was not sufficient yet.

Another set of challenges was related to the implementation of our interactive-knowledge-to-action methodology. Using a cooperative planning approach that builds on voluntary collaboration, had implications regarding its potential to overcome the inertia of established structures (King et al., 1987; Peters, 2005; Rütten & Gelius, 2013). For example, "political support" and "participation" were identified as two important key components of successful approaches. Nevertheless, involving policymakers in cooperative planning practice remained a challenge in most participating communities. Among other things, lack of time or urgent involvement of relevant policymakers in other policy issues have been named as potential reasons for non-participation. In some cases, due to negative experiences from previous processes or out of concerns regarding potential conflicts, responsible contact persons found it inappropriate to involve decision-makers in cooperative planning procedures.

Although strongly emphasized by the KOMBINE research team, the participation of people from disadvantaged groups in cooperative planning was a challenge as well. In most communities, only representatives and multipliers with contact to people with social disadvantages were involved. Reasons were manifold. One common concern from community stakeholders was that people with social disadvantages might not have benefits from participating in the process and at worst might be demotivated and stressed. It was also suggested to involve people with social disadvantages later in the process (when PA measures are already developed). Although methods and techniques to reach and involve people with social disadvantages were frequently discussed, community stakeholders expressed the need for more support and knowledge in this area.

Intersectoral collaboration was identified as another evidence-based key component of our implementation framework. Thus, participation of stakeholders from different sectors (e.g. sport, health, transport, urban planning, social services) in cooperative planning was necessary but led to challenges because of the different interests and policy agendas involved (Faling et al., 2018). For example, the overall priority of PA promotion differed between domains: in most communities, the sport and health sectors showed a high commitment while other relevant sectors were more reluctant. Moreover, some sectors mainly focused on individually-based PA programs and were struggling with the structural, population-based approach of KOMBINE.

The COVID pandemic also became a big challenge for KOMBINE in all pilot communities having the largest impact on activities led by the health sector. However, with a delay of five months, the pilot communities resumed their collaboration and the implementation of the developed measures.

44.9.2 Achievements

Strategies of "issue promotion" and "networking" were relevant during the earlier steps of policy entrepreneurship in our case study and led to the important policy outcome that federal policies acknowledged the national PA recommendations and proposed their implementation (Faling et al., 2018). Corresponding interactive research activities also initiated first links between practices of relevant national and local stakeholders for promoting processes to approach the issues of physical inactivity and health inequalities at the community level. Moreover, such research-driven networking and issue promotion activities helped to place those issues on policy agendas of relevant institutions (e.g. national/federal health and sports ministries and their authorities, local communities, umbrella organizations of health insurances).

The early steps prepared the ground for the pilot project KOMBINE. An important first outcome of bridging national policy with the practices of local communities was a co-produced framework including key components for implementing PA promotion with a special focus on health equity (KOMBINE phase 1). We further initiated the implementation of this framework in six pilot rural and urban communities (KOMBINE Phase 2). Within this systematic and stepwise procedure, researchers, in co-operation with local stakeholders (1) assed local needs regarding PA promotion and health equity, (2) formed steering committees and cooperative planning groups in each community with participants across a variety of domains, and (3) developed measures to promote PA and health equity in each pilot community.

In the KOMBINE implementation process, "Issue promotion" regarding PA and addressing health equity as well as "issue linking" were used in different meetings and bilateral communications with several stakeholders from different domains to help raise attention (Faling et al., 2018). For example, policy stakeholders in rural communities were especially interested in promoting quality of life and social cohesion for the rural population, improving the attractiveness of the rural area, or addressing the vanishing of sports clubs due to low member rates. Using the cross-boundary strategy, "building coalitions" (Faling et al., 2018) supported the participation of stakeholders from different sectors (e.g. health, sports, urban planning) and led intensified mutual discussions and formed new coalitions in some pilot communities. As a structural outcome, in four out of six pilot communities, new staff positions (initially for three years) were created to foster the sustainable implementation of the PA promoting measures. Overall, within 18 months, first bridges between policies, resources, stakeholders, and social practices of different levels/domains were built, and accordingly, first results indicating structural changes towards an improved health promotion practice could be reported.

However, due to ongoing project activities and since the main parts of outcome and impact evaluation are missing, an in-depth analysis of structural achievements will be part of further research.

KOMBINE and its preliminary outcomes helped to prepare important next steps of research-driven policy entrepreneurship in Germany. VERBUND (German acronym for "Dissemination and Implementation of Community-Based PA Promotion") has started in autumn 2020. Based on KOMBINE, this project will develop a scaling-up approach that allows the involvement of more communities with a specific focus on developing intermediary structures.

44.10 Conclusions

Studies on the development and implementation of healthy public policies are a key action area for health promotion research. An active role of researchers as health promotion policy entrepreneurs facilitates the production of new scientific insights on relevant mechanisms of such policy processes. As our study indicates, researchers as policy entrepreneurs also find a variety of opportunities for the transformation of scientific knowledge into policy and practice.

Funding Statement The development and dissemination of National recommendations for Physical Activity and Physical Activity Promotion was funded by the German Federal Ministry of Health (ZMVI 52514FSB-200).

KOMBINE was funded by the Federal Center of Health Education (BZgA) on behalf of and with funds from the statutory health insurances according to § 20a SGB V in the context of the GKV Alliance for Health (www.gkv-buendnis.de). Grant number: Z2/1.01 G/18.

References

Abel, T., & Frohlich, K. L. (2012). Capitals and capabilities: Linking structure and agency to reduce health inequalities. *Social Science & Medicine, 74*, 236–244. https://doi.org/10.1016/j.socscimed.2011.10.028

Abu-Omar, K., Rütten, A., Burlacu, I., Messing, S., Pfeifer, K., & Ungerer-Röhrich, U. (2017). Systematischer Review von Übersichtsarbeiten zu Interventionen der Bewegungsförderung: Methodologie und erste Ergebnisse. *Gesundheitswesen, 79*, S45–S50. https://doi.org/10.1055/s-0042-123502

Bakir, C., & Jarvis, D. S. L. (2017). Contextualising the context in policy entrepreneurship and institutional change. *Policy and Society, 36*, 465–478. https://doi.org/10.1080/14494035.2017.1393589

Baum, F., MacDougall, C., & Smith, D. (2006). Participatory action research. *Journal of Epidemiology and Community Health, 60*, 854–857. https://doi.org/10.1136/jech.2004.028662

Béland, D., & Katapally, T. R. (2018). Shaping policy change in population health: Policy entrepreneurs, ideas, and institutions. *International Journal of Health Policy and Management, 7*, 369–373. https://doi.org/10.15171/ijhpm.2017.143

Bergmann, M., Jahn, T., Knobloch, T., Krohn, W., Pohl, C., & Schramm, E. (2012). *Methods for transdisciplinary research: A primer for practice*. Campus Verlag.

Brouwer, S., & Biermann, F. (2011). Towards adaptive management: Examining the strategies of policy entrepreneurs in Dutch water management. *Ecology and Society*. https://doi.org/10.5751/ES-04315-160405

Brown, A. F., Ma, G. X., Miranda, J., Eng, E., Castille, D., Brockie, T., et al. (2019). Structural interventions to reduce and eliminate health disparities. *American Journal of Public Health, 109*, S72–S78. https://doi.org/10.2105/AJPH.2018.304844

Brownson, R. C., Fielding, J. E., & Green, L. W. (2018). Building capacity for evidence-based public health: Reconciling the pulls of practice and the push of research. *Annual Review of Public Health, 39*, 27–53. https://doi.org/10.1146/annurev-publhealth-040617-014746

Bundesgesetzblatt Teil I Nr. 31. (2015). §20 Präventionsgesetz SGB *V*.

Chambers, D. A., Glasgow, R. E., & Stange, K. C. (2013). The dynamic sustainability framework: Addressing the paradox of sustainment amid ongoing change. *Implementation Science, 8*, 117. https://doi.org/10.1186/1748-5908-8-117

Faling, M., Biesbroek, R., Karlsson-Vinkhuyzen, S., & Termeer, K. (2018). Policy entrepreneurship across boundaries: A systematic literature review. *Journal of Public Policy, 39*, 393–422. https://doi.org/10.1017/S0143814X18000053

Frisch-Aviram, N., Beeri, I., & Cohen, N. (2020). Entrepreneurship in the policy process: Linking behavior and context through a systematic review of the policy entrepreneurship literature. *Public Administration Review, 80*, 188–197. https://doi.org/10.1111/PUAR.13089

Frohlich, K. L., & Potvin, L. (2008). Transcending the known in public health practice: The inequality paradox: The population approach and vulnerable populations. *American Journal of Public Health, 98*, 216–221. https://doi.org/10.2105/AJPH.2007.114777

Gainforth, H. L., Berry, T., Faulkner, G., Rhodes, R. E., Spence, J. C., Tremblay, M. S., et al. (2013). Evaluating the uptake of Canada's new physical activity and sedentary behavior guidelines on service organizations' websites. *Translational Behavioral Medicine, 3*, 172–179. https://doi.org/10.1007/s13142-012-0190-z

Glasgow, R. E., & Riley, W. T. (2013). Pragmatic measures: What they are and why we need them. *American Journal of Preventive Medicine, 45*, 237–243. https://doi.org/10.1016/j.amepre.2013.03.010

Glasgow, R. E., Green, L. W., Taylor, M. V., & Stange, K. C. (2012). An evidence integration triangle for aligning science with policy and practice. *American Journal of Preventive Medicine, 42*, 646–654. https://doi.org/10.1016/j.amepre.2012.02.016

Green, L. W. (2006). Public health asks of systems science: To advance our evidence-based practice, can you help us get more practice-based evidence? *American Journal of Public Health, 96*, 406–409. https://doi.org/10.2105/AJPH.2005.066035

Guldbrandsson, K., & Fossum, B. (2009). An exploration of the theoretical concepts policy windows and policy entrepreneurs at the Swedish public health arena. *Health Promotion International, 24*, 434–444. https://doi.org/10.1093/heapro/dap033

Haire-Joshu, D., & McBride, T. D. (2013). *Transdisciplinary public health: Research, education, and practice* (1st ed., Jossey-Bass Public Health). .l.: Jossey-Bass.

Hawe, P. (2015). Lessons from complex interventions to improve health. *Annual Review of Public Health, 36*, 307–323. https://doi.org/10.1146/annurev-publhealth-031912-114421

Hawe, P., Shiell, A., & Riley, T. (2004). Complex interventions: How “out of control” can a randomised controlled trial be? *BMJ (Clinical research ed.), 328*, 1561–1563. https://doi.org/10.1136/bmj.328.7455.1561

Holmes, B. J., Best, A., Davies, H., Hunter, D., Kelly, M. P., Marshall, M., et al. (2017). Mobilising knowledge in complex health systems: A call to action. *Evidence & Policy: A Journal of Research, Debate and Practice, 13*, 539–560. https://doi.org/10.1332/174426416X14712553750311

King, P., Roberts, J., & Nancy, C. (1987). Policy entrepreneurs: Catalysts for policy innovation. *Journal of State Government, 60*, 172–179.

Kingdon, J. W. (1997). *Agendas, alternatives, and public policies* (2nd ed.). Pearson.

Kohler, S., Helsper, N., Dippon, L., Rütten, A., Abu-Omar, K., Pfeifer, K., Semrau, J. (2021). Co-producing an action-oriented framework for community-based Physical Activity Promotion in Germany. *Health Promotion International 36 (Supplement_2),* ii93-ii106. https://doi.org/10.1093/heapro/daab159

Lindblom, C. E., & Woodhouse, E. J. (1993). *The policy-making process* (Prentice-Hall foundations of modern political science series) (3rd ed.). Prentice Hall.

Meijerink, S., & Huitema, D. (2010). Policy entrepreneurs and change strategies: Lessons from sixteen case studies of water transitions around the globe. *Ecology and Society*. https://doi.org/10.5751/es-03509-150221

Messing, S., & Rütten, A. (2017). Qualitätskriterien für die Konzipierung, Implementierung und Evaluation von Interventionen zur Bewegungsförderung: Ergebnisse eines State-of-the-Art Reviews. *Gesundheitswesen (Bundesverband der Arzte des Offentlichen Gesundheitsdienstes (Germany)), 79*, S60–S65. https://doi.org/10.1055/s-0042-123378

Mintrom, M. (2019). So you want to be a policy entrepreneur? *Policy Design and Practice, 2*, 307–323. https://doi.org/10.1080/25741292.2019.1675989

Mintrom, M. (2020). *Policy entrepreneurs and dynamic*. Cambridge University Press. https://doi.org/10.1017/9781108605946

Mintrom, M., & Norman, P. (2009). Policy entrepreneurship and policy change. *Policy Studies Journal, 37*, 649–667. https://doi.org/10.1111/j.1541-0072.2009.00329.x

Moloughney, B. (2012). *The use of policy frameworks to understand public health-related public policy processes: A literature review. Final Report.*

Nutbeam, D. (2003). How does evidence influence public health policy? Tackling health inequalities in England. Health promotion journal of Australia, 14(3), 154-158. *Health Promotion Journal of Australia, 14*, 154–158. https://doi.org/10.1071/HE03154

Peters, G. B. (2005). The problem of policy problems. *Journal of Comparative Policy Analysis: Research and Practice, 7*, 349–370. https://doi.org/10.1080/13876980500319204

Rochefort, D. A., & Cobb, R. W. (1993). Problem definition, agenda access, and policy choice. *Policy Studies Journal, 21*, 56–71. https://doi.org/10.1111/j.1541-0072.1993.tb01453.x

Rochefort, D. A., & Cobb, R. W. (Eds.). (1995). *The politics of problem definition: Shaping the policy agenda (Studies in government and public policy)*. University Press of Kansas.

Rütten, A., & Gelius, P. (2013). Building policy capacities: An interactive approach for linking knowledge to action in health promotion. *Health Promotion International, 29*, 569–582. https://doi.org/10.1093/heapro/dat006

Rütten, A., & Pfeifer, K. (Eds.). (2016). *National recommendations for physical activity and physical activity promotion*. FAU University Press.

Rütten, A., Abu-Omar, K., Gelius, P., & Schow, D. (2013). Physical inactivity as a policy problem: Applying a concept from policy analysis to a public health issue. *Health research policy and systems, 11*, 9. https://doi.org/10.1186/1478-4505-11-9

Rütten, A., Wolff, A., & Streber, A. (2016). Nachhaltige Implementierung evidenzbasierter Programme in der Gesundheitsförderung: Theoretischer Bezugsrahmen und ein Konzept zum interaktiven Wissenstransfer. *Gesundheitswesen (Bundesverband der Arzte des Offentlichen Gesundheitsdienstes (Germany)), 78*, 139–145. https://doi.org/10.1055/s-0035-1548883

Rütten, A., Frahsa, A., Abel, T., Bergmann, M., de Leeuw, E., Hunter, D., et al. (2017). Co-producing active lifestyles as whole-system-approach: Theory, intervention and knowledge-to-action implications. *Health Promotion International, 34*, 47–59. https://doi.org/10.1093/heapro/dax053

Rütten, A., Abu-Omar, K., Messing, S., Weege, M., Pfeifer, K., Geidl, W., et al. (2018). *How can the impact of national recommendations for physical activity be increased?* Experiences from Germany. Health research policy and systems. https://doi.org/10.1186/s12961-018-0396-8

Schell, S. F., Luke, D. A., Schooley, M. W., Elliott, M. B., Herbers, S. H., Mueller, N. B., et al. (2013). Public health program capacity for sustainability: A new framework. *Implementation science : IS, 8*, 15. https://doi.org/10.1186/1748-5908-8-15

Söderberg, E., & Wikström, E. (2015). The policy process for health promotion. *Scandinavian Journal of Public Health, 43*, 606–614. https://doi.org/10.1177/1403494815586327

Stokols, D. (2006). Toward a science of transdisciplinary action research. *American Journal of Community Psychology, 38*, 63–77. https://doi.org/10.1007/s10464-006-9060-5

Tremblay, M. S., Rollo, S., & Saunders, T. J. (2020). Sedentary behavior research network members support new Canadian 24-hour movement guideline recommendations. *Journal of Sport and Health Science, 9*, 479–481. https://doi.org/10.1016/j.jshs.2020.09.012

Unwin, N., Samuels, T. A., Hassell, T., Brownson, R. C., & Guell, C. (2017). The development of public policies to address non-communicable diseases in the Caribbean country of Barbados: The importance of problem framing and policy entrepreneurs. *International Journal of Health Policy and Management, 6*, 71–82. https://doi.org/10.15171/ijhpm.2016.74.

Wilkinson, R. G. (1996). *Unhealthy societies: From inequality to well-being*. Routledge.

Chapter 45
Reflections on Mainstreaming Health Equity in a Large Research Collaboration: "If I can't dance it is not my revolution"

Ana Porroche-Escudero and Jennie Popay

45.1 Introduction

The concept of health promotion emerged largely in the context of the Ottawa Chapter. This term was an alternative within public health to integrate "action at the levels of individuals, communities and society" (Wold & Mittelmark, 2018, p. 21). This was quite a radical shift. It acknowledged that socio-economic and political factors and inequalities shape health (Woodall et al., 2018). But there are concerns that health promotion has been co-opted by the individualistic machinery of positivism that dominates much public health and biomedicine in general (Smith, 2014). This creates a host of challenges for health promotion practice, including the way in which research is conducted and its potential impact on policy and practice.

This chapter focuses on contemporary health promotion research. The purpose is three-fold. First, to remind readers that a health equity lens adds an invaluable dimension to health promotion practice and research in particular, and public health in general. Getting "equity" right into research can not only save lives and unnecessary suffering, it also saves money. The inequalities exposed by COVID-19 are a reminder that researchers have a critical role to play in eliminating inequalities by producing high-value relevant evidence. Research evidence, along with other types of knowledge and ideas (Smith, 2014), can then be used to develop better-tailored recommendations for policy and practice.

A. Porroche-Escudero (✉)
Lancaster Environment Centre, Lancaster University,
Lancaster, UK
e-mail: a.porroche-escudero@lancaster.ac.uk

J. Popay
Division of Health Research, Lancaster University,
Lancaster, UK

L. Potvin, D. Jourdan (eds.), *Global Handbook of Health Promotion Research, Vol. 1*,
https://doi.org/10.1007/978-3-030-97212-7_45

Second, this chapter aims to highlight one way in which a health equity lens can be organisationally embedded to improve health promotion research cultures and practices. A process that we describe as health equity mainstreaming. In what follows, we analyse the experience of a large English Research Collaboration as it sought to operationalise an equity focus by systematically integrating it in the institutions that govern research: its culture, processes, systems, projects, funding policies and individual practices.

The third objective is around methodology. In this chapter, we draw on our experiences as researcher-implementators in a large English partnership organisation. Our role was to design and oversee an organisational response to the lack of equity focus in much-applied health research, including health promotion. We want to underscore that reflective practice by us was essential to understand better how health equity mainstreaming could work (or not) in practice. The reflective process ran throughout our almost seven years of work with the Leadership in Applied Health Research and Care North West Coast (CLAHRC NWC).

Reflexions included examination of informal and formal discussions with colleagues and observations from attending meetings and delivering capacity-building activities. In addition, we were tasked with leading the internal evaluation of CLAHRC NWC. One of the strategic objectives of the evaluation was to assess whether embedding a health equity focus was achieved. This provided a brilliant opportunity to collect richer and nuanced data on progress. In addition to data from reflections, the evaluation collected data from internal documents (e.g. policies, strategies and minutes of management and SB meetings), monitoring data and data from feedback forms completed by people using the Health Inequalities Assessment Toolkit (HIAT), face-to-face interviews (n = 58) and focus group /workshops (n = 73). These included staff from CLAHRC NWC's partner organisations explained below. Information sheets and consent forms emphasised that participation was voluntary.

45.2 The Setting: CLAHRC NWC

The CLAHRC-NWC was one of 13 such collaborations established across England by the NIHR. They aimed to accelerate the translation of research findings into health policy and practice. Funded from 2014 to 2019, CLAHRC NWC included 36 partners from 3 universities, 5 NHS Clinical Commissioning Groups (CCG), 9 Local Authorities (LA), 17 NHS Provider Trusts and the NW Innovation Agency. In addition, 170 members of the public contributed as Public Advisers (PA). Some of these public partners were residents of 10 relatively disadvantaged neighbourhoods by 8 third sector organisations to join a Community Research and Engagement Network supporting place-base research.

The CLAHRC NWC operated within an English region with some of the starkest inequalities in mortality and other health outcomes. Since 1965, there have been 1.5 million excess premature deaths in the North of England compared with the rest of the country (M. (Chair) Whitehead et al., 2014). This geographical divide has been increasing, driven in part by England's public expenditure reductions and "the systematic dismantling of social protection policies since 2010" (Alston, 2018, p. 23). In this context, CLAHRC NWC acknowledged that the primary causes of health inequalities are not within the gift of researchers to act on. However, it was committed to increase the equity dimension of all its research portfolio to maximise the relevance of findings for front-line practice and policy aimed at reducing these inequalities.

The organisational architecture of CLAHRC-NWC is shown in Fig. 45.1. The Steering Board (SB) included representatives from the NHS, LAs, University Partners and PA with an independent chair. A subcommittee of the SB reviewed project proposals and made recommendations on funding. The Management Team comprised: Director; Programme Manager; Operations Manager; Director of Engagement; Director of Capacity Development and Theme Leads. There were four thematic programme and three cross-cutting themes. In addition, a Public Advisers Forum, open to all members of the public registered as Public Adviser (PA), oversaw the public involvement policy and sent representatives to the SB and the CLAHRC management group.

45.3 The Grand Challenges Faced by CLAHRC NWC

The World Health Organisation (WHO) sponsored Commission on the Social Determinants of Health's report in 2008 triggered a rapid expansion of both research and policy interest worldwide. (European Portal for Action on Health Inequalities, n.d.; WHO, 2018). More recently, the UN Sustainable Development Goals, endorsed by 193 nations in 2015 prioritised action to reduce health inequalities (Strand et al., 2009; Crombie et al., 2005). Many national health strategies now focus on these goals including the WHO's Health in All in Policies framework; the European Union (EU) Health Programme (2014) and the EU/WHO Health 2020.

Today, in the UK, multiple tools, funding streams and policies focus on health inequalities (Department of Health and Social Care, 2019; NHS Health Scotland, 2018; NIHR, 2018; Toleikyte & Colwell, 2020). They all aim to integrate action on health inequalities within planning and services redesign cycles, from assessment prior to implementation, through service design to quality assurance, audit and evaluation of existing services. Yet, they have not been systematically implemented or adopted. Indeed, our previous research did not find any initiatives that sought to embed a health equity focus across a research organisation (Porroche-Escudero et al., 2021). These findings are confirmed by a forthcoming review of English-language papers/resources aiming to strengthen the equity focus in health research, which has found that with notable exceptions (Eslava-Schmalbach et al., 2019; Plamondon & Bisung, 2019) published evidence on the processes and effectiveness of attempts to integrate a health equity focus across research organisations are lacking (Halliday et al., personal communication). Four main reasons for this absence of

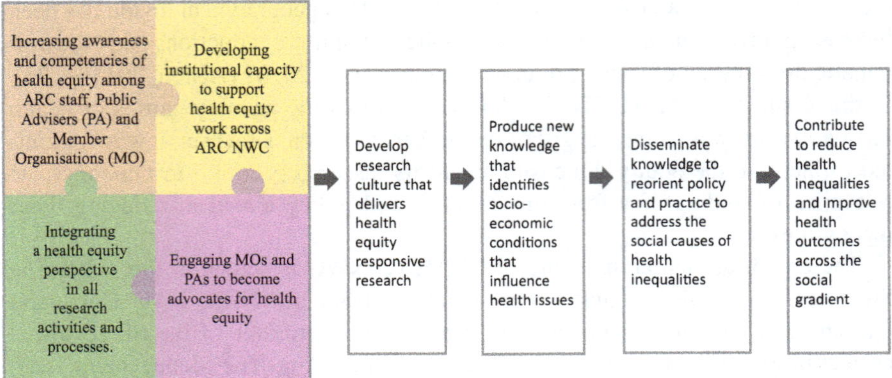

Fig. 45.1 Pathways to health equity mainstreaming

an equity focus in much public health and health promotion research have been highlighted in the literature.

45.3.1 Individualisation of Disease

Some scholars argue that public health's primary focus on the material, physiological body creates a false separation between the biological body and the wider determinants of health and neglects issues of agency and socio-economic well-being. (Pérez, 2019). The body is also viewed in terms of risks and disease. Thus, a considerable amount of public health practice and research focuses on how to modify people's behaviours without consideration of the wider social determinants of health that shape these behaviours (Wold and Mittelmark 2018:21; Scott-Samuel and Smith 2015) – a process that has been described as Lifestyle Drift (Popay et al. 2010).

45.3.2 Epistemic Violence: Lack of Meaningful Involvement of Members of the Public

Recently, feminist activists in Latin America have reinvigorated debates about public health definitions of risk. For instance, Paz and Ramírez Paz and Ramírez 2019) argue that the concept of risk is concerned with "acting in the present to modify the future and reach a desired situation". The problem, they point out, is the unexamined implicit and explicit assumptions underlying definitions of "what a desirable future should look like". Thus, they encourage public health researchers to confront the following questions:

> who desires *that* future? What actors speak? Which ones are voiceless? For whom is it desirable? Who benefits? Who loses out if interventions are undesired and enforced without consent? (Paz and Ramírez 2019:91–92, our own translation)

This lack of representation and involvement of those who will be affected by health-related research constitutes a clear example of what Spivak calls "epistemic violence" (Spivak, 1994, p. 76). It goes against the very foundational values of health promotion (Woodall et al., 2018) and health research in general (Fundación Soberanía Sanitaria et al., 2019; NIHR, 2019).

45.3.3 A Lack of Equity Focus Is a Form of Violence

Corbin raises an additional, yet interlinked challenge (Corbin, 2016). Although equity is integral to public health practice and research, the focus on behaviour/lifestyle change draws attention away from the need to generate local evaluative evidence for what is working for health equity and what is not. In other words, research and evaluation research often fail to assess "the negative impact of implementing new interventions or technologies on health inequalities" (Eslava-Schmalbach et al., 2019, p. 3) for specific socio-economic groups.

Similarly, research designs often fail to produce evidence to support and influence decision-makers and practitioners to act on the causes of health inequalities that are amenable to local action and to avoid actions that may increase inequalities. Thus, it is not surprising that Corbin asks whether researchers are part of the problem by not actively and explicitly considering equity in their projects (Corbin, 2016, p. 740) and, wonders whether we "are reproducing the exact inequity we seek to mitigate?". As Elie Wiesel reminded us in his acceptance speech for the Nobel Prize in 1986 in Oslo "We must always take sides. Neutrality helps the oppressor, never the victim. Silence encourages the tormentor, never the tormented".

45.3.4 Lack of Expertise to Design Equity-Sensitive Research

Another reason for the absence of an equity focus in health research is the lack of local expertise and confidence on how to include a health equity framework throughout the research process, from the ideas phase through research design and implementation to dissemination and how to do this in ways that involve relevant communities and professionals working with those communities.

This situation is in part caused by the paralysing idea that the upstream socio-economic causes of health inequalities are "too hard" or "too complex" to tackle by researchers, and can only be addressed by political action (Metzl & Hansen, 2014) and by different understandings of health inequalities and its causation (McMahon, 2021a, 2021b).

45.4 The CLAHRC NWC Equity Lens Journey

45.4.1 Beginnings

A recognition of the complex factors discussed above shaped the CLAHRC NWC's early strategy for action to integrate a routine health equity focus in their work. The collaboration started with four well-defined actions. First, it articulated an explicit commitment to reduce health inequalities in the official funding bid and related documents such as promotional materials and the website. This is important because what gets said, gets counted and accounted for (Sen et al., 2007).

Second, it endorsed a definition that recognised that inequalities in health cannot be tackled without fully understanding and addressing their wider social determinants. This marked a shift from the dominant framings of health inequalities in the health sector as individualised "lifestyle-centric" to recognise how "organisation and structural factors are the cause of social inequalities that affect health outcomes" (NIHR CLAHRC NWC, 2013, p. 8).

Third, it appointed a "specialist team". This included a senior researcher (JP) with an international track record of work on health inequalities to take responsibility for the health inequalities agenda from the point the original funding bid was developed, and a researcher (APE). Their role was to develop and implement a method to support the integration of equity into all CLAHRC's work and establish systems for monitoring progress.

The Health Inequalities Assessment Tool or HIAT (www.hiat.org.uk) was developed as the vehicle to support its strategic aim of embedding a health equity. The HIAT was novel in several important ways. Its development was informed by findings from a rapid review to identify interdisciplinary resources, tools and theoretical papers that could support researchers to integrate equity in their work. It had a strong focus on social determinants of health and public involvement throughout the research process. It provided guidance for a wide range of research activities (e.g. evidence synthesis, applied health research, implementation, knowledge mobilisation and capacity-building). It aimed to stimulate self-reflection in teams with a series of questions to foster debate. And finally, it was co-developed with members of the public and staff from its partner organisations including Universities, the NHS and local authorities as well as experts with international experience of health inequalities (Porroche-Escudero & Popay, 2020).

Fourth, the CLAHRC Steering Board (SB) requested mandatory HIAT assessments for all activities seeking funding support from CLAHRC, including interns and PhD students in an attempt to systematise the use of the tool.

45.4.2 Awakenings

Halfway through the CLAHRC 5-year funding term, the team took stock of progress made on the core objective of integrating the equity lens across the collaboration. The limitations of the approach were becoming apparent. The team started recognising that a focus on health inequalities was the golden thread that must run through the CLAHRC – a cultural change agenda as much as a technical endeavour. Elaboration of some of these limitations may provide important insights/lessons for others wishing to integrate health equity in research collaborations.

When CLAHRC NWC submitted its application to the funder it stated that it would "tackle health inequalities through improvements in excellent applied research and implementation to enhance quality of health, care, patient experience and outcomes" (bid p.4). The successful proposal suggested that health equity would be a cross-cutting issue and a CLAHRC-wide responsibility. It identified management of the four research themes as the primary site for monitoring and assessing the impact of activities on inequalities. But four factors that diluted the message that health inequalities were a CLAHRC-wide responsibility were apparent.

First, the location of the equity lens plans in the funding proposal may have been problematic. Work on health inequalities was described within the Public Health Theme alone, potentially suggesting that it was the primary responsibility of this theme. Second, although health inequalities were mentioned at several other points in the funding proposal, its prominence varied significantly across the descriptions of specific themes. Third, there was no explicit strategy or road map developed by the CLAHRC management group on how the focus on reducing health inequalities would be embedded across the organisation. Fourth, CLAHRC's conceptualisation of the requirement for embedding a health equity focus across an organisation was too narrow, focusing solely on a technical approach: awareness raising through training and developing a toolkit and rolling out its use across the collaboration.

The combination of these factors resulted in a fragmented and reactive approach to the equity integration "project" with mixed results and frustrations. For instance, the first wave of research projects that began before the HIAT was developed had to "retro-fit" a focus on health equity. There was an understandable reluctance amongst some research staff to engage in this process with enthusiasm. In addition, the two-member HIAT team did not have the capacity to contact, support and chase every single project to carry out a HIAT assessment, let alone to assess whether the assessment was a ticking box exercise or a valuable learning process.

Senior management in CLAHRC tried to address these issues by taking a more proactive approach. Significantly, the health inequalities team was required to provide training and individual advice to all staff, PhD students and PAs. They were allocated a dedicated budget for training, dissemination activities and the development of resources such as a HIAT website and training materials. Alongside these attempts were made to strengthen the degree of transparency and accountability in the HIAT reporting and monitoring processes. For example, the SB requested that quarterly progress report templates be modified to include a section for reporting on the extent to which a focus on health inequalities had been integrated into activities following an initial HIAT assessment.

45.4.3 The Epiphany: Why Didn't We "Walk the Talk"?

As CLAHRC NWC matured over the first five years, the official line was that it took health inequalities seriously. To its credit, we witnessed a remarkable increase in health equity values and sensitivity over the years. Yet, we did not see parallel increases in actions to integrate a systematic health equity focus throughout research projects and activities. But after three and a half years this was a feeling without evidence.

The team was forced to think again about its progress eighteen months before the end of the five years funding period when progress on integrating an equity lens became a key element of an internal evaluation of CLAHRC NWC. The evaluation process provoked an epiphany. We began thinking of the problems described by professionals working in the arena of gender mainstreaming and we could relate to them. Then, we began thinking of the problems we had with the single technical focus on training/capacity-building and mandatory use of tools. Why was it that so few teams "walked the talk" (without being chased or lured by us)? What would it take to close the gap between CLAHRC's values and researchers' practices?

Of course, some of the answers to these problems lie in the complex social dynamics discussed earlier that reach well beyond the CLAHRC. But we discovered that CLAHRC had the power to address some of these. As we drew on a rich body of work on gender mainstreaming, normalisation process theory and implementation science our understanding of the internal triggers for change grew. Our definition of progress expanded to included consideration of "what was done" and "how things had to be done" to mainstream an equity focus into the fabric that binds a research organisation together: its culture.

The evaluation helped us to see in full technicolour that we were trying to navigate this minefield blindfolded, without a clear roadmap of how the health equity integration objective had to be operationalised. Our suspicions were confirmed. Technical fixes based on training and mandatory HIAT assessments and reports were not enough to transform people's readiness to "walk the talk". We realised that delivering health equity responsive studies required a systematic approach to transform the very roots of the "institutional context of research".

From that point on, CLAHRC NWC started using the language of "mainstreaming": first amongst senior management but slowly it has filtered through to all parts of the organisation. The partners in the CLAHRC received further funding under the new name of the Applied Research Collaboration (ARC) NWC and are taking forward a new "mainstreaming" approach to the health equity integration. The ARC NWC has produced a Health Equity Mainstreaming Strategy and Action Plan, the first roadmap of its kind for a collaborative health research organisation. Important stepping stones to mainstreaming an equity lens at institutional level are highlighted in Fig. 45.1. They include: (i) building knowledge, competencies and capabilities to support health equity work amongst all groups in the organisation (ii) building and communicating a body of expert knowledge to influence policy and practice; (iii) strengthening mechanisms for health equity mainstreaming within the organisation and in all research activities; and (iv) engage member organisations and members of the public to become health equity champions and co-produce research. However, this new approach is not without its own challenges – as we discuss elsewhere (Porroche-Escudero et al., 2021).

45.5 Conclusions – Into the Future

We have taken the title of this chapter from US feminist anarchist Emma Goldman's famous quote, "If I can't dance, it's not my revolution". Because a health equity focus, like dance, is essential to develop public health research that has the potential to be revolutionary. Our understanding of revolutionary is captured in the Oxford English Dictionary definition: "a dramatic and wide-reaching change in conditions, attitudes, or operation" to greater social justice.

Equity-sensitive research is revolutionary because it gives priority to the voices and experiences of those who will be affected by the implementation of research-based evidence. These are primarily the communities of interest and place that are bearing the brunt of social inequalities in health, but it also includes many front-line practitioners working with these communities. The practical wisdom they accumulate from the lived experience of oppression and powerlessness has much to offer health research yet it is routinely ignored. It is revolutionary because it would always assess whether interventions, trials, policies and practices are having differential impacts across social groups and include an assessment of negative as well as positive impact. And it is revolutionary because it is designed to produce evidence to influence decision makers and practitioners to act on the structural causes of health inequalities that are amenable to local action. The revolutionary potential of equity in research aligns well with the health promotion ethos.

All those involved in health promotion research need to move beyond limited technical approaches to strengthening the equity focus of research: primarily capacity-building initiatives and tool usage. We need to recognise that this is a mainstreaming agenda aimed at transforming the very roots of the "institution of research" (i.e. researchers, research organisations and research funding bodies) which dictates what constitutes appropriate research, including preferred methods and issues. (McQueen, 1991). The global health research community has to embrace a systematic approach to effect change in the culture of institutions of research, ensuring that we build expertise and confidence so that thinking and actions on the wider structural determinants of health are integrated into all activities involved in all stages of the research process from prioritisation to knowledge mobilisation.

We hope that our reflective lens offers two interlinked examples of how this may be done. First, our reflective journey showed the complex steps that led the CLAHRC NWC collaboration to where they are today in relation to health equity mainstreaming. Second, our work highlights the importance of reflexivity in the practice of applied health promotion research as it strengthens methodological designs and data interpretation. Reflexivity was critical for us to understand the nature and diversity of disciplinary assumptions and values around health inequalities and to attend to context, language. It helped us to recognise and enquire into what we did not know, what we could improve and what information we needed to monitor and evaluate progress in embedding a health equity.

Acknowledgements This chapter is research funded by the National Institute for Health Research Applied Research Collaboration North West Coast (ARC NWC). The views expressed in this publication are those of the author(s) and not necessarily those of the National Institute for Health Research or the Department of Health and Social Care.

References

Alston, P. (2018). *Statement on visit to the United Kingdom, by Professor Philip Alston*, United Nations Special Rapporteur on extreme poverty and human rights. OHCHR. United Nations Human Rights Office of the High Commissioner. https://www.ohchr.org/en/NewsEvents/Pages/DisplayNews.aspx?NewsID=23881&LangID=E

Corbin, J. H. (2016). Health promotion research: Thinking critically about knowledge production. *Health Promotion International, 31*(4), 739–741. https://doi.org/10.1093/heapro/daw095

Crombie, I. K., Irvine, L., Elliott, L., & Wallace, H. (2005). *Closing the health inequalities gap: An international perspective*. WHO European Office for Investment for Health and Development.

Department of Health and Social Care. (2019). *DHSC single departmental plan*. GOV.UK. https://www.gov.uk/government/publications/department-of-health-single-departmental-plan/dhsc-single-departmental-plan

Eslava-Schmalbach, J., Garzón-Orjuela, N., Elias, V., Reveiz, L., Tran, N., & Langlois, E. V. (2019). Conceptual framework of equity-focused implementation research for health programs (EquIR). *International Journal for Equity in Health, 18*(1), 80. https://doi.org/10.1186/s12939-019-0984-4

European Portal for Action on Health Inequalities. (n.d.). *Health Inequalities in the EU*. Retrieved 25 January 2019, from http://www.health-inequalities.eu/about-hi/in-the-eu/

Fundación Soberanía Sanitaria. (2019). In S. Balaña, A. Finielli, C. Giuliano, A. Paz, & C. Ramírez (Eds.), *Salud feminista Soberanía de los cuerpos, poder y organización Fundación Soberanía Sanitaria*. Tinta Limón.

McMahon, N. (2021a). *Promoting 'structural' perspectives on the problem of health inequalities: How far does the 'upstream-downstream' story get us?* Manuscript Submitted for Publication.

McMahon, N. (2021b). *What shapes how health professionals and decision-makers understand and work to address social inequalities in health? A meta-ethnography*. Manuscript Submitted for Publication.

McQueen, D. V. (1991). The contribution of Health promotion research to public Health. *European Journal of Public Health, 1*(1), 22–28. https://doi.org/10.1093/eurpub/1.1.22

Metzl, J., & Hansen, H. (2014). Structural competency: Theorizing a new medical engagement with stigma and inequality. *Social Science & Medicine, 103*, 126–133.

NHS Health Scotland. (2018). *Health inequalities impact assessment*. NHS Health Scotland. http://www.healthscotland.scot/tools-and-resources/health-inequalities-impact-assessment/hiia-case-studies

NIHR. (2018). *Policy Research Programme*. https://www.nihr.ac.uk/funding-and-support/funding-for-research-studies/funding-programmes/policy-research-programme/

NIHR. (2019). *NIHR adding value in research framework*. National Institute for Health Research. https://www.nihr.ac.uk/documents/nihr-adding-value-in-research-framework/20147

NIHR CLAHRC NWC. (2013). *NIHR collaborations for leadership in applied Health Research and care application form*. Reference: CLAHRC-2013-10040. https://www.clahrc-nwc.nihr.ac.uk/media/Info%20Hub/CLAHRC%20NIHR%20Application%20Final.pdf

Paz, A., & Ramírez, C. (2019). Riesgo(s) en disputa: El poder de definir el futuro deseable. In S. Balaña, A. Finielli, C. Giuliano, A. Paz, & C. Ramírez (Eds.), *Salud. Soberanía de los cuerpos, poder y organización* (pp. 89–100). Tinta Limón.

Pérez, M. (2019). Salud y soberanía de los cuerpos: Propuestas y tensiones desde una perspectiva queer. In S. Balaña, A. Finielli, C. Giuliano, A. Paz, & C. Ramírez (Eds.), *Salud feminista. Soberanía de los cuerpos, poder y organización* (pp. 31–48). Tinta Limón.

Plamondon, K. M., & Bisung, E. (2019). The CCGHR principles for Global Health research: Centering equity in research, knowledge translation, and practice. *Social Science & Medicine, 239*, 112530. https://doi.org/10.1016/j.socscimed.2019.112530

Popay J., Whitehead, M., Hunter, D. J. (2010). Injustice is killing people on a large scale—but what is to be done about it? *Journal of Public Health, 32*(2), 148–149. https://doi.org/10.1093/pubmed/fdq029

Porroche-Escudero, A., & Popay, J. (2020). The Health inequalities assessment toolkit (HIAT): Supporting integration of equity into applied health research. *Journal of Public Health, fdaa047*.

Porroche-Escudero, A., Popay, J., Ward, F., Ahmed, S., Akeju, D., Cloke, J., Gabbay, M., Hassan, S., Khan, K., & Khedmati-Morasae, E. (2021). From fringe to Centre-stage: Experiences of mainstreaming health inequalities through in a collaborative health research organisation. *Health Research Policy and Systems.*

Scott-Samuel, A., & Smith, K. E. (2015). Fantasy paradigms of health inequalities: Utopian thinking? *Social Theory & Health, 13*(3–4), 418–436. https://doi.org/10.1057/sth.2015.12

Sen, G., Ostlin, P., & George, A. (2007). *Unequal, unfair, ineffective and inefficient: Gender inequity in health – Why it exists and how we can change it, final report to the WHO Commission on social determinants of Health*. Women and Gender Equity Knowledge Network. http://www.who.int/social_determinants/resources/csdh_media/wgekn_final_report_07.pdf

Smith, K. E. (2014). The politics of ideas: The complex interplay of health inequalities research and policy. *Science and Public Policy, 41*(5), 561–574. https://doi.org/10.1093/scipol/sct085

Spivak, G. C. (1994). Can the subaltern speak? In P. Williams & L. Chrisman (Eds.), *Colonial and postcolonia theory. A reader* (pp. 66–111). Columbia University Press.

Strand, M., Brown, C., Torgersen, T. P., & Giæver, Ø. (2009). *Setting the political agenda to tackle health inequity in Norway*. WHO Regional Office for Europe.

Toleikyte, L., & Colwell, A. (2020). *Health equity assessment tool (HEAT)*. Public Health England. https://www.gov.uk/government/publications/health-equity-assessment-tool-heat/health-equity-assessment-tool-heat-executive-summary#what-are-health-inequalities

Whitehead, M. (Chair), Bambra, C., Barr, B., Bowles, J., Caulfield, R., & Doran, T. (2014). *Due North: Report of the inquiry on health equity for the North*. University of Liverpool and Centre for Local Economic Strategies.

WHO. (2018). *Social determinants of health progress report at 68th WHA*. WHO-| Mandate by Member States on Social Determinants of health. WHO. https://www.who.int/social_determinants/implementation/en/

Wold, B., & Mittelmark, M. B. (2018). Health-promotion research over three decades: The social-ecological model and challenges in implementation of interventions. *Scandinavian Journal of Public Health, 46*(20_suppl), 20–26. https://doi.org/10.1177/1403494817743893
Woodall, J., Warwick-Booth, L., South, J., & Cross, R. (2018). What makes health promotion research distinct? *Scandinavian Journal of Public Health, 46*(20), 118–122. https://doi.org/10.1177/1403494817744130

Chapter 46
Studying the Case de Santé de Toulouse (France) as a Propaedeutic Step

Jean-Charles Basson, Nadine Haschar-Noé, Thierry Lang, Laurence Boulaghaf, and Fabien Maguin

46.1 Introduction

The Ottawa Charter was a critical milestone in health promotion and is a constitutive text in the field. It provides useful information on its object: "Health promotion is the process of enabling people to increase control over, and to improve, their health". However, the emphasis is placed on what is understood as "health" rather than on what "health promotion" exactly entails. The charter does, however, provide a foundation on which health promotion research can be established. In a passage that is sometimes overlooked but which we view as essential, it is specified that

J.-C. Basson (✉)
Institut Fédératif d'Etudes et de Recherches Interdisciplinaires Santé Société (IFERISS), Toulouse, France

Centre de Recherches Sciences Sociales Sports et Corps (CreSco), Toulouse, France

Centre d'Epidémiologie et de Recherche en Santé des Populations (CERPOP), Toulouse, France

Laboratoire des Sciences Sociales du Politique (LaSSP), Toulouse, France
e-mail: jean-charles.basson@univ-tlse3.fr

N. Haschar-Noé
Institut Fédératif d'Etudes et de Recherches Interdisciplinaires Santé Société (IFERISS), Toulouse, France

Centre de Recherches Sciences Sociales Sports et Corps (CreSco), Toulouse, France

Laboratoire des Sciences Sociales du Politique (LaSSP), Toulouse, France

T. Lang
Institut Fédératif d'Etudes et de Recherches Interdisciplinaires Santé Société (IFERISS), Toulouse, France

Centre d'Epidémiologie et de Recherche en Santé des Populations (CERPOP), Toulouse, France

L. Potvin, D. Jourdan (eds.), *Global Handbook of Health Promotion Research, Vol. 1*,
https://doi.org/10.1007/978-3-030-97212-7_46

"health promotion action aims at making these conditions favourable [to health] *through advocacy for health*" (our emphasis). Since health promotion was inaugurated by the charter, the associated research has been inextricably tied to it from the beginning. As determined representatives and advocates of investigations that are sensitive and open to their social and political environment, we should therefore feel free to explore this territory!

"Health promotion must advocate against social inequities in health [and, even more so] [...], be a driving force in the reassessment" of these inequities (Ridde, 2013). We are therefore keen to put health promotion research to the test by studying the processes that our partner and study site, the Case de Santé in Toulouse, designed and implemented to reduce social inequities in health. Through this example, we want to contribute to the edification of health promotion research. This contribution falls within the scope of Toulouse-France's *Institut Fédératif d'Etudes et de Recherches Interdisciplinaires Santé Société* (IFERISS). It is in line with the institute's primary, constant, persistent, and renewed ambition and is an embodiment of its ongoing mission.

This chapter builds on the principles and practices of ongoing research and argues that health promotion research must be based on three scientific conditions (I) and three singular empirical fields (II) as it aims to present a heuristic purview wherein knowledge is objectivised, conceptualised, paradigmatically reflected upon, coproduced methodically, disseminated, and shared in an effort to thwart the relentless unfolding of social inequities in health.

46.2 Three Scientific Conditions

We do not claim to set *The Rules of the Method* for health promotion (we can't all be like Durkheim!). But based on our experience, we have identified three conditions that seem beneficial to lay rational foundations to the field and to contribute to its scientific legitimisation. These three conditions are: the systematic use of a collaborative and partnership-based method that is open to interdisciplinary discussions; a method also served by the precise delimitation of a specific object of investigation; and finally, a method sustained by the rudiments of an epistemology of scientific practices.

L. Boulaghaf
Institut Fédératif d'Etudes et de Recherches Interdisciplinaires Santé Société (IFERISS), Toulouse, France

Centre de Recherches Sciences Sociales Sports et Corps (CreSco), Toulouse, France

F. Maguin
Case de Santé, Toulouse, France

46.2.1 An Interdisciplinary Method Based on Partnership and Collaboration

In order to build the field of health promotion research, we consider the first condition to be imperative: committed partnerships and effective collaborations must drive the research. The first objective is therefore to give a key role to the people in the field: the professionals, who come from different sectors, and the users, who are socially tied to various contexts and who present multiple trajectories marked by one or several forms of precariousness and vulnerability. In our case, the Case de Santé presented the initiative. Its coordinator (who, in accordance with our partnership principles, has co-written and co-signed the present text) sought out the research team to respond to a call for projects from the French Ministry for Health and Social Affairs. Once elected as a research partner, the Case de Santé led the project. In choosing this configuration, we avoided the pitfalls of a research process in which we could have been tempted to alter the investigated empirical field in order to corroborate pre-established research hypotheses. We went against the tide and did not affix any artificial scientific guarantee to the project, choosing instead a collaborative approach and including the different people in the field in a symmetrical relationship.

This methodological ambition isn't self-evident since it means that all protagonists share binding conditions such as: engaging in discussions before conducting the actual research; keeping an open mind; having a relatively homogenous set of social, intellectual, or even political dispositions; wanting to shake up the established order in the field of health; and having a taste for reflexivity. While such prerequisites are hard to guarantee, they make it possible to analyse the project in its entirety (its design, its agenda, its implementation, the social ways in which the targeted populations take hold of it, its assessment framework, and the conditions of its potential replication, modification, or interruption). Since the ability to investigate is not reserved to academics, the interesting aspect of this approach resides in confronting points of view, which in turn helps to ensure that health promotion practices improve and are properly analysed.

Since boundaries between the researchers and the people in the field are blurred, all protagonists must come together to find solutions to the various problems that arise throughout the study. Differences are to be respected since they give a meaning to a collaboration in the process of being invented. It is therefore important to attempt to create connections and to encourage confrontations at the risk of exposing divergences, tensions, or disruptive antagonisms. Such is the price to pay when co-designing health promotion research that includes all of the people involved in the various stages of the project. In our research, we ensure that everyone at each step gets a chance to share and challenge knowledge derived from scientific works and from field practice, as well as skills and worldviews in the field of health. Such exchange spaces have included cycles of national seminaries with the ministry and regular meetings with a local monitoring committee composed of many partners active in the area.

A plurality of methods are used to foster intersecting views and usages and to guarantee that participants can engage. We utilise a combination of semi-structured interviews, biographical interviews and life stories; ethnographic field notes; observations – sometimes participant observations – of various scenes at the Case de Santé; user satisfaction surveys; in-depth studies of documents created for internal use and/or meant to be shared externally; participating in and sometimes leading interactive training sessions. In addition to the methods we just outlined, the project leader and the main field workers meet in the context of formal and informal encounters (the main field workers include facilitators, professionals, employees, volunteers, activists, and users). The thoughts and the observations made by the researchers are closely based on a close insight of the populations presenting health vulnerabilities. These works and reflections are therefore collected, presented and discussed collectively in order to measure whether the research succeeds in reporting on the current situation of the Case de Santé. Issues related to the users' quest for autonomy are also objectified since autonomy is an imperative condition to fight efficiently against social inequities in health.

The methods are mostly – albeit not entirely – qualitative, and the variety of approaches is linked to the research team's deliberately interdisciplinary makeup (the members also have diverse backgrounds relative to gender, age, social origins, and professional status). The participating researchers and the project leader bring their respective analytical frameworks to the collaborative effort. Their four main fields of study are therefore combined, thus leading to fruitful exchanges: political science, sociology, ethical and social philosophy, and public health are summoned for their intrinsic qualities and used together to cover topics at the heart of the investigated context. We believe that this "intellectual adventure [is] needed in the field of health, given how knowledge is mainly to be gained at the margins of the disciplines" (Haschar-Noé & Lang, 2017). Health promotion is known for its imbalance in disciplinary resources (the biomedical model and evidence-based medicine prevail). However, objective alliances can still take shape and last around boundary objects (Trompette & Vinck, 2009). This is precisely the case for social inequities in health, as there can be an interdisciplinary conversation and a manner of producing questions and knowledge at the heart of social demands in which the civic dimension of scientific activity is developed (Fabiani, 2013).

46.2.2 A Specific Object: Innovative Measures in Health Aimed at Social Change

The second scientific condition we wish to add to the ongoing health promotion research debate comes as follows: this field should become instrumental in the study and the advancement of the many innovative measures in health aimed at social change that are developing worldwide. In so doing, these innovations would become the specific object of investigation of health promotion research (Basson & Vallereau, 2020). Viewed as "tools to drive social change" (Blum, 1981; Ridde,

2013), the themes covered by health promotion research share the same aspirations as the beliefs stated in the Ottawa Charter: "Health promotion action aims at reducing differences in current health status". In its own way, the Case de Santé project focuses on this same object.

The Case de Santé was created in Toulouse in 2006. Its health promotion approach is inspired by the founding charter and by Quebec and Belgian traditions of community health. It is composed of a primary care health centre and of a unit dedicated to help vulnerable people access their health rights. In the latter, 3 200 users are received every year (Haschar-Noé & Basson, 2019). The non-profit organisation is located in one of the last working-class neighbourhoods in downtown Toulouse and consists of a territorialised system of social innovation in health that is both inclusive and participatory. The neighbourhood went through several waves of immigration and is now undergoing a process of gentrification. At the Case de Santé, health is approached globally; all social determinants of health are taken into account. The organisation views itself as a part of its immediate environment. It campaigns for local, integrated and participatory health care based on different professions and sectors working together. Through self-management and the users' active participation in the association's internal structure, the aim is to increase users' individual and collective abilities to carry out actions that improve their health and overall living conditions.

To do so, about twenty people are employed: general practitioners, psychologists, midwives, social workers, health mediators who engage with the population, members of the administrative and financial coordination centre as well as a variety of supporting staff members and interns, medical residents and volunteer legal experts. The French Ministry for Health and Social Affairs is funding over five years (2017–2021) the Case de Santé as an experimental project for a total of 1, 025, 000 euros. All the services provided by the Case de Santé are free of charge. The project is articulated around three interdependent dimensions: community health care viewed as accelerating health autonomy; health mediation viewed as the main tool toward autonomy; training and participating in building a framework around the profession of "primary health mediator". Finally, our team of researchers is in charge of the project's assessment.

This initiative based in Toulouse is a voluntarist experiment in social and political mobilisation in the field of health (Laverack & Manoncourt, 2016). Other examples have flourished in other French cities and connections between organisations exist. This dimension, as well as all of the factors mentioned above, explains why this project has become a case study for health promotion research. The characteristic on which we choose to focus is "the reduction of inequalities, which constitutes a goal in its own right for health promotion" (Kickbusch, 1986). The project and its accompanying research are devoted to fighting against social inequities in health. Their aim is, on the one hand, for the most vulnerable populations to be included in the access and defence of their rights and to increase their health autonomy, and, on the other hand, for la Case de Santé to gain legislative recognition of the merits of its activities. The organisation, therefore, uses scientific advances on the topic to promote its project.

In this arrangement, the researchers get access to a rich sociological field of study through the Case de Santé while the leaders in la Case de Santé use the research results to further argue that socially constructed inequities in health (Lang et al., 2016) are biologically incorporated (Krieger, 2001) throughout a person's life. While we know that the bedrock of social inequities in health and the root of their reproduction are to be found in the structure of the social organisation in which they operate (Basson et al., 2013a, b), studying them means that we must closely examine the political dimension of social relations. Tenants of socialisation, power struggles, processes of domination, mechanisms of stigmatisation, and the production standards by which health is governed (Basson & Honta, 2018, 2019; Honta & Basson, 2015, 2017; Honta et al., 2018): all of these elements contribute to the perpetuation of social inequities in health, and shape individual behaviours and collective practices. We join our efforts with the Case de Santé, our special partner and co-producer of the investigation, to include these elements in our analysis.

46.2.3 From Research Practises to Research About Practices

The third scientific condition is an epistemological reflection, as we attempt to navigate from research practices to researching these same practices through a dialectical process. In sociology, two essential requirements are needed to constitute a specific scientific field: having a specific object of investigation and creating a rigorous research method to move away from "prenotions" (Durkheim, 2013). Social science practitioners find themselves caught between involvement and distancing (Elias, 1993). They must critically examine their scientific approach and track down any passions, values, or interests related to their social position as the latter threatens to subjugate them to the investigated object. This position is all the more necessary for sociologists who aim to study questions related to health and to the body, and who collaborate with individuals who are, in turn, reflexive about their own practices and conducts. To find a form of distance, sociologists must break away from subjective, irrational, and imagined ways, all the while remembering that the scientific process itself is not immune to social construction.

The structure of scientific revolutions, as identified by Thomas Kuhn, acts as a theoretical basis to our considerations. The philosopher and historian of sciences encourages the blurring of scientific and non-scientific processes. He calls us to move beyond agreed-upon scientific activity and to challenge acquired knowledge in order to produce and adopt a new paradigm. Furthermore, he is convinced of the social context's manifest influence on the production of scientific knowledge. We agree with Kuhn in saying that, on the one hand, the history of science has not been a simple, clearly legible, linear, and essentially cumulative progression, and that, on the other hand, the scientific process is a long, complex, and bumpy affair prone to potentially violent transformations. We therefore know that "normal science" does not aim "to call forth new sorts of phenomena". Innovation is made possible when there is a crisis, a radical break from scientific conformism and routine. The failure of the normal regime of science is its essential mechanism of transformation: "discovery commences with the awareness of anomaly". We are therefore tempted to view social inequities in health as a series of fundamental anomalies in the health system which, once brought to light, can trigger new types of scientific efforts in an attempt to understand the anomalies' underpinning logic and to combat them more effectively. In fact, we remind the reader of the considerable social cost of the biomedical bias when interpreting phenomena linked to social inequities in health. Since the crisis affecting health is as paradigmatic as it is inherently social, this means that social pressures can be used to bypass internal debates in the scientific world, with the aim of moving beyond the contradiction and overcoming resistance to conceptual and political changes.

46.3 Three Singular Empirical Fields

Now that we have elaborated a method, clearly defined an object, and developed a propensity for reflexivity, we have yet to identify three singular empirical fields on which to focus and on which to add an evaluative section dealing with central issues. We, therefore, consider that participation, mediation, and social innovations merit our utmost attention, especially since these notions and all of their implications cannot be fully understood via evidence-based clinical research.

46.3.1 Participation

Once again, the Ottawa Charter is relevant in reminding us that "health promotion works through concrete and effective community action in setting priorities, making decisions, planning strategies and implementing them to achieve better health". In our case, the Case de Santé depends on users' participation as it actively encourages and works towards individuals achieving autonomy. Participation in health is a collective process that depends on the members' involvement and on grassroots initiatives. It is a tool that promotes learning, socialisation, and the activation of social change as advocated by participants that are the users and the front-line workers of the Case de Santé. The systems introduced and upheld by the Case de Santé shape a multitude of participatory practices, and working-class people are likely to take ownership of some of these initiatives, including political appropriation. However, we are aware of the highly unequal nature of social distribution when it comes to participating in collective enterprises that involve the body and that interrogate health practices (Basson & Génolini, 2021).

Our ambition is to shed light on a series of participatory forms of health promotion that have developed in impoverished urban areas. To achieve this, we endorse an open-ended political sociology of citizenship fuelled by the perceptive, regular, and continuous observation of a variety of scenes and participatory interactions. We are searching for effective traces and tangible signs of the slow, progressive, and gradual effects of civic training since it is clear that "policies [...] exist concretely through the work of agents on the ground" (Dubois, 2012). The classificatory ethnography of participation in health is prevalent at the Case de Santé. Through it, the various provisions for the social construction of a health democracy that is open to vulnerable individuals can be qualified and organised. The civic and even political scope of the organisation's project and its results can then be observed. More specifically, we make note of: the voluntarism of the professional-activists; the strategic management of mobilisation and its effects on the users' self-esteem and confidence; the process of reinforcement and the activation of dispositions among the more emancipated users; the escalating power of a publicised action and the emergence of a collective consciousness which recognises broader issues and goes beyond individual interests.

46.3.2 Mediation

Mediation is one of the three "main strategies" identified by the Ottawa Charter. It is a "prerequisite" for health promotion research. This is unequivocally stated by the text: "The prerequisites and prospects for health cannot be ensured by the health sector alone. More importantly, health promotion demands coordinated action by all concerned". At the Case de Santé, the mediators' professional practices are derived from a "contractual process of building or repairing the social bond" (Faget, 2015). They operate from the standpoint of a third party which "goes towards" the public, the institutions, and the professionals in the social and health sectors and "acts with" people in a spirit of empowerment. Professionals in the Case de Santé with whom we collaborate do not limit mediation to the agreed-upon role of the local interface that informs, guides, and supports vulnerable populations and that discloses challenges to the actors of the health system. Their aim is more fundamental: they want poor populations to gain access to rights, prevention, and health care; they want these people to cement their autonomy and their ability to act on their health. They have therefore added two principles to their system: "being with" the people and "acting together" (Haschar-Noé & Basson, 2019). The first principle aims to expand health mediation to the population as a whole and not only to vulnerable groups. The actors of the Case de Santé explain it this way: mediation "*is a way of responding to the health system's general dysfunction*". The second principle serves to indicate their firm and unabashed opposition to "*the neutrality of health mediation*". They intend to be "*on the side of the people we accompany to counter the power imbalance that exists between them and the institutions*".

This professional stance takes effect in many individualised and collective mediation systems implemented by the Case de Santé. The mediators are personally committed to finding ways to "join with someone and go where he's going, at his pace" (Paul, 2012). They draw on the experience of the people they accompany, value and promote, and, in so doing, become socialising agents of health. All mediators have also experienced social and healthcare challenges at some point in their own lives, so the fact that they view their relationship with users as "*equalitarian*" shows that they are committed to involving users in a contractual process of mutual trust, as peers. They pass on their experience since they "know how to deal with domination" (Demailly, 2014). The mediators use proven popular education methods with users, some of whom do not master the French language. They listen without judging, they encourage users to speak out and express themselves, to tell their stories, to access new information, and to make use of resources which were previously unfamiliar and unexploited. This is all done in an effort to increase the user's power to take action and to ensure they are in control of their life. The mediators do more than work on autonomy; they work on restoring the person's self-confidence, the latter being a prerequisite for self-respect and to ensure one's own self-care (Paul, 2012)

There are therefore many opportunities to mediate: through a participatory health diagnosis of the neighbourhood, by sharing knowledge and experiences in health, by helping with applications to access rights, by supporting the creation of collective projects and finding users to lead and participate in events, by forming demands and appealing to public institutions in writing, by organising convivial moments that strengthen social ties with residents. All of these experiences are characterised by "the mediators' professional stance which speaks to values of community health care, ethical principles and personal commitment. This stance is coupled with a political positioning aimed at social change and anchored in alternative practices, in opposition to traditional medicine and to the compartmentalisation of the social worlds of health and social work" (Haschar-Noé & Basson, 2019). It is interesting to note that health promotion research has been produced by objectifying the practices of these innovators, our non-profit partners. Mediation, as practiced, expanded, and advocated by community activists, is an original social and professional experiment. It lends itself to deconstruction, thus leading us to think intellectually about the ways in which two new ethical and political principles can broaden and strengthen the conceptual spectrum of health mediation. This has been one of the clear results of the collaboration between researchers and field actors, and health promotion research was instrumental in these results. Its aim now is to finalise the enrichment of the mediation process by referencing the profession of "primary health mediator".

46.3.3 Innovation

The mediation practices and systems upheld by the actors of the Case de Santé foster the collective expression of demands based on democratic and inclusive versions of health care (Laville, 2014). To the extent allowed by public networks, these innovative practices can be instrumental in reshaping the field of public health (Basson et al., 2013a, b). The activation of the innovation-assessment duo (Okbani, 2014; Serverin & Gomel, 2012) brings into sharper focus the social and health issues of vulnerable populations which, in turn, facilitate the emergence of social innovations that can renew the handling of public health (Fassin, 2008). The Case de Santé uses mediation as a support tool for more health autonomy. It acts according to an ascending, non-governmental, inclusive, collective, and cooperative logic where the different people involved work together in a shared field of action (Richez-Battesti et al., 2012). It manages to "take advantage of civil society's ability to innovate [...] in order to formalise and extend some of the new practices developed by local actors" (Chevallier, 2005). These innovations fulfil unmet social needs or needs that the market, the state, or other collective entities have not yet perceived. They are designed to change social relations and institutional arrangements.

The Case de Santé shares the characteristics of innovative spaces (Grenier & Denis, 2017). It sets itself apart from dominant health practices by de-compartmentalising professional boundaries, by relying on heavily instrumented methodological and collective engineering, and by consolidating its connections with the context it wants to change to reduce social inequities in health. It has therefore positioned itself as a laboratory for social innovations and expertise in health mediation, promoting ways to accompany people towards more health autonomy, to get access to rights and health care, and to encourage the professional training of mediators. The organisation, therefore, maintains a political stance, while also seeking efficiency and wanting its modes of action to be recognised by institutions. Through our health promotion research, we intend on reporting these elements and on objectifying this innovation. When compared with other similar endeavours, we believe that promising forms of generalisation will emerge. "The main stakes of innovation are to be found at the limits of disciplinary fields" (Fabiani, 2013). In our health promotion research, we must be wary of the ways in which disciplines are divided since these divisions are conventional ways of structuring knowledge. We can instead work toward transgressing boundaries, thus promoting the emergence of disorder that is conducive to creation and discoveries (Besnier, 2013). We are convinced that this is an answer to ambitious health promotion research.

46.4 Conclusions

Health promotion research must go from elaborating research practices to codifying the research on these practices, the latter of which are the work of the people on the ground, of the users, and of the associated researchers. We believe that health promotion research should be based on collaborative and partnership-based methods, devoted to experimental measures in health aimed at social change using an interdisciplinary approach, and geared toward assessing its three major empirical fields: participation, mediation, and social innovation. If practiced in this way, we postulate that it can contribute to the slow and progressive emergence of a new framework of observation, analysis, interpretation, and objectification, all in an effort to curb the increasing social inequities in health, our main preoccupation. We intend to ensure that in "a time of globalisation, health promotion should allow each person and each group to avoid being crushed by the excesses of those who argue in favour of individual performance and of the search for profit as one's sole objective in life [...] benefitting the few while accepting that the majority becomes dependent or is excluded" (Deschamps, 2003). The Case de Santé is dedicated to this at its own level, with its own means and with a latitude that depends on the dominant players of the health sector. Our research stance supports it in this endeavour.

References

Basson, J.-C., & Génolini, J.-P. (2021). Ethnographie classificatoire de la participation citoyenne en santé. Une innovation sociale majeure ? Le programme *Ciné ma santé* des quartiers nord de Toulouse (France). *Innovations Revue d'Économie et de Management de l'Innovation / Journal of Innovation Economics & Management, 65*, 163–187.

Basson, J.-C., & Honta, M. (2018). Se bien conduire dans une ville saine. La fabrication politique du gouvernement urbain de la santé de Toulouse. *Terrains & Travaux, 32*, 129–153.

Basson, J.-C., & Honta, M. (2019). The paradoxical dynamic of urban health government. A case in Toulouse. Editorial. *Journal of Health Science & Education, 3*(1), 1.

Basson, J.-C., & Vallereau, M. (2020). Jours tranquilles à la maison de retraite. Velléités de changements autour du projet de création d'un parcours de santé dans un établissement d'hébergement pour personnes âgées dépendantes (EHPAD). *Empan, 118*, 73–80.

Basson, J.-C., Haschar-Noé, N., & Honta, M. (2013a). Toulouse, une figure urbaine de la santé publique. A propos de l'action publique municipale de lutte contre les inégalités sociales de santé / Toulouse, an urban figure of public health. Dealing with public local struggles against health social differences. *Revue d'Épidémiologie et de Santé Publique / Epidemiology and Public Health, 61S2*, 81–88.

Basson, J.-C., Haschar-Noé, N., & Theis, I. (2013b). Territorial translation of the National health and nutrition program in Midi-Pyrénées, France / La traduction territoriale du Programme national nutrition santé (PNNS) en Midi-Pyrénées, France. *Healthcare Policy / Politiques de Santé, 9*, 26–37.

Besnier, J.-M. (2013). Seul le désordre est créateur. Pour en finir avec les bataillons disciplinaires. *Hermes, 67*, 25–31.

Blum, H. (1981). *Planning for health, Generics for the eighties*. Human Science Press.

Chevallier, J. (2005). Politiques publiques et changement social. *Revue Française d'Administration Publique, 115*(3), 383–390.

Demailly, L. (2014). Les médiateurs pairs en santé mentale. Une professionnalisation incertaine, *La Nouvelle Revue du Travail* [En ligne], 5, mis en ligne le 11 novembre 2014, consulté le 14 mai 2017, URL: http://journal.openedition.org/nrt/1952

Deschamps, J.-P. (2003). Une « relecture » de la Charte d'Ottawa. *Santé Publique, 15*, 313–325.

Dubois, V. (2012). « Ethnographier l'action publique ». Les transformations de l'État social au prisme de l'enquête de terrain. *Gouvernement et Action Publique, 1*(1), 83–101.

Durkheim, E. [1895] (2013). *Les règles de la méthode sociologique*. Presses Universitaires de France.

Elias, N. (1993). *Engagement et distanciation*. Fayard.

Fabiani, J.-L. (2013). Vers la fin du modèle disciplinaire ? *Hermes, 67*, 90–94.

Faget, J. (2015). *Médiations. Les ateliers silencieux de la démocratie*. Éditions Érès.

Fassin, D. (2008). *Faire de la santé publique*. éditions de l'EHESS.

Grenier, C., & Denis, J.-L. (2017). S'organiser pour innover : espaces d'innovation et transformation des organisations et du champ de l'intervention publique. *Politiques et Management Public, 34*(3-4), 191–206.

Haschar-Noé, N., & Basson, J.-C. (2019). Innovations en santé, dispositifs expérimentaux et changement social. Un renouvellement par le bas de l'action publique locale de santé. La Case de Santé de Toulouse (France). *Innovations. Revue d'Économie et de Management de l'Innovation, 60*, 121–144.

Haschar-Noé, N., Lang, T., & (dir.). (2017). *Réduire les inégalités sociales de santé. Une approche interdisciplinaire de l'évaluation*. Presses Universitaires du Midi.

Honta, M., & Basson, J.-C. (2015). Healthy cities: A new political territory. An analysis of local health care governance in the city of Bordeaux. *French Politics, 13*(2), 157–174.

Honta, M., & Basson, J.-C. (2017). La fabrique du gouvernement métropolitain de la santé. L'épreuve de la légitimation politique. *Gouvernement et Action Publique, 6*(2), 63–82.

Honta, M., Basson, J.-C., Jaksic, M., & Le Noé, O. (2018). Les gouvernements du corps. Administration différenciée des conduites corporelles et territorialisation de l'action publique de santé. Introduction. *Terrains & Travaux, 32*, 5–29.

Kickbusch, I. (1986). Health promotion: A global perspective. *Canadian Journal of Public Health, 77*(5), 321–326.

Krieger, N. (2001). Theories for social epidemiology in the 21st century: An ecosocial perspective. *International Journal of Epidemiology, 30*, 668–677.

Lang, T., Kelly-Irving, M., Lamy, S., Lepage, B., & Delpierre, C. (2016). Construction de la santé et des inégalités sociales de santé : les gènes contre les déterminants sociaux ? *Santé Publique, 28*, 169–179.

Laverack, G., & Manoncourt, E. (2016). Key experiences of community engagement and social mobilization in the Ebola response. *Global Health Promotion, 23*(1), 86–94.

Laville, J-L. (2014). Innovation sociale, économie sociale et solidaire, entrepreneuriat social. Une mise en perspective historique. In J.-L. In Klein, J.-L. Laville, F. Moulaert, & (dir.), *L'innovation sociale* (pp. 45–80). Éditions Érès.

Okbani, N. (2014). Le rôle de l'évaluation dans l'expérimentation sociale, entre instrumentation et instrumentalisation : le cas de l'évaluation des expérimentations du RSA. *Politiques et Management Public, 31*(1), 31–50.

Paul, M. (2012). L'accompagnement comme posture professionnelle spécifique. L'exemple de l'éducation thérapeutique du patient. *Recherche en Soins Infirmiers, 110*(3), 13–20.

Richez-Battesti, N., Pettrela, F., & Vallade, D. (2012). L'innovation sociale, une notion aux usages pluriels : quels enjeux et quels défis pour l'analyse ? *Innovations, 38*, 15–36.

Ridde, V. (2013). *À quoi sert la promotion de la santé ? Essai introductif sur la réduction des inégalités sociales de santé*. Harmattan Burkina.

Serverin, E., & Gomel, B. (2012). L'expérimentation des politiques publiques dans tous ses états. *Informations Sociales, 174*(6), 128–137.

Trompette, P., & Vinck, D. (2009). Retour sur la notion d'objet frontière. *Revue d'Anthropologie des Connaissances, 3*, 5–27.

Chapter 47
Brazilian Experiences in Interdisciplinary Networks: From Advocacy to Intersectoral Participatory Research and Implementation

Samuel Jorge Moysés, Rosilda Mendes, Julia Aparecida Devidé Nogueira, Dais Gonçalves Rocha, Maria Cristina Trousdell Franceschini, and Marco Akerman

47.1 Introduction

This chapter reflects on the experience of a Brazilian group that established an interdisciplinary network in participatory research, aimed at producing and sharing knowledge, building capacity, and promoting advocacy and sustainable development in health promotion. Structuring different sciences from the perspective of networks shows that theoretical and practical knowledge can coexist and influence each other (Cavalcanti, 2018).

S. J. Moysés
Pontifícia Universidade Católica do Paraná, Escola de Ciências da Vida (PUCPR, School of Life Sciences), Curitiba, Paraná, Brazil

R. Mendes
Universidade Federal de São Paulo-UNIFESP, campus Baixada Santista (Federal University of São Paulo- Baixada Santista campus), São Paulo, SP, Brazil

J. A. D. Nogueira
Universidade de Brasília, Faculdade de Educação Física (UNB – Physical Education College), Brasília, Brazil

D. G. Rocha
Universidade de Brasília, Faculdade de Ciências da Saúde (UNB - Health Sciences College), Brasília, Brazil

M. C. T. Franceschini
CEPEDOC – Centro de Pesquisa e Documentação em Cidade Saudáveis (CEPEDOC Healthy Cities – WHO/PAHO Collaborating Center), São Paulo, SP, Brazil

M. Akerman (✉)
Universidade de São Paulo, Faculdade de Saúde Pública (USP, School of Public Health), São Paulo, SP, Brazil
e-mail: marcoakerman@usp.br

L. Potvin, D. Jourdan (eds.), *Global Handbook of Health Promotion Research, Vol. 1*,
https://doi.org/10.1007/978-3-030-97212-7_47

We are part of a Working Group (WG) that integrates the Brazilian Collective Health Association, *Abrasco* (GT Promoção da Saúde – Abrasco). The WG has been materializing since 2002, with the adoption of a potent conceptual-methodological framework that serves as a device to activate the engagement for social justice and to fight inequality. It was born with the ambition of articulating, congregating, mobilizing, and promoting the principles and assumptions of health promotion, in the production of knowledge, practices, and public policies in Brazil.

Then, the WG's mission is to support the formulation of health promotion policies and programs. We are committed to fulfilling this mission through education, research, community services, and support for the management of public policies in general, and to the public health system, in particular. Thus, we encourage the development of networks and partnerships with national and international researchers, as well as with managers/teams at the municipal, state, and federal levels. Unequivocally, we form alliances with popular movements that dispute communicational narratives and struggle in the search for a healthier life. The networks with which we relate have contributed to the consolidation of a structured field of research, based on the paradigms of social justice, intersectorality, and full democracy – now and beyond rhetorical democracy.

These networks operate as connections between subjects, knowledge, and practices so different, and, at the same time, inseparable in the production of the meaning of life. They can be understood as "collectives" who bring a variety of conceptions about the subjects that unite them – the objectives, the territories, and the very role that each actor occupies in this network. This also fits the central idea of protagonist actors, generators of knowledge, who use the reflexivity underlying the action to become political subjects when they create and articulate themselves in broad socio-political groups (Alexander et al., 2020).

We share the idea that health promotion should be a field of action-reflection-action, pursuing practices that transform the oppressive and exploitative living conditions of vulnerable population groups, victimized by historical inequities – one of our main "diseases" (Buss & Pellegrini Filho, 2006). Our work embodies critical elements of social reality, anchored in international references common to the Health Promotion community, but without renouncing our Iberian, Latin American, Brazilian, tropical culture and traditions, which so well illustrate the possibilities of the southern epistemologies (Porto, 2019b). Thus, our work includes our own semantics of language – beyond the abysmal dividing lines of neo-colonial thought – and claims an ecology of knowledge (Santos, 2014).

47.2 Standpoint on Paradigms

The expression Epistemologies of the South is a metaphor for coping with the suffering, exclusion, and silencing of peoples and cultures that have been dominated by capitalism and colonialism in recent centuries (Tavares, 2009). Colonialism impressed a historical dynamic of political and cultural domination, submitting to its ethnocentric vision the knowledge of the world, the meaning of life, and social practices. In short, the imposition of "a" unique ontology, of "an" epistemology, of "an" ethics, of "an" anthropological model, as if they were universal truths. For another epistemological invention, there is a need for a return to places and peoples in search of their meanings and understandings of the world, inseparable from their realities – something that is also intertwined with the cultural competence of communities, a concept highly valued by Paulo Freire (Freire, 1980, 1996a, 2014).

The colonialist, capitalist, and neoliberal version of modernity drained the wealth of meanings from the world in the global North and South. Boaventura Souza Santos calls for the return of the stolen "objects" to create a new pattern of interculturality (Santos, 2014; Santos & Meneses, 2013). Coming back to these places with a different look will allow the reinvention of what has been marginalized, silenced, and forgotten. We must collaborate for a new type of intercultural and inter-epistemological relations that contribute to the decolonization of knowledge.

This theoretical conception, to become a social struggle, could have "cognitive justice" as an ally. This concept is a normative principle for the respectful treatment of all forms of knowledge (Leibowitz, 2017; Santos, 2014). This does not mean that all forms of knowledge are equal, but that the equality of knowers forms the basis of dialogue between knowledges, and that what is required for democracy is a dialogue amongst knowers and their knowledges. Just as the concept of cognitive injustice problematizes the recurring failure to recognize the different ways of wisdom creation, by which people around the world lead their lives and give sense of its existence (Santos, 2014). Injustice and discrimination persist across the world and socioeconomic gaps in access and privilege continue to expand the binary division – an abyssal line – between the valued and the not (or under) valued world. The historical processes of colonization in the West have strongly marginalized the knowledge and wisdom that may exist (or be instituted) in the global South. To overcome the epistemicide against many peripheral societies, we must rescue and value the epistemological diversity of the world.

It is not convenient to romanticize innovative possibilities, but southern epistemologies pursue a new type of intellectual, academic, and popular cosmopolitanism, from the bottom up, in which conviviality, solidarity, and life triumph against the logic of rapacity dominated by the predatory market and cynical and indifferent individualism. This approach brings a creative force of resistance and re-existence, encouraging detachments from the colonial power matrix and its "universals". Then, arguments and struggles for dignity and life unfold against death, destruction, and civilizational despair (Mignolo & Walsh, 2018).

Such struggles result from the confrontation of capitalism in its most ubiquitous forms, which are (i) platform and surveillance capitalism, (ii) unburied colonialism, and (iii) patriarchy revitalized by extreme right-wing forces, the three main forms of modern conflicts (Porto, 2019a, b; Santos & Meneses, 2019). Emancipatory movements clearly challenge the status quo by championing a variety of provocative claims that address political, economic, social, scientific, and historical issues. Therefore, without naiveté, we are familiar with the difficulty for the dominant and stabilized academic world to endorse the central questions on the agenda of the philosophy of science about the role that science can play in promoting – or weakening – cognitive and social justice. Santos asks us to "dismiss" all our most deeply held bias (Santos & Meneses, 2013). He thus outlines a truly different possible future to build. In doing so, it creates inevitable tensions within our intercultural spaces. These are not just geopolitical, but epistemological issues, whose resolution at the level of practices, disciplines, experiences, and affections has the potential to shape a new Humanity in a new Environment. We are all invited to see the world from a non-Eurocentric perspective and to propose counter-hegemonic understandings for emancipatory action. This would be a "pluriverse" – a world consisting of many worlds, each with its own ontological and epistemic basis establishing productive dialogues (Escobar, 2020).

47.3 Applying Paradigms in Our Research Production

Tensions and devaluations discussed above do not only exist between North and South, but also among academic and laypeople. Brazil is a country painfully influenced by social inequalities that reflect in health (Viacava et al., 2019). The Brazilian movement for health promotion is oriented towards the production of sound evidence and the support for social transformation guided by principles deeply rooted in an "emancipatory view" of Paulo Freire's pedagogy (Brass & Macedo, 1985; Paulo Freire 1996a, b; Horton et al., 1990). Moreover, its knowledge foundation is engrained in the framework of socio-environmental determinants of health-disease-care and is based on the evidences of successful interventions, adjusted to our reality (Akerman & Fischer, 2014; Akerman et al., 2016).

In the last two decades, powerful tools for health promotion practices such as advocacy (Gould et al., 2012; Masuda et al., 2010) and network collaboration (Belza et al., 2017; Hogg & Varda, 2016) in participatory approaches have marked health promotion in the Brazilian milieu, nuanced by different loco-regional contexts (Akerman & Mendes, 2006). In our dialogue, we emphasize the adoption of a strategic orientation that unfolds from an original ethical-political and epistemological postulation, derived from the values and canons fed mainly by the Federal Constitution of Brazil of 1988, a landmark in the country's re-democratization.

Paulo Freire's philosophy of "reading the world" is an appeal to respect for the knowledge of the laity, so that they can critically assume the conditions that affect their lives and their communities. These are ideas for co-building knowledge with participatory partners. It is a simple fact that academic knowledge alone is insufficient to support health promotion strategies or social movements that can make a sustainable difference to health. The knowledge that comes from the practices and culture of the community is essential and, often, the most important to direct research and use the findings both for community actions, and for new public policies and social changes. It means not doing research "about" a community; and not doing research "in" a community environment, but literally doing research "with" community partners – social actors and groups to facilitate the most important principle of co-creation and the equal value of each partner's knowledge (Wallerstein, 2018).

Participatory research requires a central commitment to "participation in the research stages". From problem identification, through co-creation of the study, co-development tools, data collection, co-analysis and interpretation, and finally, through the dissemination of results, so that community members or social actors can understand and use the data to create new programs, practices, or influence public policies (Wallerstein, 2018; Wallerstein et al., 2017a, b, 2019). The use of the Freirean framework results from dialogic meetings developed in the so-called "culture circles". They translate into the dialectic of (i) thematic research (thematization); (ii) encoding and decoding (problematization); (iii) critical unveiling for political conscience (clarity and purpose to overcome impasses and practical action to solve problems with critical autonomy of those involved). This provides for complementarity between scientific and popular knowledge, in an effort to collectively build contextualized knowledge of a local reality. Here, then, is the philosophical difference between the idea of talking "to people" with that of talking "with people", where the second overcomes the first through the interaction of knowledge between the subjects (Heidemann et al., 2010, 2014, 2019).

Allied to this, we have used and encouraged other research groups to use participatory research methods, and to include different actors and stakeholders (Wallerstein et al., 2017a, b, 2018; Heidemann et al., 2014; Rice & Franceschini, 2009). For instance, we inevitably consider the relationships and production chains of different sectors, especially in the public, but also philanthropic and private sectors, which affect the Sustainable Development Goals and, consequently, health promotion of the population. This requires combining quantitative, qualitative, or hybrid approaches (Creswell, 2014; Pluye et al., 2018), by triangulation of methods and using extensive systematic critical reviews, tailoring a research itinerary that legitimately typifies health promotion research at national level.

Specifically, the authors of this chapter participated in the years 2004–2006 in one of the first convergent, networked exercises to conduct research projects with a participatory approach in Brazil. The aim was to assess and validate the "Guide for participatory evaluation for healthy municipalities and communities / *Guía de evaluación participativa para municipios y comunidades saludables*" (Perú. Ministerio de Salud et al., 2006; Rocabado et al., 2005), in different Brazilian contexts. Subsequently, between 2007 and 2009, we took part in a multi-centre investigation in different regions of the country related to local development agendas that had emerged in previous years, including Agendas 21, Healthy Cities/Municipalities, and Integrated Sustainable Local Development (*Desenvolvimento Local Integrado e Sustentável - DLIS*) (Nascimento et al., 2014; Westphal et al., 2013; Sperandio et al., 2016). We also played a decisive role throughout 2013–2015, in the revision of the National Health Promotion Policy (*Política Nacional de Promoção da Saúde - PNPS2006*) in Brazil (Brasil et al., 2009; Minowa et al., 2017; Rocha et al., 2014; Sa et al., 2016). More recently, from 2017 onward, the network consolidated its national role in community-based participatory research (CBPR) by disseminating teaching, researching, and conduction extension work in a multi-centric movement called "Multiple Seeds" (Wallerstein et al., 2017a, b).

The chapter will present some relevant aspects of these Brazilian experiences, highlighting evidences and lessons learned from our work in the field of health promotion, particularly those related to intersectoral approaches and participatory methods, which are a hallmark of our practice and research projects.

47.4 Forming an Interdisciplinary Network

The first block of experiences contemplates the objective of applying and assessing the participatory evaluation guide of healthy municipalities and communities – hereinafter referred to as "the Guide" (Perú. Ministerio de Salud et al., 2006; Rocabado et al., 2005). This was the basis for a multi-centre evaluation study in Health Promotion, carried out in eight singular contexts, in different regions of the country (Akerman & Mendes, 2006). We come together on the perception of the differences inherent to the realities of application of the Guide. For instance, the propositional/programmatic scope of each experience; its maturation time; the objectives pursued; the contextual influences and conditions related to the sustainability of ongoing operations.

47.4.1 "Go Shine!"

The experience with the Guide in *"Rio de Janeiro, Vila Paciência, CEDAPS"* (Akerman & Mendes, 2006; Becker et al., 2004) is characterized as a territorial intervention based on the conceptual framework of Integrated and Sustainable Local Development. The central concept highlighted in the experience was that of the "empowerment" of the subjects achieved through participation. The strategy focused on building shared solutions based on the concrete demands of the community's dwellers, with the creation of social intervention networks, strongly supported by local society and the third sector. The fundamental message was that empowerment is an intricate strategy, but it can occur within complex and apparently very unfavourable social environments – mostly affronted by the cruel experience of exclusion and low individual, family, and community esteem. Effective strategies can depend a lot on the agency and leadership of the people involved, under the influence of the context in which they take place.

47.4.2 "Settlements in the Healthy Municipality"

The experience with the Guide in *"São Paulo, Motuca - Healthy Municipality, CEPEDOC"* (Westphal & Franceschini, 2016; Mendes & Falvo, 2007; Akerman & Mendes, 2006) is emblematic. Possibly, it reflects the urban "ethos" of hundreds of small Brazilian cities, with their difficulties related to population size, power, political visibility, and access to resources. However, the experience of Motuca was surprising, because it partially contradicts the very common situation described in the strategic planning literature about Brazilian local governments (Andrews et al., 1999). Often, a fragile government triangle prevails: (i) absence of a "Government Project" previously discussed with the local society, generating uncertainty regarding the desired future; (ii) low or no "Government Capacity", related to technical, administrative, and organizational knowledge and skills; (iii) little "Public Governance", related to the control of material, political or symbolic resources. The *Motuca Healthy Municipality* is an experience whose central axis of intervention was on the binomial "participation" and "intersectoriality". A Commission, comprising about 60 members, developed the city's future vision, through awareness-raising workshops. In addition to rescuing the municipality's history and producing what has been called "biomapping" (how does the city make us feel, and how can we use our feelings to make cities), people helped to diagnose and determine urban spaces which should be subject to improving urban assets and logistics. One important aspect of this project was the emphasis on including residents of existing settlements in the group conducting the participatory assessment and seeking strategies to overcome difficulties related to the low level of education of those residents. This experience highlights the importance of the communicative process when the question of participation is problematized, which points to a need to reframe the concepts used in academic language (health literacy).

47.4.3 "Healthy People, in the Plasticity of Leminski's[1] Land"

The experience *"Paraná, Healthy Environments in Curitiba, PUCPR / Curitiba City Hall"* is engaging (Moysés et al., 2004; Akerman & Mendes, 2006; Bueno et al., 2013). It highlights how to address the political, methodological, and strategic challenges in the formulation and implementation of healthy public policies and sustainable development in a large metropolis, Curitiba – the capital of the state of Paraná. There were interventions with clear guidelines in the search for socio-environmental and institutional changes, to reduce situations of vulnerability, tackle inequalities, and incorporate participation and social control in the management of public policies. One of the chief concepts of the proposal was, explicitly, government accountability (in a broader sense, taken as a dimension that induces interventions that promote health), which highlights the centrality of the concept of "health in all public policies", and, therefore, the intersectorality in the political basis of the proposal. The interventions were multidimensional, including the ingredient of complex thinking. The choice of an environment-oriented approach (settings

[1] *Paulo Leminski, local poet whose work has national/international repercussions. (http://www.paulolerminski.com.br/)*

approach) embodies this complexity, framing different scenarios, institutional cultures, and political configurations, such as a network of public schools and universities, as well as corporations in the productive private sector, with about 140 institutions and hundreds of individuals involved.

47.4.4 "The School as a Transcendent Space, Beyond Its Educative Mission"

The "*Tocantins, Health-promoting Schools, SESAU*" experience involves a scaling up project, initially covering 10 municipalities and a network of 205 schools and 96 health units (Akerman & Mendes, 2006; Brasil. Ministério da Saúde and Organização Pan-Americana da Saúde, 2006). The central concept that appears in this experience was intersectorality, as a structuring operation of an integral school health policy, seeking to produce local autonomy. In this case, the teams already constituted for the integrated management of the project, at either the state or municipal level, were catalysts for the process of intersectoral implementation of the policy. It should be noted that the Health-promoting Schools initiative was disseminated internationally as an effective way to promote the health of children, adolescents, and the broader school community. Yet, only in recent times, systematic evaluative experiences have been published (Hung et al., 2014; Mukamana & Johri, 2016).

47.4.5 "Our Place Is with Local Agenda 21"

The team report "*Mato Grosso do Sul, Local Agenda 21, City Hall of Campo Grande*" (Akerman & Mendes, 2006; Akerman et al., 2016) was another experience aimed at strengthening public policies at the municipal level and tackling the social determinants of health, through integrated management with the Social Councils. Strategically, a momentous intervention in the logic of management and social valorization was decided, focusing on urban violence and opening space for intra- and intersectoral integration. A new perspective was developed, redefining assessment from a basis on which policymakers set goals to a commitment to all stakeholders regarding the value and meaning of their practices. Approachable assessment is especially appropriate in health promotion contexts characterized by a high degree of ambiguity, as in the case of political change or contradictory interpretations of "what for, what can or what should be done, when and where...". Ambiguity is high in the case of non-routine programs, where there is a lack of knowledge about success indicators, the uncertainty of the role of collaborators, and an absence of consensus among stakeholders.

47.4.6 "Feliz Cidade (Happy City) Is Achieved by Understanding the Population's Life Cycles"

The report from *"Goiás, NascerFeliz, Municipal Health Department of Goiânia"* (Akerman & Mendes, 2006; Akerman et al., 2014) described yet another experience of great latitude, within the scope of a Brazilian state capital, Goiânia, seeking to evaluate the integrated management of public policies. Here, too, the central concept was intersectorality. Once again, power relations, political dispute over projects, and the temporal impermanence of public actors characterized the urban management of a Brazilian city. It is positively surprising to note that, despite the political changes that took place and the dissolution of the original teams linked to the evaluated project, twenty-six intersectoral strategic actions were still accounted for. The procedural assessment in response to contextual aspects, such as politics/ideology changes over time, was used to monitor the implementation of projects/programs, helping to understand the relationship between specific elements of the intervention proposals and the results achieved. In this sense, the importance attributed to process evaluation increased along with the intricacy of conducting one, while its complexity escalates. Some dimensions have been suggested for the formulation of an evaluative approach that addresses this complexity, such as dependability, scope, adherence, appropriation, subjectivation, autonomy, and change of context.

47.4.7 "Between the Forest and the Hinterland, the Wild Can Also Be Healthy"

The *"Pernambuco, A Network of Healthy Municipalities in Northeast Brazil, UFPE-NUSP / SEPLAN / JICA"* (Moysés & Sá, 2014; Akerman & Mendes, 2006; Freire et al., 2016) experience was encouraging, in all aspects. The application of the Guide, in an aggregate of five municipalities in the semi-arid countryside of Pernambuco, brought the underlying concept of "social capital" as a background of the reported experience. The predominance of the materialist-structural use of the social capital concept, since its translation from the social sciences to the health field, has neglected its importance and influence with regard to the formation of networks in the subjective relational encounters of individuals. Gradually, its logical formulation, decoded on the cognitive as well as on the emotional dimension was achieved with the participation of the community to define levels of intervention, under the logic of the life cycle. The applicability of abstract concepts such as cognitive social capital (micropolitical space of the community involved) and structural social capital (municipal and regional level) was no longer unintelligible and questionable by ordinary people in the communities. Just to emphasize the point, this experience included a "Local Implementation Committee", by which some conceptual deficiencies in the Guide were considered, for example, criticisms that it was markedly bureaucratic or "perfunctory", dispersing the energy that would be used as a resource for change in the political sphere. It was also noted that the Guide did not facilitate the observation of a paramount component, which was the cultural competence of the community, as well as popular skills and assets to promote change. An evaluation design of health promotion interventions, which intends to be transdisciplinary, must use the available knowledge in a way to contribute to the construction of an interactive/relational process necessary to analyze the assessed situation.

47.4.8 *"Thinking/Acting in a Network Arouse Reflection on the Question of Power"*

Finally, the report *"São Paulo, Network of Potentially Healthy Municipalities, UNICAMP"* (Akerman & Mendes, 2006; Sperandio et al., 2016) presented a realistic portrait of the political fluctuation that appears when trying to work in an expanded network, with many municipalities and political wills involved. Researchers in the fieldwork found a situation of great political instability, related to the electoral period in the municipalities. However, they note that it is necessary to negotiate with parties and candidates committed to change in political campaigns, inducing a programmatic platform that includes Health Promotion strategies, that is, agreeing public commitments with eventual winners. Thus, government plans gain transparency and accountability.

47.5 Expanding the Interdisciplinary Network

The second block of experiences that we describe relates to several local development agendas that have emerged in recent years, including: Agenda 21, adopted by the Brazilian Ministry of the Environment; Healthy Cities/Municipalities, promoted by the Pan-American Health Organization; and Integrated Sustainable Local Development, supported by the federal government.

The United Nations Organization agreed with some countries, including Brazil, on the Millennium Development Goals (MDG) with the objective of reassuring the development of nations, states, and municipalities (Akerman, 2005). The objective of the research was to identify how these comprehensive agendas had been influencing the living and health conditions of the population in the five macro-regions of the country. This multi-centre evaluative study was carried out between 2007 and 2009 by seven Brazilian universities: The School of Public Health of the University of São Paulo, and CEPEDOC Healthy Cities; Goiás Federal University; Federal University of Pernambuco; Federal University of Tocantins; University of the

Amazon; Pontifical Catholic University of Paraná and Catholic University Dom Bosco of Campo Grande, Mato Grosso do Sul.

The methodology considered mixed methods – qualitative and quantitative – and used an explanatory sequential design, comprised of three phases: (i) mapping of the social agendas; (ii) retrospective, longitudinal, comparative study – case-control – with secondary data from various sources; (iii) qualitative case studies of municipalities with different population sizes, with better results in relation to the MDG.

As for the results, 105 identified municipalities in phase I were developing at least one of the studied social agendas. In phase II, a grid of 29 indicators was built to monitor the MDG. The statistical tests carried out showed that, three years after the implementation of the agendas, there was no statistical significance between their existence and the performance of the MDG indicators. Obviously, it must be considered that the time elapsed was also short in the evaluation temporal cut-off. On the other hand, the results of phase III demonstrated that Agenda 21 and Healthy Cities presented different configurations in relation to the process of diagnosis and involvement with the local government, as well as differences regarding local sustainability. In some cases, it had become an innovative public management model, inspiring local governance.

The participation of civil society in the diagnostic and planning processes was the value most frequently identified in the cases studied. This finding suggests effects on the empowerment of the local population, indicating that these local social agendas resulting from federal initiative have collaborated with the improvement of living conditions of populations (Baltar et al., 2014; Nascimento et al., 2014; Westphal et al., 2013).

47.6 Strengthening the Interdisciplinary Network

The third block of innovative and participatory experiences in health promotion includes multiple approaches and participatory research at the revision of the National Health Promotion Policy. This focuses on the main results related to advocacy, public transparency, political activism, and institutional change.

> Since 2002, there have been movements in Brazil to formulate a National Health Promotion Policy (NHPP). This intent happened when the Brazilian government promulgated this policy on March 30, 2006. Six broad themes were defined for the PNPS, unfolding in many programs, actions, services and goals. Healthy food; Body practice/Physical activity; Smoking prevention and control; Reduction of morbidity and mortality due to the abuse of alcohol and other drugs; Reduction of morbidity and mortality from traffic accidents; Prevention of violence and stimulation of a culture of peace, promoting sustainable development. For the ABRASCO WG, the operationalization of these themes gave the PNPS a more introverted preventive biomedical orientation and, therefore, subject to a persuasive narrative dispute, in the epistemological and political perspective of an expanded health promotion revision. In 2013–2014, the PNPS was revised with the support of our network of researchers. The previous themes of the first edition are published in the new Policy with

a formulation more in line with the accumulation of research in the field of health promotion. In the 2014 document there was the inclusion of "capacity building and continuing education" in HP as a public policy; also, we highlight the inclusion of the themes "Safe Mobility", and "Human Rights".

Public policy can be understood as a translation of the purposes of governments and the wishes of society. However, historically, Brazil has a developmental model that promotes the concentration of political, economic, and social resources and power which, consequently, increases social disintegration and health inequities. Furthermore, interaction of the multiple actors involved in the construction of a public policy does not occur automatically. It requires institutionalization of arrangements and mechanisms deliberately fostered to strengthen social participation.

Again, given the need to integrate agendas and overcome the small social participation in the preparation of the first edition of the Brazilian National Health Promotion Policy (Brasil. Ministério da Saúde, 2006), the WG was deeply provoked. It conducted multiple approaches to the *PNPS2006* review and update process (Albuquerque et al., 2016; Guerra et al., 2015; Magalhaes, 2016; Minowa et al., 2017; Rocha et al., 2014; Sa et al., 2016), leading to its new publication in 2015 (Brasil. Ministério da Saúde, 2015). Many simultaneous movements aiming at social representation were used as a strategy for mobilizing and listening to emerging voices, views, and syntheses. Information was collected through five regional workshops with participation of representatives of the population and health councils; intra- and intersectoral Delphi technique with University groups; and an electronic questionnaire (*Form-SUS*) that considered heterogeneous sources, different local contexts (the five macroregions in Brazil), and peer validation (systematization and consensus workshops). This model of public policy analysis made it possible to apply the principles of Health Promotion and participatory research in the collective elaboration of the *PNPS2006* revision.

Results were systematized and triangulated using an analysis matrix (organized around objectives, principles, guidelines, themes, and actions) and resulted in a draft of the new *PNPS2006*, which was presented and validated at a national seminar. Regional workshops and systematization meetings showed that interregional, intersectoral, and intergenerational learning achieved by collective work and the validation movement was an important legacy of the process. The whole process contributed to knowledge production, dissemination, subsidized guidelines, and mechanisms for research, training, and permanent education on health promotion.

Social participation was expanded in the *PNPS2015* reviewed version, guaranteeing democratic representativeness in policy formulation. The research led during the revision process was a way to tackle intra- and interregional inequities. For instance, to: (i) overcome the deficit of the approximation with regional realities; (ii) problematize implementation of health promotion practices in different contexts; and (iii) identify convergences and singularities of the policy implementation and characterization of the socio-spatial diversity of the five Brazilian regions. Moreover, it contributed to the formation of a network of commitments and interests mobilized in the regions that favours its sustainability.

The expansion of regional participation and capillarity in the policy formulation process resulted in partnerships, established among the community, non-governmental representatives, and the government team (representatives of the Ministry of Health), mediated by the Pan American Health Organization (PAHO). These results signal the potential for new advocacy and good governance arrangements by creating spaces for intergovernmental and intersectoral coordination to strengthen the doctrinal and organizational principles of health promotion and the Unified Health System (*Sistema Único de Saúde - SUS*). Finally, they favour the continuity of the political, communicative, and strategic agendas supportive of including guidelines, principles, and values for health promotion in the action plans of regional and local governments.

47.7 Multiplying the Interdisciplinary Network

The last block of initiatives that well represent a way of acting/researching in the field of health promotion, with empowered population groups, is a multi-centric partnership ("Multiple Seeds") formed in 2019. It included the Faculty of Population Health, Centre for Participatory Research, University of New Mexico (USA) and several Brazilian Education Institutions from all regions of the country: the School of Public Health, University of São Paulo; Federal University of São Paulo; Federal University of ABC; University of Brasília; Federal University of Minas Gerais; Federal University of Pernambuco; Community University of Chapecó; Pontifical Catholic University of Rio de Janeiro; Federal University of Paraíba; State University of Maringá; State University of Bahia; Federal University of Goiás; University of Franca.

The main references used are the experience and studies of the "*Engage for Equity: Advancing Community Engaged Partnerships*" initiative (Wallerstein et al., 2017a, b, 2019, 2020), whose authors have worked in research to advance participatory methodologies and evaluate the results of partnerships among universities and communities. In addition, its scope is the creation and implementation of workshops, training tools, and resource development to strengthen the practices of participatory methodologies in various locations to accomplish equity in health through interdisciplinary, intersectoral educational practices, devoted to critical learning.

In 2020, the Group organized five nationwide upgrading courses – Southeast (2), South (1), Northeast (1), and Midwest (1) for around 120 professionals, teachers, and students. The Group's objectives are to (i) share tools and reflections on CBPR and empowerment (formative); (ii) foster a collaborative network of multipliers (collaborative); (iii) nurture CBPR nuclei for local development and democratization of knowledge; and (iv) expand a network of training and research, tutoring multipliers to develop the course in their regions in the semi-presential modality (Wallerstein, 2018; Mendes, 2019; Wallerstein et al., 2018).

47.8 Discussion

At the outset, the analysis of these experiences points to the understanding that each intervention presents disputes and consensus about the direction that the projects should follow. In a word, the material is heterogeneous. To deal with heterogeneity, in the research perspective, requires recalling that such a situation presents methodological complexities, in addition to the epistemological problems related to the indexability of the results to any external reality. This is not exactly new in the field of Health Promotion. Similar international initiatives have generated a vast body of publications, pointing out the plurality of theories and methods as a central element of the field (Pan American Health Organization, 1996; McQueen et al., 2007; Akerman et al., 2014; Arroyo, 2016; Super et al., 2016; Gelius & Rutten, 2018; Fernandez et al., 2019).

The Report of the Working Group on the theme of health promotion evaluation, promoted by the World Health Organization (WHO Europe, 1998) established four aspects that should, necessarily, be part of health promotion evaluation initiatives: (a) participation; (b) multiple methods; (c) capacity building; (d) appropriateness. Unfortunately, the critical information needed to judge the quality of a health promotion intervention, and whether it is useful as a reference for the recommendation of "good practices", are vague or lacking in most studies (Schwarzman et al., 2019).

In any case, cultural change provides insights into why it can be difficult to maintain the dynamics of change processes (Alvesson & Sveningsson, 2015). There are many questions imposed by the hermeneutic task. For an evaluation of participatory research/action, using hybrid methods, to provide a demonstration of its quality, some questions must be underway: Is it contributing to the creation process of knowledge? Is it credible in the sense of the rationale and arguments it presents? Is it defensible from a methodological point of view? Is it rigorous in research driving?

Innovative and skilled approaches to account for this complexity must consider that populations are defined by size, density, diversity, and complexity. The health of these populations is a function of individual living conditions, which interacts with the social determinants of health, local environment, and national and/or global trends – a "glo-cal" phenomenon (Kickbusch, 1999; de Leeuw et al., 2006; Akerman et al., 2016; Galvão et al., 2016). In consequence, it is necessary to consider the different meanings of the "judgement of effects", and to avoid the influence of the neo-positivist paradigm in this field, since it does not include the polysemy of the terms "quality/quantity" and its close overlapping with human subjectivity.

A challenge for the health promotion field remains the development of high quality, widely recognized, and acceptable standards for assessing evidence of effectiveness (Victora et al., 2004; Li et al., 2015; Meyer et al., 2018). The openness to methodological plurality cannot ignore the fact that the use of hybrid methods can lead to different and, at times, contradictory results due to the precariousness of the data or methodological flaws. Each database, whether from a qualitative or quantitative point of view, must be thoroughly examined and methodological/analytical approaches be compatible with such data. The contemporary challenge is to enlarge the theoretical ground, underpinned on the robustness of the methods used to generate a greater degree of confidence in the processes triggered and the results achieved. The more widespread use of hybrid methods in complex interventions is likely to increase the overall quality of the evidence-based health promotion (Wallerstein & Duran, 2006; Jolley, 2014). On the other hand, attempting to seek evidence from randomized experimental designs, which have high internal validity and low external validity, is inappropriate in complex circumstances. In this case, the notion of "best evidence" from gold standard randomized trials ignores the complexity involved in the decision-making process for health promotion interventions in practical situations (Victora et al., 2004; Li et al., 2015).

Our societies demand an urgent commitment from policymakers, decision-makers, researchers, and professionals, as well as popular movements and civil society in general, in order to face and overcome misery, exclusion, and distress (Horton et al., 1990). We see the advance of neo-fascist, obscurantist, and denialist political regimes, perverse in their actions of necropolitics and environmental degradation, with marked setbacks in economic-based decisions that aim at austerity. As has been vividly argued, in the context of the pandemic, this worldwide calamity is not only a health crisis (Horton, 2020). It is a crisis about life itself.

Brazil has not yet an institutional culture and a permanence of actors that allow the preservation and systematic treatment of the "memories" of the interventions carried out, of their use in the present, and their projection in the future. The experiences reported in the present chapter include information related to decision-makers and beneficiaries of projects/programs, expanding the traditional assessment of evidence to incorporate the "assessment of the theory of change" underlying the action, the integrity of interventions, the context, governance and the sustainability of the projects, as well as some of their intermediate results. Such interventions are multidimensional and aimed at diverse populations, seeking to measure multiple results, mixing designs and evaluation methods, in addition to the "context effect" on the approach, implementation, and effectiveness (Sá & Moysés, 2009; Potvin et al., 2009; Tremblay et al., 2013; South, 2014; Jolley, 2014; Meyer et al., 2018). In policy formulation/implementation, evidence frequently comes from units of analysis or intervention at an ecological level, under the influence of the context.

Anchored in participatory research methods, the authors' experiences under analysis make it possible to them to establish a critique of conventional explanatory theoretical/methodological keys. They take part in the intersectoral debate that problematizes and interprets the health-disease-care processes by the counter-hegemonic side of the political spectrum. The experiences reveal the militant – but lucid – "implication" of the authors themselves with the research objects and the impact on the pressing reality of those who participated in the research, recognizing the perception of the differences inherent to the realities (Fassin, 2018).

Overall, one should keep in mind that this is a "work in progress". The mindset of the people who lead a challenging social intervention must be placed in a perspective of cultural vanguard, knowing that to galvanize the necessary changes they are likely to encounter strong resistance and risk of failure. This is a world full of uncertainties and long-range disruptions. That is why the validity for contexts of low political maturity and high dynamics in the participation of subjects, as observed in some realities worked on locally, still provides room for more future innovative and participatory research.

47.9 Conclusions

The case of the Brazilian collaboration network for Health Promotion presented here encompasses dense and thought-provoking material derived from social research and interventions made possible by the mobilization of countless political-institutional actors. The experiences were carried out by "in situation" actors, with diverse assets and who express conflicts, hopes, disappointments, desires, as well as regulatory/control tactics, seeking to spur actions oriented to change. They are permeated now and then by more unstable or more solid coalitions, in which the relations of power, ideology, and cultural porosity conflate. The co-authors converge for a consensual interpretation on the aspects that stand out from the health promotion research initiatives carried out in the interdisciplinary network.

To summarize, we have shown the key theoretical/methodological elements of our research approach (southern epistemology, participatory intersectoral research, implications of the authors). It was possible to infer a reasonable degree of horizontal participation by different subjects and institutions, the multiplicity of methods (plus the need for adaptation/diversification of phases, according to some local contexts), and the importance of the capacity building achieved by most of the interventions.

The chapter provides ideas for structuring the field of health promotion research at a global level. This multi-centric repertoire of Brazilian experiences points to the need for an epistemological and political positioning of the subjects that produce knowledge in health promotion, especially in the problematic national and international realities. Above all, nowadays, it is imperative that health promoters, internationally, face the risks of disinformation and the decline of democracy, due to the constant threats – in Brazil and elsewhere. The experiences reported here derive from realities rich in current possibilities and future developments, with a diversity of characters, theoretical approaches, and methodological arrangements. They show that we do not have to choose between militancy and political lucidity or scientific robustness. Not later, but "now" is the time to accept the historic challenge of working with those who suffer the consequences of inequalities, which are unjust and avoidable. Health promoters must more than ever "walk the talk".

References

Akerman, M. (2005). *Saúde e desenvolvimento local: princípios, conceitos, práticas e cooperação técnica (Saúde em debate)*. Editora Hucitec.

Akerman, M., & Fischer, A. (2014). Agenda Nacional de Prioridades na Pesquisa em Saúde no Brasil (ANPPS): foco na subagenda 18 - Promoção da Saúde. *Saúde e Sociedade, 23*(1), 180–190.

Akerman, M., & Mendes, R. (Eds.). (2006). *Participating evaluation of healthy cities, communities and environments: The Brazilian trajectory - memory, thoughts and experiences / Avaliação participativa de municípios, comunidades e ambientes saudáveis: A trajetória Brasileira - memória, reflexões e experiências*. Midia Alternativa.

Akerman, M., Sá, R. F., Moysés, S. T., Rezende, R., & Rocha, D. (2014). Intersetorialidade? IntersetorialidadeS! / Intersectoriality? IntersectorialitieS! *Ciência & Saúde Coletiva, 19*(11), 4291–4300.

Akerman, M., Maymone, C. C., Bógus, C., Chioro, A., Buss, P. M., & Fortun, K. (2016). New health agendas based on social determinants. In L. A. C. Galvão, J. Finkelman, & S. Henao (Eds.), *Environmental and social determinants of health* (pp. 1–15). Pan American Health Organization.

Albuquerque, T. I. P., Sá, R. F., Araújo Júnior, J. L., & d. A. C. d. (2016). Perspectives and challenges of the "new" National Health Promotion Policy: To which political arena does management point? / Perspectivas e desafios da "nova" Política Nacional de Promoção da Saúde: Para qual arena política aponta a gestão? *Ciência & Saúde Coletiva, 21*(6), 1695–1706.

Alexander, S. A., Jones, C. M., Tremblay, M. C., Beaudet, N., Rod, M. H., & Wright, M. T. (2020). Reflexivity in health promotion: A typology for training. *Health Promotion Practice, 21*(4), 499–509.

Alvesson, M., & Sveningsson, S. (2015). *Changing organizational culture: Cultural change work in progress*. Routledge.

Andrews, C. W., Comini, G., & Vieira, E. H. (1999). Continuities and change in Brazilian administrative reform. *International Journal of Public Sector Management, 12*(6), 482–500. https://doi.org/10.1108/09513559910301351

Arroyo, H. V. (Ed.). (2016). *La promoción de la salud en América Latina: apuntes históricos, estructuras y políticas nacionales*. Universidad de Puerto Rico, Centro Colaborador de la OMS para la Capacitación e Investigación em Promoción de la Salud y Educación para la Salud.

Baltar, V. T., Sousa, C. A., & Westphal, M. F. (2014). Mahalanobis' distance and propensity score to construct a controlled matched group in a Brazilian study of health promotion and social determinants. *Revista Brasileira de Epidemiologia, 17*(3), 668–679.

Becker, D., Edmundo, K., Nunes, N. R., Bonatto, D., Souza, R., & d. (2004). Empowerment e avaliação participativa em um programa de desenvolvimento local e promoção da saúde. *Ciência & Saúde Coletiva, 9*(3), 655–667.

Belza, B., Altpeter, M., Smith, M. L., & Ory, M. G. (2017). The healthy aging research network: Modeling collaboration for community impact. *American Journal of Preventive Medicine, 52*(3 Suppl 3), S228–S232. https://doi.org/10.1016/j.amepre.2016.09.035

Brasil, Ministério da Saúde. (2006). *Política Nacional de Promoção da Saúde*. Ministério da Saúde, Secretaria de Vigilância em Saúde, Secretaria de Atenção à Saúde.

Brasil, Ministério da Saúde (2015). *Política Nacional de Promoção da Saúde - PNaPS: revisão da Portaria MS/GM n° 687, de 30 de março de* 2006. Brasília: Ministério da Saúde, Secretaria de Vigilância em Saúde. Secretaria de Atenção à Saúde.

Brasil, Ministério da Saúde, & Organização Pan-Americana da Saúde (2006). *Escolas promotoras de saúde: experiências do Brasil*. Série Promoção da Saúde; n° 6. Ministério da Saúde Brasília.

Brasil, Ministério da Saúde, Secretaria de Vigilância em Saúde, & Departamento de Análise de Situação da Saúde. (2009). *Anais: I Seminário sobre a Política Nacional de Promoção da Saúde* (p. 252). Ministério da Saúde.

Brass, N., & Macedo, D. P. (1985). Toward a pedagogy of the question: Conversations with Paulo Freire. *Journal of Education, 167*(2), 7–21. https://doi.org/10.1177/002205748516700203

Bueno, R. E., Moysés, S. T., Reis Bueno, P. A., Moysés, S. J., de Carvalho, M. L., & França, B. H. S. (2013). Sustainable development and child health in the Curitiba metropolitan mesoregion, state of Paraná, Brazil. *Health & Place, 19*, 167–173. https://doi.org/10.1016/j.healthplace.2012.10.007

Buss, P. M., & Pellegrini Filho, A. (2006). Health inequities in Brazil, our most serious illness: Comments on the reference document and the work of the National Commission on social determinants of health. / Iniqüidades em saúde no Brasil, nossa mais grave doença: comentários sobre o documento de referência e os trabalhos da Comissão Nacional sobre Determinantes Sociais da Saúde. *Cadernos de Saúde Pública, 22*(9), 2005–2008.

Cavalcanti, M. (2018). Knowledge networks: Interdisciplinary thinking [Redes de saberes: Pensamento interdisciplinar]. *Periferia, 10*(1), 261–273.

Creswell, J. W. (2014). *A concise introduction to mixed methods research*. SAGE publications.

de Leeuw, E., Tang, K. C., & Beaglehole, R. (2006). Ottawa to Bangkok--Health promotion's journey from principles to 'glocal' implementation. *Health Promotion International, 21*(Suppl 1), 1–4. https://doi.org/10.1093/heapro/dal057

Escobar, A. (2020). *Pluriversal politics: The real and the possible*. Duke University Press.

Fassin, D. (2018). *Life: A critical user's manual*. Polity Press.

Fernandez, M. E., Ruiter, R. A. C., Markham, C. M., & Kok, G. (2019). Intervention mapping: Theory- and evidence-based health promotion program planning: Perspective and examples. *Frontiers in Public Health, 7*, 209. https://doi.org/10.3389/fpubh.2019.00209

Freire, P. (1980). *Pedagogia do oprimido* (8ª ed.). Paz e Terra.

Freire, P. (1996a). *Letters to Cristina: Reflections on my life and work*. Routledge.

Freire, P. (1996b). *Pedagogy of autonomy: Knowledge necessary for educational practice / Pedagogia da autonomia: Saberes necessários à prática educativa* (39 ed., Coleção Leitura). Paz e Terra.

Freire, P. (2014). *Pedagogy of Freedom / Pedagogia da autonomia: Saberes necessários à prática educativa*. Paz e Terra.

Freire, M. D. S. M., Salles, R. P. D. S., & Sá, R. F. (2016). Mapeando iniciativas territoriais saudáveis, suas características e evidências de efetividade. *Ciência & Saúde Coletiva, 21*(6), 1757–1766.

Galvão, L. A. C., Finkelman, J., & Henao, S. (Eds.). (2016). *Environmental and social determinants of health*. Pan American Health Organization.

Gelius, P., & Rutten, A. (2018). Conceptualizing structural change in health promotion: Why we still need to know more about theory. *Health Promotion International, 33*(4), 657–664. https://doi.org/10.1093/heapro/dax006

Gould, T., Fleming, M. L., & Parker, E. (2012). Advocacy for health: Revisiting the role of health promotion. *Health Promotion Journal of Australia, 23*(3), 165–170. https://doi.org/10.1071/he12165

GT Promoção da Saúde - Abrasco. WG on Health Promotion and Sustainable Development: 15 years of trajectory (2002 to 2017) / GT de Promoção da Saúde e Desenvolvimento Sustentável: 15 anos de trajetória (2002 a 2017). Available at: https://www.abrasco.org.br/site/gtpromocaodasaude/, Acessed: 21 Sept 2020.

Guerra, V. A., Rezende, R., Rocha, D. G., Silva, K. R., & Akerman, M. (2015). Workshop as an exercise of learning and collaborative listening: The case of the review of National Policy of health promotion. *ABCS Health Sciences, 40*(3), 352–359.

Heidemann, I. T. S. B., Boehs, A. E., Wosny, A. M., & Stulp, K. P. (2010). Theoretical, conceptual and methodological incorporation of the educator Paulo Freire in research. *Revista Brasileira de Enfermagem, 63*(3), 416–420. https://doi.org/10.1590/s0034-71672010000300011

Heidemann, I. T. S. B., Wosny Ade, M., & Boehs, A. E. (2014). Health promotion in primary care: Study based on the Paulo Freire method. *Ciência & Saúde Coletiva, 19*(8), 3553–3559. https://doi.org/10.1590/1413-81232014198.11342013

Heidemann, I. T. S. B., Alonso da Costa, M. F. B. N., Hermida, P. M. V., Marçal, C. C. B., Antonini, F. O., & Cypriano, C. C. (2019). Health promotion practices in primary care groups. *Global Health Promotion, 26*(1), 25–32.

Hogg, R. A., & Varda, D. (2016). Insights into collaborative networks of nonprofit, private, and public organizations that address complex health issues. *Health Aff (Millwood), 35*(11), 2014–2019. https://doi.org/10.1377/hlthaff.2016.0725

Horton, R. (2020). Offline: A global health crisis? No, something far worse. *The Lancet, 395*(10234), 1410. https://doi.org/10.1016/S0140-6736(20)31017-5

Horton, M., Freire, P., Bell, B., Gaventa, J., & Peters, J. M. (1990). *We make the road by walking: Conversations on education and social change*. Temple University Press.

Hung, T. T., Chiang, V. C., Dawson, A., & Lee, R. L. (2014). Understanding of factors that enable health promoters in implementing health-promoting schools: A systematic review and narrative synthesis of qualitative evidence. *PLoS One, 9*(9), e108284. https://doi.org/10.1371/journal.pone.0108284

Jolley, G. (2014). Evaluating complex community-based health promotion: Addressing the challenges. *Evaluation and Program Planning, 45*, 71–81. https://doi.org/10.1016/j.evalprogplan.2014.03.006

Kickbusch, I. (1999). Global + local = glocal public health. *Journal of Epidemiology and Community Health, 53*(8), 451–452. https://doi.org/10.1136/jech.53.8.451

Leibowitz, B. (2017). Cognitive justice and the higher education curriculum. *Journal of Education (University of KwaZulu-Natal), 68*, 93–112.

Li, V., Carter, S. M., & Rychetnik, L. (2015). Evidence valued and used by health promotion practitioners. *Health Education Research, 30*(2), 193–205. https://doi.org/10.1093/her/cyu071

Magalhães, R. (2016). Evaluation of the National Health Promotion Policy (PNPS): Prospects and challenges / Avaliação da Política Nacional de Promoção da Saúde: Perspectivas e desafios. *Ciência & Saúde Coletiva, 21*(6), 1767–1776. https://doi.org/10.1590/1413-81232015216.07422016

Masuda, J. R., Poland, B., & Baxter, J. (2010). Reaching for environmental health justice: Canadian experiences for a comprehensive research, policy and advocacy agenda in health promotion. *Health Promotion International, 25*(4), 453–463. https://doi.org/10.1093/heapro/daq041

McQueen, D. V., Kickbusch, I., Potvin, L., Pelikan, J. M., Balbo, L., & Abel, T. (2007). *Health and modernity: The role of theory in heath promotion*. Springer.

Mendes, R. (2019). Abordagens participativas em pesquisa: agir em favor do diálogo e da inclusão. *O social em questão (on line), 21*, 341–344.

Mendes, R., & Falvo, F. (2007). Motuca healthy municipality project: Building together a better future. *Promotion & Education, 14*(2), 81–82. https://doi.org/10.1177/10253823070140021703

Meyer, S. B., Edge, S. S., Beatty, J., Leatherdale, S., Perlman, C., Dean, J., et al. (2018). Challenges to evidence-based health promotion: A case study of a food security Coalition in Ontario, Canada. *Health Promotion International, 33*(5), 760–769. https://doi.org/10.1093/heapro/dax011

Mignolo, W. D., & Walsh, C. E. (2018). *On decoloniality: Concepts, analytics, praxis*. Duke University Press Books.

Minowa, E., Watanabe, H. A. W., Nascimento, F. A., Andrade, E. A., Oliveira, S. C., & Westphal, M. F. (2017). Contribution of universities to the revision of the National Health Promotion Policy / Contribuição das universidades na revisão da Política Nacional de Promoção da Saúde. *Saúde e Sociedade, 26*(4), 973–986.

Moysés, S. T., & Sá, R. F. (2014). Planos locais de promoção da saúde: intersetorialidade(s) construída(s) no território. *Ciência & Saúde Coletiva, 19*(11), 4323–4330.

Moysés, S. J., Moysés, S. T., & Krempel, M. C. (2004). Avaliando o processo de construção de políticas públicas de promoção de saúde: a experiência de Curitiba. *Ciência & Saúde Coletiva, 9*(3), 627–641.

Mukamana, O., & Johri, M. (2016). What is known about school-based interventions for health promotion and their impact in developing countries? A scoping review of the literature. *Health Education Research, 31*(5), 587–602. https://doi.org/10.1093/her/cyw040

Nascimento, P. R., Westphal, M. F., Moreira, R. S., Baltar, V. T., Moysés, S. T., Zioni, F., et al. (2014). Impact of the social agendas-agenda 21 and healthy cities-upon social determinants of health in Brazilian municipalities: Measuring the effects of diffuse social policies through the dimensions of the millennium development goals. *Revista Brasileira de Epidemiologia, 17*, 01–14.

Pan American Health Organization. (1996). *Health promotion: An anthology*. PAHO.

Perú. Ministerio de Salud, Dirección General de las Personas, & Proyecto AMARES (Eds.). (2006). *Participatory evaluation guide for healthy municipalities and communities / Guía de evaluación participativa para municipios y comunidades saludables*. MINSA.

Pluye, P., Bengoechea, E. G., Granikov, V., Kaur, N., & Tang, D. L. (2018). A world of possibilities in mixed methods: Review of the combinations of strategies used to integrate qualitative and quantitative phases, results and data. *The International Journal of Multiple Research Approaches, 10*(1), 41–56.

Porto, M. F. (2019a). Crisis of utopias and the four justices: Ecologies, epistemologies and social emancipation for reinventing public health. *Ciência & Saúde Coletiva, 24*(12), 4449–4458. https://doi.org/10.1590/1413-812320182412.25292019

Porto, M. F. (2019b). Emancipatory promotion of health: Contributions from Brazil in the context of the global South. *Health Promotion International, 34*(Supplement_1), i56–i64. https://doi.org/10.1093/heapro/day086

Potvin, L., McQueen, D. V., Hall, M., Salaza, L., Anderson, L. M., & Hartz, Z. M. A. (Eds.). (2009). *Health promotion evaluation practices in the Americas*. Springer.

Rice, M., & Franceschini, M. C. (2009). The participatory evaluation of healthy municipalities, cities and communities initiatives in the Americas. In L. Potvin, D. V. McQueen, M. Hall, L. D. Salaza, L. M. Anderson, & Z. M. A. Hartz (Eds.), *Health promotion evaluation practices in the Americas* (pp. 221–236). Springer.

Rocabado, F., Cambría, C., & Ruiz, R. (2005). *Guía de evaluación participativa para municipios y comunidades saludables*. Organización Panamericana de la Salud.

Rocha, D. G., Alexandre, V. P., Marcelo, V. C., Rezende, R., Nogueira, J. D., & Franco de Sá, R. (2014). The review process of the National Health Promotion Policy: Simultaneous multiple movements/ Processo de revisão da Política Nacional de Promoção da Saúde: múltiplos movimentos simultâneos. *Ciência & Saúde Coletiva, 19*(11), 4313–4322.

Sá, R. F., & Moysés, S. T. (2009). O processo avaliativo em promoção de saúde como estratégia de empoderamento e de desenvolvimento de capacidades / The evaluation process in health promotion as a strategy for empowerment and capacity development. *Boletim Técnico Do Senac, 35*(2), 28–35.

Sá, R. F., Rezende, R., Akerman, M., Freire Mdo, S., Salles, R. P., & Moyses, S. T. (2016). Author-actors and organizational and relational processes in the review of the National Health Promotion Policy. *Ciência & Saúde Coletiva, 21*(6), 1707–1716. https://doi.org/10.1590/1413-81232015216.06742016

Santos, B. S. (2014). *Epistemologies of the South: Justice against epistemicide*. Routledge.

Santos, B. S., & Meneses, M. P. (Eds.). (2013). *Epistemologies of the South [Epistemologias do Sul]*. Cortez.

Santos, B. S., & Meneses, M. P. (Eds.). (2019). *Knowledges born in the struggle: Constructing the epistemologies of the global South (Epistemologies of the South)*. Routledge.

Schwarzman, J., Bauman, A., Gabbe, B. J., Rissel, C., Shilton, T., & Smith, B. J. (2019). Understanding the factors that influence health promotion evaluation: The development and validation of the evaluation practice analysis survey. *Evaluation and Program Planning, 74*, 76–83. https://doi.org/10.1016/j.evalprogplan.2019.03.002

South, J. (2014). Health promotion by communities and in communities: Current issues for research and practice. *Scandinavian Journal of Public Health, 42*(15 Suppl), 82–87. https://doi.org/10.1177/1403494814545341

Sperandio, A. M. G., Francisco Filho, L. L., & Mattos, T. P. (2016). Política de promoção da saúde e planejamento urbano: articulações para o desenvolvimento da cidade saudável. *Ciência & Saúde Coletiva, 21*(6), 1931–1938.

Super, S., Wagemakers, M. A., Picavet, H. S., Verkooijen, K. T., & Koelen, M. A. (2016). Strengthening sense of coherence: Opportunities for theory building in health promotion. *Health Promotion International, 31*(4), 869–878. https://doi.org/10.1093/heapro/dav071

Tavares, M. (2009). Epistemologies of the South [Epistemologias do Sul]. *Revista Lusófona de Educação, 13*, 183–189.

Tremblay, M. C., Richard, L., Brousselle, A., & Beaudet, N. (2013). How can both the intervention and its evaluation fulfill health promotion principles? An example from a professional development program. *Health Promotion Practice, 14*(4), 563–571. https://doi.org/10.1177/1524839912462030

Viacava, F., Porto, S. M., Carvalho, C. C., & Bellido, J. G. (2019). Health inequalities by region and social group based on data from household surveys (Brazil, 1998-2013). *Ciência & Saúde Coletiva, 24*(7), 2745–2760. https://doi.org/10.1590/1413-81232018247.15812017

Victora, C. G., Habicht, J.-P., & Bryce, J. (2004). Evidence-based public health: Moving beyond randomized trials. *American Journal of Public Health, 94*(3), 400–405. https://doi.org/10.2105/AJPH.94.3.400

Wallerstein, N. (2018). Prefácio. In R. F. D. Toledo, T. E. D. C. Rosa, T. M. Keinert, & C. T. Cortizo (Eds.), *Pesquisa participativa em saúde: Vertentes e veredas / participatory research in health: Slopes and paths* (pp. 11–26). Instituto de Saúde.

Wallerstein, N., & Duran, B. (2006). Using community-based participatory research to address health disparities. *Health Promotion Practice, 7*(3), 312–323. https://doi.org/10.1177/1524839906289376

Wallerstein, N., Duran, B., Oetzel, J. G., & Minkler, M. (2017a). *Community-based participatory research for health: Advancing social and health equity*. Jossey-Bass Wiley.

Wallerstein, N., Giatti, L. L., Bogus, C. M., Akerman, M., Jacobi, P. R., de Toledo, R. F., et al. (2017b). Shared participatory research principles and methodologies: Perspectives from the USA and Brazil-45 years after Paulo Freire's "Pedagogy of the oppressed". *Societies (Basel), 7*(2). https://doi.org/10.3390/soc7020006

Wallerstein, N., Duran, B., Oetzel, J. G., & Minkler, M. (Eds.). (2018). *Community-based participatory research for health: Advancing social and health equity*. Jossey-Bass.

Wallerstein, N., Calhoun, K., Eder, M., Kaplow, J., & Wilkins, C. H. (2019). Engaging the community: Community-based participatory research and team science. In *Strategies for team science success* (pp. 123–134). Springer.

Wallerstein, N., Oetzel, J. G., Sanchez-Youngman, S., Boursaw, B., Dickson, E., Kastelic, S., et al. (2020). Engage for equity: A long-term study of community-based participatory research and community-engaged research practices and outcomes. *Health Education & Behavior, 47*(3), 380–390.

Westphal, M. F., & Franceschini, M. C. T. (2016). A contribuição do CEPEDOC Para a construção da Política de Promoção da Saúde no Brasil / the contribution of CEPEDOC to the development of the Brazilian health promotion policy. *Ciência & Saúde Coletiva, 21*(6), 1819–1828.

Westphal, M. F., Fernandez, J. C. A., Nascimento, P. R., Zioni, F., André, L. M., Mendes, R., et al. (2013). Práticas democráticas participativas na construção de agendas sociais de desenvolvimento em municípios do sudeste brasileiro. *Ambiente & Sociedade, 16*(2), 103–128.

World Health Organization Regional Office for Europe, W. H. O. (1998). *Health promotion evaluation: Recommendations to policymakers*. WHO, European Working Group on Health Promotion Evaluation.

Chapter 48
Researching a Diverse Epistemic Social Movement: The Challenges and Rewards of European Healthy Cities Realist Synthesis

Evelyne de Leeuw

48.1 Introduction: Engaged Health Promotion Research in Dynamic Epistemic Communities

When the Ottawa Charter for Health Promotion was developed in the early 1980s and formalised at the eponymous conference in 1986, two global networks of systems change for health had already started to emerge. One was Health Promoting Schools with its roots in the European Health Behaviour in School Children effort (e.g., Currie et al., 2009) and the Americas health education in schools programmes (e.g., Connell et al., 1985). The other was Healthy Cities, a focus variously attributed to 1960s pioneering work by Len Duhl (1963) and 1980s celebrations in Toronto (Hancock, 2017). They both saw the urban social, human, and ecological environment as systems in their own right, with an ability to take on health promotion endeavours much better than other jurisdictions and institutions. Simultaneously, an emphasis on local primary health around the world (from barefoot doctors in Asia to *Sistemas Locales de Salud SILOS* in the Americas – e.g., Paganini & Chorny, 1990) facilitated a more diverse and bespoke re-casting of appropriate levels of health promotion. In this chapter, we will illustrate the consequences of the very nature of these endeavours for the quintessence of the research enterprise. Neither Health Promoting Schools, Healthy Cities, nor the premises of the Ottawa Charter were conceived as traditional experiments or trials. Rather, they were – and remain – dynamic networks that connect vast groupings of diverse institutions, actors, the events that they shape, and their contexts. Scholarship is part of these networks, but

E. de Leeuw (✉)
University of New South Wales, Liverpool, NSW, Australia

Healthy Urban Environments Collaboratory of Maridulu Budyari Gumal SPHERE, Sydney, NSW, Australia
e-mail: e.deleeuw@unsw.edu.au

L. Potvin, D. Jourdan (eds.), *Global Handbook of Health Promotion Research, Vol. 1*,
https://doi.org/10.1007/978-3-030-97212-7_48

so are activism, practice, and politics. The result of this dynamic complexity for health promotion research is that many scholarly efforts struggle to 'get things right': they reduce the immense interconnected landscape of the field to separate, disconnected elements that fit a more traditional (Cartesian) research paradigm.

Let's provide some context. The launch of the European Healthy Cities network in 1986–1987 was based on a tradition in social movement-driven urban health. It was originally conceived as a mere small-scale demonstration project of the Ottawa Charter for Health Promotion. The European Office of WHO anticipated to find a handful of cities across the region prepared to be challenged and show the benefits of a new approach to health promotion. Very soon, though, the enthusiasm and membership for the European effort exploded and was copied by cities and networks around the world. In the late 1980s and early 1990s, cities and networkS of cities adopting the European standards (e.g., Hancock & Duhl, 1986; Kickbusch, 1989; WHO, 1988) emerged from Australian states and territories and their cross-Tasman neighbors Aotearoa to Canadian provinces, Japan, Malaysia, and beyond.

A current count (de Leeuw, 2017; de Leeuw & Simos, 2017) claims over 15,000 'cities' around the world – from very small (~200 inhabitants at l'Isle-Aux-Grues) to very large (~24 million, Shanghai) – that in some way or other have signed up to the Healthy City vision. In Europe, the European Healthy Cities Network (HCN) consists of 'designated' cities (following a process of meeting specific membership requirements) and 'accredited' National Networks (supporting larger groups of mostly nation-based local governments). HCN operates in Phases since its inception in 1986. Each Phase lasts ~5 years and pursues specific, commonly agreed, objectives and parameters. Phases have been evaluated with increasingly sophisticated methodological and theoretical toolboxes (de Leeuw & Green, 2017). Here we present the perspective of Phase V (2009–2013).

48.2 Healthy Cities: Urban Health Promotion as an Epistemic Repository and Resource

48.2.1 Situating Healthy Cities

European Healthy Cities Phase V – like the previous and following phases – are communities of local governments and their constituent agents and communities, across WHO/EURO's 53 member states. Each of these (social; policy; epistemic) communities has its own unique jurisdictions, responsibilities, accountabilities, and governance arrangements for health. For instance, Goumans (1998) compared five Dutch with five United Kingdom networks in Healthy Cities and found radically diverging network shapes and connections. This is of course no surprise. Like wine, cities have their unique 'terroir' and are driven by ecologically, historically, socially, culturally, and politically unique developments. To account and control for some of this diversity, in Europe for each HCN Phase cities with WHO and their elected representatives jointly establish a set of designation and accreditation criteria. These align with the priorities set for the European Region of WHO – which generally apply to the international level. Our case study concerns Healthy Cities in their Phase V (2009-2013); by the close of this Phase in 2013, there were 99 designated European Healthy Cities.

The priorities of the WHO in each region, and therefore in Europe too, are set by its governance arrangement – in Europe and most other regions called the 'Regional Committee' (in the Americas, PAHO, it is the 'Pan American Sanitary Conference' and the 'Directing Council'). This regionalisation allows for a more direct response to unique issues and opportunities, and also creates different speeds and directions for priority policies. Within regions, there can be distinctive flavours to the priorities. For instance, in PAHO there are separate emphases on Latin America and the Caribbean. In WPRO (the Western Pacific) there is a focus on Pacific Islands in the Pacific Division – which therefore emphasises '*Healthy Islands*' over Healthy Cities. Where 'Healthy Cities' has consistently been a priority in Europe, it has been oddly absent from the agenda of the South-East Asian region (where densely urbanising population growth is a critical phenomenon for human and ecosystems health), and emerged as 'healthy urbanization[1]' in the Western Pacific region.

The dynamic nature of health and well-being in communities and local governments is both an intriguing policy, research, and practice area, as well as a cause of considerable headaches when one is trying to map and understand them – particularly comparatively.

In itself, the fact that WHO works directly with local governments is an ongoing governance challenge to the organisation. Cities, local and sub-national governments are not members of WHO – nation-states are. The interests of lower-level jurisdictions may therefore not necessarily be represented well by their national overlords (i.e., Ministries of Health). Fortunately, for most of the more than three decades of Healthy City operations in Europe, the WHO and its member states have seen a focus on lower levels of government and governance (including Healthy Regions)[2] as a beneficial strengthening of the reach of the agency. There is, however, nothing 'natural' about a global focus on local matters. At the time of writing this, the WHO European office seems to be retreating from its urban priority focus, though.

48.2.2 European Healthy Cities Priorities and Governance

The WHO European HCN shares vision, values, and an explicit commitment to good governance for health by local councils and their executive arms. Phase V had three core themes set within a framework of four overarching priorities and six strategic goals (Table 48.1).

[1] https://iris.wpro.who.int/handle/10665.1/6772

[2] https://www.euro.who.int/en/about-us/networks/regions-for-health-network-rhn

Table 48.1 Strategic priorities for the WHO European Healthy Cities Network Phase V (2009–2013)

Core themes	Priorities	Strategic goals
Caring and supportive environments	• To address the determinants of health, equity in health and the principles of health for all; • To integrate and promote European and global public health priorities; • To put health on the social and political agenda of cities; and • To promote good governance and integrated planning for health.	To promote policies and action for health and sustainable development at the local level and across the WHO European region, emphasising the determinants of health, people living in poverty, and the needs of vulnerable groups
		To strengthen the national standing of Healthy Cities in the context of policies for health development, public health, and urban regeneration, emphasising national-local cooperation
Healthy living		To generate policy and practice expertise, good evidence, knowledge and methods that can be used to promote health in all cities in the region
		To promote solidarity, cooperation, and working links between European cities and networks and with cities and networks participating in the Healthy Cities movement
Healthy urban environment and design		To play an active role in advocating for health at the European and global levels through partnerships with other agencies concerned with urban issues and networks of local authorities
		To increase the accessibility of the WHO European Healthy Cities Network to all Member States in the European region.

Based on the experience of the previous four Phases, there were also ten operational standards for managing and developing Healthy Cities successfully (Fig. 48.1) – they are part of the designation process assessment, and candidate cities have to demonstrate that they have resources, principles, and governance in place to meet the ten directives. Some of these were deeply pragmatic (such as a designated Healthy City having access to appropriate ICT facilities), others enforcing some of the essential elements of engagement (a requirement to attend Mayoral meetings) or aspirational (network development and capacity building). As de Leeuw and Skovgaard (2005) have observed the designation process itself possibly set the parameters for the success of a Healthy City more than the actual work as a member of the particular Phase.

Considering the diversity of governance for health arrangements across 53 European countries, and differences even between sub-national entities (e.g., oblasts in Russia; autonomous regions in Spain; conglomerates of local authorities in Sweden, cf. Green, 1998) an evaluation of the accomplishment and impacts of European Healthy Cities required a novel approach.

In earlier Phases, the network of cities and their governance arrangements, as well as WHO, had agreed to a more permanent framework to record and account for local priorities, changes, impacts, and outcomes. This MARI (Monitoring;

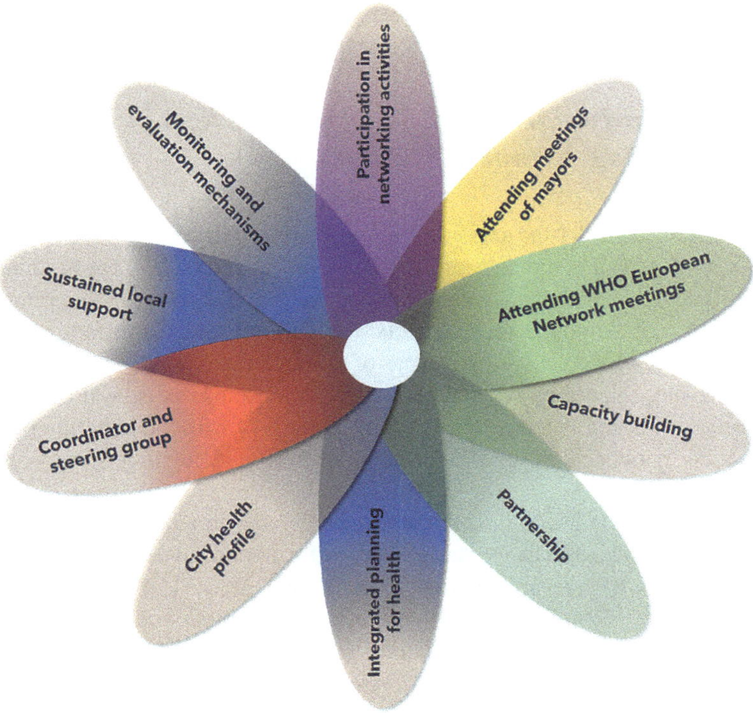

Fig. 48.1 Operational requirements ('prerequisites') for designation as a European WHO Healthy City. Reprinted from *Healthy cities: Promoting health and equity – evidence for local policy and practice. Summary evaluation of Phase V of the WHO European Healthy Cities Network*, de Leeuw, et al. (ed). p. 2, © World Health Organization 2014

Accountability; Reporting; Impact) approach consisted of a grid with about 140 questions that hinged on designation parameters and established models of good practice (cf. Table 48.1 and Fig. 48.1) and allowed member cities to self-select emphases in their assessments. A shorter, snappier, and between WHO and city delegates mutually negotiated, version of the MARI system was the Annual Reporting Template (ART) with twelve items that each city committed to address each year (the full system, its background, and development parameters is reported in de Leeuw, 2009).

Heritage and Green (2013) reviewed these mechanisms and identified the European Healthy Cities Network at the supranational as well as local level as an elite epistemic community. Combined with findings from research into Phase III of the effort (that city networks produce superior policy outcomes – Camagni & Capello, 2004) the design of an assessment mechanism for Phase V had to recognise the strength and importance of dynamic networking at every glocal level of Healthy City activity.

48.3 Context, Conflict, and Comparison: The Birth of Healthy City Realist Synthesis

48.3.1 Driven Toward a New Research Paradigm in Inclusive Epistemic Networks

The research team, under the aegis of WHO and with the blessing of cities and their networks, engaged in some substantial innovation in research – not on cities and their health processes, but in generating meaningful knowledge. Stepping away from the Cartesian paradigm that connects sets of distinctive variables in causal and final ways, we embraced evolving notions of research meaning and scope in a local, context-relevant, and policy-responsive way. We connected realist evaluation and an empirically networked version of it ('realist synthesis') with the adoption of policy and practice networks as co-producers and users of intelligence ('epistemic communities').

Let's start with the latter. In the last section, we described the foundation principles and umbrella governance arrangements for European Healthy Cities. Each (Healthy) City is unique and part of an epistemic network. Haas (1989, 1992) defined epistemic communities as "*networks of professionals with recognised expertise and competence in a particular domain and an authoritative claim to policy relevant knowledge within that domain or issue-area.*" In our conversations with a broad spectrum of stakeholders, we saw that WHO Healthy Cities are much more than an elite professional knowledge community. The tenets and governance drivers of European Healthy Cities demonstrate and sustain a view of the epistemic community as embracing an inclusive view of policy process engagement. Not only professionals lay authoritative claims on managing a subject domain, but rather citizens, enterprises, interest groups, and institutions have a key role in shaping, validating, and sustaining network knowledge generation and utilisation (in this case, for health promotion). There is a vast suite of commitments, pursuits, and prerequisites for the European network of cities. A critical part of the network is a highly bureaucratic, chronically underfunded, and politically embroiled World Health Organization (Lee, 2014).

Member cities hail from political and governance systems that cover anything on the welfare state typology spectrum (Esping-Andersen, 1990) and beyond, and they have varying degrees of control over the social, political, and commercial determinants of health (e.g., some cities run hospital systems; others do not have control over hospitals but run public transport; etc.). Some of these cities were very early adopters of the Healthy City paradigm and joined in 1986 thus becoming 'seasoned operators'. Others were actively pursued by (national or language based) city networks and WHO to sign up, for geopolitical or other reasons. Within this dynamic context, there also was a rolling system of 'old' cities being re-designated and 'new' cities designated throughout the life of the Phase (Fig. 48.2).

Our conceptualisation of epistemic community therefore also includes dynamic policy context and its shifting (interest and policy framing) networks.

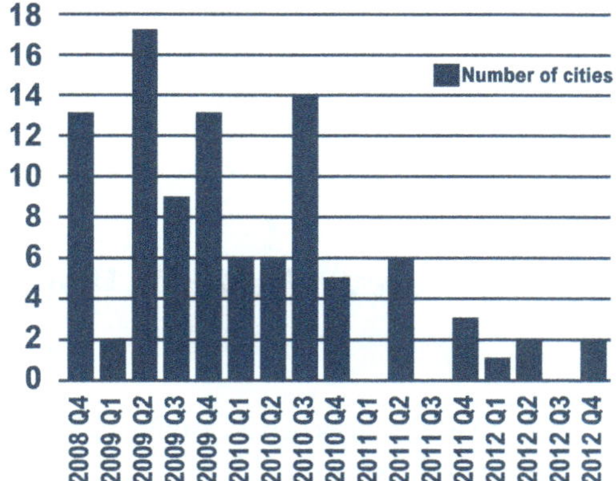

Fig. 48.2 Designation of members: a continuous process (number of cities designated in Phase V, by quarter) (Reprinted from de Leeuw et al., 2014, p. 3, © World Health Organization 2014)

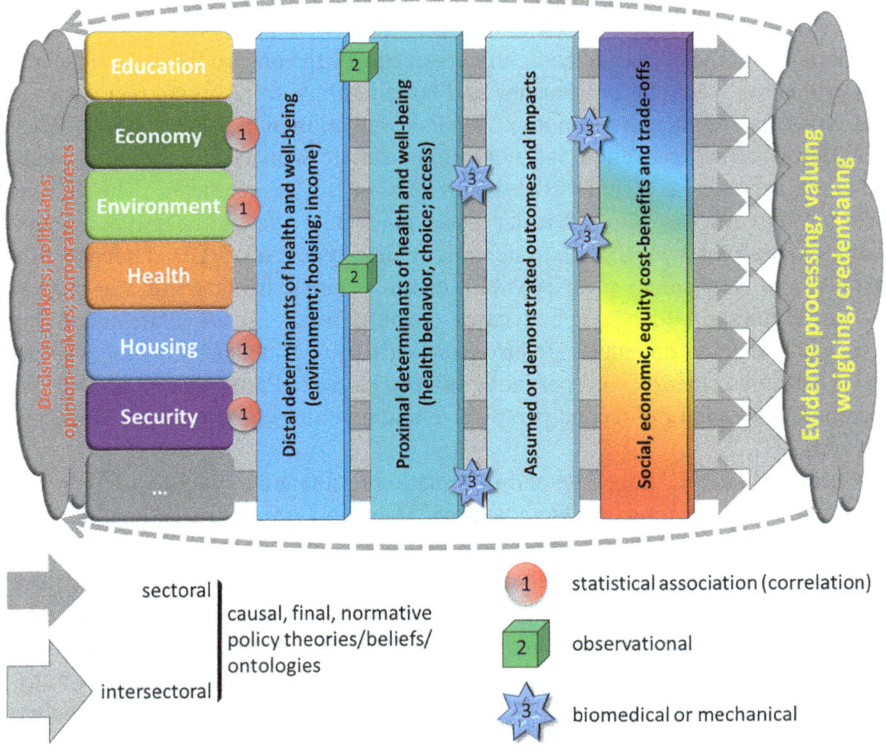

Fig. 48.3 Developing an evidence-based approach to city public health planning and investment in Europe (DECiPHEr) adapted programme logic (Adapted from Whitfield et al., 2013. CC BY 2.0)

Unlike a research paradigm where everything is accounted for, and where a specific moment in time is designated to be the official start point (T_0) of a particular intervention which is then measured at T_1 and so on, our research necessarily became looped, iterative and dynamic.

48.3.2 *"We Don't Want More Problems; We Want More Solutions."*

'Realist synthesis' as a methodological heuristic aligns with our view of epistemic communities. WHO/EURO and the network of cities agreed to a process in which the terms of reference and projected outcomes and outputs of an evaluation effort were transparently negotiated and responsively framed. The dynamic nature (and rolling designation process) of priorities, values, themes, and strategic expressions required a deeply responsive and negotiated evaluation paradigm. Over a period of 2 years, an immersed team of 15 WHO advisors negotiated with and trained city-based operators who attended so-called Business Meetings (these include lead local politicians, technical personnel, and members of the community).

Members of the epistemic community voiced a deep concern that more research and evaluation would be burdensome and not contribute to resolving real issues in real cities for real health promotion. Realist evaluation as per Pawson and Tilley (1997) was considered alien and not commensurate with Healthy City agendas. Common ground was found in the deployment of 'realist synthesis'. This term is used in two ways: first, as a particular method in meta-evidence generation (synthesising existing knowledge in a systematic review-type manner), and second as a technique to amalgamate primary (field) research with existing sources of contextual and empirical evidence. In both cases, the purpose is '…to articulate underlying programme theories and then to interrogate the existing evidence to find out whether and where these theories are pertinent and productive' (Pawson et al., 2004). We specifically adopted the second perspective that combines field research with desk research.

Cities had been feeding data and information to a range of agencies within and outside the network for a considerable time. They were tired of repeating that exercise. They told the evaluation team that they'd love to be evaluated, but only on issues that mattered, and not for the sake of data crunching. Also, they let the team know in no uncertain terms that for health committed workers at the coalface a lot of the evidence was already crystal clear. For instance, physical activity is healthy. Facilities to promote active transport (e.g., bicycle lanes and parking; public transport with appropriate shelters; canopy for shade and protection against weather; etc.) would therefore be reasonably clearly linked to health outcomes. The questions that Healthy Cities struggled with had very little to do with these (health and disease) epidemiological evidence bases, but everything with political expediency and values such as equity, access, and universal proportionate policy. Or, as expressed

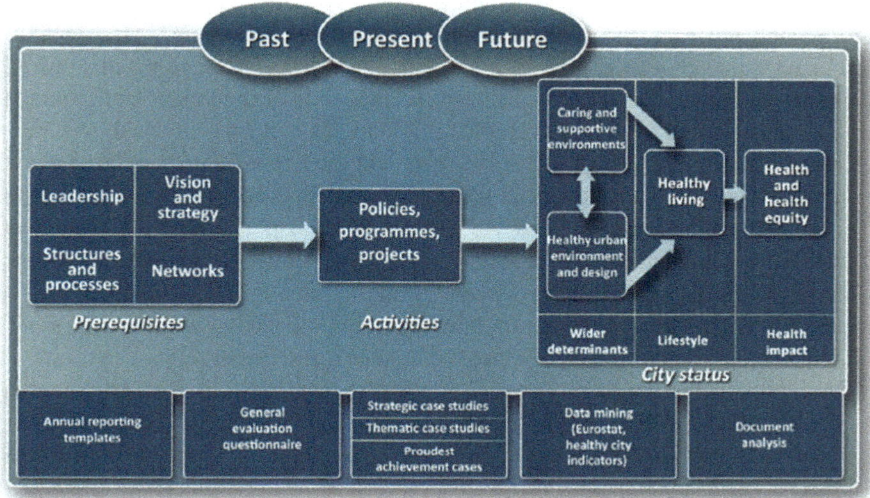

Fig. 48.4 Programme logic and data sources/processes for Healthy Cities Phase V realist synthesis (Reprinted from de Leeuw et al., 2014, p. 4, © World Health Organization 2014)

by Healthy City officials: "*We do not want more data. We want to know how to generate change for better health.*" They asked our mantra to be "We don't want more problems; we want more solutions."

The team, with WHO and cities, then considered that an effort needed to be made to (**a**) identify existing data and databases on health and its determinants at a most proximal geospatial level to city governance arrangements; and (**b**) to record and exploit those data in addition to other 'evidence' in order to support cities in relevant policy and political processes for better and more equitable health. We compiled a fact file from existing documentary evidence (de Leeuw et al., 2015a). We adapted the DECiPHEr (*Developing an evidence-based approach to city public health planning and investment in Europe*) programme logic (Whitfield et al., 2013) to allow for the 'plugging in' of pre-existing context-relevant evidence.

Our version of the full programme logic of the ultimate realist synthetic approach is found in Fig. 48.4.

48.4 Negotiated Realist Synthesis Leads to Ultra-High Response Rates

The negotiation of evaluation parameters is not a new thing. In fact, Guba and Lincoln (1989) see negotiated evaluations as a necessarily superior next evolutionary step in evaluation approaches. In our case, the model that we landed on (a) respected the needs of different stakeholders locally, nationally, in Europe, and globally; (b) addressed the complex interrelations between local realities and needs, existing evidence base, varied local policy priorities, and high-level aspirations; (c) minimised the need of local original quantitative health research and yet maximised community engagement and 'stories from the field side of the binoculars'; and (d) served management needs of WHO/EURO, and the network of Healthy Cities against evidence needs of local communities and their representatives. De Leeuw et al. (2015a) report validated quality measures on the larger project – aggregate response rates are shown in Table 48.2. Such high response rates in, and user-friendliness assessments of, the negotiated approach validate these four dimensions of the model. But this type of realist synthesis also means that we spent as much time talking with, listening to, and appreciating local knowledge and practices as we did in actual data collection from a range of sources, and constructing deliverables.

Conceptually and practically the effort was a gargantuan task. Recognising that we would not have budget for fieldwork in nearly 100 cities across Europe we had to make best use of opportunities at annual 'Healthy City Network Business Meetings'. These are sessions integral to the designation prerequisites (Fig. 48.1) – Healthy City political leadership (typically Mayors or otherwise elected Councillors), bureaucrats and managers, and often community representatives attend these large gatherings and mix with expert keynote speakers. At these Business Meetings, the evaluation team ran data and evaluation capacity-building workshops and case-study writing master classes. We negotiated local government data access through Eurostat and other sources and combined these with analyses from other already available hard and soft data. Together (in a process of virtual stakeholder, conceptual and methodological triangulations) they shaped a new, utilitarian, evidence base.

The return on these investments was overwhelming. Response rates for the various data collection mechanisms were 65% and above, and on some parameters in the highest percentile (See Table 48.2; for the different data tools, see lowest row in Fig. 48.4; de Leeuw et al., 2015b). We were conscious of the possibility that these responses might be rigged, or biased in a number of ways (e.g., toward social desirability; in a type of trade-off prisoners' dilemma; or as a mechanism in delayed gratification with a perception that participation would create favourable conditions for WHO perks). In order to assess the quality and truthfulness of the response packages, we performed a range of quality assessments. These included analyses by geopolitical dimension, welfare state type, membership of the network, city size, and network density (de Leeuw et al., 2015b). In none of these we found any

Table 48.2 Response rate (%) for three data collection tools

Annual reporting template		General evaluation questionnaire	Case studies	
2010	87	72	Thematic	67
2011	79			
2012	67		Strategic	69
2013	72			

Reprinted from de Leeuw et al., 2014, p. 5, © World Health Organization 2014 untoward aberrations, suggesting that not only data *quantity* was high, but also that there was a significant degree of *quality* (reliability).

48.5 A High-Intensity Effort

In the negotiated realist synthesis process, we made it clear that all stakeholders explicitly were considered members of the research team. City elected representatives, managers, members of civil society, local academics, stray statisticians, and others were invited to actively engage in data production and processing. Within this very large group, there was a smaller team (cf. the full authorship of de Leeuw et al., 2015c) that coordinated data collection, maintained integrity of databases, and provided feedback to individual city stakeholders. General oversight of the effort was provided by EdL under the guidance of the WHO Healthy Cities Officer Mariana Dyakova, two full-time research assistants, a data manager, and a WHO executive administrator (the incomparable Connie Petersen). Together, they generated large 'Mother Reports' in the general domains of the Phase V Programme Logic – the upper part of Fig. 48.4. These 'Mother Reports' contained all data (and where necessary hyperlinks to external databases) for a particular domain of interest (Table 48.1 and Fig. 48.1). Such encyclopaedic Mother Reports were developed for, for instance, *Caring and Supportive Environments*, but also around *Integrated Planning for Health*. The formulation of bespoke and context-rich research question was then developed with cities and WHO and then, research staff. This involved discussion of data availability and resource requirements, and feedback to/with the epistemic community on how stakeholders might assist.

For instance, one team responded to cities' request to focus on age-friendly environments, and brought on board an Italian Healthy City operator, a WHO bureaucrat, a scholar in the area of ageing, and a Phase V evaluation team member. The team subsequently formulated a research question and interrogated the Mother Reports for relevant data. This led to the drafting of a manuscript for peer-reviewed publication (Jackisch et al., 2015).

In this process once again, we were concerned about any data manipulation, blind spots, inconsistencies, etc. For that reason, we cross-assessed the reporting and analysis process with each of the teams. No significant issues were found, although every single participant in the process observed that the wealth of data did not do full justice to the frugality of just one published output. It appears that our approach to realist synthesis may have created a relatively vast data cemetery.

48.6 Data Generation, Diversity, and Episteme

Data from 99 cities in the WHO European Healthy Cities Network and 31 national networks of Healthy Cities[3] were collected on all elements of the programme logic by means of five instruments.

Cities' ongoing reporting requirement on designation criteria is implemented through ART (the Annual Reporting Template). In the wrap-up of the Phase, WHO/EURO had a need to explore and document strengths and weaknesses of its urban efforts in Europe. For internal management and leadership quality assurance, they needed to know whether their operations were compliant with WHO internal processes. To generate information on its management of the programme, responses at city level, and gauging local dynamics that might have influenced active participation in the network, a General Evaluation Questionnaire was developed (and validated through pre-testing) based on a theory-based programme logic (cf Birckmayer & Weiss, 2000). Theory-based evaluation does not just allow for identification *that* a change has occurred in the phenomenon under study, but in its optimum form also *why* and *how*. Interestingly, this was also a critical request by cities that the programme responded to.

Finally, in original data generation, we formulated a framework for compiling case studies from cities that enabled the theory-based documentation of stages of development in the life of Healthy Cities – but with recognition of the unique contexts and expectations of each. Ideally, the team would have immersed itself and taken time to craft these case studies. Across 99 cities in Europe, this was, understandably, an effort that was beyond the available resources. We took advantage of the annual Business Meetings and spent time with city delegations and trained them to compile their own case study material in a standard, staged, programmatic and responsive format (i.e., they could send in the material and the team would reflexively engage with the city representatives to more fully detail the case). Two broad areas were to be covered: thematic case studies (columns 1 and 2 in Table 48.1), and strategic case studies (column 3), where 'thematic' intended to explore a particular health or population *issue or intervention*. 'Strategic' case studies were to look at longer-range *systems change, policy development, and political and social agenda setting*. Training sessions at the Business Meetings allowed for fine-tuning and clarification, also because many city delegations did not speak English (the lingua franca of the HCN and therefore our evaluation effort). Translation efforts to identify and validate critical constructs followed a standard protocol (e.g., Behr & Shishido, 2016).

As reported before, response rates for each of these tools were considerable, particularly against acceptable norms in qualitative research (see Cook et al. (2000), although these authors also argue – in line with our approach – that representativeness is more important than response).

[3] Processed and reported separately in Janss Lafond, 2015

The team compiled large data sets with quantitative indicators mined from Eurostat and other national statistics collections not included in the Eurostat database. These include WHO/EURO member states beyond the European Union, but not many Central-Asian nation-states which emerged out of the demise of the Soviet Union, see Alastalo, 2018. We also re-assessed 'designation packages' (the materials candidate Healthy Cities sent to WHO/EURO for assessment of membership eligibility). Where necessary and/or prudent, we pursued additional clarification material that was either actively sought in online repositories, or provided voluntarily (as progress reports) by designated cities.

Data were entered in standard software packages for quantitative (SPSS) and qualitative (NVivo) analysis. The raw and semi-processed material was made available to research partners for further investigation on a secure website that had a wide search operability. We negotiated and established six interdisciplinary data analysis and writing teams to interrogate the overall data set; they composed six Mother Reports (policy and governance; healthy urban environment and design; caring and supportive environments; health and active living; national Healthy Cities networks in Europe; and health and equity) which were then presented and benchmarked during a 2-day workshop in the WHO Office in Copenhagen.

It was our every intent to also develop bespoke reports on the entire Phase V designation criteria and prerequisites suite of information to each individual city. This is what they requested, and the team felt that it was a moral and functional obligation to support their efforts toward achieving Phase V goals through the provision of a unique document that was tailored to particular local needs. Unfortunately, the team ran out of time, capacity and resources to provide this important last stage in the realist synthesis evaluation cycle (de Leeuw et al., 2015c).

48.7 Discussion: Five Dimensions of Realist Synthesis Health Promotion Research

What can be learned from this lengthy and complex case study in realist synthesis?

We deployed a vast and complex, negotiated research programme across 99 cities in Europe on a shoestring budget. There have been successes and failures in the work. In wrapping up, I focus on (a) resourcing of realist synthesis; (b) the *deployment and fidelity of methods* in a realist synthesis approach; (c) some *moral and ethical* considerations; (d) considerations of *outcome and impact*; and (e) the *future of the epistemic community*.

It is clear that the negotiated process of realist synthesis requires significant resources. However, there was no remuneration for any of the team members directly from WHO or Healthy Cities for this work. Designated Healthy Cities themselves provide an annual payment into the network to finance practical coordination capacity; yet, this was not necessarily earmarked for supporting evaluation. The evaluation officer dedicated by WHO was on a public health secondment supported by the UK National Health Service; her workload included other commitments in WHO policy development and programme support; although a keen and intelligent thinker she did not necessarily avail of the required theoretical and methodological mindset for high-level realist synthesis management, and (intellectual) capacity-building necessarily became part of the research process. Three interns (Australian La Trobe University Master of Public Health students; one Deakin University medical student) provided unpaid research support above and beyond what could have been expected. Evaluation coordination and engagement were provided through in-kind compensation by WHO of travel and accommodation costs; no per diem payments or honorariums could be provided. Essentially, this massive evaluation exercise was run out of the goodness of heart of a bunch of committed individuals that had known most of each other for many years, feeling obliged to support evidence-based evolution of Healthy Cities values.

These 'soft' commitments (as opposed to research-institutionally funded and accountably managed research positions) naturally created particular issues in the research process. First of all, there was little or no opportunity to steer the process through the allocation of incentives, and research organisation (concordant with realist synthesis values) mostly consisted of 'management by substance' rather than directive governance. In a 'management by substance' research approach the unique content expertise of the team member is acknowledged and supported – it is then up to the team member's personal style and preferences to craft the reporting. For instance – in the collection of peer-reviewed papers published in https://academic.oup.com/heapro/issue/30/suppl_1 all papers are co-authored by interdisciplinary team members, bar one (Grant, 2015). In the spirit of realist synthesis, we had not anticipated single-authored pieces to come out of the process. Also, with an absence of distinct remuneration and (resource and bureaucratic) accountability, projectitis affected programmatic continuity. Once the internal brief for WHO was published (de Leeuw et al., 2014) and the collection of peer-reviewed papers delivered, the project ceased.

Through realist synthesis, and driven by evaluees' – negotiated – expectations, we deployed a rich toolbox of methods and data collection mechanisms. Some of the personnel involved had greater strength in some areas than in others. There was a significant challenge in maintaining a good overview of the entire process and the activities that its elements were involved in. Oversight of the project was based in Australia, with the operational management in Europe. A data management arm was run out of California. Not only the difference in time zones but also the diversity of scholarly, socio-cultural, bureaucratic, and even seniority grounding of the team members created research management challenges. Ultimately, the effort delivered on important parts of the realist promise. However, the negotiated and evolutionary nature of the exercise continuously challenged overall integrity, direction, and maintenance of scholarly momentum. In hindsight, stricter operational monitoring and control mechanisms might have been useful and would have delivered even better outcomes.

The team and diverse stakeholders (WHO, cities' networks, member states) felt they jointly advanced knowledge significantly. The evidence base and methodologies for Healthy Cities were meaningfully enhanced. Drawbacks were that, although we had an enormous data set, we only scratched the surface of what is possible in Big Data synthesis. There is a server somewhere in Copenhagen, backed up somewhere in the cloud, that still vibrates with the promise of much more elegant processing of the raw data that the effort compiled. One reason that we could embark on this enormous research adventure is found in the availability of faster and more efficient ICT systems. A next step, by necessity, is to bring the capacities of Big Data processing and dynamic dashboarding to the process. Good algorithms and data management should allow for this diverse network of stakeholders to instantly and real-time appreciate their status. This ought to create front-end visualisation ('infographics') of quantities and qualities. Boulos and Al-Shorbaji (2014) provide a first – perhaps overly technocratic – glance at what may be possible.

The above two observations (the dynamic and complex nature of research management; and data challenges) must be placed into another context that I have not discussed: moral and ethical considerations of such vast, negotiated processes across many stakeholders, jurisdictions, and data mines. A critical reader of the outputs from the Phase V realist synthesis evaluation will note that nowhere there is mention of an approval by a research ethics office. Guided by WHO bureaucrats and the implicit approval of Healthy City operators, the evaluation team worked on the assumption that the research exercise was ethically and morally sound. WHO/EURO's position, furthermore, suggested that as we were engaged in a quality improvement process, rigorous ethics clearance might not have been required. Such assertions can, and should, of course be challenged. Edwards et al. (2012) have documented the problems, barriers, and unconscionable differences in achieving ethics clearance for research across different jurisdictions. The realist synthesis approach across different levels and types of stakeholders adds an additional challenge.

Did we accomplish the impact that we aimed for? We ran this project mostly for a practice-oriented audience (WHO; cities; communities). We published twelve papers in the international peer-reviewed literature, and three public records through WHO. The realist synthesis approach, and its process and outcomes, has been the subject of at least half a dozen conference sessions. There is, however, very little '*evidence*' that the effort has made any difference. 'Did it make a difference?' has been elevated as the key research question in recent perspectives on impact evaluation (Vaessen et al., 2016). Praise from Healthy Cities and the high participation rates suggest we did make a difference. There is, however, not a shred of measurement and evidence that our realist synthesis evaluation has made a difference, without undertaking another round of assessment.

Establishing the relevance, value, output, and impact of – co-produced – research remains the Holy Grail of current academia. Many academies and their sponsors maintain a dangerously navel-staring attitude to these issues. Impact Factors, authorship, competitive grant income are the presumed hard proxies of 'good research'. But impact cannot and should not be measured by dud metrics such as 'impact factor', or 'H-value'– all rather incestuous measures within elite epistemic communities (Leydesdorff et al., 2016). Greenhalgh et al. (2016) present a comprehensive narrative review of research impact models and their metrics – including a realist synthesis approach. But surprisingly, almost all of the models are generated and maintained by the professionals in the elite epistemic communities that dominate scholarship. 'Those affected', or the local institutional and individual agents where impact is needed, are hardly ever party to the establishment of impact parameters. There is a 'Google Scholar' to document scientific output – but when will the 'Google Policy' be launched that shows how, and how many, policies are adopting the evidence and impact generated by high-quality, joined-up, relevant, and responsive synthetic (social) research?

Finally, a reflection on the notion of 'epistemic communities'. In this piece I more or less casually adopted this concept to describe a network of actors, agents, and structures (even virtual ones) that share sets of normative values and principles; share beliefs about the causal relations in their world; trust that there is purpose and validity to their actions; and are willing to create and deploy knowledge for a 'higher' policy or social change purpose (Haas, 1989). Antoniades (2003) has dug deep into defining and critiquing different levels of these epistemic communities. He traces the origin of the idea to a Foucauldian perspective on 'episteme'. But Foucault, in line with tenets of ancient Greek philosophers, also advocated the use of parrhesia ('truth-telling', cf Dyrberg, 2014). Episteme and parrhesia are but two of five ancient 'ways of knowing' (the others are techne (mastery of art and skill); phronesis (good judgment); and sophia (wisdom). As such the idea of 'epistemic' community is at the potential detriment of other forms of knowing and knowledge activism. Parrhesic communities should be as prominent as the mere epistemic ones – let's legitimise 'speaking truth to power' and not merely claim episteme (factfulness – cf Rosling et al., 2018) as the purview of professional knowledge entrepreneurs. Impact and action ought to be our end game.

48.8 Synthetic Health Promotion

We described a highly complex and dynamic situation that merited a particular, and strongly conceptualised, health promotion research methodology. Healthy City networks (and other very large health promotion efforts across different jurisdictions) seem exquisitely well suited to realist synthesis. Does this mean that this must be the 'go-to' paradigm for research in our field?

No. It clearly is an essential set of approaches in our overall toolbox. But landing on a particular approach like realist synthesis must be the result of clear reasoning and logical navigation of ontologies in research needs, opportunities, and sought-for outcomes. We mentioned Guba and Lincoln's Fourth Generation Evaluation (Guba & Lincoln, 1989) approach that stood at the basis of our work. It asserts that it is important to negotiate research and evaluation at every stage with all stakeholders. If European cities had landed on a consensus that more epidemiological research was needed into the drivers of obesity – this was precisely what we would have delivered. But they insisted on a sophisticated lens to learn from a vastly diverse network that is unified in a number of values and principles. Realist synthesis, both as a process and a deliverable, was the outcome of this particular negotiated reality.

We do not claim that such a lens or paradigm is necessarily the easiest to deploy, or that it delivers easy impact. Part of this problem lies in the very nature of the phenomenon that is under investigation. We constituted WHO European Healthy Cities as a particular form of epistemic community. By necessity, then, we had to respect and exploit the constituent parts of that network – the players, their roles, preferences, and histories. And their connections and ambitions. This complicated matters, but made the effort also much more enjoyable and rewarding. I wish on every researcher that they can be the immersed activist realism entrepreneur that we were allowed to be during our adventures.

References

Acuto, M. (2016). Give cities a seat at the top table. *Nature, 537*(7622), 611–613.

Alastalo, M. (2018). Eurostat: Making Europe commensurate and comparable. In *Policy design in the European Union* (pp. 87–110). Palgrave Macmillan.

Antoniades, A. (2003). Epistemic communities, epistemes and the construction of (world) politics. *Global Society, 17*(1), 21–38.

Behr, D., & Shishido, K. (2016). The translation of measurement instruments for crosscultural surveys. In C. Wolf, D. Joye, T. W. Smith, & Y. Fu (Eds.), *The SAGE handbook of survey methodology* (pp. 269–287). Sage.

Birckmayer, J. D., & Weiss, C. H. (2000). Theory-based evaluation in practice: What do we learn? *Evaluation Review, 24*(4), 407–431.

Boulos, M. N. K., & Al-Shorbaji, N. M. (2014). On the Internet of Things, smart cities and the WHO Healthy Cities. *International Journal of Health Geographics, 13*, 10.

Camagni, R., & Capello, R. (2004). The city network paradigm: theory and empirical evidence. *Contributions to Economic Analysis, 266*, 495–529.

Connell, D. B., Turner, R. R., & Mason, E. F. (1985). Summary of findings of the school health education evaluation: Health promotion effectiveness, implementation, and costs. *Journal of School Health, 55*(8), 316–321.

Cook, C., Heath, F., & Thompson, R. L. (2000). A meta-analysis of response rates in web-or internet-based surveys. *Educational and Psychological Measurement, 60*(6), 821–836.

Currie, C., Gabhainn, S. N., Godeau, E., & International HBSC Network Coordinating Committee. (2009). The Health Behaviour in School-aged Children: WHO Collaborative Cross-National (HBSC) study: Origins, concept, history and development 1982–2008. *International Journal of Public Health, 54*(2), 131–139.

Davidson, P., Bradbury, B., Wong, M., & Hill, T. (2020). *Inequality in Australia, Part 1: Overview*. Australian Council of Social Service and UNSW.

De Leeuw, E. (2009). Evidence for healthy cities: Reflections on practice, method and theory. *Health Promotion International, 24*(suppl_1), i19–i36.

De Leeuw, E. (2017). Cities and health from the neolithic to the anthropocene. In E. de Leeuw & J. Simos (Eds.), *Healthy cities – the theory, policy, and practice of value-based urban planning* (pp. 3–30). Springer.

De Leeuw, E., & Green, G. (2017). The logic of method for evaluating healthy cities. In E. de Leeuw & J. Simos (Eds.), *Healthy cities – the theory, policy, and practice of value-based urban planning* (pp. 463–487). Springer.

De Leeuw, E., & Simos, J. (2017). Healthy cities move to maturity. In E. de Leeuw & J. Simos (Eds.), *Healthy cities – the theory, policy, and practice of value-based urban planning* (pp. 75–86). Springer.

De Leeuw, E., & Skovgaard, T. (2005). Utility-driven evidence for healthy cities: Problems with evidence generation and application. *Social Science and Medicine, 61*, 1331–1341.

De Leeuw, E., Tsouros, A. D., Dyakova, M., & Green, G. (2014). *Healthy cities. Promoting health and equity – evidence for local policy and practice. Summary evaluation of Phase V of the WHO European Healthy Cities Network.* World Health Organization Regional Office for Europe.

De Leeuw, E., Palmer, N. & Spanswick, L. (2015a). *City fact sheets: WHO European Healthy Cities Network.* World Health Organization Regional Office for Europe, . http://www.euro.who.int/__data/assets/pdf_file/0006/280842/CityFactSheetsBook_12-06.pdf?ua=1. Accessed 2 June 2021.

De Leeuw, E., Green, G., Dyakova, M., Spanswick, L., & Palmer, N. (2015b). European healthy cities evaluation: Conceptual framework and methodology. *Health Promotion International, 30*(suppl_1), i8–i17.

De Leeuw, E., Green, G., Tsouros, A., Dyakova, M., Farrington, J., Faskunger, J., Grant, M., Ison, E., Jackisch, J., Janss Lafond, L., Lease, H., Mackiewicz, K., Östergren, P.-O., Palmer, N., Ritsatakis, A., Simos, J., Spanswick, L., Webster, P., Zamaro, G., … on behalf of the World Health Organization European Healthy Cities Network. (2015c). Healthy cities phase V evaluation: further synthesizing realism. Health Promotion International. In E. de Leeuw, A. Tsouros, & G. Green (Eds.), *Intersectoral governance for health and equity in european cities – healthy cities in Europe*, Supplement, 30(Suppl) (pp. i118–i124).

Duhl, L. (1963). *The urban condition: People and policy in the metropolis*. Simon and Schuster.

Dyrberg, T. (2014). *Foucault on the Politics of Parrhesia*. Springer.

Edwards, N., Viehbeck, S., Hämäläinen, R. M., Rus, D., Skovgaard, T., van de Goor, I., Valente, A., Syed, A., & Aro, A. R. (2012). Challenges of ethical clearance in international health policy and social sciences research: Experiences and recommendations from a multi-country research programme. *Public Health Reviews, 34*(1), 11.

Esping-Andersen, G. (1990). *The three worlds of welfare capitalism*. Princeton University Press.

Goumans, M. J. B. M. (1998). *Innovations in a fuzzy domain: Healthy cities and (health) policy development in the Netherlands and the United Kingdom*. Universiteit Maastricht. https://cris.maastrichtuniversity.nl/files/727120/guid-4a2762cd-9fd4-4a8c-9a7d-b4a2d713e30c-ASSET1.0.pdf. Accessed 2 June 2021.

Grant, M. (2015). European healthy city network phase V: Patterns emerging for healthy urban planning. *Health Promotion International, 30*(suppl_1), i54–i70.

Green, G. (1998). *Health and governance in European cities: A compendium of trends and responsibilities for public health in 46 member states of the WHO European Region*. European Hospital Management Journal.

Greenhalgh, T., Raftery, J., Hanney, S., & Glover, M. (2016). Research impact: a narrative review. *BMC Medicine, 14*(1), 78.

Guba, E. G., & Lincoln, Y. S. (1989). *Fourth generation evaluation*. Sage.

Haas, P. M. (1989). Do regimes matter? Epistemic communities and mediterranean pollution control. *International Organization, 43*(3), 377–403.

Haas, P. M. (1992). Introduction: Epistemic communities and international policy coordination. *International Organization; Knowledge, Power, and International Policy Coordination, 46*(1), 1–35.

Hancock, T. (2017). Healthy cities emerge: Toronto–Ottawa–Copenhagen. In E. de Leeuw & J. Simos (Eds.), *Healthy cities – the theory, policy, and practice of value-based urban planning* (pp. 63–73). Springer.

Hancock, T., & Duhl, L. (1986). *Promoting health in the urban context* (WHO Healthy Cities Papers No. 1). FADL Publishers.

Heritage, Z., & Green, G. (2013). European national healthy city networks: The impact of an elite epistemic community. *Journal of Urban Health, 90*(1), 154–166.

Jackisch, J., Zamaro, G., Green, G., & Huber, M. (2015). Is a healthy city also an age-friendly city? *Health Promotion International, 30*(suppl_1), i108–i117.
Janss Lafond, L. (2015). *National healthy cities networks in the WHO European Region. Promoting health and well-being throughout Europe*. World Health Organization Regional Office for Europe, . https://www.euro.who.int/en/publications/abstracts/national-healthy-cities-networks-in-the-who-european-region.-promoting-health-and-well-being-throughout-europe-2015. Accessed 2 June 2021.
Kickbusch, I. (1989). *Good planets are hard to find*. WHO Healthy Cities papers No. 5, FADL Publishers, .
Lee, K. (2014). *World Health Organization*. Ch 27, pp 504–518 in: Sperling, J. (2014) Handbook of governance and security. Edward Elgar Publishing, .
Leydesdorff, L., Bornmann, L., Comins, J. A., & Milojević, S. (2016). Citations: Indicators of quality? The impact fallacy. *Frontiers in Research Metrics and Analytics, 1*, 1.
Mitroff, I. I., & Featheringham, T. R. (1974). On systemic problem solving and the error of the third kind. *Behavioral Science, 19*, 383–393.
Paganini, J. M., & Chorny, A. H. (1990). Los sistemas locales de salud: desafíos para la década de los noventa. *Boletín de la Oficina Sanitaria Panamericana (OSP), 109*(5-6) nov.-dic.
Pawson, R., & Tilley, N. (1997). *Realist evaluation*. SAGE.
Pawson, R., Greenhalgh, T., Harvey, G., & Walshe, K. (2004). *Realist synthesis: An introduction*. ESRC Research Methods Programme, University of Manchester.
Rosling, H., Rosling, O., & Rosling Rönnlund, A. (2018). *Factfulness: Ten reasons we're wrong about the world – and why things are better than you think*. Flatiron Books.
Vaessen, J., Raimondo, E., & Bamberger, M. (2016). Impact evaluation approaches and complexity chapter 4. In M. Bamberger, J. Vaessen, & E. Raimondo (Eds.), *Dealing with complexity in development evaluation: A practical approach* (pp. 62–87). Sage. https://doi.org/10.4135/9781483399935.n4
Whitfield, M., Machaczek, K., & Green, G. (2013). Developing a model to estimate the potential impact of municipal investment on city health. *Journal of Urban Health, 90*(1), 62–73.
WHO. (1988). *Five-year planning framework*. WHO Healthy Cities papers No. 3, FADL Publishers, .
Yamatani, H., Mann, A., & Feit, M. (2013). Avoiding type III, IV, and V errors through collaborative research. *Journal of Evidence-based Social Work, 10*(4), 358–364.

Chapter 49
Researching Health for All in South Australia: Reflections on Sustainability and Partnership

Fran Baum, Helen van Eyk, Colin MacDougall, and Carmel Williams

49.1 Introduction

This chapter presents a reflection on the theoretical and methodological lessons from a five-year research project (2012–2016) funded by the Australian National Health and Medical Research Council which evaluated South Australia's Health in All Policies (HiAP) approach. The research involved a collaboration between University researchers and public servants who were involved in implementing HiAP in South Australia. During the research, we made advances in understanding the ways in which HiAP works and the value of different methodological and theoretical approaches. Drawing on our published work about this research, our chapter describes the contribution our work has made to knowledge, to the implementation of HiAP, and to methodological and theoretical approaches for studying complex policy interventions.

F. Baum (✉) · H. van Eyk
Stretton Health Equity, University of Adelaide, Adelaide, Australia
e-mail: fran.baum@adelaide.edu.au

C. MacDougall
College of Medicine and Public Health, Flinders University, Adelaide, Australia

University of Melbourne, Melbourne, Australia

C. Williams
Centre for Health in All Policies Research Translation, Health Translation SA, SAHMRI, Adelaide, Australia

L. Potvin, D. Jourdan (eds.), *Global Handbook of Health Promotion Research, Vol. 1*,
https://doi.org/10.1007/978-3-030-97212-7_49

49.1.1 HiAP in South Australia

HiAP is a horizontal, cross-sectoral, policy approach that facilitates intersectoral relationships and policy development to address health, well-being, and equity issues while also contributing to other sectors' policy goals. It is well recognised that many of the factors that contribute to health and well-being sit outside of the control of the health system, such as access to housing, education, employment, and transport. The intersectoral focus of HiAP recognises the importance of these factors to population health, well-being and equity, and positions health as a shared goal across government.

A HiAP approach was adopted in South Australia in 2008 following a recommendation by Professor Ilona Kickbusch as part of her South Australian Thinker in Residency. Initially, HiAP was linked closely to South Australia's Strategic Plan which called explicitly for "joined-up" government approaches to act on the social determinants of health (Baum et al., 2017). The initial approach of the HiAP initiative centred on undertaking Health Lens Analysis which is similar to Health Impact Assessment but differs in the ways in which it is directly linked to policymakers' actions (Delany et al., 2014). We show how the HiAP approach survived because it has been constantly adapted to South Australia's changing political context to ensure that it remains relevant and useful. This included adapting to new government priorities and a change of government. Under the new government, HiAP became part of the mandate of a newly established government agency – Wellbeing SA in 2019. The evolution of the South Australian HiAP approach is shown in Table 49.1.

49.2 Focus of Research

Our research covered the period from 2012 until 2016 and included retrospective and concurrent analysis. We examined the reasons HiAP was established, the contextual and policy factors that made this possible, and the ways in which the initiative navigated a changing policy context. We used program theory to determine the likely impacts on health and equity.

Our research questions were as follows:

- To what extent is the South Australian Health in All Policies (HiAP) approach an effective method of building healthy public policy in order to modify the determinants of population health, well-being, and health equity?
- To what extent does the application of policy agenda-setting and implementation theory explain the strengths and weakness of the HiAP model as a means of bringing about action on the determinants of health, well-being, and health equity across sectors of government?
- How effective is the combination of a program logic and action research as a framework for determining the impact of a complex multi-sectoral policy initiative on population health?

Table 49.1 Evolution of South Australian HiAP

Phase	Authorising environment	Policy opportunities	Adaptive HiAP action/response	Supportive structures
Proof of Concept & Emerging Practice 2007–2008	State government Cabinet "Thinkers in residence" program	Draft recommendations	Intersectoral policy makers' workshop	Informal intersectoral network: Commence work on policy opportunities. HiAP catalyst – Prof Ilona Kickbusch with researcher support
Establish & apply methodology 2008–2009	State government – Cabinet sub-committee (ExComm chief executives' group) Memorandum of understanding between central government and health department	South Australia's strategic plan – Whole of government targets	HiAP unit formed Develop South Australian approach to HiAP Including health lens analysis. International meeting on HiAP Adelaide statement on HiAP	Informal intersectoral network: Begins to formalise in authorising environments (vertical and horizontal). Builds capacity. Workshops. Applies South Australia's approach to HiAP, including health lens analysis. Develops resource on HiAP Links with WHO Develops National Health & Medical Research Council research grant application

(continued)

Table 49.1 (continued)

Phase	Authorising environment	Policy opportunities	Adaptive HiAP action/response	Supportive structures
Consolidation & growth 2009–2013	Central government champions Advocacy. Reinforce the value of HiAP to health and whole of government.	South Australia's strategic plan version 2.0	WHO/South Australian government HiAP Summer School National Health & Medical Research Council Grant – HiAP research	South Australian HiAP "Community of Practice" forums: Broad recognition of outcomes and purpose. Emerging advocates and champions. Implementation of action research
Adaptive / renewal 2013–2014	Cabinet taskforce Senior government officers groups	7 Cabinet strategic priorities Renewal phase – Reframed health Department's purpose in government Vulnerabilities. Reframe. Renew. Explore new opportunities.	HiAP approach mapped against 7 Cabinet strategic priorities Public Health Act 2011 – enacted	South Australian HiAP Community of Practice is maintained Linking our joined-up approach to others across government Legislative and regulatory support for HiAP in South Australia Action research continues

(continued)

Table 49.1 (continued)

Phase	Authorising environment	Policy opportunities	Adaptive HiAP action/response	Supportive structures
Strengthen / systematise 2015–2020	Renewed memorandum of understanding between central government and health department Systematise HiAP across government. Designation of WHO Collaborating Centre (WHO CC) for advancing HiAP implementation. Linking 4-year work plan of WHO HiAP CC with Flinders University WHO CC on the Social, Political & Commercial Determinants of Health Equity.	Premier's priorities, including: Focus on "one government". Planning reform. Links with economic priorities. Identified as a flagship program. HiAP is a key strategy in Wellbeing SA's 5-year strategic plan.	Public Health partner authorities Formalised partnerships to achieve co-benefits through action on the social determinants of health. Section 17 of Public Health Act Rapid health lens analysis assessment. Desktop analysis. 90 day projects Health lens analysis. WHO HiAP CC 4 year agreed work operationalised through Wellbeing SA	South Australian HiAP Community of Practice expanded Actively participates in strengthening and systematising HiAP across government, WHO HiAP CC advisory committee. Links between HiAP and researchers continue.

Adapted from South Australian Government (2017) with permission of Wellbeing SA.

49.3 Methodology and Methods

Our research was conducted within an action research framework which we adopted with the knowledge that public services are prone to restructures and policy change and must adapt to changing political mandates. Action research is a collaborative methodology that is well-suited to working in partnership with public servants. We used the framework of the Commission on the Social Determinants of Health (2008) which explains why social determinants are so influential. We also used several theories from political science to improve our understanding of intersectoral action for population health and equity: Kingdon's (2014) theory of agenda setting; Giddens on trust; Howlett, Ramesh and Perl (2009) and Exworthy et al., (2003; Exworthy and Hunter 2011) on policy processes and implementation; Finnemore and Sikkink (1998) on norms; and Scott (2014) on institutional theory. Our data were collected using the following methods:

- 144 in-depth interviews
- Two program logic design workshops.
- Two electronic surveys of public servants.
- Five case studies to examine the HiAP Health Lens Analysis processes in detail.
- Document analysis of project plans, reports, meeting papers and briefings, and a log of observations of key policy events.

We examined governance structures, the fine detail of intersectoral working, including the major enablers and obstacles to implementing HiAP in a state government. The use of program logic enabled us to determine the ways in which HiAP could be argued to have affected population health and equity (Lawless et al., 2018).

49.4 Contribution to Knowledge and Understanding About HiAP Implementation and Impact

In this section, we discuss six aspects of our 5-year research program: 1) how it enabled a detailed understanding of the factors that contributed to the adoption of HiAP in South Australia; 2) its contribution to the understanding of intersectoral collaboration; 3) how links can be made from a complex policy intervention to longer-term health and equity outcomes; 4) how methods can be adapted to accommodate changing bureaucratic and political environments; 5) how we used a range of theories to assist in the analysis of our data; 6) the policy recommendations we were able to make on the basis of the research and the nature of our research partnership. These aspects were selected following a review of the papers published over the five years of the project and through a process of distillation of the key points that had emerged. This distillation was done through group discussion among the authors. Each factor is meaningful because they explain how HiAP was promoted on to the policy agenda (point 1); the main methods used by HiAP to achieve a contribution to improved health (point 2); how the research processes were able to link the HiAP actions to health outcomes (point 3) and how both method and theory are vital to understanding the processes and means by which outcomes are achieved (points 4 and 5); and how the research provides a basis for policy recommendations (point 6).

49.4.1 Detailed Description of the Processes by Which HiAP Came to Be Adopted in South Australia

Our research enabled a description of the ways in which HiAP came to be adopted in South Australia. The enabling factors we identified are listed in Box 49.1.

Box 49.1 Enabling Factors for Adoption and Early Success of HiAP in South Australia (Delany et al., 2016)

- A rich history of health promotion and community health, which meant public servants understood the importance of social determinants and intersectoral action.
- The role of policy entrepreneurs.
- The provision of a resourced, centrally mandated unit that is easy for other sectors to work with
- Governance and mandate – a central mandate
- Establishing and maintaining trust and credibility
- Aligning HiAP with core business and strategic priorities
- Collaborators require clearly defined timelines and achievement milestones to support HiAP feasibility

One crucial factor was the rich history of health promotion and community health in South Australia which provided very fertile ground for HiAP. This meant there was a cadre of public servants and academics who were deeply imbued with an understanding of health promotion and especially committed to implementing the WHO Ottawa Charter for Health Promotion in their state. A resourced HiAP unit with a mandate from the centre of government was also crucial. A senior public servant from a sector other than health we interviewed noted: "I don't think any of this would have happened unless there was a dedicated unit and the resources to go with it". The central government mandate was reinforced in several ways. Legislative frameworks that legitimise collaboration across government to work on shared targets, such as South Australia's Strategic Plan, the State Government's Seven Strategic Priorities, and the South Australian Public Health Act, add power to mandates from the central government. Similar findings have come from other research (St-Pierre, 2009; Merkel, 2010; Gawith, 2012; Storm et al., 2014). Also crucial were the ways in which intersectoral working was facilitated and these are discussed below. Trust was also important, and we discuss the ways in which we have added to the understanding of how trust works within public sectors below.

An important kick-start to HiAP in South Australia was the appointment of Ilona Kickbusch as a Thinker in Residence (Baum et al., 2015). She recommended that South Australia adopt HiAP in her final report (Kickbusch, 2008). The Adelaide Thinkers in Residence scheme was an initiative of the then Labor Premier Mike Rann. Between 2003 and 2013 it brought 24 internationally recognised experts to South Australia each spending between two and six months in Adelaide and many establishing long-term links. The intention of the scheme was to encourage the state of South Australia to be "flexible, responsive and adaptive". While Kickbusch made the recommendation about HiAP, many of the other thinkers also emphasised the value of cross-government action and the role other sectors could play in health promotion (Baum et al., 2015). Examples include Alexandre Kalache who advocated for government, universities, and older people to work together in the creation of age-friendly policy and services. Fraser Mustard's residency on early childhood stressed the need to work intersectorally to highlight the importance of the early years in developing a healthy and productive population. He emphasised how work in all sectors impacts on, and can benefit from, healthy child development. Stephen Schneider advocated for greater intersectoral collaboration at the state and local level to manage climate change and offset risks. He stressed that measures to reduce the progression of climate change may also have health benefits. For example, improving public transport systems will reduce air pollution and may reduce social isolation. This latter residency together with work from the HiAP team made a significant contribution to South Australia's world-leading transition to renewable energy which we have documented as an excellent case of energy transition (McGreevy et al., 2021).

The result of this activity was to highlight the potential for cross-government action to create and support actions to address difficult issues and provide a supportive authorising environment for collaborative strategies such as HiAP to proceed.

49.4.2 *Improved Understanding of the Processes of Intersectoral Collaboration*

Our research enabled us to unpack the processes of intersectoral collaboration and examine how HiAP was received and adapted in sectors other than health. We used institutional theory to examine how a mix of ideational, institutional, and actor factors combined to make the intersectoral action initiated by HiAP effective (Baum et al., 2017) (Fig. 49.1). Below we examine these factors in detail using three cases

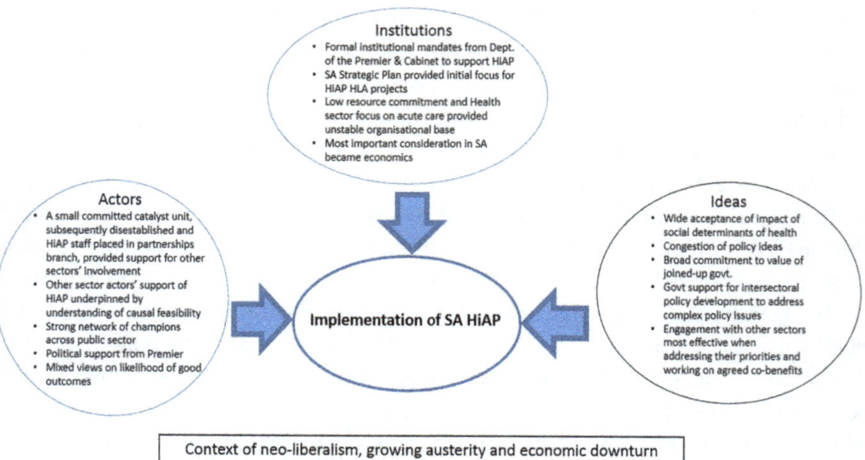

Fig. 49.1 Intersection of actors and institutional and ideational factors in South Australian HiAP (Reprinted from Baum, et al., (2017), CC BY 4.0)

of HiAP action – parental engagement in children's literacy, a healthy weight initiative, and an Aboriginal driver's licensing project. All were intersectoral, and involved a Health Lens Analysis facilitated by the HiAP unit.

An important part of the approach of the HiAP team was to ensure that their work addressed the core business of the other partnering department as well as contributing to improving health. The HiAP team called these situations in which a win-win was possible a co-benefits approach. Their experience was that progress was only made with departments outside health if "health imperialism" was avoided. While health benefits were expected, the HiAP team was always determined to ensure clear gains for the partnering department (co-benefits), and sought to put the other department's priorities and interests first, "to be seen to be useful". The HiAP team placed great importance on relationship establishment and maintenance with partnering departments and saw this as crucial to engaging with them on cross-sector collaborative initiatives. The ways this was done are exemplified in a partnership with the Education Department to improve children's literacy (van Eyk et al., 2019b) described in Box 49.2.

Box 49.2 Parental Engagement in Children's Literacy (van Eyk et al., 2019b)

HiAP and Education Department staff collaborated to identify potential areas of work that would advance both health and education goals and so achieve co-benefits. The agreed aim of the Health Lens Analysis project was to investigate how parents could be more effectively engaged in the co-creation of literacy-rich environments for their children at home and school. A concern was ensuring that any policy recommendations could be readily operationalised and implemented under real-world conditions and be acceptable to the schools and teachers involved. Four schools categorised as low socio-economic status with culturally diverse school communities participated in shaping and trialling strategies that would form the basis of policy action. The project included focus groups of parents in the four schools which explored their views and experiences of engagement in their children's schooling. A working group of HiAP staff, teachers, and the regional project officer identified areas of activity to support child literacy development.

Each school developed its own suite of activities in response to its context, and policy recommendations were developed for schools, the region, and the state. The involvement of the four schools led to tangible resources and examples of structural changes, and resources that were widely disseminated, including a DVD resource for parents.

The parental engagement initiative was successful because it embedded the changes in real-life practice as well as encouraging change in the ways in which the Education Department engaged parents. A similar co-benefits approach was adopted in the Healthy Weight initiative (see Box 49.3). Our analysis of this initiative (van

Eyk et al., 2019a) found that a combination of economic and systemic framing, in conjunction with a co-benefits approach, facilitated intersectoral engagement. Economic framing enabled a focus on the economic consequences for the state of the "obesity epidemic" and was consistent with the growing concern within the South Australian Government about population obesity trends and implications for the health budget. Combining economic framing with a systemic framing of healthy weight supported the HiAP unit's arguments for population-based intersectoral responses (Khayatzadeh-Mahani et al., 2018).

Box 49.3 Healthy Weight (van Eyk et al., 2019a)

Many factors that influence body weight are beyond the scope of health sector activity and the choices of individuals. Diet and opportunities for physical activity are strongly influenced by income, transport, education, food supply systems, and the local built and natural environments.

HiAP fostered relationships with other departments to develop a whole of government approach to healthy weight. These departments included: the Office for Recreation and Sport; the Education Department; the Department for Communities and Social Inclusion; the Housing Department; the Transport Department; the Primary Industries Department; the Environment Department; and the Department of Correctional Services.

The HiAP unit's co-benefits approach was critical to their effective engagement with other sectors (Khayatzadeh-Mahani et al., 2018; Baum et al., 2017) and achieved the historical and political goals of advancing understanding of how to act intersectorally. However, it was also recognised that a co-benefits approach has limitations and is not suitable for all policy problems. For example, the absence of a government policy and therefore commitment to equity as a policy goal made it difficult for HiAP to engage with partner agencies to consider the equity dimensions of overweight and obesity (in particular the impact of poverty). The co-benefits approach is useful when working to influence and strengthen health considerations within existing government priorities. It is less useful when health agencies want to alter or change government policy positions (Chaufan et al., 2015; van Eyk et al., 2017). Similarly, it is difficult for any sub-national HiAP to expand from its strong mandate of state-based intersectoral government action to focus, for example, on the influence on rising obesity rates resulting from international trade and the growth of a transnational food industry which markets and produces ultra-processed products through high fat and sugar food and beverages (Otero, 2018). Even the measures a state government might have within its control, such as a tax on sugary drinks, can require a political rather than public service decision, and HiAP's role may be to work to create the political will for such a measure. These reflections suggest rethinking health promotion strategies when solutions to problems are clearly beyond the scope of sub-national or state governments, for example, in relation to national and international policy response and regulation (Duckett et al., 2016).

Our detailed interviews also enabled us to examine the role of trust in relationship building, which emerged as vital to HiAP (Delany-Crowe et al., 2019). We integrated Giddens' theoretical perspectives on trust (1991a, b) with existing typologies of trust in order to understand how trust operates as a resource within non-traditional joined-up government working relationships, serving to bridge the gap between the known and unknown, and acting as a productive resource to stimulate action within government systems that are perceived to feature high levels of risk. In Box 49.4 we discuss how trust enabled and distrust impeded an Aboriginal Road Safety initiative.

Box 49.4 Aboriginal Road Safety (Delany-Crowe et al., 2019)
The analysis of trust can be seen by highlighting its role in an initiative which aimed to increase the number of Aboriginal and Torres Strait Islander Australians who can obtain and retain their driver's licence. Trust is vital in any relationship between Aboriginal and Torres Strait Islander peoples given the history of dispossession and lack of cultural respect which characterised Australian colonialism. Possessing a driver's licence is important to employment, education, socialisation, and access to services. A driver's licence also provides proof of identity, which is important in many areas of life. Improving access to driver's licences is also likely to reduce road crash-related morbidity and mortality, while reducing incarceration as punishment for driving while unlicensed. The driver's licencing system, and Aboriginal Australians' engagement with it, is influenced by decisions made in multiple departments, including the Transport Department, the Attorney-General's Department, the Department of Correctional Services, the Health Department, the Department for Further Education, Employment, and Training, and the Police Department. HiAP led a collaboration involving representatives from all these departments to review and improve the South Australian driver's licensing system. The views of different departments about system changes and how they framed issues varied, making the development of strong intersectoral relationships and communication both difficult and essential. The history of dispossession and persecution of Aboriginal people since colonisation means that having trust in governments is hard for Aboriginal people. In this exercise trust was important. It supported the functioning of the large group and was a facilitator for open, honest communication.

We found that trust is a dynamic aspect of collaborative intersectoral relationships, which must be nurtured (Fig. 49.2). This nurturing included guarding against practices that threaten trust and maintaining shared understandings and goals (Scott & Bardach, 2019), remaining empathetic to the workloads and departmental contexts of collaborators, adapting timelines to reduce pressure when required, and sharing ownership of projects and credit for positive outcomes. In this regard, our findings support Giddens' (1991a: 33) argument about the value of a "reflexive

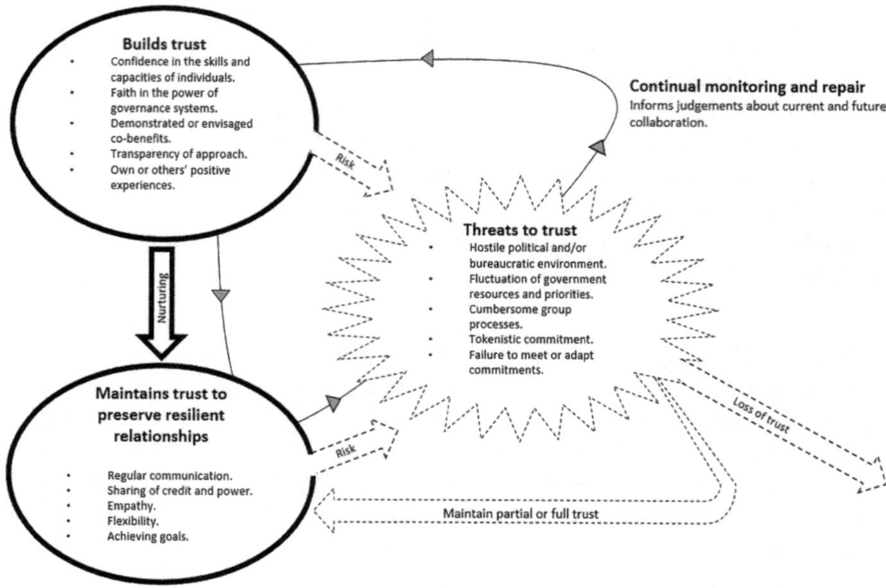

Fig. 49.2 Dynamics of trust within joined-up government relationships formed under the South Australian HiAP initiative (Reprinted from Delany-Crowe, et al., (2019) with permission of John Wiley and Sons. © 2019 Institute of Public Administration Australia)

monitoring of action", which facilitates ongoing assessment of behaviour and context in order to prevent or minimise the impact of potential threats.

49.4.3 Linking HiAP Action to Health and Equity Outcomes

When we began this research, we recognised that demonstrating that HiAP could lead to health and equity outcomes was conceptually and methodologically fraught. This is because much of the action of HiAP would be expected to have an impact in the future, and for some interventions, the long-term future. Additionally, it is difficult to directly attribute the change to HiAP in a situation where there is no possibility of a control or comparison group. Consequently, our methodological approach was to articulate the theory of change that underpins the actions selected and map the path from the HiAP action to likely health and equity impacts in the future. Thus, we constructed a narrative argument much like that used in legal proceedings. This narrative draws on existing literature to predict that if certain measures were adopted then they were likely to lead to improvements in health. For example, there is a significant literature which predicts that if a population has a healthy weight then this will contribute to reducing the prevalence of chronic disease. A further example is that if HiAP were able to influence the planning of new suburbs so that they encouraged walking, this would be predicted to result in a

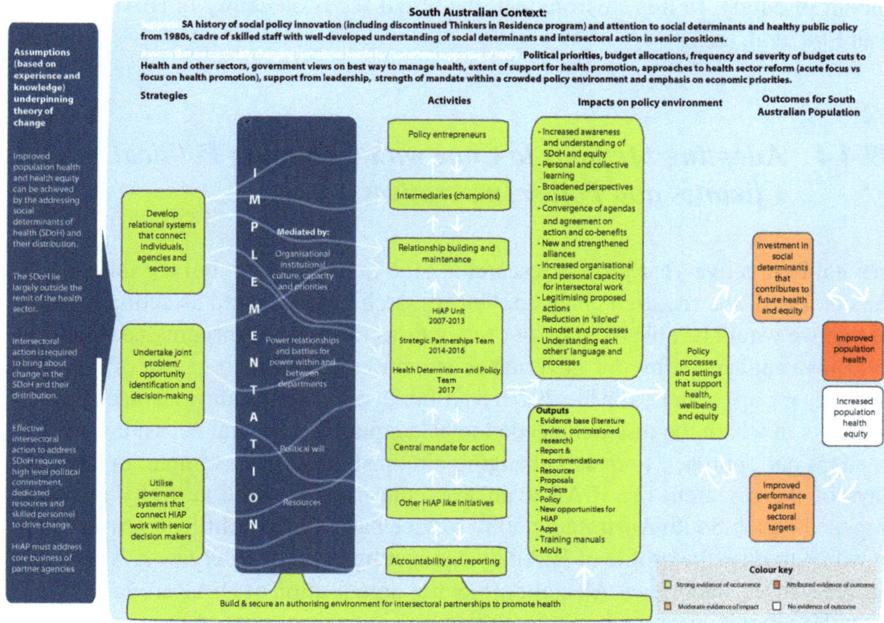

Fig. 49.3 Program theory used to frame the South Australian HiAP research (Reprinted from Baum, et al., (2019a). CC BY 4.0)

healthier population, other things being equal. On this basis, we were able to predict that HiAP was likely to improve health in some ways (Baum et al., 2019a). Our program theory model (see Fig. 49.3) enabled us to demonstrate the ways in which HiAP created the conditions for progress towards health improvements. The model considers the impact of context, the processes of implementation, how these affected the policy environment, and then the likely sum impact on health and equity outcomes. Using this program theory model, we were able to identify why little progress was made on equity goals. While government agencies readily understood HiAP as improving the process of intersectoral policy development, the more distal intent of improving equity was not well understood and gained less traction. Public servants in other departments understood well that their actions affected health but struggled, when asked, to explain how they might contribute to health equity. While some early rhetorical support existed for progressing an equity agenda through South Australian HiAP, subsequent economic pressures resulted in the government narrowing its priorities to economic goals which did not stress equity. The HiAP team emphasised relationship maintenance and working on partner agencies' agendas (the co-benefits approach) to build trust and collaboration of partner agencies. Because the equity agenda was not promoted by successive governments and did not resonate with partner agencies, the process goal of establishing and maintaining relationships – as the critical political goal of HiAP- had to be privileged over the pursuit of equity. In this environment, the initial focus on equity in HiAP was lost (van Eyk et al., 2017).

49.4.4 Adapting Methods to Cope with Changing Political Climates and Policy Imperatives

Inevitably in a five-year project researching the implementation of a public policy, the context of the research changed. Our research was designed as action research so that we would be able to adapt our methods as the research progressed. Our flexibility was enhanced by our governance structures (including our use of a project advisory group) (van Eyk et al., 2020) (see Table 49.3), which allowed discussion of the ways in which the research needed to be adapted. On several occasions, we had to adapt our approach to match changing circumstances. For example, in the early days of the research, the HiAP team was concerned that the austerity measures imposed on the South Australian public service had created a difficult environment in which to raise the profile of HiAP by conducting research interviews. As a result, we delayed the interviews. Also, the structural organisation of HiAP around a "dedicated HiAP unit" was originally identified as a key component of the program theory. After 2013, an organisational restructure led to the integration of the unit into a group with a wider public health remit, and a change in their activities. This provided us with an opportunity to adapt the program theory and document ways in which this change manifested itself in terms of policy-making processes and the actions that arose from them.

The political support for HiAP did wax and wane over the period of our research and subsequently. At the high points, HiAP was promoted strongly by the Department of the Premier and Cabinet and given a very high profile. In 2019, it again was more in the spotlight with the formation of a new government agency – Wellbeing SA – which welcomed the HiAP approach. In between, we documented periods when HiAP had to go "under the radar" to maintain its role and function. It did this successfully even at a time when the Department of Health's division of health promotion was abolished. Our research suggested part of the reason for this was its high profile internationally and the fact it was the subject of a five-year research program from the premier Australian funding body (the National Health and Medical Research Council). The research partnership has also contributed to the establishment of two WHO Collaborating Centres in South Australia one located in Wellbeing SA on Health in All Policies, and one at Flinders University on the Social, Political and Commercial Determinants of Health Equity.

Table 49.2 Examples of how the application of social and political science theory helped our HiAP research

Research questions	Theory	Focus
Why was HiAP successful in reaching the government agenda? Why did particular HiAP projects succeed in reaching the agendas of multiple government departments? How did HiAP continually realign to accommodate changing government agendas?	Agenda setting theory (Kingdon, 2014)	Proposes that policy action requires a policy window to become available through linkage of problems, policy, and politics.
Why and how did other agencies and departments engage with HiAP? What was the role of actors, such as champions, in diffusing HiAP ideas across sectors? How did the political and bureaucratic systems support or impede HiAP's focus on health equity and why did equity fail to get on the government agenda or drop from it?	Institutional theory (Howlett et al., 2009; Scott, 2014)	Describes influence of actors, ideas, and institutions in increasing acceptability of particular initiatives
How can expectations of competence and goodwill inform new intersectoral relationships? How is trust lost in intersectoral relationships and what are the impacts?	Trust theory (Giddens, 1991a, b)	Explains how trust serves to bridge the gap between the known and unknown in non-traditional ways of working, such as intersectoral action, to facilitate effective relationships
Understanding how ideas were translated into norms.	Norm theory (Finnemore & Sikkink, 1998)	We used the idea of a norm life cycle to see how ideas of intersectoral action and the importance of social determinants emerged and then, through a "norm cascade", were institutionalised. The idea of a norm entrepreneur enabled us to understand the role of the thinkers in residence scheme in making international ideas locally relevant and politically acceptable

(continued)

Table 49.2 (continued)

Research questions	Theory	Focus
Why and how do particular HiAP activities and outputs lead to distal health outcomes for the South Australian population? How can intersectoral action influence health and why is an intersectoral approach important in addressing health and its distribution (health equity)?	Social determinants of health theory (Solar & Irwin, 2010)	Prompts analysis of the impacts of upstream distal factors on health and well-being
How does advocacy operate to strengthen or marginalise health promotion as a priority in health policy? How do relational networks and the interactions of policy actors support policy change across sectors?	Advocacy Coalition Theory (Sabatier, 1988)	Describes interaction between policy actors in bringing about policy change
How have different types of learning occurred during the development and implementation of HiAP? – Instrumental learning, conceptual learning and social learning. What is the nature of the learning that has occurred within the government and what impacts has learning produced on policy and practices?	Policy networks and policy learning (Sabatier & Jenkins-Smith, 1993)	Considers how learning occurs over time within policy networks and how it produces changes in values, goals, processes, and meanings

Adapted from Lawless et al., (2018), Table 2. CC BY 4.0

49.4.5 Applying and Assessing the Usefulness of Different Policy Theories

The HiAP research has enabled us to apply a range of theories to assist the interpretation of our data. The theories we used included the Commission on Social Determinants of Health theoretical framework on why social determinants have a substantial impact on both overall population health and health equity; Kingdon's (2014) theory of agenda setting; Giddens (1991a, b) on trust; Howlett, Ramesh and Perl (2009) and Exworthy and Hunter (2011) on policy processes and implementation; Scott on institutional theory (2014); and Finnemore and Sikkink (1998) to explain how norm changes supported HiAP, to improve our understanding of intersectoral action. Their contributions are described in Table 49.2. Our HiAP research

Table 49.3 Formal governance structures

Structure	Formal role	Participants	Contribution to reflexivity and rigour
Project advisory group Met 7 times between 2014 and 2016	Project direction and feedback on findings. Higher-level oversight and endorsement linked research to senior executives. Learning about changing political and bureaucratic contexts (context mapping). Knowledge transfer. Provision of authorising environment for the evaluation	Chaired by a public servant. Public servants from health department, Department of the Premier and Cabinet, representatives of partner sectors, and chief and associate investigators	Credibility and transferability. Organisational learning and knowledge exchange. Context mapping, especially for political and structural changes. Public servants provided regular reports at each project advisory group meeting on developments in changing political context. University researchers presented early findings for discussion
Executive Met three monthly, 13 times between 2012 and 2015	Discussed research design, timing of research, context mapping. Site to openly negotiate power and control	Chaired by a public servant. Core group of university researchers and public servants	Collaborative space to plan data analysis and debate publication plans and authorship
Public events: Research fora Three held, in 2013, 2016, and 2017.	Three research fora, each attended by 70–100 researchers, policy actors, practitioners, and advocates to present emerging findings and obtain feedback on emerging themes and theories. The first focused on emerging findings from an international perspective, the second on local government and the third on policy implications and international application of HiAP. Public servants chaired key sessions at the research fora and an external "critical friend" was engaged to reflect on learnings from the day and to contribute to the agenda for further data analysis	Chaired by senior external academics and involving a senior external academic or senior former public servant as critical friend at each forum	Credibility and transferability. Knowledge exchange. Importance to the action research principles of continually releasing and discussing findings to improve confirmability and relevance and to enhance dissemination

(continued)

Table 49.3 (continued)

Structure	Formal role	Participants	Contribution to reflexivity and rigour
Public events: Policy clubs	Addressed topics of interest to academics, policymakers, and practitioners within government and not-for-profit sectors. A wide range of perspectives brought both a depth and a practicality to policy agendas in relation to health, society, and equity	Two Policy clubs with attendances of approximately 30 people each to discuss topics of interest and policy implications	Transferability

team included time in each of our research meetings to discuss the relevance and application of theoretical ideas to our emerging analysis. This process was helped by an Academy of Social Sciences in Australia two-day workshop (Baum et al., 2019b) on how social and political theory can help understand public health policy. At this workshop, we presented much of the HiAP research and were able to analyse the utility and fit of different theories.

Our use of these theories enabled us to make our research relevant beyond South Australia by highlighting the underlying mechanisms at work, such as trust (using Giddens (1991a, b)) or Finnemore and Sikkink's (1998) theory on how ideas become institutionalised norms.

49.4.6 Deriving Broader Lessons for Policymakers and Knowledge Exchange

Health promotion research should be about improving the conditions which determine the equitable distribution of health within a population. Our research enabled us to derive general lessons for policymakers about how their work might improve population health and equity. The governance structures we established for the project were designed to ensure both research rigour and transfer. The roles of the different structures that contained actors other than researchers are detailed in Table 49.3. We conducted forums for policymakers to share emerging findings and gain feedback. We also summarised lessons for policymakers in a policy brief titled: "Does a Health in All Policies Approach Improve Health, Wellbeing and Equity in South Australia?" (https://www.adelaide.edu.au/stretton/our-research/stretton-health-equity) which recommended that:

- A systematic and mandated response to promoting health and well-being in other sectors is required to protect and build on HiAP gains.
- Equity should become a prominent aspect of the government's agenda, with a strong focus on closing the life expectancy gap between Aboriginal and Torres

Strait Islander Australians and other Australians and on reducing the socio-economic status gradient.
- Government should give greater priority attention to addressing health equity and flattening the social gradient in health.

Public servants said that well-timed discussions of emerging findings from our data led directly to improvements in the HiAP approach and the operation of the dedicated HiAP team. For example, the research findings indicated that because some HiAP projects took longer than was considered desirable by some of HiAP's policy partners they were less likely to inform the government's agenda or attract further funding. As a result of these findings, HiAP staff adapted their approach to include rapid reviews, including mechanisms to identify and manage delays.

During research fora (Table 49.3), the research team presented emerging results to an audience comprising academics and policy experts outside the team, thereby contributing to credibility and transferability. Public servants told us how there were few opportunities and significant disincentives for them to engage in advocacy arising from research. They found the partnership useful because university researchers experienced fewer constraints and could advocate on the basis of the data via social media, publications and government agencies directly. This also extended to comments and public submissions about government policy which, while arising from the evaluation of HiAP, strategically only included the names of university researchers.

49.5 Conclusions

Our experience of our 5-year HiAP action research program provides a rich example of how research, which combines flexible methods with a range of theoretical interpretations, can inform health promotion practice. The application of theory is particularly useful in that it makes it easier for those wishing to learn from a situation in one context to see the transferrable lessons from a particular case. Our experience also highlights the value of research partnerships between health promotion actors and researchers. While such partnerships are challenging for both parties, when done well they do enable a critical examination of practice. In our study, they enabled us to track the development of HiAP from its earlier stages through its evolution into a Health Partnerships Branch within the Department of Health. The use of a multi-method study enabled us to document both the processes by which HiAP works and the likelihood that the initiatives HiAP conducted would result in health gains over the coming decades. The use of program theory enables researchers to extrapolate from short- and medium-term achievements to longer-term outcomes by using existing evidence to indicate the contribution health promotion actions are likely to make to population health over the long term. This research was conducted over five years and includes in-depth data which enables a much clearer understanding of what made initiatives work or impeded their implementation. It also provides a good basis for extrapolation to other jurisdictions.

Acknowledgements We acknowledge the input of all Chief and Associate Investigators who have contributed to the design of this research: Angela Lawless, Jennie Popay, Elizabeth Harris, Dennis McDermott, Danny Broderick, Ilona Kickbusch, Kevin Buckett, Sandy Pitcher, Andrew Stanley, and Deborah Wildgoose. We acknowledge the significant role and contribution of Toni Delany-Crowe, who was the project manager for this research from 2012–2016.

This work was supported by the Australian National Health and Medical Research Council (grant number 1027561).

The views expressed in this paper do not necessarily reflect those of the South Australian Government.

References

Baum, F., Lawless, A., MacDougall, C., Delany, T., McDermott, D., Harris, E., & Williams, C. (2015). New norms new policies: Did the Adelaide thinkers in residence scheme encourage new thinking about promoting well-being and Health in All Policies? *Social Science & Medicine, 147*, 1–9. https://doi.org/10.1016/j.socscimed.2015.10.031

Baum, F., Delany-Crowe, T., MacDougall, C., Lawless, A., van Eyk, H., & Williams, C. (2017). Ideas, actors and institutions: Lessons from South Australian Health in All Policies on what encourages other sectors' involvement. *BMC Public Health, 17*(1), 811. https://doi.org/10.1186/s12889-017-4821-7

Baum, F., Delany-Crowe, T., MacDougall, C., van Eyk, H., Lawless, A., Williams, C., & Marmot, M. (2019a). To what extent can the activities of the South Australian Health in All Policies initiative be linked to population health outcomes using a program theory-based evaluation? *BMC Public Health, 19*(1), 88. https://doi.org/10.1186/s12889-019-6408-y

Baum, F., Graycar, A., Delany-Crowe, T., de Leeuw, E., Bacchi, C., Popay, J., Orchard, L., Colebatch, H., Friel, S., MacDougall, C., Harris, E., Lawless, A., McDermott, D., Fisher, M., Harris, P., Phillips, C., & Fitzgerald, J. (2019b). Understanding Australian policies on public health using social and political science theories: Reflections from an Academy of the Social Sciences in Australia workshop. *Health Promotion International, 34*(4), 833–846. https://doi.org/10.1093/heapro/day014

Chaufan, C., Yeh, J., Ross, L., & Fox, P. (2015). You can't walk or bike yourself out of the health effects of poverty: Active school transport, child obesity, and blind spots in the public health literature. *Critical Public Health, 25*(1), 32–47. https://doi.org/10.1080/09581596.2014.920078

Commission on Social Determinants of Health. (2008). *Closing the gap in a generation: Health equity through action on the social determinants of health*. World Health Organization.

Delany, T., Harris, P., Williams, C., Harris, E., Baum, F., Lawless, A., Wildgoose, D., Haigh, F., MacDougall, C., Broderick, D., & Kickbusch, I. (2014). Health Impact Assessment in New South Wales & Health in All Policies in South Australia: Differences, similarities and connections. *BMC Public Health, 14*(1), 699. https://doi.org/10.1186/1471-2458-14-699

Delany, T., Lawless, A., Baum, F., Popay, J., Jones, L., McDermott, D., Harris, E., Broderick, D., & Marmot, M. (2016). Health in All Policies in South Australia: What has supported early implementation? *Health Promotion International, 31*(4), 888–898. https://doi.org/10.1093/heapro/dav084

Delany-Crowe, T., Popay, J., Lawless, A., Baum, F., MacDougall, C., van Eyk, H., & Williams, C. (2019). The role of trust in joined-up government activities: Experiences from Health in All Policies in South Australia. *Australian Journal of Public Administration, 78*(2), 172–190. https://doi.org/10.1111/1467-8500.12383

Duckett, S., Swerissen, H., & Wiltshire, T. (2016). *A sugary drinks tax: Recovering the community costs of obesity*. Grattan Institute.

Exworthy, M., & Hunter, D. J. (2011). The challenge of joined-up government in tackling health inequalities. *International Journal of Public Administration, 34*(4), 201–212. https://doi.org/10.1080/01900692.2011.551749

Exworthy, M., Blane, D., & Marmot, M. (2003). Tackling health inequalities in the United Kingdom: The progress and pitfalls of policy. *Health Services Research, 38*(6 Pt 2), 1905–1921. https://doi.org/10.1111/j.1475-6773.2003.00208.x

Finnemore, M., & Sikkink, K. (1998). International norm dynamics and political change. *International Organization, 52*(4), 887–917.

Gawith, L. (2012). *Information sheet 1: Background information on health in all policies (HiAP)*. Canterbury Health in All Policies Partnership (CHIAPP).

Giddens, A. (1991a). *The consequences of modernity*. Stanford University Press.

Giddens, A. (1991b). *Modernity and self-identity: Self and society in the late modern age*. Stanford University Press.

Howlett, M., Ramesh, M., & Perl, A. (2009). *Studying public policy: Policy cycles and policy subsystems* (3rd ed.). Oxford University Press.

Khayatzadeh-Mahani, A., Ruckert, A., & Labonté, R. (2018). Obesity prevention: Co-framing for intersectoral 'buy-in'. *Critical Public Health, 28*(1), 4–11. https://doi.org/10.1080/09581596.2017.1282604

Kickbusch, I. (2008). *Healthy societies: Addressing 21st century health challenges*. Adelaide Thinkers in Residence.

Kingdon, J. (2014). *Agendas, alternatives, and public policies* (updated 2nd ed., Longman Classics in Political Science ed.). Longman.

Lawless, A., Baum, F., Delany-Crowe, T., MacDougall, C., Williams, C., McDermott, D., & van Eyk, H. (2018). Developing a framework for a program theory-based approach to evaluating policy processes and outcomes: Health in All Policies in South Australia. *International Journal of Health Policy and Management, 7*(6), 510–521. https://doi.org/10.15171/ijhpm.2017.121

McGreevy, D. M., MacDougall, C., Fisher, D. M., Henley, M., & Baum, F. (2021). Expediting a renewable energy transition in a privatised market via public policy: The case of South Australia 2004-18. *Energy Policy, 148*, 111940. https://doi.org/10.1016/j.enpol.2020.111940

Merkel, B. (2010). *European Union experience and perspectives*. Adelaide 2010 – Health in All Policies international meeting. Adelaide, South Australia.

Otero, G. (2018). *The neoliberal diet: Healthy profits, unhealthy people*. University of Texas Press.

Sabatier, P. A. (1988). An advocacy coalition framework of policy change and the role of policy-oriented learning therein. *Policy Sciences, 21*(2), 129–168. https://doi.org/10.1007/BF00136406

Sabatier, P. A., & Jenkins-Smith, H. (1993). *Policy change and learning: An advocacy coalition approach*. Westview Press.

Scott, W. (2014). *Institutions and organizations, ideas, interests and identities*. Sage.

Scott, R. J., & Bardach, E. (2019). A comparison of management adaptations for joined-up government: Lessons from New Zealand. *Australian Journal of Public Administration, 78*(2), 191–212. https://doi.org/10.1111/1467-8500.12348

Solar, O., & Irwin, A. (2010). *A conceptual framework for action on the social determinants of health*. World Health Organization.

South Australian Government (2017) *How the governance and practice of Health in All Policies has changed over time in South Australia: Exploring the evolution 2007–2017*. Government of South Australia.

Storm, I., Harting, J., Stronks, K., & Schuit, A. J. (2014). Measuring stages of Health in All Policies on a local level: The applicability of a maturity model. *Health Policy, 114*(2–3), 183–191. https://doi.org/10.1016/j.healthpol.2013.05.006

St-Pierre, L. (2009). *Governance tools and framework for Health in All Policies*. National Collaborating Centre for Healthy Public Policy.

van Eyk, H., Harris, E., Baum, F., Delany-Crowe, T., Lawless, A., & MacDougall, C. (2017). Health in All Policies in South Australia – did it promote and enact an equity perspective? *International Journal of Environmental Research and Public Health, 14*(11), 1288. https://doi.org/10.3390/ijerph14111288

van Eyk, H., Baum, F., & Delany-Crowe, T. (2019a). Creating a whole-of-government approach to promoting healthy weight: What can Health in All Policies contribute? *International Journal of Public Health, 64*(8), 1159–1172. https://doi.org/10.1007/s00038-019-01302-4

van Eyk, H., Delany-Crowe, T., Lawless, A., Baum, F., MacDougall, C., & Wildgoose, D. (2019b). Improving child literacy using South Australia's Health in All Policies approach. *Health Promotion International, 35*(5), 958–972. https://doi.org/10.1093/heapro/daz013

van Eyk, H., Friel, S., Sainsbury, P., Boyd-Caine, T., Harris, P., MacDougall, C., Delany-Crowe, T., Musolino, C., & Baum, F. (2020). How do advisory groups contribute to healthy public policy research? *International Journal of Public Health, 65*(9), 1581–1591. https://doi.org/10.1007/s00038-020-01504-1

Part V
Conclusion: An Appraisal of Health Promotion Research Practices

Chapter 50
Markers of Ethical References in Health Promotion Research

Didier Jourdan and Louise Potvin

50.1 The Pervasiveness of Ethical Discussions

Ethical issues are discussed in one way or another in all contributions. In 16 out of 54 contributions, the authors devote at least one paragraph to the ethical underpinnings of their work and describe explicitly and in depth the values and principles that inform their research. Values and principles are the roots of their work (O'Hara and Taylor, Chap. 36). In some cases, an ethical reflection is considered as an objective of the research program. "This study was part of a theoretical inquiry that was also intended to be an ethical reflection with a view to developing analytical tools that avoid labelling individuals according to attributes such as smoker, obese, drug user, diabetic"(Adam et al., Chap. 6).

Many researchers do not assume that all health promotion research is inherently good. That's why they detail what legitimises their research. They take seriously that failure to be explicit about definitions and values leads to conceptual confusion (Seedhouse, 2009). The importance given to explicit ethical choices appears to be a key feature of health promotion research even if the way in which the ethical issues are described differ significantly across chapters. The values and principles of health promotion shape the research programmes, which may lead one to consider the field as primarily value-based or values-driven (McQueen, 2007).

D. Jourdan (✉)
UNESCO Chair and WHO Collaborating Centre in Global Health & Education, University of Clermont Auvergne, Clermont-Ferrand, France
e-mail: didier.jourdan@uca.fr

L. Potvin
School of Public Health, University of Montreal, Montréal, QC, Canada

Centre de recherche en santé publique (CReSP), Université of Montreal and CIUSSS du Centre-Sud-de-l'Île-de-Montréal, Montreal, QC, Canada

L. Potvin, D. Jourdan (eds.), *Global Handbook of Health Promotion Research, Vol. 1*,
https://doi.org/10.1007/978-3-030-97212-7_50

Our analysis identifies four markers that describe the way in which the ethical dimension shapes health promotion research.

The first relates to the values and principles mentioned by the authors, and which set the ethical scene of their work. In relation to the values and principles underlying the Ottawa Charter for Health Promotion (Potvin & Jones, 2011), these values and principles are often formulated in reference to values of justice and equity, or principles such as participation or empowerment. We call this first marker the ethical horizon of the research.

The second marker is more specific. It is linked to the way in which researchers justify and legitimise their work. It does not refer to general principles but provides more concrete references to mechanisms likely to facilitate social transformations in favour of social justice and participation of vulnerable people and groups, highlighting the relevance of an individual's and a population's knowledge. Therefore, research has a broader purpose, one that goes beyond the mere production of knowledge. It aims at contributing to social transformations. We call this second marker the source of legitimacy of the research.

The third marker is related to the status of the participants in the research process. In almost every chapter, mention is made of the role of people and groups as participants, as subjects and not objects of research. There is a strong tendency to do research with people instead of doing research on people. In this respect, research becomes a means to make the voices of vulnerable groups, such as homeless youth (Chap. 5) or people living in poverty (Chap. 6), heard and articulated in the context of broad social circumstances. We call this third marker the status of the people involved in the research.

Finally, these principles lead to a specific ethical position as the foundation for the approaches and methods used (Jourdan, 2012). This is the fourth marker.

50.2 Marker 1: The Ethical Horizon of Health Promotion Research

The reference to the Ottawa Charter (World Health Organization, 1986) is central to the way researchers define the ethical foundations of their studies. In 13 chapters, the Charter is put forward as the foundation of health promotion research. "Since health promotion was formalized by the charter, the associated research has been inextricably tied to it from the beginning" (Basson et al., Chap. 46). It is seen as the tie that links all research partners. "The partners operated from a common-values base derived from the Ottawa Charters' principles of empowerment and community action" (Gibson et al., Chap. 14). Sharing ethical references among those involved is considered a prerequisite to the research. "Adoption of knowledge-based strategies as well as the involvement of citizens, stakeholders, and multi-sectoral governance are recommended in order to achieve international and national objectives for promoting population health, quality of life, and health equity. This demands new skills and changes in the coordination of activities. It also requires development of

Table 50.1 Descriptors of the ethical horizon of health promotion research

Marker	Descriptors
The ethical horizon of the research	Values and principles derived from the Ottawa charter
	Salutogenesis ethical framework
	Critical pedagogy of Paulo Freire
	Contemporary social struggles

trust and the establishment of shared ethics and goals among those involved" (Lillefjell et al., Chap. 26). Some authors also point out that the principles governing health promotion intervention and policies are also those that structure research (Ali and Cunningham, Chap. 10).

The translation of the Ottawa Charter into values and principles for research is variously interpreted by researchers. Although they all share the view that health promotion is grounded in humanist values based on a positive orientation towards health and action-oriented, they emphasise different dimensions. Values such as equity, social justice, and human rights, as well as principles like participation and empowerment, respect, accountability, collaboration, co-production, community development, authenticity, consistency, recognition, openness, and credibility are mentioned by researchers. This list of principles is similar to the one stemming from the IUHPE study (Bull et al., 2012).

The ethical dimensions of salutogenesis (Lillefjell et al., Chap. 26) or of the work of Paolo Freire are also referred to. "The work was underpinned by principles of critical pedagogy (Paulo Freire), co-production and community development and placed the young person at the centre" (Moysés et al., Chap. 47).

Reference to social struggles is also widely present: the regulation of transnational corporations (Anaf et al., Chap. 33), decolonizing (Tremblay and Echaquan, Chapter 9), adultism (MacDougal and Gibbs, Chap. 7)… Table 50.1 summarizes the four descriptors of the first marker.

50.3 Marker 2: The Sources of Legitimacy of the Research

Based on these values and principles, researchers refer to four sources of legitimacy for their research (see Table 50.2). The first source is the research's contribution to the common good through the production of knowledge on the mechanisms likely to facilitate social transformations towards increased social justice. Transformations are sought at various levels. At the local level Franceschini et al. (Chap. 15) explain: "This study focused on the interfaces between the sectors that integrated the Network 'Guarulhos, the City that Protects' – education, health, social and development assistance and public safety – with a view to promote a culture of peace and non-violence, having public schools of a large Brazilian municipality, as the starting point". An example at the national level can be found in Owusu-Addo (Chap. 31): "This chapter presents a case study of a research focused on understanding how a

Table 50.2 Descriptors of the source of legitimacy of the research

Marker	Descriptors
The source of legitimacy of the research	Facilitating social transformations in favour of more justice
	Transforming settings or services in order to make them healthpromoting
	Empowering people and groups living in vulnerable conditions
	Considering the social and environmental determinants

social policy intervention called the Livelihood Empowerment Against Poverty works to influence the social determinants of health and the factors that influence health sector involvement in the programme in Ghana". Less frequent are transformation efforts oriented towards the global levels. "Transnational corporations are part of a wider economic system of global capitalism that functions within a neoliberal regime… Regulating their activities to reduce their harmful human health and environmental impacts is therefore an important task for health promotion" (Anaf et al., Chap. 33). In many cases, researchers take the position of enablers of social change: "By acting as 'policy entrepreneurs,' researchers can orient and support a change of such structures towards health equity. At the same time, this enables researchers to co-produce new knowledge on these fundamental processes" (Rütten et al., Chap. 44).

The second source of legitimacy is linked to the production of knowledge on mechanisms aimed at transforming settings or services in order to make them health promoting. This is the case for schools as described by Bartelink et al. (Chap. 12): "Health promotion in school has therefore the potential to decrease the gap in health disparities among children… system-wide change is a complex task to fulfil". It also quite frequently targets health services. "Respectful Maternity Care research was envisaged to understand the behaviours of service providers, advocating with the policy makers to review and revise the policies and programs and engaging with service providers" (Kaur, Chap. 11). It is much less frequent that researchers address commercial services. "Supermarkets account for a large proportion of all food and grocery spending, and therefore represent a key setting for promoting healthy diets. Eat Well @ IGA was a collaboration between a supermarket retailer, local government, researchers, and government funding partners to improve the healthiness of the supermarket food environment" (Blake et al., Chap. 24).

The third source of legitimacy lies in the possibility of the research process giving a voice to people and populations living in conditions of vulnerability. For example, in Chap. 5, Rodriguez's research rationale is explicitly formulated in terms of fulfilling the needs of people experiencing homelessness. "On the other side, those affected by homelessness do not feel welcomed when accessing services. We presented a research process that addressed the need of improving young people's participation in the design of interventions to promote health". Various groups living in situations of vulnerability were given a voice throughout the research projects presented in this volume. A non-exhaustive list of these includes: disadvantaged young people in Barry et al. (Chap. 19), children and young people experiencing chronic condition or handicap in Dugas et al. (Chap. 4), indigenous people in Tremblay and Echaquan (Chap. 9), and unemployed people in Hollederer (Chap. 8).

The fourth source of legitimacy relates to considerations of the structural constraints, such as the social and environmental determinants, in prevention and healthcare approaches. This means going beyond the individual dimension of health to address people's context and life circumstances from a systemic perspective. The social determinants of health are systematically mentioned as a legitimate ethical perspective on the research. "To enable implementation of relevant interventions, the oral health inequalities have first to be described and understood within the local context, to highlight social injustices and support stakeholders' political decisions" (Tubert-Jeannin et al., Chap. 29). Some authors put forward the socio-cultural determinants (Tremblay and Echaquan, Chap. 9). Some also include consideration of environmental determinants such as housing. "There is a need to use multidisciplinary, multi-phase, mixed method research to bring change in the social and physical environment for changing the behaviour of individual" (Kaur, Chap. 11).

50.4 Marker 3: The Status of the People Involved in the Research

The active involvement of those whose practices are studied is another marker that characterises health promotion research (Table 50.3). For most researchers, this is not simply a methodological issue but an ethical position. When they argue that they conduct "research with" instead of doing "research on", it is because they value study participants' knowledge about health and their capacity to influence the determinants of their own health and that of their communities. Values and principles such as citizen participation, partnership, open communication, sustainability, and empowerment have been highlighted (Mittelmark, 2008).

Researchers consider people, especially those living in the most vulnerable conditions (e.g. socio-economic status, origin, age, chronic condition), as being able to take control over their health. About young people experiencing homelessness, Rodrigues et al. write: "This work permitted young people having the role of active participants, becoming agents of social change, with increased health learning capacity, and critical consciousness. Future follow-up projects with young people to implement progressive change on health policies and practice can make a

Table 50.3 Descriptors of the status of the people involved in health promotion research

Marker	Descriptors
The status of the people involved in the research	People are able to take control of their health
	People's experience is valued in the research
	People's participation is a prerequisite
	People's knowledge is valued in the research

substantial difference to their lives" (Chap. 5). Children are considered as citizens whose rights need to be respected. "We introduce a theoretical and ethical framework building on rights approaches and conceptualising children as citizens in the making who are capable of providing critical perspectives on their lives and futures" (MacDougall and Gibbs, Chap. 7).

Researchers value experience andknowledge of individuals and communities. "Health leaders among the rural dwellers were encouraged to become aware of their own knowledge and the impact that their practices have on the people in their community. … The researchers adopted the role of learners" (Damus et al., Chap. 12). This is true at an individual or community level, but also at a network level. For example, de Leeuw (Chap. 48) considers the WHO network of healthy cities as an "epistemic repository".

For many authors, citizens involved in change processes and activists are considered members of the research communities. "Interdisciplinary networks for participatory, translational, sustainable, and militant research are foundations applied to the health promotion experiences reported here. Proactively, our research group has been working with resources that operate as social catalysts for the implementation of health promotion" (Moysés et al., Chap. 47).

This conception of people's capabilities is not blind to power relationships and the influence of structural socioeconomic factors. It is not aligned with a neoliberal rationality, which considers that people are entirely responsible for their health. This trust in people's ability to take control over their health as rightful citizens is coupled with a meticulous consideration of the contextual determinants that affect health. "Power relations also play an important role within the health care system, irrespective of the clamour for ethics and rights. The health service providers often use the power of knowledge and fail to provide space to the health service users for expressing their needs" (Kaur, Chap. 11).

Consequently, researchers often design their research to highlight and understand people's experience. "To be clear, the aim of the research was not to determine the outcomes of programs rather the focus was on participants' experiences of school food programs. The project was about understanding how different program imperatives impacted on their everyday school/family food practices and their lives in general" (Leahy, Chap. 40). Some focus on people's perceptions and emotions. "Like any other human practice, scientific research is deeply linked and influenced by participants' reactions. Emotions reveal how knowledge develops. Emotions are closely related to all phases of the research process particularly when this occurs collaboratively" (Garista and Pocetta, Chap. 37).

Almost all authors consider participation of individuals and groups an essential condition for research. "Involvement and participation constitute an essential health promotion principle. Sustainable health promotion change can only take place if the target group has the opportunity to develop ownership – and ownership and internalisation are more likely to be achieved if the target group is actively involved in the participatory processes from the start" (Grabowsky et al., Chap. 3).

50.5 Marker 4: The Ethical Foundations of Research Approaches and Methods

The paradigms and methods used by researchers are discussed in detail in the section dedicated to the analysis of the epistemological frameworks (Chap. 52). However, it appears that researchers take particular care to closely align their research approaches with their ethical assumptions. Choices of research methods are often justified by ethical arguments. It becomes relevant to examine how research methods are aligned with the values and ethical principles held by researchers (MacDonald & Mullet, 2008).

Two elements can be highlighted (Table 50.4): 1) researchers fit into the ethical framework for the responsible conduct of research, and 2) they draw the methodological consequences of their ethical presuppositions in terms of participatory approaches and contribution of their work to the political change agenda.

First, researchers emphasise the fact that they meet the criteria of research ethics through the reference to the Helsinki declaration on Ethical Principles for Medical Research Involving Human Subjects. "Ethical considerations are of vital importance in health promotion research. The main ethical standards that should guide any project are to do no harm, ensure informed consent and confidentiality, and secure anonymity (Helsinki declaration). The COMPLETE project fulfilled these standards, but some were at times challenged, mainly due to the collaborative and co-creation nature of the project that involved different stakeholders representing practice and research" (Larsen et al., Chap. 18). General principles are also mentioned. "Methodological questions are answered by documenting the processes of knowing and discovering what we seek to know, bearing in mind issues of ethics, appropriateness, legitimacy, and acceptability" (Amo-Adjei and Tenkorang, Chap. 28). In addition, when particular ethical issues such as interactions with commercial interests are raised, researchers detail the ethical framework of the research in a precise and transparent manner. "Eat Well @ IGA was a collaboration between a supermarket retailer, local government, researchers, and government funding partners to improve the healthiness of the supermarket food environment… The conflict of interest was managed by a clear delineation of partner roles, the provision of external funding to maintain researcher financial independence, the inclusion of local government in a liaison role, and acknowledging multiple stakeholder priorities and outcomes. Analysis of the results were conducted independently without involvement from the retailers" (Blake et al., Chap. 24).

Table 50.4 Descriptors of the ethical foundations of research approaches

Marker	Descriptors
The ethical foundations of research approaches	Research protocols meet guidelines and standards of research ethics
	An explicit normative framework informs research approaches

Second, researchers explicitly justify the approaches and methods used in their research on the basis of their ethical references. In most cases, there is a rejection of the evidence-production model that treats study participants as mere research objects (Dugas et al. Chap. 3). Study participants are conceived of as agents in their own lives, navigating their unique social circumstances as shaped by broader social forces. "The design of this study was based on the aforementioned ethical principle to develop a method that would provide access to individuals' actions without dissociating them from their contexts" (Adam et al., Chap. 6). Considering people as actors in their own right leads to the implementation of participatory approaches that value their experience. "The hegemony of the positivist research paradigm has dominated Nepali higher education for a long time. As a contrast … we adopted Participatory Action Research … [that] assumes that knowledge is based on experience and people's real life... This method empowers both the researchers and the research participants" (Ghimire and Devkota, Chap. 20).

Contributing to social change is an ethical position that leads researchers to consider that research inquiry needs to be intertwined with a political-change agenda to confront the social oppression that leads to health inequities (see, for example, Dugas et al., Chap. 4; Adam et al., Chap. 6; and Moyse et al., Chap. 47). The underlying idea is that producing relevant data is a way to contribute to social change for health. "The motivation of the research endeavour is to more meaningfully engage governmental and community agencies and stakeholders in knowledge co-production and real-world application of such findings. Ultimately, an embedded approach to health promotion research has the potential to increase localized understanding of organisational/systems culture, and awareness of social, political, and economic realities in which research findings would be actualized" (Torres et al., Chap. 17). For research to be useful for transformations, its co-production with the concerned groups and individuals appears to be necessary. "The research program described in this chapter offers a promising example of how health promotion research can contribute to meaningfully transforming health services and promoting culturally safe health care, through respectful, equitable and reciprocal partnerships with Indigenous communities" (Tremblay and Echaquan, Chap. 9).

50.6 Conclusions

This analysis highlights the centrality of ethical arguments in the description and analysis of their own research practices by health promotion researchers. Ethics here are not just a set of principles to ensure compliance with the rules of the responsible conduct of research. Ethics are the *primum movens* of research. They are what justify research, define its ambitions, and shape its approaches. For Creswell (2009), this prominence of values and principles is one of the main characteristics of the transformative worldview. Following Creswell, we consider this to be a major emerging paradigm of research, together with the postpositivist, constructivist, and pragmatic worldviews. According to Mertens and Ginsberg (2009) insert reference in the list Mertens, D. M., & Ginsberg, P. E. (2009). The handbook of social research ethics. Thousand Oaks,CA: Sage., the transformative research paradigm is a set of assumptions and procedures used in research including:

- Underlying assumptions that rely on ethical stances of inclusion and challenging oppressive social structures.
- An entry process into the community that is designed to build trust and make goals and strategies transparent.
- Dissemination of findings in ways that encourage use of the results to enhance social justice and human rights.

There is no doubt that the ethical framework determines the objects of enquiry, the approaches, and the methods of health promotion research. Health promotion research appears to be based on a value-driven transformative paradigm.

References

Bull, T., Riggs, E., & Nchogu, S. N. (2012). Does health promotion need a code of ethics? Results from an IUHPE mixed method survey. *Global Health Promotion, 19*(3), 8–20. https://doi.org/10.1177/1757975912453181

Creswell, J. W. (2009). *Research design qualitative, quantitative, and mixed methods approaches* (3rd ed.). Sage Publications.

Jourdan, D. (2012). *La santé publique au service du bien commun ? : Politiques et pratiques de prévention à l'épreuve du discernement éthique*. Éditions de Santé.

MacDonald, M., & Mullet, J. (2008). Dilemmas in health promotion evaluation: Empowerment and participation. In L. Potvin & D. McQueen (Eds.), *Health promotion evaluation in the Americas: Values and research* (pp. 149–178). Springer.

McQueen, D. (2007). Critical issues in theory for health promotion. In I. D. V. McQueen, I. Kickbusch, L. Potvin, J. Pelikan, L. Balbo, & T. Abel (Eds.), *Health and modernity. The role of theory in health promotion* (pp. 21–42). Springer.

Mittelmark, M. B. (2008). Setting an ethical agenda for health promotion. *Health Promotion International, 23*(1), 78–85. https://doi.org/10.1093/heapro/dam035

Seedhouse, D. (2009). *Health promotion: Philosophy, prejudice and practice* (2nd ed.). Wiley. https://www.wiley.com/en-us/Health+Promotion%3A+Philosophy%2C+Prejudice+and+Practice%2C+2nd+Edition-p-9780470847336

World Health Organization (1986). Charte d'Ottawa pour la promotion de la santé. World Health Organization (1986). Ottawa Charter for Health Promotion. https://www.euro.who.int/__data/assets/pdf_file/0004/129532/Ottawa_Charter.pdf

Chapter 51
Markers of the Objects Studied in Health Promotion Research

Didier Jourdan and Louise Potvin

The aim of this chapter is to analyze the practices studied in health promotion research, i.e., what the researchers want to produce knowledge about. Before describing these objects, it is critical to mention that there is a wide variety of conceptions about what constitutes health promotion across the chapters comprising this volume. Broadly, health promotion is conceived of as:

- What individuals and groups do to promote their own health
- A comprehensive framework encompassing non-medical health interventions
- An approach to design interventions to address the social determinants of health
- Interventions and policies aiming to influence the levers of social transformation toward better health and more generally the empowerment of populations

The fact that there is no universally accepted definition and theory for health promotion has been known for a long time (McQueen, 1996). It is, in part, what makes it difficult to define precisely a field of practice for health promotion.

Practices studied in the various chapters in this volume are not always health promotion practices in the sense of the Ottawa Charter. This could be seen as paradoxical. In fact, all are practices that seemingly contribute to promoting the health of the population, even if they do not have all the attributes of health promotion. This leads to the distinction between health promotion and health-promoting practices. Health promotion practices are interventions, programmes, and policies

D. Jourdan (✉)
UNESCO Chair and WHO Collaborating Centre in Global Health & Education, University of Clermont Auvergne, Clermont-Ferrand, France
e-mail: didier.jourdan@uca.fr

L. Potvin
School of Public Health, University of Montreal, Montréal, QC, Canada

Centre de recherche en santé publique (CReSP), Université of Montreal and CIUSSS du Centre-Sud-de-l'Île-de-Montréal, Montreal, QC, Canada

L. Potvin, D. Jourdan (eds.), *Global Handbook of Health Promotion Research, Vol. 1*,
https://doi.org/10.1007/978-3-030-97212-7_51

classified in the category of health promotion using an objective set of criteria based on the Ottawa Charter. Health-promoting practices (Jourdan et al., 2021) are everyday practices of individuals and groups: practices of traditional healers, disease prevention practices, and health education practices that contribute to promoting the health of individuals and groups. In addition, the people who implement these practices are not necessarily aware that they are "doing" health promotion.

A large proportion of the practices studied in health promotion research are public health, educational, or social interventions. We define interventions as sequential processes of physical, human, financial, or symbolic means organized in a particular context to disrupt the natural course of things or a sequence of foreseeable events. These processes aim at preserving or transforming a state of health in populations, or modifying its foreseeable trajectory of evolution, by acting on a certain number of its determinants (Trompette, 2017). This broad understanding of intervention encompasses health promotion practices that deliberately attempt to transform the distribution of health and its determinants.

Few research programmes study what people and groups do in relation to their own health. Within these health-promoting practices, we further distinguish spontaneous practices that are not related to, or modified by, an intervention. Following Goigoux (2007), we call the former ordinary practices as opposed to practices modified by interventions.

Sometimes, health-promoting practices (ordinary or modified by an intervention) are used as a support for research. They are not studied as such. A problematization process is needed to make them researchable. For example, the work of Grabowski et al. (Chap. 3) is seemingly about an intervention aiming at the co-creation of a toolbox to facilitate interactions between families of children living with diabetes and healthcare professionals. However, the research focuses on a single element of the system, the participation of families at all stages of the intervention. Research projects studying the implementation of health-promoting school programmes (see, e.g., Chaps. 20 and 21) could have different foci, such as, for instance, professionals and school management.

To characterize the practices studied in health promotion research, we identified three markers. The first concerns the actors involved in the practices. In reference to health promotion interventions, the second marker relates to the purpose of the intervention. The third marker concerns the nature of the intervention. By nature, we mean the approach implemented in the intervention.

Like all classifications, the present one has limitations. Some interventions relate to a diversity of actors, others involve different approaches. This classification represents a first attempt to describe the objects of health promotion research.

Table 51.1 Descriptors of the categories of actors engaged in practices

Marker	Descriptors
The categories of actors engaged in practices	Individuals' and populations' health-promoting practices
	Professionals' health promotion practices
	Politicians' and decision-makers' health promotion practices
	Researchers' and innovators' health promotion practices

51.1 Marker 1: The Categories of Actors Engaged in Practices

We have already described in detail (see Chaps. 1 and 2) practices that can be categorized according to the actors involved (see Table 51.1). The practices of individuals and populations may be related to the involvement of people in the design or development of dedicated services (Dugas et al., Chap. 4), the creation of resources not only for but also with people (Grabowsky et al., Chap. 3), or capacity-building (Hollederer, Chap. 8).

The activity of the professionals are often linked to thematic programmes, for example in the field of mental health (Barry et al., Chap. 19), comprehensive-setting approaches to health promotion (Larsen et al., Chap. 18) or interventions focused on the professional development of educators (Ghimire & Devkota, Chap. 20) or health professionals (Gibson, Chap. 14). Also included as the practices of professionals are those enacted in intersectoral coalitions (Franceschini et al., Chap. 15; Gelius & Pfeifer, Chap. 16).

The interventions aimed at influencing the organization of structures and systems such as schools (Sormunen, Chap. 22), NGOs (Richmond et al., Chap. 23), supermarkets (Blake et al., Chap. 24), local policies (Breton et al., Chap. 27), or national social protection programmes (Owusu-Addo, Chap. 31) can be considered as examples of the practices of policy-makers and institutions.

Examples of the practices of innovators are knowledge co-production and transfer programmes (Bilodeau et al., Chap. 35), collaborative research practices and ways of promoting paradigm changes (Porroche-Escudero & Popay, Chap. 45), or the activity of "interdisciplinary networks for participatory, translational, sustainable, and militant" (Moyses et al., Chap. 47).

51.2 Marker 2: The Relationship to Social Change

Health promotion is essentially a transformative project pursued through interventions (Potvin & Jones, 2011). In general, health promotion practices have the ambition to put forward and support people's health-promoting practices, to contribute to the creation of healthy environments, and/or to empower people. However, health-promoting interventions do not all aim at the same type of change (Table 51.2). This marker differentiates intervention practices based on the levels of social organization that are the focus of change. Health promotion interventions are focused on individual action, the physical and social organization of settings, and broader societal and institutional processes. Although these levels of social organization are nested, they involve different social processes.

Some practices do not aim at modifying people's practices or social organization. In some cases, the intervention aims to give people a voice. "Exploring children's perspectives about how the places, spaces and communities in which they live influence their experiences of, and engagement in, play and physical activity" (MacDougall & Gibbs, Chap. 7). Other practices seek to give people and groups the means to make explicit and to recognize their ordinary practices. "Holders of local knowledge, most of them matrons, took part in a dialogue workshop on the state of local knowledge related to health promotion held in rural communities of Jean-Rabel in Haiti. This research was rooted in the beliefs and practices of the rural actors" (Damus et al., Chap. 12).

Most interventions described in this volume aim to contribute to social change. Following Swerissen and Crisp (2004), we distinguish two types of change that social and health interventions may produce: first- and second-order changes. First-order changes occur within a system that remains stable and does not change. Examples are interventions that seek to change individuals (or their immediate environment) so that they are better able to adapt to the existing settings and institutions. In contrast, second-order changes transform the fundamental rules and processes of social systems. Often this requires changing the rules for the allocation and distribution of access, information, and resources (Swerissen & Crisp, 2004).

Practices aimed at implementing comprehensive sexuality education (Amo-Adjei & Tenkorang, Chap. 28), increasing the relevance of interventions through an assessment of their viability (Decroix et al., Chap. 41), or contributing to the professional development of community health workers (Gibson et al., Chap. 14) fall into the category of first-order change.

Many initiatives aimed at generating second-order changes are described throughout this volume. These interventions seek changes at various levels. An example of an attempt to transform conditions at the local level can be found in Franceschini et al.: "the study focused on the interfaces between the sectors that integrated the Network – education, health, social and development assistance and

Table 51.2 Descriptors of the relationship to social changes

Marker	Descriptors
The relationship to social change	The ordinary health-promoting practices of individuals and groups
	The interventions and policies that seek to build the capacities of individuals or groups
	The interventions and policies that seek to produce change in the fundamental rules and processes of social systems

public safety – with a view to promote a culture of peace and non-violence" (Chap. 15). At the other end of the spectrum, Anaf et al. present a research program about transnational corporations (TNCs) using "critical theory to develop and test a corporate health impact assessment framework in order to document the health and environmental harms of the practices and products of TNCs" (Chap. 33).

As an element to be further investigated, most interventions, programmes, and policies described in this volume are culturally sensitive and oriented to increase equity, and many target vulnerable populations.

51.3 Marker 3: The Types of Interventions Studied

The analysis of the contributions shows that there is a great diversity of intervention approaches in the practices studied in health promotion research. These cover almost the entire socio-health field (Jourdan et al., 2012). Some of them are clearly related to public health functions other than health promotion (disease and risk prevention, health protection), while others are mostly focused on supporting the social dynamics of transformation at various levels from the local to the global (Table 51.3). In between these two types, there is a wide range of interventions, programmes, and policies that aim to act on health determinants through the creation of healthy environments and/or people's capacity-building (Jourdan, 2021) (Fig. 51.1).

Some studied practices reported in this volume fall into the category of disease prevention. "In this chapter we will look at the role of research and health promotion in a project for intensive engagement for hepatitis C diagnosis and treatment in high-risk occupational groups of hepatitis C in urban Pakistan" (Ali & Cunningham, Chap. 10); "Prevention Tracker aimed to describe, guide and monitor system change efforts in the chronic disease prevention systems of four communities across Australia" (Riley et al., Chap. 42).

Others are health education programmes. "Breastfeeding practices of mothers in developing countries emerge as relevant subject in health promotion research" (Iellamo et al., Chap. 8); "Classroom implementation of a comprehensive sexuality education curriculum faces diverse challenges, ranging from teacher preparedness to community and parental acceptance of certain topics" (Amo-Adjei & Tenkorang, Chap. 28).

Table 51.3 Descriptors of the types of interventions studied

Marker	Descriptors
The types of interventions studied	Disease prevention
	Health education
	Setting approach
	Community development

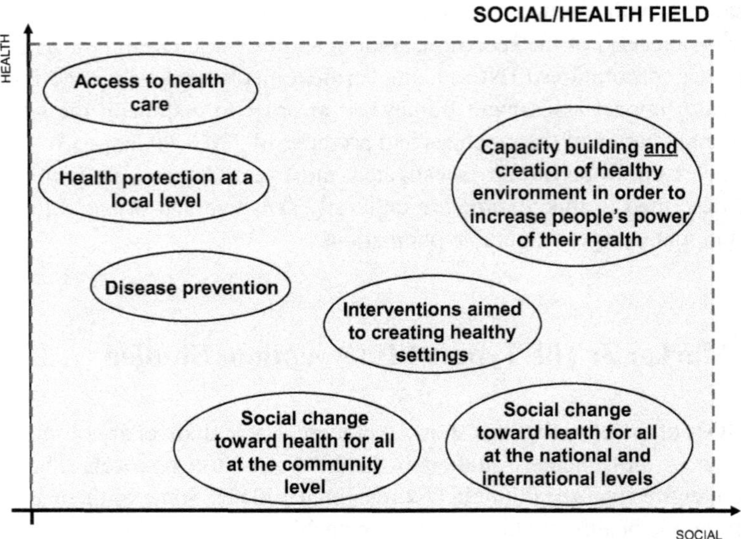

Fig. 51.1 Distribution of the practices studied within the socio-health field (Adapted and translated from Jourdan, D. (2021). La prévention (Les mots pour comprendre): Éditions Sciences Humaines. https://editions.scienceshumaines.com/la-prevention_fr-796.htm. Used with permission from Sciences Humaines Communication)

The setting approach to health promotion, especially in schools but also in communities, sport settings, and health services, is the most common among interventions described by the researchers. "Improving health promotion in the school setting is challenging. To create a meaningful impact, it requires introducing, managing and sustaining health promoting changes in all aspects of the school including individual health behaviour, school environment, policies and curriculum and even in families and the local community" (Bartelink et al., Chap. 21). "The setting approach is a relevant and useful conceptual framework for developing intervention-based initiatives aimed at sustainable impacts in community health promotion" (Lillefjell et al., Chap. 26).

Health promotion research also studies different features of community development programmes. "Community-based participatory research is a critical approach to health promotion practice, grounded in recognition of the importance of addressing power dynamics in the process of promoting health equity" (Franceschini et al., Chap. 15). "This chapter presents a case study of a research focused on understanding how a social policy intervention called the Livelihood Empowerment Against Poverty works to influence the social determinants of health" (Owusu-Addo, Chap. 31).

51.4 Conclusions

The field of health promotion research cannot be simply defined as the research done on health promotion practices. In fact, the objects of research are not always health promotion practices in the sense of the Ottawa Charter. This is not surprising since health promotion has become an umbrella concept for a diversity of interventions, programs, and policies addressing the non-medical determinants of health. What is common to the practices studied is the normative framework of health promotion. This framework is action-oriented. It defines the social determinants of health as targets for changes; proposes advocacy, enabling, and mediation as the main strategies of action; and suggests values and principles to orient the change process, such as participation, empowerment, equity, intersectoral action, holism, sustainability, multiple strategies, and contextualism. Like all classifications, the present one has limitations. Some interventions relate to a diversity of actors, others involve different approaches. This classification represents a first attempt to describe health promotion research objects.

This analysis of the research objects confirms what has been shown in the chapter about the ethical references of health promotion research. "The ethical framework determines both the objects of enquiry, the approaches, and the methods of health promotion research. Health promotion research appears to be based on a values-driven transformative paradigm" (see Chap. 50).

References

Goigoux, R. (2007). Un modèle d'analyse de l'activité des enseignants. *Éducation et didactique, 1*(3), 47–69. https://doi.org/10.4000/educationdidactique.232

Jourdan, D. (2021). *Les mots de la prévention.* https://editions.scienceshumaines.com/la-prevention_fr-796.htm

Jourdan, D., et al. (2012). Quarante ans après, où en est la santé communautaire ? *Santé Publique, 24*(2), 165–178.

Jourdan, D., et al. (2021). Supporting every school to become a foundation for healthy lives. *The Lancet. Child & Adolescent Health, 5*(4), 295–303. https://doi.org/10.1016/S2352-4642(20)30316-3

McQueen, D. V. (1996). The search for theory in health behavior and health promotion. *Health Promotion International, 11*, 27–32.

Potvin, L., & Jones, C. M. (2011). Twenty-five years after the Ottawa Charter: The critical role of health promotion for public health. *The Canadian Journal of Public Health, 102*, 244–248.

Swerissen, H., & Crisp, B. R. (2004). The sustainability of health promotion interventions for different levels of social organization. *Health Promotion International, 19*(1), 123–130. https://doi.org/10.1093/heapro/dah113

Trompette, J. (2017). Complexité des interventions en santé publique et en promotion de la santé : Exploration de son appréhension par les chercheurs et par les acteurs de terrain (Ph.D. diss., Université de Lorraine). http://www.theses.fr/2017LORR0335

Chapter 52
Markers of an Epistemological Framework in Health Promotion Research

Louise Potvin and Didier Jourdan

The chapters in this book illustrate the great diversity of research methods featured in health promotion research practices. Research approaches, methods, and designs are ways to codify the interactions between researchers and the phenomena under study in order for research conclusions to be replicated, confirmed, or contested. They are derived from an epistemological position associated with a disciplinary tradition. Epistemology is generally defined as the study of how valid knowledge is produced (Piaget, 1967). Researchers' epistemological positions relate to their conceptions and assumptions about scientific knowledge, the conditions of its production, and its relations to other types of knowledge.

Despite the diversity of the health promotion research practices reported in this volume, a certain number of descriptors of the ways in which researchers address the knowledge-related issues emerge. In turn, these descriptors inform markers of use in a possible epistemological framework for the field of health promotion research. These markers indicate recurring themes presented in various forms across the various health promotion research practices described in this volume. They do not indicate uniformity in designing and conducting health promotion research. Instead, they represent knowledge-related issues that influence the ways in which health promotion research is carried out and vis-à-vis which research practices can be positioned. Many descriptors are linked to one another and across markers,

L. Potvin (✉)
School of Public Health, University of Montreal, Montréal, QC, Canada

Centre de recherche en santé publique (CReSP), Université of Montreal and CIUSSS du Centre-Sud-de-l'Île-de-Montréal, Montreal, QC, Canada
e-mail: louise.potvin@umontreal.ca

D. Jourdan
UNESCO Chair and WHO Collaborating Centre in Global Health & Education, University of Clermont Auvergne, Clermont-Ferrand, France

L. Potvin, D. Jourdan (eds.), *Global Handbook of Health Promotion Research, Vol. 1*,
https://doi.org/10.1007/978-3-030-97212-7_52

possibly leading to a limited number of configurations distinctive of the field of health promotion research.

52.1 Marker 1: The Recognition of Diverse Forms of Knowledge

Many research practices reported in this book underscore the importance of the individual and collective experience of study participants as a valid source of knowledge regarding their own health-promoting and health promotion practices and their context (Table 52.1). Participants are conceived of as agents in their own life, capable of making decisions, and knowledgeable experts about their own experience.

In addition to the scientific knowledge introduced by researchers into the research process, two other types of knowledge are frequently incorporated and valued in health promotion research: the experiential knowledge of those whose health-promoting practices are being studied, and the professional knowledge of those who intervene to promote health. There are variations in the ways in which participants' experiential knowledge is mobilized and integrated into the research process. A high level of integration is explicit and at the core of research practices in participatory action research such as the one reported by Rodriguez and collaborators (Chap. 5) to co-design interventions for marginalized homeless youth in Scotland: "Participants are encouraged to raise their voices on issues that affect their lives recognizing connections between their individual problems and social contexts of inequalities in which they are embedded." The experiential knowledge of those who are at the receiving end of a professional practice is also a central element for projects aimed at making the practices of health professionals more health-promoting, as exemplified in the research on hepatitis C with a high-risk occupational group in Pakistan (Chap. 10), or in the respectful maternity care project in India (Chap. 11). This is emphasized in Tremblay and Echaquan's project (Chap. 9) on the cultural adaptation of health care professional practices to make them safe for Indigenous people. "In a decolonization approach to research, the purpose of research goes beyond producing new knowledge; it allows the research process to refocus on the specific knowledge, worldviews and methodologies of Indigenous peoples, in order to counteract the power relationships that are inherently embedded in Western knowledge production." Concerning professional knowledge, it is also centrally

Table 52.1 Descriptors of the recognition of diverse forms of knowledge

Marker	Descriptors
The recognition of diverse forms of knowledge	Valuing and legitimizing experiential, professional, and scientific knowledge
	Co-creating knowledge and interventions
	Creating the conditions for collaboration
	Regulating the interactions among stakeholders

positioned in health promotion research as shown in the Capital4Health project in Germany (Chap. 16), or Franceschini's study of intersectoral networks in Sao Paulo, Brazil (Chap. 15). In the latter: "The Network's actors were involved in all phases of the research. In 2016, the project was presented to the Coordinating Committee to assess its interest and gather inputs. These included representatives from all sectors involved, which was particularly interesting since the group's different perspectives on intersectorality quickly came into view, sparking reflections about intentions and motivations that the group had not contemplated until then."

Research projects are sometimes conceived of as a way of creating a dialogue between various ways of experiencing a situation. This was true in the respectful maternity care project in India (Chap. 11), wherein the researchers created numerous forums and workshops that allowed diverse stakeholders to share their knowledge about maternity care. The valuing of participants' own experience is the radical epistemological proposition that underlies Damus and collaborator's study (Chap. 12). Their work with traditional healers in remote Haitian communities highlights how the epistemological domination of western science led to the marginalization and elimination of locally adapted health-promoting knowledge, and in this case, without an appropriate replacement. The authors use the term "epistemicide" in reference to those deliberate attempts to discredit and discard local knowledge. Their chapter illustrates how research is a means to expose and value traditional, local knowledge, and its custodians. Another radical epistemological proposition is exemplified in the work of Montero and Kelly (Chap. 43), which brings art to the forefront of the innovation-development process, introducing and valuing the unconscious, symbolic dimension of behaviour into the research space.

Throughout the numerous research practices described in this volume, there is an underlying proposition on the legitimacy of various forms of knowledge. This multiplicity of ways of knowing and their necessary complementarity is particularly striking in several chapters about researching professional practices. Innovative knowledge and intervention result from a co-creation process emerging from the research-oriented dialogue between the professional knowledge of practitioners, the experiential knowledge of those who benefit from the professional practice and interventions, and the scientific knowledge derived from theories and previous studies. These efforts to conjugate various types of knowledge and transcend the power differentials inherited from the domination of western science in a co-creation process are visible in a variety of projects that aim to co-develop and implement new health promotion interventions. This is the case in the Capital4Health project (Chap. 16), and in others that aim at improving existing health services. For example, Torres and collaborators (Chap. 17) describe their approach as embedded research: "Embedded research has gained traction in recent years, as a form of acknowledging implementation actors as important stakeholders in knowledge creation on the health programs in which they work and for which they are ultimately responsible."

Many research practices described in this book aim at creating the conditions and circumstances for the various actors relevant to the practices under study to meet and account for their experience in a safe and respectful way. There is a genuine concern to use the dynamics of those encounters between the various stakeholders to create knowledge that will contribute to a more general body of knowledge, make a difference in people's lives locally, and support the sustainability of innovative interventions. In reference to the French concept of *collectif épistémique* (Lhoste, 2019), we apply the label "epistemic forums" to research-oriented temporary gatherings of people from different horizons who legitimately share their knowledge about a given situation in order to enhance their understanding of the situation and inform action. Such forums may or may not evolve into epistemic communities.

Many chapters in this book describe various forms of regulating structures for these epistemic forums to ensure a pluralist and equitable governance of the research process. Assembling the conditions of success for these epistemic forums requires deliberately planned strategic work that is described in detail in several chapters (see, e.g. Chaps. 25, 26, and 27). There are additional difficulties and even potential conflicts of interest when some of the stakeholders' primary interests may not be directly compatible with the public good, as in the case of the private sector. The Eat Well @IGA project (Chap. 24) is a case in point: the various compromises resulting from intense and extensive negotiations between a supermarket retailer and the research team allowed the former to align commercial interests with improving the healthiness of the consumers' experience and the latter to test a series of hypotheses in a controlled study. "The conflict of interest was managed by a clear delineation of partner roles, the provision of external funding to maintain researcher financial independence, the inclusion of local government in a liaison role, and acknowledging multiple stakeholder priorities and outcomes."

52.2 Marker 2: The Embeddedness of Research Practices in Context

There is one aspect of research practice common to all contributions in this volume. Health promotion research is always conducted in a real-life context. Social practices cannot be isolated from their context (Table 52.2). This is true for ordinary practices as well as practices modified by intervention, programs, and policies, and this is true for health promotion practices. Therefore, the space of research and knowledge production always intersects and interacts with the social circumstances of the practices under study (Mantoura et al., 2007). They constantly influence each other. Two epistemological consequences follow from these constant interactions. First, the knowledge produced by health promotion research is always contingent, meaning that the influence of context cannot be controlled for or ruled out. The

Table 52.2 Descriptors of the embeddedness of research practice in context

Marker	Descriptors
The embeddedness of research practice in context	Emphasis on complex causal mechanisms
	Use of a systems lens to address complexity
	Methodological pluralism

complexity and pervasiveness of the practice-context interactions (Poland et al., 2008) are part of the effective mechanisms that affect the phenomenon under study. They should be included in a comprehensive explanation of the situation. Second, from a practical perspective research design must adapt to the changing context and circumstances of the practice under study.

This brings to the forefront the question of the nature of the knowledge produced in health promotion research. Given the critical role of context in health promotion practices and research, the positivist quest for evidence "all else being equal" is most often impractical and even mainly irrelevant to the production of knowledge aimed at closing the research-practice gap. As exemplified by Riley and collaborators (Chap. 42), the necessary reductionist approach that requires isolating effective mechanisms or controlling for local conditions "fails to grapple with the complexity of health promotion practice." A more pragmatic perspective on the nature of knowledge is needed. In this sense, Decroix and collaborators (Chap. 41) discuss an alternative to the Campbellian model of validity that puts more weight on the internal validity of scientific evidence (the capacity to attribute an observed effect to a specific cause or treatment) compared to external validity (the capacity to generalize observed causal relationships to a broader class of events). Adding viable validity (the capacity of the research results to produce evidence helpful in real-world conditions) as a criterion for valid knowledge highlights the pragmatic and contingent nature of health promotion evidence.

Throughout this volume, system thinking and complexity have been referred to as lenses to appraise the mutual influences of health promotion interventions and context (Hawe, 2015). Increasingly health promotion interventions are conceived as systems of events that trigger (health-promoting) mechanisms in the broader systems in which they are implemented (Hawe et al., 2009), or as socio-technical networks embedded in larger systems (Bilodeau & Potvin, 2018; Minary et al., 2018). Frohlich and collaborators (Chap. 32) clearly address the contingent nature of knowledge about interventions. "The capacity of an intervention to change a system's dynamic relies on the interaction between the resources it offers and the pre-existing configuration of the system. By coupling and embedding with the pre-existing configuration, therefore changing it, health promotion interventions create opportunities to trigger new mechanisms and generate different events (outcomes)." The role of research is not to predict the trajectory of a system in an implausible controlled environment, but to explain and understand the mechanisms that produced observable outcomes as argued by Riley and collaborators (Chap. 42). The only way to understand how changes result from the complex intervention-context interactions is through in-depth knowledge of the context and focussed research on the intervention-context interactions. Even in a randomized trial as in the COMPLETE project presented by Larsen and collaborators (Chap. 18), there is a recognition that the implementation context needs to be documented and its effect on the intervention implementation process taken into account, leading to epistemological tensions. "There is an inherent contradiction between the RCT as a deductive method and the process evaluation as an inductive approach. Researchers need to balance the extent to which the analyses will be guided by theory and the extent to which the analyses can pursue findings that emerge during discussions among the parties of the project." Addressing the complexity of these interactions requires intense and close collaboration between researchers and the intervention stakeholders, in context, to document the transformative processes at play.

The changing nature of context and the necessity to embed and adapt research in context lead to two consequences for health promotion research: the importance of methodological pluralism to capture the various relevant features of context, and research design flexibility to adapt to changing contexts. Methodological pluralism involves the integration of data from various sources as well as taking into account the perspective of the various stakeholders and participants as equal partners in the research project. There are many examples of such requirements throughout this book. Basson and collaborators (Chap. 46) go as far as to propose that "an interdisciplinary method based on partnership and collaboration" constitutes one of the scientific conditions for health promotion research. To operationalize this condition, many research programmes or projects presented in this volume have discussed the role and functioning of research governance instances in which researchers and the relevant stakeholders in the phenomenon under study make decisions about the conduct of the research. Such governance instances take diverse forms and perform various tasks. In most cases, researchers insist that their governance structure reflects a partnership in which all partners are equal and all partners' expertise is valued and recognized. The Project Council described by Larsen for the COMPLETE project is an example of such a governing structure. "The Project Council was the arena in which the complexity of the project was discussed and where different interests emerged most clearly. It was also a forum where challenges associated with the project were addressed and discussed. The Project Council was important in the continuous anchoring of the various parties´ engagement and ownership. It was also the forum where the tension between the considerations of the RCT design, the process evaluation and the dynamics of practise was most clearly expressed" (Chap. 18).

52.3 Marker 3: The Relationship Between Researchers and Other Stakeholders

A great deal of health promotion research is about programmes and policies that attempt to change the context that shapes health. This is generally referred to as structural interventions that aim to change the distribution of health by addressing broader determinants of health (McLaren et al., 2010). The settings approach, a recognized hallmark of health promotion that deals with settings as whole systems, and attempts to change the health-promoting properties of those systems, has generated a large amount of research on how to intervene to change these properties to improve health (Dooris, 2009). In this book, this research is mostly found in the parts about the practices of policymakers and institutions and about the practices of researchers and innovators.

There are generally two models of research on these interventions and innovations (Table 52.3). On the one hand, there are research programs in which researchers take the lead in the design and implementation of the intervention. This is the case for the Smart Eating project in India (Chap. 30), in the CARA model for school health promotion (Chap. 22), and in many others. On the other hand, there is research conceived of as studies to support, and derive knowledge from, innovations planned and implemented by non-research organizations. This is the case for La Case de Santé (Chap. 46) in Toulouse; the CLoterreS project undertaken by Breton and collaborators on the Local Health Contracts, a national program implemented in French municipalities to foster prevention (Chap. 27); and the Livelihood Empowerment Against Poverty (LEAP) programme in Ghana (Chap. 31).

Both innovation development models coexist in the field of health promotion research. However, whether or not they take the lead in the intervention, researchers are deeply involved in collaborative arrangements with local actors and decision-makers. Such collaborations are obviously critical to accessing data about the intervention and intervention participants in the cases where research accompanies innovations designed and implemented by others. However, even in the case where researchers are driving the project definition and the gathering of the necessary intervention resources, as in the Capital4Health project (Chap. 16) or in the Levelling the playing field project (Chap. 32), intervention implementation responsibilities are generally shared with local organizations in a collaborative arrangement. Such collaborations are necessary not only to ensure the sustainability of the intervention but even more fundamentally to enable its successful implementation. Frohlich and collaborators (Chap. 32) explain why the gap between an intervention idea and its implementation needs to be filled with the means of partnerships with local actors. "Indeed, the implementation of pilot projects to transform the built environment using innovative ideas such as Play and School Streets, in two entirely different cities, is complex. It requires a clear articulation of the idea and the development of collaborative relationships with municipal decision-makers, professionals and local community members. It also requires the adoption of a language of operationalization already mastered by urban planning professionals, something that researchers do not always have within their skill set. Our research team at the École de Santé

Table 52.3 Descriptors of the relationship between research and practice as a structuring dimension of the research design

Marker	Descriptors
The relationship between researchers and other stakeholders	Researchers lead the innovation development model
	Researchers support intervening institutions
	Researchers and stakeholders negotiate collaborative agreement
	Researchers hold a critical perspective on the status of a control group

Publique, Université de Montréal (ESPUM) turned to a non-governmental organization, the Montreal Urban Ecology Center (MUEC), to accompany us in the development, implementation and research process we foresaw as being critical to success." Such collaborative arrangements lead generally to the co-ownership of the intervention and the blurring of the frontiers between research and practice. Ruetten describes in great detail an example of the creation and functioning of such a collaborative arrangement, the Cooperative Planning Process implemented in the Kombine project to foster an active lifestyle in Germany (Chap. 44).

A fourth descriptor associated with this epistemological marker concerns the critical perspective that researchers hold about the usefulness of using a control group in their research design. To the extent that in many instances research aims at explaining how practices are shaped by, and in turn, influence context instead of predicting outcomes, the use of a counterfactual in the form of a control group appears to be much less critical than in other forms of research. This is true even in the case where the practice under study is a programme or a policy. For example, Sormunen (Chap. 22) clearly links the relevance of using control schools in her study of the participatory development of health promotion research in schools to a specific research question about the predictability of the outcome. The outcome of the 2-year intervention was estimated using a non-equivalent control group design with a pre-test and post-test. But this was one among four research questions. The other questions concerned the development of collaborative programs in schools, for which a control group was not necessary. Furthermore, even in the case where intervention outcome is of interest, the mere use of a control group is insufficient to explain the results. An in-depth understanding of the intervention implementation process and how it interacts with context is required to track how the observed outcome is produced, for whom, and in what conditions. In a randomized cluster trial evaluation of the Eat Smart India intervention, Kaur and collaborator (Chap. 30) also implemented an extensive process evaluation to support the improvement of the intervention implementation as it unfolds and to explain the variation of outcomes across clusters. In many cases, the use of a control group is simply impractical.

Two main strategies were used to allow an assessment of the intervention outcome. Using single or multiple case study design, some researchers have implemented a range of methods to follow more closely the programme implementation in a small number of units and thus to document how the various activities implemented are linked, or not, to observable transformations. This is the case of the study about the Malvik Path in Norway (Chap. 26), a 3-km biking and walking path connecting two residential areas. Through the meticulous and continuous documentation of the implementation and utilization of the path, coupled with a population survey and various methods to collect residents' experience of this new infrastructure, the researchers were able to connect the implementation of the path with various outcomes in the exposed communities. This process is well described in Chap. 49 on the research program about health impact assessment in Southern Australia. "It is difficult to directly attribute changes to HIAP in a situation where there is no possibility of a control or comparison group. Consequently, our methodological approach was to articulate the theory of change that underpins the actions selected and map the path from the HiAP action to likely health and equity impacts in the future."

Another strategy is to gather implementation and outcome information on a large number of instances in which a policy or program is implemented and to link implementation variation with variations in outcomes. This was the case reported by de Leeuw for the evaluation of the European Network of Healthy Cities (Chap. 48) that uses the massive amount of data provided by local projects through annual reports to codify various types of actions undertaken by cities and link them with observed transformations.

52.4 Marker 4. The Articulation of Knowledge Production and Sharing

Throughout the various accounts and analyses of research projects and programmes presented in this volume, knowledge translation and its capacity to inform the transformative practices of decision-makers and professionals stands out as a distinct epistemological marker of health promotion research (Table 52.4). Over and above the requirements for knowledge co-production, knowledge transfer and exchange appear as an integral part of the knowledge produced in context. We identified three descriptors for this marker.

Some authors have made a convincing argument that scientific knowledge about practice is not the equivalent of practical knowledge of the professionals. There is a reciprocal epistemic relationship between these two forms of knowledge. Professional practices and interventions are not directly transferable into scientific, more generalizable, knowledge. To do so, researchers need theoretical frames and methodological devices to link local observations to more general knowledge. Conversely, the scientific knowledge derived from research is not directly actionable by practitioners. Scientific knowledge is decontextualized and codified in more general and abstract notions that can be more freely associated to contribute to a larger body of knowledge and to inform action in contexts other than the one it has been produced (Latour, 1999). Reciprocally, abstract scientific knowledge needs to be re-contextualized in an empirical reality to be meaningful for professional practice and interventions. Bilodeau and collaborators (Chap. 35) explain in great detail the work involved in translating scientific abstractions about practices into instruments that encapsulate this knowledge and make it usable by practitioners. "The

Table 52.4 Descriptors of the articulation of knowledge production and sharing

Marker	Descriptors
The articulation of knowledge production and sharing	A reciprocal epistemic relationship between practical and scientific knowledge
	Knowledge translation as a form of validation
	Solution and action-oriented knowledge

researchers' work consists in producing an interpretation of who the practitioners are and what they do, based in an explicit theoretical reference and the data derived from their observations. The added value of this work is to put forward a theoretically informed perspective (…) to draw generic knowledge out of singular realities. Then, by submitting this reading of their reality and practices to actors from the field, we can translate theory and experience into an instrumentation that is both contextualized because it is anchored in empirical observations and generalizable through its derivation from a broader theory."

Another marker of the critical role of knowledge sharing in health promotion research is the use of the various collaborative arrangements between researchers and practitioners to validate research results in terms of "cultural fit." This process documents to which extent the researchers' interpretation captures the complexity of the practice-in-context. The process of doing collaborative research reaches its full potential when the outcome of the process is reintroduced as data that enrich the initial results. The detailed account of the collaborative data analysis process implemented by Franceschini and collaborators (Chap. 15) provides an example of its value and how it comes full circle when, in turn, these results impact on practices. "Analyzing the results with the actors was rich and insightful. Their interpretations filled in gaps not previously seen in the research process, redirected the initial analysis and helped to shape the research conclusions. These discussions provided insights for the group to rethink through their own actions and led to a reorientation of strategies related to the GCP Network's development."

Finally, several chapters in this volume provide compelling evidence that giving a central role to knowledge sharing between researchers and practitioners and decision-makers in the research process is a condition for research results to lead to solution- and action-oriented knowledge. Bilodeau and collaborators (Chap. 35) have shown the limitations of researchers in reintroducing context into their abstract interpretations so as to make their results "actionable." Likewise, through a detailed account of the functioning of a multi-stakeholder research steering committee, Beaulieu and her team (Chap. 38) were able to link the action-oriented output of the research to specific actions undertaken by practitioners, decision-makers, and community partners in the steering committee. "How the knowledge was used differed according to the committee members' profiles. For example, there were more instrumental and strategic uses of the research results among community partners, which suggests that they could play an active part in closing the gap between research and practice."

52.5 Conclusions

The inductive analysis of the rich contextualized descriptions of health promotion research practices provided by the authors of the various chapters in this volume identified 11 descriptors related to four markers that may serve as a basis for an epistemological framework for health promotion research. These four markers are as follows.

1. The recognition of the various forms of knowledge that need to be combined in a regulated dialogue to explain and illuminate health-promoting and health promotion practices.
2. The embeddedness of research practice in context, embracing complexity and using a systems perspective to produce explanations that answer the questions: How does this health-promoting or health promotion practice come about; and what kinds of outcomes can be expected for whom, and under which circumstances?
3. The relationship between researchers and other stakeholders involved in the research and in the practice under study. Although this relationship takes various forms, there is a critical examination of how it shapes the knowledge produced.
4. The articulation of knowledge production and sharing, recognizing that closing the science-practice gap requires different work from the various stakeholders, including the researchers, involved in the research.

These markers are not prescriptions. They are elements of health promotion research practices that researchers explicitly consider in the planning and conduct of their research. They do not lead to ready-made solutions and pre-determined research method choices. Interestingly, these markers are related to the ethical references as discussed in Chap. 50. They represent the epistemological consequences of the normative frames that health promotion researchers explicitly refer to in reflecting on their research practices. Also, not all researchers consider all these markers and in those exact terms. Some research projects or programmes lend themselves to specific markers instead of others. Some researchers may be more or less explicit in their respective positions on several or all of these markers. Nonetheless, taken together these markers provide a distinctive epistemological landscape for health promotion research that needs to be further investigated.

References

Bilodeau, A., & Potvin, L. (2018). Unpacking complexity in public health interventions with the actor-network theory. *Health Promotion International, 33*(1), 173–181.

Dooris, M. (2009). Holistic and sustainable health improvement. The contribution of the settings-base approach to health promotion. *Perspectives in Public Health, 129*, 29–36.

Hawe, P. (2015). Lessons from complex interventions to improve health. *Annual Review of Public Health, 36*, 307–323.

Hawe, P., Shiell, A., & Riley, T. (2009). Theorising interventions as events in systems. *American Journal of Community Psychology, 43*, 267–276.

Latour, B. (1999). *Pandora's hope*. Harvard University Press.

Lhoste, E. (2019). Innover pour inclure: apprendre à faire ensemble. hal-02518944

Mantoura, P., Gendron, S., & Potvin, L. (2007). Participatory research in public health: Creating innovative alliances for health. *Health & Place, 13*, 440–451.

McLaren, L., McIntyre, L., & Kirkpatrick, S. (2010). Rose's population strategy of prevention need not increase social inequalities in health. *International Journal of Epidemiology, 39*, 372–377. https://doi.org/10.1093/ije/dyp315

Minary, L., et al. (2018). Addressing complexity in population health intervention research: The context/intervention interface. *Journal of Epidemiology and Community Health, 72*(4), 319–323. https://doi.org/10.1136/jech-2017-209921

Piaget, J. (1967). L'épistémologie et ses variétés. In J. Piaget (Ed.), *Logique et connaissance scientifique* (pp. 3–61). Gallomard. Encyclopédie de la Pléiade, Vol 22.

Poland, B., Frohlich, K. L., & Cargo, M. (2008). Context as a fundamental dimension of health promotion program evaluation. In L. Potvin & D. V. McQueen (Eds.), *Health promotion evaluation practices in the Americas: Values and research* (pp. 299–317). Springer.

Chapter 53
Conclusion: Characterising the Field of Health Promotion Research

Didier Jourdan and Louise Potvin

With this handbook, our project is to map out health promotion research practices using a bottom-up approach. This is why we invited experts from the different research traditions that coexist in the field to contribute chapters. Throughout the chapters of this volume, individuals and groups who self-identify as health promotion researchers have reflected on their research practices, describing what they actually do, how they work, the activities they put in motion, and with whom they produce, co-produce, and/or share health promotion knowledge. We cannot pretend that this collection is exhaustive, or even representative of all the research practices implemented to create a knowledge base about, and for, health promotion. However, taken together, these practices illustrate the diversity of research objects, approaches, methods, and epistemological and ethical positions that can be found in health promotion research. This diversity closely mirrors that of research articles published in scientific health promotion journals. It involves qualitative and quantitative data collection and analysis, observational and experimental methodologies, integration or not of previous theoretical knowledge, a more or less radical integration of contextual knowledge, and so on. In this conclusion, it is important to look back at the contributions we have received and our way of drawing out principles for structuring the field and to summarise what we have learned throughout this process.

A snapshot of the geographical locations of the contributing research teams shows that the collection in this volume is truly global, with contributions from 27

D. Jourdan (✉)
UNESCO Chair and WHO Collaborating Centre in Global Health & Education, University of Clermont Auvergne, Clermont-Ferrand, France
e-mail: didier.jourdan@uca.fr

L. Potvin
School of Public Health, University of Montreal, Montréal, QC, Canada

Centre de recherche en santé publique (CReSP), Université of Montreal and CIUSSS du Centre-Sud-de-l'Île-de-Montréal, Montreal, QC, Canada

L. Potvin, D. Jourdan (eds.), *Global Handbook of Health Promotion Research, Vol. 1*,
https://doi.org/10.1007/978-3-030-97212-7_53

countries and territories from five continents (Fig. 53.1). Although the number of contributions differs across countries, both the global North and the global South are represented. Not surprisingly, the underlying conceptions of health promotion and the practices investigated appear to be influenced by the historical, cultural, political, and socio-economic context of the countries in which the research is conducted. In some countries, health promotion is institutionalised, anchored in a well-defined policy framework encompassing a wide range of activities. In other countries, health promotion is more a matter of activism and community dynamics fuelling social transformations. Although these differences in context influence the research activity, it was possible to identify some common features in the research configurations. These were presented as markers of the research's ethical references (Chap. 50), objects (Chap. 51), and epistemological framework (Chap. 52) of the field of health promotion research.

For this mapping exercise, our ambition was not to define the "right way" to do health promotion research but instead to identify its distinctive features on the basis of the research practices collated in this book. We sought to make the framework explicit rather than to try to achieve consensus about the relevant paradigms, tools, and methods in health promotion research. Each research project is a unique, singular, original activity in a specific context. However, each can be described by a set of characteristics that reflect the different dimensions of the research. At this point

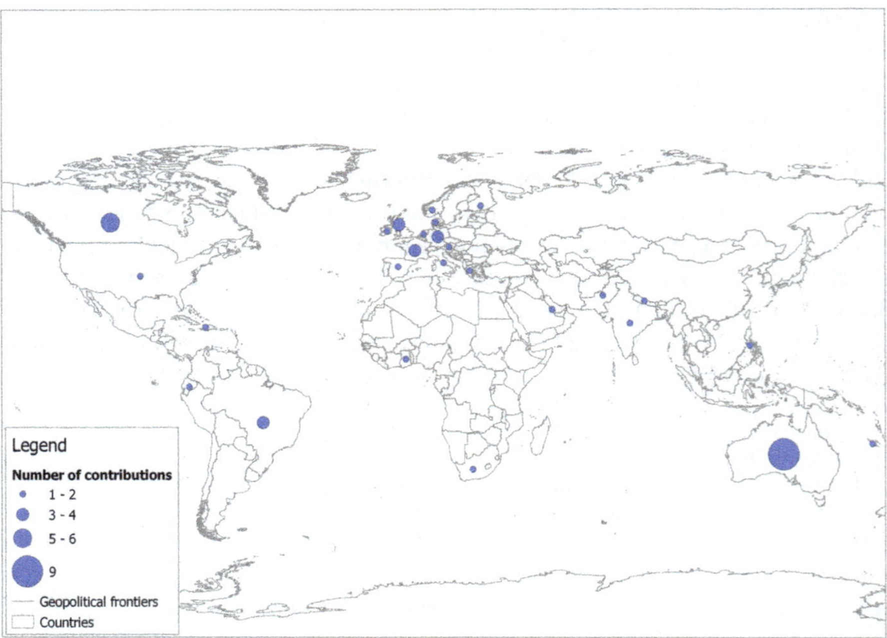

Fig. 53.1 Geographical distribution of the contributions to the handbook (Source: Original creation made with open data furnished by Natural Earth. Free vector and raster map data @ naturalearthdata.com)

in the development of the health promotion research field, identifying possible configurations in the various dimensions of research practice appears more relevant than trying to define typologies of research (Tomamichel & Clerc, 2005). Our approach was to look for markers to characterise the field. In their description of their research practices, authors have discussed, sometimes extensively, how their research addresses some of these different markers; we have identified 39 different descriptors. There exist probably more, but at this point, this collection is sufficiently comprehensive to account for the diversity of the field.

The analysis of the contributions to this handbook (45 complete chapters and 9 short reports grouped in Chaps. 8 and 34) shows a real diversity of research practices. It led us to identify 11 markers that fall under the three structuring dimensions we used to define the field of health promotion research: the ethical references, the objects of enquiry, and the epistemological configurations (Potvin & Jourdan, 2021).

Our analysis led us to identify four markers that describe the way in which the ethical references shape health promotion research. The ethical references relate to the principles and values that justify and guide the research process and how researchers translate these values and principles into their research practices. It allows for the development of a common understanding among the different actors in the research process, by defining meaningful values that guide action. The first marker concerns the ethical horizon and relates to the values and principles mentioned by the authors. These clearly set the ethical scene of their work. The second marker is more specific; it is linked to the way in which researchers justify, legitimise their work: the source of legitimacy of their work. It does not refer to general principles. Instead, it provides concrete references to mechanisms likely to facilitate social transformations in favour of social justice and the empowerment and participation in the research process of people living in conditions of vulnerability. It also highlights the relevance of individuals' and populations' knowledge. The third marker that characterises the ethical references of health promotion research is related to the status of the people involved in the research. In almost every chapter, a mention was made on the role of people and populations as participants, active subjects in the research and not research objects. Finally, these principles lead to a specific ethical position regarding the approaches and methods used. The fourth marker supposes the ethical foundations of research approaches (Jourdan, 2012). These ethical markers are specified by 14 descriptors (see Chap. 50).

We also identified three markers that characterise the objects of health promotion research. These are always social practices. They are either the health-promoting practices of individuals and groups or the health promotion practices of those who intervene to transform them or the systems that shape them. The practices studied (the research objects) differ across projects. They fall into the classical categories of disease prevention, health education, setting approach to health promotion, and community development (community health). Our analysis identified three markers to describe the way in which the objects studied shape health promotion research. The first marker concerns the categories of actors that practices relate to. These are the practices of individuals and populations, of professionals, politicians, an institution's decision-makers, researchers, and innovators. The second marker concerns the relation between a practice and social change. Some of the practices studied aimed to enable people and groups to make explicit and recognise their ordinary health promotion practices. Others seek to build the capacities of individuals or groups to adapt to existing settings and institutions (first-order change) or to produce changes in the fundamental rules and processes of social systems (second-order change). Finally, the third marker characterises the types of interventions studied. These markers related to health promotion research objects are specified by 11 descriptors (see Chap. 51).

Health promotion researchers come from a broad range of epistemological horizons, creating epistemological tensions. Altogether, the chapters in this book illustrate the diversity of research paradigms, approaches, and methods used by health promotion researchers. Despite this diversity, a number of descriptors of ways of dealing with knowledge emerge that inform four epistemological markers for the field of health promotion research. These markers indicate recurring themes presented in various forms across chapters, and across the various health promotion research practices. The first is the recognition of diverse forms of knowledge relevant for producing new, valid health promotion knowledge. The second marker is linked to the embeddedness of research practices in context. Health promotion practices cannot be isolated from their context. This is true for ordinary practices as well as for policies and programs. Thus, health promotion research appears to be always conducted in a real-life context. The third marker is about the relationship between researchers and stakeholders. Many research practices described in the handbook are about interventions that attempt to change the context that shapes health. Researchers can lead the innovation development model, accompany intervening institutions, or be part of a consortium organised through a collaborative agreement. In all instances, the regulation of those spaces appears as a key feature of the methodological device. The fourth marker relates to the articulation of knowledge production and sharing. Throughout the accounts and analysis of various research projects and programmes presented in this volume, knowledge sharing and its capacity to inform the transformative practices of decision-makers and professionals stands out as a distinct epistemological marker of health promotion research. Over and above the requirement for knowledge co-production, knowledge sharing appears as an integral part of knowledge produced in context (Fig. 53.2). These markers related to the epistemological framework of health promotion research are specified by 14 descriptors (see Chap. 52).

These three dimensions, 11 markers, and 39 descriptors could be considered as a first attempt to characterise the field of health promotion research (Potvin & Jourdan, 2021). This work is mainly descriptive and preliminary, as the database is not exhaustive. Its interest lies in the fact that it is based on a bottom-up analysis. This rich source of data and the analysis we conducted form the basis for further development.

Volume 2 of the handbook, *Framing Health Promotion Research*, proposes a framework for a distinct field of health promotion research. It is composed of short chapters with a didactic aim that describe and discuss what we consider as the fundamental elements for structuring the field and their specific configurations that

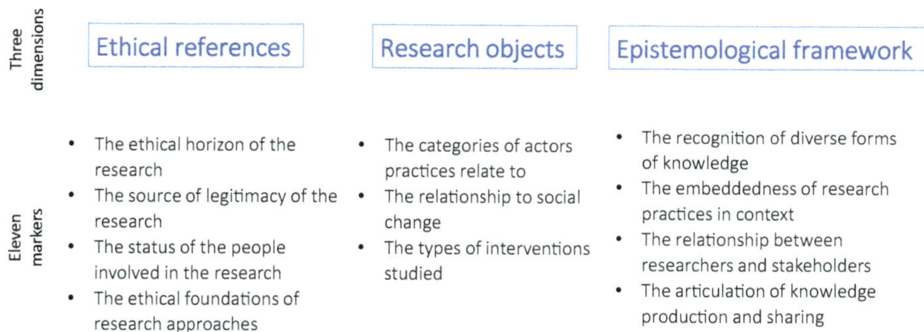

Fig. 53.2 Dimensions and markers to describe the field of health promotion research

make this field of research distinct. The argument is organised into four parts. The first part defines what constitutes a research field and why it is relevant and useful to distinguish health promotion research from other related fields of research. The second part discusses the values and the ethical references underlying health promotion research. The third part examines the range of social practices that comprise the objects of health promotion research. The fourth part proposes a pluralist epistemological framework for health promotion research.

Finally, Volume 3 of the Global Handbook, *Doing Health Promotion Research*, provides introductory-level presentations of paradigms, strategies of inquiry, and methods associated with, and contributing to, health promotion research. It is composed of short chapters written by authors who have developed a recognised expertise with regard to either a paradigm, strategy of inquiry, or method associated with health promotion research. These chapters are written as introductions to these paradigms, approaches, or methods in relation to the specific health promotion research challenge they address. The volume is structured in three parts. Part I addresses the various paradigms as sets of beliefs, worldviews, or epistemologies that guide health promotion research practices. Part II presents strategies of inquiry that are implemented in health promotion research and provides specific directions for designing studies. Part III discusses the various methods that are used in, or adapted to, the conduct of health promotion research. These are related to the collection, analysis, and interpretation of the empirical material used in a study.

Recognising that we cannot pretend to be an exhaustive coverage of all relevant paradigms, strategies of inquiry, and methods for health promotion research, and that the field of health promotion research evolves rapidly, this handbook, especially the third volume, is conceived of as an opening for the future and a steppingstone for an ongoing global initiative. In collaboration with the Editorial Board of *Global Health Promotion*, the official journal of the International Union for Health Promotion and Education (IUHPE), we will create a section in the journal entitled "Doing health promotion". This section will publish introductory-level presentations of paradigms, approaches, and methods relevant for health promotion research and written by health promotion researchers.

Characterising the field of health promotion research is a collective endeavour. We hope that this volume will be a milestone on the road to establishing health promotion research as a recognised field. We also invite all people interested in health promotion research to contribute to the framing of the field. Scientific events in the field such as the IUHPE conferences provide opportunities for further interaction on these initial proposals.

References

Jourdan, D. (2012). *La santé publique au service du bien commun ? : Politiques et pratiques de prévention à l'épreuve du discernement éthique*. Éditions de Santé.

Potvin, L., & Jourdan, D. (2021). Health promotion research has come of age! Structuring the field based on the practices of health promotion researchers. *Global Health Promotion, 17579759211044076*. https://doi.org/10.1177/17579759211044077

Tomamichel, S., & Clerc, F. (2005). La recherche en sciences de l'éducation. État des lieux et points de vue. *Recherche en soins infirmiers, 83*(4), 4–17.

Appendix

Overview of the Chapters

Introduction
This first volume is dedicated to mapping the field of health promotion research. In order to guide the reader within the content of the chapters, we have written short summaries of each of the contributions. This will help the reader to navigate the rich material in this book. Of course, the handbook can be read from beginning to end, but it also can be used as a working tool for researchers, students, and practitioners. It is possible to read the introduction and then explore chapters according to needs and interests. It is also possible to read the conclusion and then follow the cross-references to the chapters that illustrate the markers and configurations that shape the field of health promotion research.

Part I: Researching the Practices of Individuals and Populations

Chapter 3: Design-Based Research on Active Family Involvement: Developing a Family Toolbox to Support Health Care Professionals Working with Diabetes Management

Dan Grabowski, Jens Aagaard-Hansen, Bjarne Bruun Jensen
Denmark

This chapter describes a comprehensive design-based research project on promoting family health. The project – referred to as the Family Toolbox intervention – involved a comprehensive, integrated health promotion approach, including a set of

L. Potvin, D. Jourdan (eds.), *Global Handbook of Health Promotion Research, Vol. 1*,
https://doi.org/10.1007/978-3-030-97212-7

five evidence-based principles. This research and its outcomes have been instrumental in the development of a family-oriented approach to health promotion.

Chapter 4: Action Research with People Being Treated for Cancer or a Rare Disease: Health Mediation Central to Their Experiences and Inclusion

Éric Dugas, Zoé Rollin, Lucas Sivilotti, Karyn Dugas
France

Knowledge production in health promotion research is intimately linked to and shaped by its social and ethical aims. It requires the creation of contextually based approaches and methods that ensure the genuine participation of such people. This chapter analyzes such a process, reporting on an action research on an innovative life-course support and health-mediation intervention for students with cancer or a rare disease.

Chapter 5: Critical Health Promotion and Participatory Research: Knowledge Production for and with Young People Experiencing Homelessness in Scotland

Andrea Rodriguez, Sabrina Galella, Shea Moran, Ruth Freeman
United Kingdom

This chapter presents an inclusive, participatory, and multidisciplinary research process based on the principles of Paolo Freire's critical pedagogy to promote the right to health of marginalized groups. It highlights the need to place young people at the centre of the process, recognizing their expertise and seeking to put into dialogue the various types of knowledge involved in projects.

Chapter 6: Acting-in-Context: A Methodological and Theoretical Approach to Understanding the Actions of People Living in Poverty

Caroline Adam, Sylvie Gendron, Louise Potvin
Canada

Acting on the social determinants of health requires that health promotion research produce methodological approaches and theoretical tools to study and understand the interactions between individuals and their contexts, especially contexts unfavourable to health. This chapter describes the aims and value of acting-in-context, an approach that makes it possible to consider and analyze the relationships between the social context and the actions of individuals without slipping into individualistic or deterministic approaches.

Chapter 7: Participatory Health Promotion Research with Children

Colin MacDougall, Lisa Gibbs
Australia

This chapter describes an approach to research health practices of children through the analysis of four studies. The researchers present a theoretical and ethical framework that builds on rights approaches and conceptualizes children as citizens in the making. It shows how qualitative and ethnographic research methods are relevant for research with children underpinned by participation and empowerment.

Chapter 8: Engaging with People and Populations in Health Promotion Research: A Snapshot on Participatory Processes

Valérie Ivassenko, Andrew J. Macnab, Danilo Di Emidio, Alfons Hollederer, Efrelyn A. Iellamo, Jimryan Ignatius B. Cabuslay, Ivan Rene G. Lim, Shannen G. Felipe, Bridget Ira C. Arante, Andy Sharma

Research on the practices of individuals and populations involves specific methods, approaches, and objectives that need to be constantly interpreted and adapted to their utilization context. Through five snapshots of promising programmes, this chapter shows how participation of various stakeholders is a common thread of health promotion research and redefines the very questions, methods, and aims of research.

Part II: Researching the Practices of Professionals

Chapter 9: Fostering Cultural Safety in Health Care Through a Decolonizing Approach to Research with, for, and by Indigenous Communities

Marie-Claude Tremblay, Sandro Echaquan
Canada

Based on a two-eyed seeing approach and co-developed with Indigenous partners, this work proposes research strategies for enacting the established values of health promotion of participation, empowerment, social justice, and equity. Its approach and processes make it possible to combine multiple types of knowledge to co-develop a new intervention model reorienting health care with the aim of increasing cultural safety.

Chapter 10: Doing Research with People: Hepatitis C and Intensive Engagement with High-Risk Occupational Groups in Karachi, Pakistan

Tassawar Ali, Nance Cunningham
Pakistan

This chapter describes how knowledge production can be a springboard for developing a health promotion programme. This intervention aimed at tackling the critical issue of the spread of the hepatitis C virus and promoting community engagement in diagnosing and treating hepatitis C among high-risk occupational groups in urban Pakistan. The research highlights the importance of community engagement in the research process, which can yield a rich harvest of knowledge for sharing with all stakeholders, thereby bolstering the database and project success.

Chapter 11: Respectful Maternity Care: A Methodological Journey from Research to Policy and Action

Manmeet Kaur
India

The Respectful Maternity Care Project describes the challenges and issues in changing the behaviour of individuals, specifically maternity care professionals in India. It clearly brings out the need for complex multilevel, mixed method of evolving research, combining multidisciplinary and participatory approaches to understand, and initiate a sustainable change process. This chapter describes how the research project was developed to adapt to the context and develop advocacy for professional change.

Chapter 12: Valuing Indigenous Health Promotion Knowledge and Practices: The Local Dialogue Workshop as a Method to Engage and Empower Matrons and Other Traditional Healers in Haiti

Obrillant Damus, Maude Vézina, Nicola J. Gray
Haiti

This chapter presents an original research project about the beliefs and practices of traditional healers in Haiti. It describes the techniques used to value their knowledge and support their empowerment in communities isolated from official public health promotion policies. The dialogue workshop technique allowed the research team to critically reflect on the hierarchies of knowledge and local knowledge destruction.

Chapter 13: Aligning Research Practices with Health Promotion Values: Ethical Considerations from the Community Health Worker Common Indicators Project

Noelle Wiggins, Kenneth Maes, Leticia Rodriguez Avila, Keara Rodela, Edith Kieffer
United States of America

In this chapter, the authors reflect on how they used a participatory epistemology approach to identify constructs and indicators for the practices, working conditions, and outcomes of a group of health promotion practitioners, referred to as the Community Health Workers. Articulating scientific knowledge with experiential and professional knowledge, they suggest how wider use of this approach could support and expand the deeply held values and goals in the field of health promotion.

Chapter 14: Investing in Health Promotion Research Among Community Health Workers in Semi-rural Uganda Using a Partnership Approach

Linda Gibson, Deborah Ikhile, Mathew Nyashanu, David Musoke
United Kingdom

This chapter explores the challenges and the benefits of an interdisciplinary partnership approach to undertaking research in Uganda. Informed by the key health promotion principles of listening to and working with and in communities, this partnership approach provides an ethical framework for research practice and contributes to improving and strengthening the capacity of community health workers and bringing about real-world change.

Chapter 15: Intersectoriality and Health Promotion Research: The Perspective of Practitioners from a Brazilian Experience

Maria Cristina Trousdell Franceschini, Marcia Faria Westphal, Marco Akerman
Brazil

Moving from words to action and making intersectoriality not just a concept but a tangible and achievable approach remains a challenge. This research on the practices of actors involved in the "Guarulhos, the City that Protects" intersectoral network fuels the discussion on how intersectoriality is brought about, how it connects with other health-promoting concepts, and what its contributions are to policies and programmes that ultimately affect people and communities.

Chapter 16: Capabilities and Transdisciplinary Co-production of Knowledge: Linking the Social Practices of Researchers, Policymakers, Professionals, and Populations to Promote Active Lifestyles

Peter Gelius, Klaus Pfeifer
Germany

This chapter reports on the experience of Capital4Health, a transdisciplinary German research consortium composed of four intervention projects involving researchers from different disciplines and non-academic actors. This research provides unique and valuable insights on how knowledge co-creation and sharing can be used effectively to implement physical-activity promotion interventions in various real-world settings across the course of life.

Chapter 17: Conducting Embedded Health Promotion Research: Lessons Learned from the Health-on-the-Go Study in Ecuador

Irene Torres, Daniel López-Cevallos, Fernando Sacoto
Ecuador

Based on an experience of implementing embedded research in Quito, Ecuador, this chapter identifies the values, opportunities, challenges, and limitations of conducting research with health care professionals. The research approach is based on recognizing the importance of local knowledge and capacity. The design provided for knowledge co-production with the various actors involved in health promotion programmes. It offers a promising approach for informing sustainable changes in health practices and policies.

Chapter 18: Doing Collaborative Health Promotion Research in a Complex Setting. Lessons Learned from the COMPLETE Project in Norway

Torill Larsen, Ingrid Holsen, Helga B. Urke, Cecilie Høj Anvik
Norway

This chapter describes the development of multi-tier collaborative research within schools as complex health-promoting settings. It illustrates how genuine partnerships between academics, NGOs, and health and education professionals can be built and maintained throughout an intensive research process. Intervention evaluation appeared to be much more relevant with parallel evaluations of the implementation process closely involving the various stakeholders.

Chapter 19: Researching the Process of Implementing Mental Health Promotion: Case Studies on Interventions with Disadvantaged Young People

Margaret M. Barry, Tuuli Kuosmanen, Katherine Dowling
Ireland

This chapter presents two case studies on the implementation of mental health promotion programs. The authors argue how the systematic study of implementation can strengthen not only the body of knowledge but ultimately contribute to more effective practice and policy as well as to sustainable population health and well-being. A number of key characteristics of implementation research – supported by a literature review – are discussed, including employing participatory research methods.

Chapter 20: Skills-Based Health Education for Health Promotion Among School Adolescents Through Participatory Action Research: A Case from Nepal

Sudha Ghimire, Bhimsen Devkota
Nepal

This chapter reflects on the process, challenges, and lessons learned while conducting participatory action research (PAR) in government-funded schools in Nepal. This novel approach involved all the stakeholders (students, teachers, parents, outside agencies, and health professionals) as co-researchers in the research process. The outcomes of this study outline how this co-production of knowledge can inform research questions and practices as well as strengthen the sustainability of programmes and the skills acquired.

Part III: Researching the Practices of Policymakers and Institutions

Chapter 21: Evaluating Health Promotion in Schools: A Contextual Action-Oriented Research Approach

Nina Bartelink, Patricia van Assema, Maria Jansen, Hans Savelberg, Stef Kremers
Netherlands

The contextual action-oriented research approach takes into account the complexity of the school system and identifies the nature of the interactions between the intervention and its context. This chapter describes one use of this approach and discusses the methods used and the insights gleaned from the evaluations. It also sets down the consequences for researcher positioning, the study design, data collection, and research analysis.

Chapter 22: Developing School Health Promotion Through Research: An Example of a Participatory Action Research Project

Marjorita Sormunen
Finland

Schools are ideal settings for health promotion but are also challenging social environments for conducting research. This chapter describes a two-year school intervention study applying a combination of methodologies and a participatory action research approach to understand and collectively develop health-promoting practices with the school as a wider community.

Chapter 23: Fourth Generation Realist Evaluation: Research Practice to Empower the NGO. A Reflection on the Case of Sport for Social Change

Alex Richmond, Evelyne de Leeuw, Anne Bunde-Birouste
Australia

Researching international non-governmental community-based organizations involves a number of challenges. This chapter presents the conceptual and methodological foundations of Fourth-Generation Evaluation (4GE), which structures evaluation as a negotiated conversation between the researcher and stakeholders. This process of ongoing negotiation raises the question of ethical and social responsibility in health promotion research and highlights the need for research to engage in participatory processes that closely involve various stakeholders.

Chapter 24: A Successful Intervention Research Collaboration Between a Supermarket Chain, Local Government, Non-governmental Organization, and Academic Researchers: The Eat Well @ IGA Healthy Supermarket Partnership

Miranda R. Blake, Gary Sacks, Josephine Marshall, Amy K. Brown, Adrian J. Cameron
Australia

Is it possible to collaborate with a supermarket retailer despite its commercial priorities to improve the healthiness of the supermarket food environment? The research team used a co-design approach to the intervention and multi-sector collaboration to create retail interventions for a healthy supermarket that were effective, feasible, and acceptable to all partners. The mixed-methods device used to produce knowledge, underpinned by a strong theoretical basis and program logic with a controlled study design, made it possible to capture a holistic range of outcomes relevant to each partner.

Chapter 25: Participatory Approaches to Research Intersectoral Actions in Local Communities: Using the Theory of Change, Systems Thinking, and Qualitative Research to Engage Different Stakeholders and Foster Transformative Research Processes

Viola Cassetti, Joan J. Paredes Carbonell
Spain

Based on a case study of a local intersectoral partnership to promote health, this chapter presents an approach to researching community-based intersectoral partnerships and actions, using participatory methods informed by systems thinking, theory-based evaluation, and qualitative research paradigms. This participatory research process combines both "epistemic" (knowledge production) and "transformative" (empowerment of different actors) aims, specific to health promotion while strengthening the production of practice-based evidence.

Chapter 26: A Salutogenic, Participatory and Setting-Based Model of Research for the Development and Evaluation of Complex Interventions: The Trøndelag Model for Public Health Work

Monica Lillefjell, Kirsti Sarheim Anthun, Ruca Elisa Katrin Maass, Siw Tone Innstrand, Geir Arild Espnes
Norway

This chapter proposes an analytic framework and research approach to strengthen the capacities of municipalities to work more systematically and to integrate knowledge and multi-sectoral actors in promoting health and health equity in the population. Attention is paid to crucial research elements that should be considered when implementing and evaluating complex health-promoting initiatives.

Chapter 27: The Contribution of Health Promotion Research in Advancing Local Policies: New Knowledge, Lexicon, and Practice-Research Network

Eric Breton, Yann Le Bodo, Dieinaba Diallo, William Sherlaw, Cyrille Harpet, Hervé Hudebine
France

How can research address the issue of local health policies and practices, and what contributions can it make to informing and improving them? Based on the study of a policy innovation, this chapter analyzes the conditions and challenges of research on/with local health policies. It describes the different types and processes of producing knowledge to inform and support the development of local policies and practices to promote health.

Chapter 28: Implementation Research on Comprehensive Sexuality Education in Ghana: Lessons for Health Promotion Research

Joshua Amo-Adjei, Eric Y. Tenkorang
Ghana

Implementing sexuality education policy in schools entails a variety of challenges as highlighted by the research programme discussed in this chapter. The programme revealed that through collaboration and the development of strong partnerships with various interest groups, research on sensitive public health topics can generate evidence that broadly mirrors the opportunities and challenges of translating sexuality education policies and curricula into classroom realities.

Chapter 29: Oral Health Promotion Intervention Research: A Pathway to Social Justice Applied to the Context of New Caledonia

Stephanie Tubert-Jeannin, Helene Pichot, Amal Skandrani, Nada El Osta, Estelle Pegon-Machat
France

Given that oral health is a component of overall health, this chapter presents an oral health promotion intervention and research program conducted in an archipelago in the Pacific Ocean. It describes the theoretical and ethical framework used to generate, collect, and analyze relevant knowledge and develop a comprehensive understanding of the issues underlying oral health inequities. The authors highlight how the knowledge produced can serve a socially transformative purpose and provide an important resource for advocacy, stakeholder engagement, and policy support to address health inequalities.

Chapter 30: Methodological Reflections on the "SMART Eating" Trial: Lessons for Developing Health Promotion Practices

Jasvir Kaur, Manmeet Kaur, Venkatesan Chakrapani, Rajesh Kumar
India

The nature of health promotion research is both complex and changing. As a result, it requires the integration of different approaches and paradigms in order to respond specifically to the needs of the populations in specific contexts. Providing a rich epistemological step back, this chapter offers a sound example of how to cross different methods with a randomized controlled trial. It describes the analysis of the research framework, paradigms, approaches, and methods used in planning, implementing, and evaluating the "SMART Eating" health promotion intervention.

Chapter 31: Researching the Practices of Policymakers in Implementing a Social Policy Intervention in Ghana

Ebenezer Owusu-Addo
Ghana

The research project discussed in this chapter aimed at understanding how a national social policy intervention affects the social determinants of health in Ghana. Moreover, the author examines the factors that influence the health sector's involvement in the programme, highlighting the dual epistemological and ethical framework of this research. The need to integrate the practices of policymakers and political actors into the design and implementation of the research programme is also explored.

Chapter 32: Capturing Complexity in Health Promotion Intervention Research: Conducting Critical Realist Evaluation

Katherine L. Frohlich, Kate St-Arneault, Mikael St-Pierre
Canada

Understanding the complex contextual conditions of health promotion intervention is a challenge that a critical realist perspective helps to overcome. Using a case study, this chapter presents the interest in and relevance of this perspective for studying the complex systems and leads to a fruitful reformulation of research questions and knowledge production.

Chapter 33: Using Critical Theory to Research Commercial Determinants of Health: Health Impact Assessment of the Practices and Products of Transnational Corporations

Julia Anaf, Matt Fisher, Fran Baum
Australia

The practices and products of transnational corporations have major impacts on population health and the environment. The research programme presented in this chapter developed and tested a corporate health impact-assessment framework based on critical theory in order to better grasp the commercial determinants of health. This framework aims to provide an evidence base to inform policies so as to regulate practices harmful to health and equity as well as to support advocacy to shift these determinants to the heart of health promotion practices.

Chapter 34: Knowledge Transfer: A Snapshot on Translation Processes from Research to Practices

Valérie Ivassenko, Ioanna Bakogianni, Jan Wollgast, Sandra Caldeira, Vanessa de Almeida Guerra, Keli Bahia Felicíssimo Zocrato, Conceição Aparecida Moreira, Daniela Souzalima Campos, Mirela Castro Santos Camargos, Eike Quilling, Maja Kuchler, Janna Leimann, Christina Plantz, Adamandia Xekalaki, Achilleas Attilakos, Alexia Prasouli, Ioanna Antoniadou-Koumatou

The transformative nature of health promotion places knowledge transfer at the very heart of the research configurations. The articulation of knowledge production and transfer is all the more crucial when it comes to guiding and supporting the practices of policymakers and institutions. This chapter presents different forms and responses to the challenge of knowledge-sharing and transfer and making scientific data available, understandable, and actionable.

Part IV: Researching the Practices of Researchers and Innovators

Chapter 35: From the Production to the Use of Scientific Knowledge: A Continuous Dialogue Between Researchers, Knowledge Mobilization Specialists, and Users

Angèle Bilodeau, Marie-Pier St-Louis, Alain Meunier, Catherine Chabot, Louise Potvin
Canada

Knowledge mobilization is an inherent dimension of health promotion practice and research. But how can researchers translate their knowledge into a meaningful form for practice settings? This foray into the topic presents a critical reflection, informed by the actor–network theory, on the knowledge translation practices from a research programme to the development and implementation of professional training tools in Canada.

Chapter 36: A Critical Health Promotion Research Approach Using the Red Lotus Critical Health Promotion Model

Lily O'Hara, Jane Taylor
Qatar

Because of its multifaceted perspectives, health promotion research must develop approaches linking research to the practices of individuals, populations, professionals, and institutions. This is the purpose of the critical research model in health promotion. This chapter explores how the application of this model can generate knowledge and address the structural determinants of health and well-being and reduce health inequalities.

Chapter 37: Making Reflexivity and Emotions Visible. The Contribution of Logbooks and Polar Semantic Maps in Health Promotion Research

Patrizia Garista, Giancarlo Pocetta
Italy

The very nature of health promotion research requires a shift away from the ideal of objectivity to explore the potential of reflexivity. Reflexive research practice can uncover implicit knowledge, challenge hypotheses, and consequently yield innovative research perspectives. Recognizing the importance of emotions in the process of knowledge production as well as the use of diaries and semantic maps are presented as tools capable of informing, evaluating, and guiding research.

Chapter 38: Steering Committee: A Participatory Device to Support Knowledge Flow and Use in Health Promotion

Marianne Beaulieu, Alix Adrien, Clément Dassa, Louise Potvin, the Comité consultatif sur les attitudes envers les PVVIH
Canada

The author bridges the gap between research and action with a promising knowledge-sharing approach focusing on the flow and use of research results. The chapter examines a case study of a participatory device (a steering committee) involving various stakeholders in a long-term dialogue throughout a project's development. This partnership challenges the traditional distinction between knowledge producers and users, leading to the co-construction of knowledge and a shared redefinition of the notion of expertise.

Chapter 39: Reflections on Health Promotion Research in the Field of Health-Promoting Health Care: The What, Why, and How of the Viennese Tradition

Daniela Rojatz, Birgit Metzler
Austria

The roots of the Vienna tradition in this field stretch back more than three decades. This chapter presents a critical reflection on the use of sociology to support the development of a global network to reorient health services, more particularly health-promoting hospitals. The authors describe how theories and concepts influenced by systems theory, the salutogenesis paradigm, and quality-development approach were combined and applied to develop models, concepts, and tools for the practical implementation of the reorientation of health services.

Chapter 40: Addressing the Complexity of School Health Promotion Through Interdisciplinary Approaches: An Invitation to Think Wildly About Research

Deana Leahy
Australia

The author takes a fully innovative outside-the-box look at this complexity, highlighting the need to adopt new theories and think more wildly about how to conduct research and plan school health programmes. This research focuses on understanding how different programme imperatives impact everyday school/family food practices as well as the lives of children and families in general. It underscores the value of social theory in making sense of complex problems with multiple contexts and actors.

Chapter 41: Fitting Health Promotion Research with Real-Life Conditions: Viability Evaluation

Charlotte Decroix, Charlotte Kervran, Linda Cambon, François Alla
France

In this chapter, the authors introduce the concept of viability validity and analyze its relevance in various contexts. They argue that viability validity should be considered as early as possible in an innovation process, starting with the pilot study. The authors offer a critical reflection on the notion of validity and the proposition of viability validity in scaling up an intervention in the real world, from a pilot project to a real intervention.

Chapter 42: A System's Approach to Research Practice in the Co-production of Evidence About Partnership-Based Health Promotion Interventions

Therese Riley, Kim Jose, Kate Garvey, Michelle Morgan
Australia

This chapter offers a critical reflection on research evidence through the lens of complexity and systems theory. The analyses of four real-world case studies highlight the critical need for researchers to engage with uncertainty and complexity, the challenges associated with doing so, and the additional insights gained when co-production and flexibility are embedded within the research process.

Chapter 43: Researching the Aesthetics of Health Promotion Interventions: Reflections on Fit to Drive, a Long-Running Road Safety Education Program

Kerry Montero, Peter Kelly
Australia

The critical reflection in this chapter – informed by the actor–network theory – introduces the notion of aesthetics in researching health promotion programs in secondary schools. This novel approach considering the unconscious and the symbolic aspect of behaviour focuses on the deeper dimensions of engagement and sense-making within health promotion programs and how this translates into innovative research approaches.

Chapter 44: Researchers as Policy Entrepreneurs for Structural Change: Interactive Research for Promoting Processes Towards Health Equity

Alfred Rütten, Jana Semrau, Natalie Helsper, Lea Dippon, Simone Kohler, Klaus Pfeifer
Germany

Studies on the development and implementation of healthy public policies are a key action area for health promotion research. The approach presented in this chapter builds on an interactive knowledge-to-action methodology systematically linking research practice with the practices of policymakers, professionals, and population groups. Drawing on a case example from the field of physical activity promotion in Germany, this work offers an analysis of the requisite conditions of policy entrepreneurship for health promotion researchers.

Chapter 45: Reflections on Mainstreaming Health Equity in a Large Research Collaboration: "If I can't dance, it is not my revolution"

Ana Porroche-Escudero, Jennie Popay
United Kingdom

This chapter is about the response of a large English partnership organization to the lack of equity focus in health research. It highlights a process described as health equity mainstreaming, a way to embed a health equity lens in the institutions governing and conducting health promotion research. This chapter also reveals how reflective practice throughout the process was essential to understanding how health equity mainstreaming could work in practice.

Chapter 46: Studying the Case de Santé de Toulouse (France) as a Propaedeutic Step

Jean-Charles Basson, Nadine Haschar-Noé, Thierry Lang, Laurence Boulaghaf, Fabien Maguin
France

The authors provide a critical reflection on the epistemological and ethical implications of health promotion research. They argue that three conditions are necessary for health promotion research to have an impact on social inequities: (1) research should be based on collaborative and partnership-based methods, (2) it should be devoted to experimental measures in health aimed at social change using an interdisciplinary approach, and (3) it should be geared towards assessing the three major intervention strategies of participation, mediation, and social innovation.

Chapter 47: Brazilian Experiences in Interdisciplinary Networks: From Advocacy to Intersectoral Participatory Research and Implementation

Samuel Jorge Moysés, Rosilda Mendes, Julia Aparecida Devidé Nogueira, Dais Gonçalves Rocha, Maria Cristina Trousdell Franceschini, Marco Akerman
Brazil

The challenges, conditions, and lessons learned from an interdisciplinary network of participatory research aimed at producing and sharing knowledge, building capacity, and promoting sustainable development and health come together in this chapter. This Brazilian experience highlights the intertwined ethical, political, and epistemological dimensions of its concrete implementation, and, more broadly, of knowledge production in health promotion, reflecting its dual epistemic and transformative purposes.

Chapter 48: Researching a Diverse Epistemic Social Movement: The Challenges and Rewards of European Healthy Cities Realist Synthesis

Evelyne de Leeuw
Australia

This chapter reports on the work done in the European Healthy Cities Network. It led to the definition of a model of realistic research synthesis, adapted to the dynamic evaluation of complex social interventions and the use of a multi-method and multidisciplinary evidence base. Based on a Fourth Generation Evaluation paradigm, this model creates a lens for research stakeholders to determine the most appropriate research questions, methods, counterparts, processes, and outcomes.

Chapter 49: Researching Health for All in South Australia: Reflections on Sustainability and Partnership

Fran Baum, Helen van Eyk, Colin MacDougall, Carmel Williams
Australia

The authors offer a critical reflection on the conduct of Health in All Policies based on an analysis of a 5-year research program on the implementation of this approach in the state of South Australia. They show how combining flexible research methods with a range of political-science theories for interpretations can yield a more sophisticated understanding of the processes of multi-sectoral governance for health and inform health promotion practice.

Index

L. Potvin, D. Jourdan (eds.), *Global Handbook of Health Promotion Research, Vol. 1*,
https://doi.org/10.1007/978-3-030-97212-7

Lightning Source UK Ltd.
Milton Keynes UK
UKHW021128130223
416809UK00001B/3

9 783030 972110

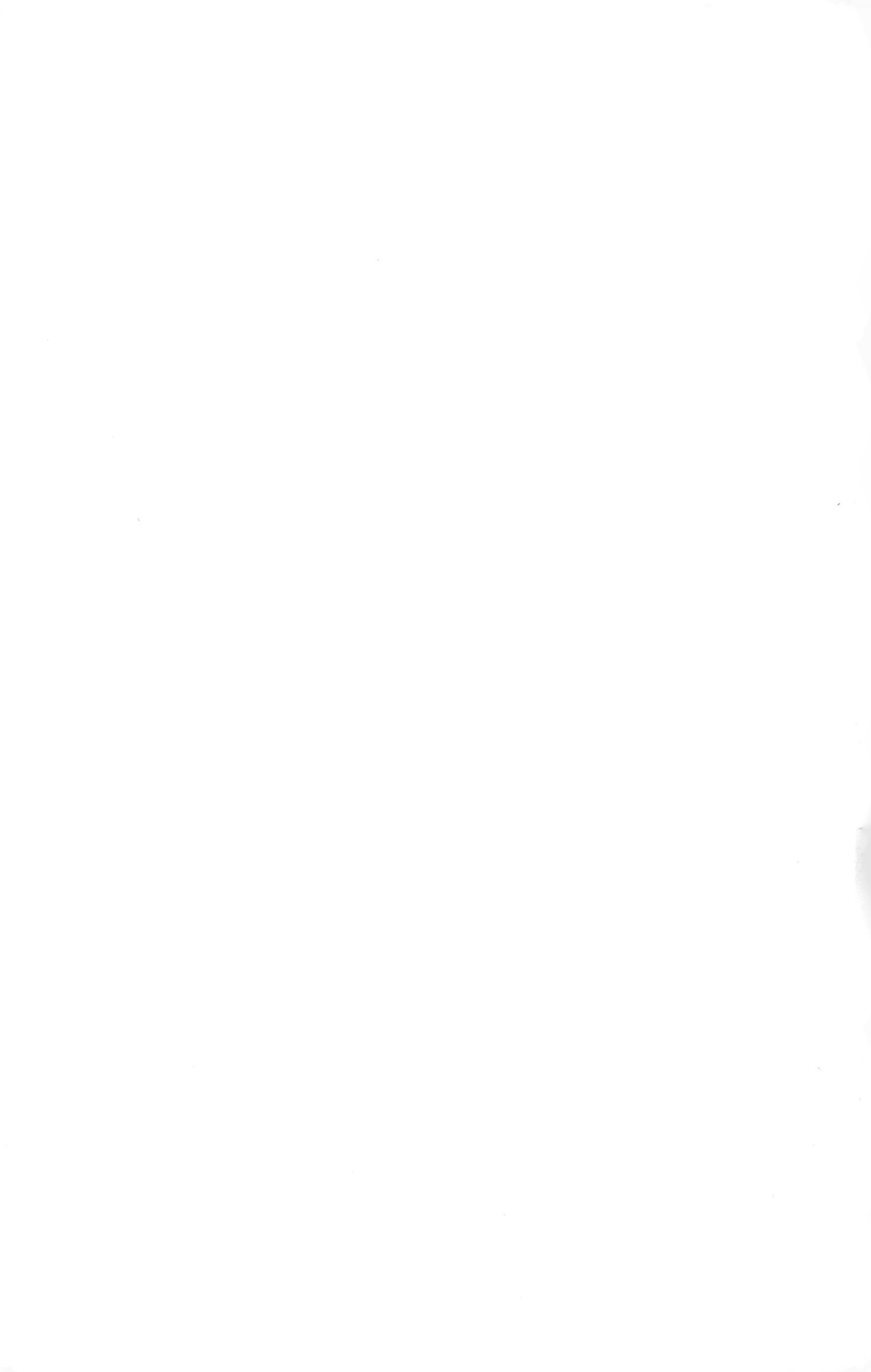